# SYNTHETIC FOSSIL FUEL TECHNOLOGIES
## Results of Health and Environmental Studies

Proceedings of the Fifth Life Sciences Symposium
Gatlinburg, Tennessee
October 24–27, 1982

Sponsored by
U.S. Department of Energy
Office of Health and Environmental Research
and
Assistant Secretary for Fossil Energy

Edited by
## K.E. Cowser
*Oak Ridge National Laboratory*
*Oak Ridge, Tennessee*

Technical Editor

Vivian A. Jacobs
*Oak Ridge National Laboratory*
*Oak Ridge, Tennessee*

BUTTERWORTH PUBLISHERS
Boston • London
Sydney • Wellington • Durban • Toronto

An Ann Arbor Science Book

Ann Arbor Science is an imprint of Butterworth Publishers.

**Library of Congress Cataloging in Publication Data**

Main entry under title:

Synthetic fossil fuel technologies.

"An Ann Arbor science book."
Proceedings of the Fifth Life Sciences Symposium, held October 24–27, 1982, Gatlinburg, Tenn.
Includes index.
1. Synthetic fuels industry—Hygienic aspects—Congresses. 2. Synthetic fuels industry—Environmental aspects—Congresses. 3. Toxicity testing—Congresses.
I. Cowser, K. E.
II. Life Sciences Symposium (5th : 1982 : Gatlinburg, Tenn.)
RA568.5.S98 1984 363.1'7 84–7616
ISBN 0–250–40624–1

Butterworth Publishers
80 Montvale Avenue
Stoneham, MA 02180

10 9 8 7 6 5 4 3 2 1

Printed in the United States of America

# CONTENTS

# PREFACE

An extensive program of research on the health and environmental consequences associated with advanced fossil energy technologies has been conducted since our first life sciences symposium in 1978. In particular, a
considerable data base on the toxicological properties of synthetic fossil fuels
and on the transport, fate, and effects of residuals occurring during the
production of these materials has evolved.

The purpose of the *Fifth Life Sciences Symposium, Synthetic Fossil
Fuel Technologies: Results of Health and Environmental Studies,* was to
review the present state of knowledge, uncertainties, and future research
requirements of these technologies and thereby assist in the development
of environmentally acceptable fossil energy processes. To achieve this objective, scientists and engineers from government, industry, universities, and
national laboratories were invited to present their most recent experimental
findings. Ample time was provided for debate. Also, a special panel of
government and industry officials considered the need and opportunities for
future research. It was within such a multidisciplinary setting that partici-
pants representing thirty-eight organizations explored the solution to presently identified problems and considered the longer-term issues related to
technology development. This book provides a compilation of the principal
research findings and interpretations for the scientists, engineers, and interested public, as well as identifies the requirements for additional research.

The efforts of the Symposium Committee are gratefully acknowledged.
Not only did they participate in the organization of the technical program,
but they also contributed in the conduct of the symposium as Session Chair-
persons. These include P.H. Buhl, U.S. Department of Energy, and M.R.
Guerin, Oak Ridge National Laboratory, Session I: Technology-Oriented
Studies; J.L. Epler, Oak Ridge National Laboratory, G.E. Stapleton, U.S.
Department of Energy, and R. Pelroy, Pacific Northwest Laboratory (who
assisted during the session), Session II: Toxicology; and C.W. Gehrs, Oak
Ridge National Laboratory, and F.J. Wobber, U.S. Department of Energy,
Session III: Transport, Transformation, and Fate. A special acknowledg-
ment is due C.R. Richmond, Associate Director, Oak Ridge National Laboratory, who served as Co-Chairman and introduced the theme of the
symposium in his opening remarks.

I am very grateful to Bonnie S. Reesor, Conference Coordinator for
Oak Ridge National Laboratory, for the superb management of symposium

arrangements and to the tireless efforts of the support staff, Lindy Norris, Sherry Haney, Deborah Shepherd, and Pamela Valliant, for their flawless handling of symposium mechanics. To Vivian Jacobs I extend a special acknowledgment for a job well done in providing editorial assistance to the authors and in coordinating the preparation of these proceedings. I hope the information contained in these proceedings will serve both the researchers and decision makers as the development of synthetic fossil fuel technologies continues.

K.E. Cowser
Chairman

# INTRODUCTION

## Life Sciences Research in Support of Fossil Fuel Technologies: Reflections and a Look Forward

### C.R. Richmond

*Associate Director for Biomedical and
Environmental Sciences
Oak Ridge National Laboratory
Oak Ridge, TN 37831*

Welcome to the Symposium on Synthetic Fossil Fuel Technologies: Results of Health and Environmental Studies. I am very pleased and honored to be able to welcome you to this Fifth Annual Oak Ridge National Laboratory (ORNL) Life Sciences Symposium. It is very appropriate that we are returning to the subject of the First ORNL Life Sciences Symposium, entitled "Synthetic Fossil Fuel Technology—Potential Health and Environmental Effects," which was held here in Gatlinburg in late September of 1978, just 5 years after the Arab oil embargo. Since that time, much has been said and written about energy policy. Let me share with you the following Presidential message concerning energy policy.

Our energy resources are not inexhaustible; yet we are permitting waste in their use and production. In some instances, to achieve apparent economies today, future generations will be forced to carry the burden of unnecessarily high costs and to substitute inferior fuels for particular purposes. National policies concerning these vital resources must recognize the availability of all of them; the location of each with respect to its markets; the costs of transporting them; the technological developments which will increase the efficiency of their production and use; the use of lower grade coals; and the relationships between the increased use of energy and the general economic development of the country.

It is difficult in the long run to envisage a national coal policy, or a national petroleum policy, or a national waterpower policy without also in time a national policy directed toward all of these energy procedures—that

1

is, a national energy resources policy. Such a broader and integrated policy toward the problems of coal, petroleum, natural gas, and waterpower cannot be evolved overnight.

Perhaps you noted several things in this quotation. Although there is no reference to nuclear power, not much has changed in the intervening years since this message was presented to the Congress of the United States by Franklin Delano Roosevelt in 1939, some 43 years ago.

In 1978 I mentioned my hope that we would be able to continue this Life Sciences Symposium series. Following the 1978 "Symposium on Synthetic Fossil Fuel Technology—Potential Health and Environmental Effects," we explored the subjects of "Atmospheric Sulfur Deposition— Environmental Impact and Health Effects" in 1979, "Health Risk Analysis" in 1980, and "The Environment and Solid Wastes: Characterization, Treatment, and Disposal" in 1981; and, as I mentioned earlier, it is fitting that we are returning to the subject of synthetic fossil fuels this year. I should emphasize that in 1978 we were interested in the *potential* health and environmental effects of synthetic fossil fuel technologies, whereas we are now examining some of the results of health and environmental studies related to synthetic fossil fuel technologies. Many of us look forward with great interest to hearing about the research activities that have taken place during the intervening 4 years.

When I introduced this symposium series in 1978, I noted that the ORNL Life Sciences Symposium series was an attempt to move away from the very specific research areas covered in the past by topical symposia covering research subjects at the forefront of biological research. The current series was established to cover broader areas of research and development, which encompass multidisciplinary programmatic research and development efforts that are typical of much of what we do at ORNL in our Life Sciences Program. At that time, I expressed my belief that we needed both kinds of symposia. In fact, I made the following statement, not fully realizing how drastic and severe some of the changes would be in the 4 years following 1978.

Times change, as do public and governmental attitudes towards research and development support and funding. No research and development institution is the same as it was 10 or 20 years ago. Times and people change, as do the nature of technical and scientific problems and their priorities on the local, national, and global scales.

In a sense, I am happy that I could not foresee the future and the very traumatic changes that have occurred in the 4 years since 1978. We have had a major change in administration of our federal government at the Washington level, which has resulted in good news for some and bad news for others. One needs only to examine the size of the U.S. Department of

Energy (DOE) Fossil Energy budgets for FY 1981 and FY 1982 and the proposed budgets for FY 1983 to get some idea of the magnitude of change expected to occur over this relatively short period of time. We have also changed from an era in which research and development should be targeted to short-term payoffs to research of a long-term, high risk, high potential payoff nature. I know many of you in this audience have tried to adapt to these drastic changes. This is particularly difficult, as they occur at a time when there is considerable uncertainty facing other technologies that in one way or another could help provide sufficient and reliable energy supplies to our country. These are, indeed, confusing times. I read in the popular press just last week that Exxon is auctioning equipment that would have been used in its shale programs in the Southwest at the same time when the Tennessee Valley Authority (TVA) is trying to sell parts to nuclear reactors that it has decided we do not need at this point in time. I guess about the only bright outlook comes, not from solar energy, but from hydropower. It appears that currently there are bountiful supplies of electricity from hydroelectric projects in several parts of the United States, and I guess we all have to admit that this is not a result of careful planning or research and development on anyone's part.

The particularly wet fall weather has contributed to this unusual situation. TVA and the Bonneville Power Administration have abundant electrical supplies from hydroelectric systems. Last month, on September 5, TVA experienced its lowest power demand since 1971. We have also experienced severe drought periods around the United States since 1971. Weather is fickle and unpredictable. How unpredictable? Well, as an example, TVA had its all-time peak demand for power in January of this year because of the extremely cold weather. No one planned for this surfeit of power. Let us not forget the other major contributor to this situation; that is the current state of our economy, which, like the weather, is also unpredictable.

Let me return to a more optimistic note. Four years ago I heard numerous comments to the effect that the synthetic fuel industries would move so rapidly that there would not be time to mount a useful life sciences supporting program. It was a time of optimism for the industry. However, the situation has changed and there has been time to mount a strong, viable, and I think useful program at numerous locations within the United States. We have been able to develop information not only on the potential health and environmental effects of synthetic fossil fuel technologies, but also on ways to reduce or even eliminate some of the potential harm or detriment to man and his environment that might otherwise result from these unwanted components of synthetic fuel technologies.

When we started our Life Sciences Program in support of synthetic fuel technologies about six years ago at ORNL, we firmly believed that there was a real opportunity to identify and possibly correct potential health and environmental problems associated with these technologies. As I stated in 1978, we firmly believed that the development and demonstration of new energy technologies should proceed in concert with research supporting engineering and process design. The research designed to ensure protection of the environment and human health should be initiated during the early stages of process conception and continued throughout the operation of the demonstration plants. I expressed my concern that in the haste of developing new demonstration units, the technologists might not consider issues related to the working environment or the off-site environment to be of significance until the licensing procedure had to be initiated. I reminded the audience that society now demands that those who develop technologies work closely together as a team to help ensure that a particular technology will not provide more stress than benefit to society. I proposed a troika approach for such a system comprised of the three components shown here.

Troika Approach to Development of New Technology

---

Determination of technical feasibility
Determination of economic viability
Determination of environmental acceptability

---

As an aside, I might mention that on one occasion the word "viability" was transcribed from a tape as "liability." One of my colleagues jokingly suggested that either word could be used.

Four years ago, it was also quite clear that we needed to develop cost effective procedures so that we could test materials efficiently and economically. Prescreening and screening tests using a tier approach were devised so that we could rapidly and economically identify those materials that most probably would present potential health and environmental problems. Once they were identified, we could then concentrate on those materials rather than others that would be of much lesser importance to man and his environment. The approach would assist us in conserving our resources, in avoiding false negatives, and in designing experiments for only those most critical compounds necessitating long-term commitments of people, money, and animal facilities for toxicity testing. I think we have learned a great deal since 1978, and there is still much to be learned.

I am very pleased that ORNL and other DOE laboratories have been a major component, not only in the research associated with the synfuels technologies, but, perhaps more importantly, in the development of an entirely new philosophy of how the life scientist can help provide useful information to the technologist as the technology is being developed. The ultimate decision of whether or not a system is socially acceptable in terms of its technical, economic, and environmental components can be made on the basis of research and development information covering many disciplines and areas of expertise. The approach we have developed helps provide the kinds of information required to make important decisions about deployment of technologies that have been developed to the stage where the net benefit to society is greater than the detriment to human health and safety.

It is abundantly clear that we must develop an adequate, reliable supply of energy. It is also clear that we must decrease our reliance on liquid fuels produced by other countries and therefore not fully under our control. Many of the confrontation attitudes between the technologist and the life scientist that were prevalent in the 1970s have given way to attitudes of collaboration, cooperation, and, where necessary, compromise among the individuals involved. Please note that I am not arguing that we compromise issues related to health, safety, or the environment. People have learned the futility of referring to systems as safe or non-safe. These words mean different things to different people. There is little question in my mind that sooner or later large commercial activities will be developed to produce synthetic fuels in the United States.

I recently had the opportunity to read a report prepared by the National Research Council's Commission on Engineering and Technical Systems, *Safety Issues Related to Synthetic Fuels Facilities*.[1] It is most interesting and I recommend it to you. To begin with, the report points out that the goal for synthetic fuel production set under the 1980 Energy Security Act will not be met. The goal was for industry to produce synthetic fuels from coal, oil, shale, peat, and tar sands at the minimum rate of 500,000 barrels per day (equivalent to crude oil) by 1987. By 1992 this rate would increase fourfold to a level of 2,000,000 bbl/d. The National Research Council (NRC) study states that it is unlikely that an industry capable of producing 500,000 bbl/d could be on line prior to the mid 1990s. The report is optimistic, as the authors think it appropriate to view the present decade as one which will witness the construction of "commercial pioneer plants" prior to the large-scale development of the synthetic fuels industry as we move into the next century.

Interestingly, the report mentions that this slow industrial development may provide the opportunity to use the first-generation plants as a means to develop effective implementation of the technology and to produce safe and environmentally acceptable designs. During the deployment of the first generation of synfuels plants, particular attention should be paid to industrial hygiene characterization of occupational hazards, medical surveillance (including biological and epidemiological monitoring), toxicological investigations (including synergisms), and development of an occupational health program to interrelate these individual items.

The report also identified the need for a committee of experts from the health field, policy makers from private industry, and experts from the universities and government agencies to develop a synfuels worker registry. The committee would determine which health and exposure data should be collected for the registry, how the data might be stored and used, and who should have access to such data. It is felt that a synfuels workers registry would be extremely useful and beneficial for accurately identifying occupationally induced diseases with long latency periods. The registry would also provide information for case control and medical studies. I strongly endorse this concept, and I would like to see this recommendation from the NRC accepted and implemented without further delay. Actually, the Life Sciences Synthetic Fuels Program at ORNL has made similar recommendations on several past occasions.

Perhaps another historical divergence is appropriate. In early 1977 I was invited to participate in a symposium on "Polynuclear Aromatic Hydrocarbons in Coal Conversion Processes." The specific symposium topics dealt with were medical surveillance and industrial experiences, including personnel protection and monitoring. The following information, which is pertinent to the question of a worker registry, is taken verbatim from my presentation at that symposium.

> I believe we need to direct more effort for the developing technologies toward man and his protection in the workplace. Much instrumentation needs to be developed—for both area and personnel monitors. Documentation of exposures will be important as will surveillance and follow-up of worker populations. An example from another technology may help illustrate this need. Men who helped build the first nuclear weapons worked in the D building at what is now Los Alamos Scientific Laboratory, and was then part of the Manhattan Project. These working conditions were such that they would be totally unacceptable by today's standards. In fact, they would be considered to be quite primitive. Incoming, not outgoing, air was filtered. Work with plutonium was performed in open hoods. So-called "portable" monitors were large, awkward, and unwieldy. Yet these were the working conditions for a new technology that was rapidly exploited under wartime conditions.
>
> About two dozen men who worked under the conditions mentioned above were identified in the mid-1940s and were kept under medical follow-up and surveillance ever since. This action has resulted in information of the most useful kind, in that it is obtained directly from man. Some might have agreed at the time that the group should not be studied because of its size and was not, therefore, adequate or acceptable for an epidemiological study. This group has provided useful information despite its small size and, in fact, provides the most relevant information concerning plutonium exposure and its effect on man. No biological effects, including cancer, have developed in these men during the more than 30 years since exposure, despite their relatively high exposures to plutonium. This information would not be available today were it not for the foresight of several individuals in the 1940s. Perhaps a lesson can be learned from this experience—that is, even small-size study groups can supply useful data and should be thoroughly studied.

We included a session on "Occupational Health Control Technology" in our 1978 Life Sciences Symposium on "Synthetic Fossil Fuel Technology." Included in that session was a paper on mortality experience of fifty workers with occupational exposure to the products of a coal hydrogenation process. This particular cohort of workers had diagnosed skin cancer or precancerous lesions that were identified between 1955 and 1959 at a coal hydrogenation plant in the United States. The purpose of the follow-up study was to attempt to establish if there was an increase in death caused by systemic cancers. I understand that DOE supports a shale worker follow-up study. There are, to my knowledge, no funded projects concerning worker registries for coal conversion facilities.

The NRC report also provides some explicit information needs related to technological, environmental, and health effects research and development. Under environmental research and development, the committee perceived a need to monitor control technologies and strategies in the first-generation synthetic fuel plants. They thought the required research would be typical of that required to monitor a first-of-a-kind system. Specific environmental research and development recommendations are shown in Table I. It is interesting to note that we will be hearing about these research and development categories during the next several days at this meeting.

Similarly, the NRC report identifies health effects research and development information needs. These also are given in Table I. The Committee felt that the health concerns associated with the development of synthetic fuel processes were of greater concern for workers in the industry than for members of the general public. They stress that ongoing programs directed towards the assessment of health effects associated with the major synthetic fuels activities (shale oil, coal gasification, and direct coal liquefaction) ". . . should continue to receive research emphasis, as should evaluations of worker training facilities and personal protective equipment." I strongly endorse this particular recommendation. We will also hear interesting reports during the next several days on some items shown in Table I.

**Table I.**   Summary of Information Needs for Environmental and Health Effects Research and Development[a]

| Type of Research and Development | Information Needed |
|---|---|
| Environmental | Solid Waste Management |
| | Transport of Pollutants |
| | Potential Effects of Pollutants on the Environment |
| Health Effects | Medical Surveillance of Workers |
| | Monitoring Worker Exposures |
| | Instituting Engineering Controls |
| | Training Competent Workers |
| | Maintaining Strict Industrial Hygiene Standards |
| | Instituting a Worker Registry for the Earliest Possible Identification of Manifest Health Effects |
| | Evaluating the Toxicity of Process Emissions and Product Streams |

[a]Source: Reference 1, this chapter.

The NRC report also discussed cost-benefit analysis. The following paragraphs are of particular interest:

> Adequate consideration of health and safety issues implies potential cost effects that could significantly influence the social benefits from the commercial production of synthetic fuels. The trade-offs that exist between the reduction of health risks and the market competitiveness of synthetic fuels should be considered. Cost analysis methodology should be developed from a solid data base. Key areas include: health effects research, research on plant performance and toxic exposure, and research on cost and performance trade-offs.
>
> Data generated from this research will provide input for developing the appropriate model. Available literature on equipment failures can help identify candidate variables to predict performance levels. Links between health effects research, regulatory policy, and product costs must be incorporated into a methodology to stimulate policy decisions.

This raises the important question of risk assessment and risk analysis and their important potential contributions to the developing synthetic fuels industry. I hope the responsible federal agencies and the private sector can continue to expand their efforts in risk assessment activities. The temptation during periods of reduced support for research and development may be to cut back in this kind of research. I do not agree. Risk analysis research is a worthwhile investment of resources that should receive strong support. As shown below, I believe it is especially important to invest in risk analysis work during austere periods of funding, because such studies can help us identify the most important areas where research needs to be done. In other words, the output of risk assessment studies can assist research managers in establishing research priorities.

Risk Analysis

---

Will assist in establishing research priorities
Important to support especially during periods of reduced R&D funding

---

I look forward to an exciting meeting here with you in Gatlinburg during this Fifth Annual ORNL Life Sciences Symposium. On behalf of Oak Ridge National Laboratory, I welcome you to this Symposium, to Gatlinburg, to the Great Smoky Mountains, and to Tennessee.


## ACKNOWLEDGMENT

This research was sponsored by the U.S. Department of Energy under contract W-7405-eng-26 with Union Carbide Corporation.

## REFERENCE

1. "Safety Issues Related to Synthetic Fuels Facilities—Final Report of the Committee on Synthetic Fuels Facilities Safety," Commission on Engineering and Technical Systems, National Research Council, DOE/EV/10659-T1 (Oak Ridge, TN: Technical Information Center, U.S. Department of Energy, 1982).

# SECTION I

# TECHNOLOGY-ORIENTED STUDIES

M.R. Guerin
*Oak Ridge National Laboratory*
*P.O. Box X*
*Oak Ridge, TN 37831*

The environmental and health aspects of synthetic fuels technologies have been investigated extensively. The intent has been to detect potential hazards sufficiently early in the development of these technologies to allow their control. This has involved the toxicological and chemical characterization of products, process streams, wastes, and by-products resulting from pilot plant and smaller facilities. Because it is not possible to quantitatively predict the hazards associated with commercial plants from data on experimental facilities, research has focused on issues fundamental to the technologies as a whole and on issues of unique concern to individual technologies. Particular attention has been given, for example, to determining whether unusual (in kind or in magnitude) toxicological hazards exist and to identifying the materials responsible for those hazards. Solid waste characteristics, occupational exposure, and environmental releases have received additional specific attention.

Summaries of current knowledge relating to the environmental and health aspects of coal liquefaction, coal gasification, oil shale retorting, and synfuels-related solid wastes are presented as status reports. An important conclusion is that the kinds of toxicological hazards associated with synfuels technologies are generally the same as those associated with current coal and/or petroleum processing technologies. The degree of hazard varies widely depending on the specific concern and specific technology considered, but tends to be more severe for synfuels technologies than for the petroleum technologies they are intended to supplement. The toxicology observed to date is readily explained by the chemical properties of the materials. As such, suitably modified versions of currently available environmental control technologies and industrial hygiene practices are thought to be adequate to control hazards.

Recommendations for further research are made throughout this section and are highlighted by chapters addressing specific issues. Results of ambient air analysis in the vicinity of a commercial coal gasification facility and of monitoring the occupational environment in a low-Btu coal gasifier plant illustrate the importance of applying fundamental research methods to larger-scale facilities. Conversely, laboratory-scale facilities are shown to be particularly useful for providing materials and data to guide fundamental research. Of special importance is the recognition that comparisons between technologies require a uniform terminology applied to operationally common materials. An example is provided for shale oil processing streams.

# CHAPTER 1

## Summary of Health and Environmental Research: Coal Liquefaction

R.H. Gray, D.D. Mahlum,
J.A. Strand, and W.C. Weimer

*Coal Liquefaction Environmental
Research Program
Pacific Northwest Laboratory
P.O. Box 999
Richland, WA 99352*

This chapter summarizes health and environmental research (1976 to present), supported by the U.S. Department of Energy, to assist in the development of environmentally acceptable coal liquefaction processes. Four major direct coal liquefaction processes have been evaluated: SRC-I and -II (solvent-refined coal), H-coal (catalytic), and EDS. Short-term bioassays were used to screen coal-derived materials for possible health and environmental effects. Longer-term bioassays were used to evaluate materials considered most representative of potential commercial practice and with greatest possibility for human exposure or release to the environment. Detailed chemical analyses were used to identify compounds and classes of compounds responsible for biological activity. Effects of process modification, control technologies, and changing operational conditions on potential health and environmental effects are also being evaluated. Significant research results are described.

## INTRODUCTION

Four major direct coal liquefaction processes have been under development by industry in cooperation with the U.S. Department of Energy (DOE). These include two solvent-refined coal processes (SRC-I and -II), H-coal (a catalytic process), and the Exxon donor solvent (EDS) process. These processes all produce liquid fuels. The SRC-I process also produces a low sulfur, low ash, solid fuel. Some of these processes may be ready for large-scale deployment by the 1990s.

Several organizations were selected by DOE to study the potential health, environmental, and safety aspects of direct coal liquefaction. Pacific Northwest Laboratory (PNL) was asked to evaluate SRC processes and prepared and initiated comprehensive health and environmental research plans for SRC-I and -II. Similar plans were prepared and initiated for H-coal by Oak Ridge National Laboratory (ORNL) and for EDS by Exxon Research and Engineering Company. The programs had the following objectives:

- Identify and evaluate the long-term health and environmental issues associated with direct coal liquefaction.
- Evaluate control technology and ameliorative options to permit the design of environmentally acceptable coal liquefaction processes.
- Assess and quantify potential risks to man and the environment from large-scale deployment of direct coal liquefaction processes.

This chapter is based on a status report[1] that PNL and ORNL prepared for DOE. The status report identified the health and environmental issues (Table I), described a research strategy, and summarized results obtained to date from DOE's environmental, health, and safety research programs on direct coal liquefaction. Additionally, results were used to define future research efforts. (Research needs in coal conversion is the subject of another chapter.[2]) The information summarized here is contained in numerous doc-

**Table I.** Health and Environmental Research Issues
Relative to Direct Coal Liquefaction

| *Issue* | *Research* |
| --- | --- |
| Health effects | Toxicology |
| |     Chemical characterization and monitoring |
| |         Obtain, store, and characterize coal liquefaction products, process streams, solid and liquid wastes, and atmospheric emissions. Determine, in coordination with biological assays, the chemical compounds/compound classes responsible for toxicological effects. |
| |     Short-term bioassay |
| |         Apply microbial, submammalian, and mammalian acute toxicity and teratogenicity assays to determine potential genotoxicity and acute hazards of exposure to coal liquefaction materials. Quantify dose-response relationships and compare to other synfuel materials and petroleum products. |

**Table I.** *(continued)*

| Issue | Research |
|---|---|
| | Chronic bioassay |

Chronic bioassay
  Evaluate, in mammalian systems, carcinogenicity, effects on juvenile development, reproduction, neurotoxicity, and other chronic effects on tissues as a function of route of exposure (inhalation, ingestion, or dermal application). Quantify dose-response relationships and compare to other synfuel materials and petroleum products. Evaluate potential synergistic action of synfuel-related pollutants with selected chemical, biological, and environmental stresses.
Occupational health
  Industrial hygiene
    Design and implement industrial hygiene programs, including identification of high-risk workers; educate workers to workplace risks and consequences; develop protective clothing, equipment, and decontamination procedures; maintain medical surveillance of workers. Use toxicological data to determine sources of potential hazards.
  Workplace and personnel monitoring
    Develop measuring and monitoring systems for work areas and personnel that define potential and actual exposure to hazardous materials.
  Epidemiology
    Conduct epidemiological studies on work forces at coal liquefaction facilities. Integrate with information relevant to exposure doses, medical histories, and surveillance.
Public health
  Determine the potential for exposure of the general populace to synfuel products, by-products, and wastes as the result of accidental and planned releases. Using toxicological and industrial hygiene data, determine the relative health risk and develop appropriate surveillance equipment and emergency response plans. Implement epidemiologic studies on selected populations.

Environmental fate and effects
  Accidental product release (a)
  Solid waste leachates (b)
  Unplanned solid/liquid release (c)
  Planned treated effluent release (d)
  Planned/fugitive atmospheric emission (e)
  [Items from here to Risk Assessment apply to (a) through (e)]

**Table I.**   *(continued)*

| Issue | Research |
|---|---|
| | Acute and chronic bioassay<br>    Test coal liquefaction materials for acute and chronic effects on aquatic and terrestrial organisms. Identify chemical compounds/compound classes responsible for effects.<br>Biological and chemical fate<br>    Determine rates of transport and transformation of coal liquefaction materials mediated by chemical and biological processes. Determine potential toxicity of transformation products identified under "Toxicology," at top of table. Measure bioaccumulation and determine potential for food chain transfer.<br>Field monitoring<br>    Accumulate baseline, operational, and post-operational data relevant to environmental fate and effects at coal liquefaction facilities. |
| Risk assessment | Health<br>    Use data from unit operations and potential plant/transportation accident scenarios to identify sources of occupational and environmental exposure, and couple with analyses of dose-effect from toxicological and appropriate epidemiological studies to identify and quantitate potential occupational and environmental health risks.<br>Ecology<br>    Use data from unit operations and potential plant/transportation accident scenarios to identify sources of aquatic and terrestrial contamination and couple with laboratory and field studies to identify and predict environmental risks and potential food chain transfer to man.<br>Amelioration (i.e., hydrotreatment, fractional distillation)<br>    Evaluate effectiveness of existing and planned ameliorative measures relative to present and anticipated regulations. Assess impact on occupational and environmental health and on potentially affected ecosystems. |
| End use | Use of coal liquefaction materials will affect the environment contingent on their specific use (e.g., combustion, use as refinery and petrochemical feedstock). Research required is identified in the preceding components of this table. |

uments, including technical reports, symposia proceedings, and open literature publications (see Ref. 1 for a complete bibliography).

## RESEARCH STRATEGY

Although the ultimate goal of DOE's research program was to evaluate long-term health and environmental effects of a large-scale coal liquefaction industry, there were no large-scale (i.e., demonstration or commercial) coal liquefaction facilities in existence. Therefore, research efforts focused on materials produced at process development units (PDUs) and pilot-scale facilities that were operated under conditions that approximated potential demonstration or commercial facility practice. Thus, health, environmental, and safety research accompanied engineering development, so that results might influence final process designs. For comparative purposes, other fossil-derived materials and selected chemicals were also evaluated. These materials, which include shale oil, crude and refined petroleums, and pure forms of known chemical mutagens and carcinogens, assist in placing results obtained with direct coal liquefaction materials in perspective.

Coal liquefaction materials were subjected to a battery of short- and long-term bioassays in conjunction with chemical fractionation and analyses to identify compounds and classes of compounds responsible for biological effects. Short-term studies provided the first indication of potential health and environmental problems associated with coal liquefaction materials. Longer-term studies evaluated materials that were considered most representative of potential demonstration or commercial practice. These materials were subjected to whole-animal and ecosystem studies relative to effects and environmental fate. Studies are also being conducted to evaluate the influence of process or operational modifications and control technology options on potential health and environmental effects of coal liquefaction materials.

## RESULTS TO DATE

This section summarizes chemical characterization and health effects data relative to worker exposure, occupational health and industrial hygiene efforts, engineering options that modify chemical composition and biological activity, and the ecological fate and effects data relative to release of coal-derived materials to the environment.

### Chemical Characterization

Coal liquids are extremely complex chemically compared with similar boiling-range crude petroleums. This complexity likely reflects chemical reactions during coal dissolution that fragment the coal structure and produce a variety of smaller molecules. Certain constituents of coal-derived materials, responsible for biological activity, are present in only ultratrace concentrations and are masked during analysis by major constituents. Thus, biologically nonactive components (generally the major components) of coal liquids must be separated from the trace quantities of biologically active agents. Separation requires special fractionation and state-of-the-art analytical techniques.

Data on chemical class distribution of various coal liquids have been compared with data on petroleum crudes and shale oils. Chemical classes compared were volatiles, insolubles, acids, bases, polynuclear aromatic hydrocarbons (PAHs), and other neutral components. Depending on boiling range (which is directly related to molecular weight), coal liquids may contain a significant amount of material that is insoluble in commonly used organic solvents (e.g., isooctane). Petroleum crudes contain essentially none of this insoluble material. Although the chemical nature of this material has not been completely characterized, the insolubles probably contain high-molecular-weight and polar, polyfunctional polycyclic aromatic materials. The acid fraction is considerably larger in coal liquids than in either crude petroleums or shale oils and contains phenols and carboxylic acids. The basic fraction is also considerably larger in coal liquids than in other fuels and is composed predominantly of nitrogen-containing molecules such as pyridines, amines, and higher-molecular-weight azaarenes. The PAH fraction constitutes a greater portion of the coal liquids than it does in shale oil or petroleum. The PAH fraction contains two- to seven-ring hydrocarbons, some heterocyclic compounds, and numerous highly alkyl-substituted polycyclic aromatics. The neutral fraction containing aliphatic, alicyclic, olefinic, and alkylated mono-aromatic materials tends to be highest in petroleum, but it also comprises a significant fraction of some lighter-boiling-range coal liquefaction materials.

In summary, synthetic coal liquids from all processes evaluated are enriched in PAH, basic, acidic, and insoluble fractions compared with petroleum. Additionally, the degree of alkylation and substitution on aromatic rings is greater in coal liquids than in natural petroleums. The degree of enrichment of the above four fractions in coal liquids appears to be a function of boiling range. The higher-boiling-range cuts appear to be enriched in PAH and nitrogen- and oxygen-containing molecules in SRC-I and -II and H-coal materials. Data for a full-boiling-range EDS material show the same enrichment in heterocyclic and PAH compounds.

## Health Effects

Health effects research has focused on process streams and materials that might affect workers or be used as commercial products, or both. Several approaches to isolate biologically active fractions from these materials have been developed. The complex coal liquid is first screened with a variety of biological assays (see below). Active materials are then fractionated chemically. Each fraction is again screened biologically, and fractions containing biologically active agents are further fractionated. Subfractions may be subjected to additional bioassay and further chemical analyses. This iterative approach has allowed researchers to concentrate on identifying chemical components responsible for biological activity in SRC-I and -II and H-coal materials.

### Cellular Screening Studies

SRC-I and -II materials have been evaluated in several microbial and mammalian cell assays. SRC-I light oil (LO, bp <380°F), wash solvent (WS, bp 380–480°F) and process solvent (PS, bp 480–850°F), and SRC-II light (LD, bp <350°F), middle (MD, bp 350–550°F), and heavy (HD, bp 550–850°F) distillates were assayed with the Ames *(Salmonella)* histidine reversion plate assay. No mutagenic activity was observed with the LO, WS, LD, or MD. In contrast, substantial activity was found in SRC-I PS and SRC-II HD, which showed, respectively, 20 and 80 times the activity of crude shale oil. In comparison, a known chemical carcinogen, benzo[a]pyrene (BaP), showed about nine times the activity of PS and three times the activity of HD. Another well-known chemical carcinogen, 2-aminoanthracene (2-AA), was about 400 times as active as PS and about 100 times as active as SRC-II HD.

High-boiling-range materials, SRC-I PS and SRC-II HD, also transformed Syrian hamster embryo (SHE) cells, whereas lower-boiling-range materials, SRC-I LO and WS, and SRC-II LD and MD, did not. SRC-II HD was as active as BaP and several times more active than 2-AA. Cells transformed by SRC-I PS and subsequently undergoing several passages in culture produced tumors when injected into nude mice.

SRC-I PS and SRC-II HD were subjected to a number of fractionation schemes, including solvent extraction, distillation, alumina and silicic acid chromatography, and high-pressure liquid chromatography. Resulting fractions were then assayed for microbial mutagenicity. Mutagenic activity was associated with relatively polar fractions. Further chemical and biological characterization of the active fractions provided evidence that primary aromatic amines (PAAs) were the major determinants of microbial mutagenesis. Several independent approaches, one that decreased mutagenic activity (chemical deactivation with nitrous acid, which eliminates the primary amine group and converts PAAs to phenols); another that enhanced mutagenic activity (selectively activates PAAs to their mutagenic form); and hydrotreatment studies (see below) confirmed this conclusion. Analyses of SRC-I PS, SRC-II HD, and an SRC-II distillate blend have identified about 70 PAAs. These amines range in size from two to six aromatic rings and include numerous alkyl-substituted compounds. Relative mutagenicities of different chemical subfractions generally correlate with concentrations of PAAs having three or more aromatic rings. Mutagenicity does not appear to correlate with any other chemical constituents. However, genetically active fractions were also enriched in azaarenes, carbazoles, and polar substituted aromatics, which may affect genetic activity. Simultaneous analyses of many of these fractions, using mammalian cell culture assays, showed that neutral PAHs were also biologically active components of coal liquids.

Ames assays with PDU-derived H-coal materials showed that the lower-boiling-range atmospheric still overheads (bp 150–650°F) were not mutagenic, whereas the higher-boiling-range crudes, atmospheric still bottoms, vacuum still overheads, and vacuum still bottoms were. Fractionation studies indicated that most mutagenic activity resides in the ether-soluble base and the neutral polyaromatic fractions of these materials. Some additional activity was found in the insoluble base (tar) and in the neutral polar fractions. Mutagenic activity of the insoluble base fraction was significant for only high-boiling-range, high-molecular-weight materials with large concentrations of tars. The mutagenically active neutral polyaromatic fractions of some coal liquids are enriched in azaarenes and substituted azaarenes, implicating these compounds in microbial activity. One additional fraction that appears to have some biological activity is the neutral polar fraction. This fraction contained numerous hydroxylated and carbonyl compounds and a series of nitrogen-containing compounds. The nitrogen compounds included azaarenes and polycyclic PAAs. Detection of activity in neutral fractions of H-coal materials, compared with lack of activity in similar fractions of SRC materials, may reflect differences in fractionation procedures. It is probable that biologically active agents in H-coal materials are similar to those in SRC-I and -II materials.

The naphtha, solvent, heavy gas oil, vacuum gas oil, and residue from the EDS process have also been assayed for mutagenic activity in the Ames system. All but the naphtha were positive. Components responsible for mutagenic activity in EDS materials have not been investigated to the same extent as those from SRC and H-coal.

## Skin Carcinogenesis

Skin tumorigenesis studies have been performed with materials derived from the SRC, H-coal, and EDS processes. Both long-term (2 years) and short-term (6 months) assays have been used. Generally these studies show that tumorigenic activity of coal liquids increases with boiling-range temperature. The SRC-II HD, H-coal atmospheric still bottoms and vacuum still overheads, and high-boiling EDS liquids were highly tumorigenic to mouse skin. In contrast, SRC-II LD, H-coal atmospheric still overheads, and EDS naphtha were inactive. Because average molecular weight increases with boiling-range temperature, there is also substantial correlation between tumorigenic activity and average molecular weight. The identity of coal liquid constituents thought to be responsible for skin tumorigenesis in mice is discussed by Pelroy et al.[3] Although other fossil fuel materials such as petroleum crudes and shale oil are also carcinogenic, these materials show less activity than do comparable high-boiling-range coal liquids.

### Acute Toxicity

SRC-II LD, MD, and HD, SRC-I LO and PS, and some PDU-derived H-coal distillates were moderately toxic ($LD_{50}$ = 2 to 3.5 g per kg of body weight) after oral administration to rats. SRC-I WS was the most toxic coal liquid tested, probably reflecting its high phenolic content. No coal liquid tested produced skin sensitization when applied intradermally. Eye irritation was noted with some H-coal and SRC materials, but it was a reversible effect.

### Teratogenesis

Effects of SRC-II LD, MD, and HD and SRC-I LO, WS, and PS on fetal development were determined after oral administration of these materials to pregnant rats at 7 to 11 and 12 to 16 days gestation (dg). Pregnant rats were also exposed to SRC-II HD aerosols at 12 to 16 dg. Although materials boiling below 450°F produced no teratisms, fetal growth and survival were decreased by all materials administered at either gestation period. Doses producing fetal effects often produced indications of maternal toxicity. In contrast to low-boiling-range materials, administration of SRC-I PS and SRC-II HD at 12 to 16 dg increased the incidence of fetal malformations, primarily cleft palate, hypoplastic (immature) lungs, and herniated diaphragms. Coal-derived materials were also teratogenic in amphibian and insect test systems (see Terrestrial Effects, this chapter).

### Mammalian Mutagenesis

Several mammalian mutagenesis assays including the male mouse dominant lethal test, female mouse reproductive capacity test, heritable translocation test, spot test, and specific locus test have been applied to coal liquids (SRC-II HD and Synthoil) and several of their fractions and two PAHs (BaP and dimethylbenzanthracene). Although some assays were positive for some materials assayed, there was no clear evidence that any of the materials studied were overly mutagenic in the whole animal. However, the coal liquids were cytotoxic, and there was some evidence that several materials may interfere with reproduction.

### Inhalation Studies

Preliminary inhalation studies have been conducted with mice, rats, and guinea pigs exposed to SRC-I PS and SRC-II HD for up to 21 d. A relatively high dose (greater than 0.6 mg/L) inhibited weight gain in mice and rats. Guinea pigs were most sensitive and required only 0.1 to 0.3 mg/L of material to inhibit weight gain by more than 10%. Although weight gain of rats and mice was reduced during exposure, it increased to normal following cessation of exposure.

SRC-I PS and SRC-II HD produced minor changes in a battery of pulmonary function tests in rats. However, guinea pigs exposed by inhalation to either PS or HD showed substantial changes in pulmonary function when challenged by a histamine aerosol. Although both compliance and resistance of guinea pig lungs were markedly altered, substantial recovery occurred within 3 d after cessation of exposure.

### Occupational Health and Industrial Hygiene

Extensive occupational health and industrial hygiene programs have been designed for coal liquefaction pilot plants and proposed demonstration facilities. These programs were based on the premise that workers at coal liquefaction facilities would be exposed to potentially toxic materials.

Occupational health and industrial hygiene programs for coal liquefaction facilities have several components: (1) engineering design and control, (2) personnel and area monitoring for pollutants, (3) education, (4) work practices, (5) personal hygiene, and (6) medical surveillance. To date, there have been no indications of unique health problems in coal liquefaction pilot plants.

### Engineering Options that Modify Chemical Composition and Biological Activity

The relative biological activity of coal liquids compared with that of shale oils and crude petroleums has generated interest in evaluating methods of modifying chemical properties to reduce or eliminate genotoxic and carcinogenic potential and systemic toxicity. Hydrotreatment (i.e., addition of hydrogen) and selective distillation have been evaluated.

#### Hydrotreatment

Studies with a PDU-derived H-coal distillate and an SRC-II blend indicate that hydrotreatment reduces or eliminates the biological activity of coal liquids. Heavy hydrotreatment eliminated the mutagenic activity of the H-coal distillate in the Ames assay; light and medium hydrotreatment had little demonstrable effect. Ames assay of the hydrotreated SRC-II distillate blend showed that moderate and severe hydrotreatment reduced mutagenicity about 100-fold. Hydrotreatment also decreased SHE cell transformation activity by 25 to 40%, and impairment of cell growth was reduced as hydrotreatment severity increased.

Hydrotreating reduced the aromatic, phenolic, PAH, nitrogen hetero-cycle, and PAA content and increased the hydroaromatic content of the SRC-II blend. Both moderate and severe hydrotreatment reduced PAA levels at least 340-fold (from 1900 ppm to concentrations below detection limits). The reduction in genotoxic activity is believed to reflect the decrease in PAA concentration.

Skin-painting studies with PDU-derived H-coal liquids showed that carcinogenicity was also substantially reduced (>50%) with minimal hydro-treatment. Similar results have been reported for shale oil. However, as levels of hydrotreatment were increased sufficiently to reduce mutagenicity in the Ames assay, mammalian systemic toxicity increased. If this effect is confirmed and extended to other coal liquids, only the minimal hydrotreat-ment needed to achieve satisfactory physical and chemical requirements and to reduce skin carcinogenic potential should be utilized.

### Selective Distillation

Biological activity of coal liquids increases with boiling-range temperature (i.e., molecular weight). H-coal heavy still bottoms showed higher muta-genic activity than still overhead materials. Chemical and biological exam-ination of different boiling ranges of SRC-I and -II full-boiling-range materials showed no mutagenic activity below 725°F. Some activity was detected from 725 to 750°F. Mutagenicity increased with temperature from 750 to 850°F and decreased slightly in still-bottoms material above 850°F. Corresponding changes in chemical composition also occurred in high-boiling-range mate-rials. SRC-I and -II materials showed decreasing concentrations of aliphatic hydrocarbons and increasing concentrations of PAHs with increasing boiling point. The increase in aromatic hydrocarbons occurred in the neutral, hy-droxylated, and nitrogen-containing PAH fractions of SRC-II material, but was seen only in the hydroxylated and nitrogen-containing PAH fractions of SRC-I material. The PAAs also increased with boiling-range tempera-ture. Treatment of high-boiling-range materials with nitrous acid reduced the concentration of PAAs and lowered mutagenicity, suggesting that mu-tagenicity was due to increasing concentration of higher-molecular-weight PAAs (with four- to five-ring systems) with increasing boiling-range temperature.

## Environmental Fate and Effects

Environmental research has focused on the fate and effects of coal lique-faction product, process, and waste materials that may be released (e.g., by accidental spills) to terrestrial or aquatic systems, or both, and the potential for food chain transfer of coal liquefaction residuals to man.

### Terrestrial Fate and Transport

A series of soil sorption studies with aniline and phenol was initiated to define the fate of coal liquid components in terrestrial habitats. These compounds account for the majority of water-soluble organics in the SRC-II distillate blend. Results suggest that soils of the eastern coal region (Westmorland silt loam) may retard the movement of organic nitrogen bases (anilines), while phenols remain relatively mobile. Thus, phenols would likely be the first compounds to affect groundwater quality. In contrast, the primary environmental impact of anilines may result from plant uptake and subsequent food chain incorporation and transport.

Studies with a petroleum crude, shale oil, and coal liquid added to laboratory soil columns suggest that phenolic or other compounds in coal liquids are highly toxic to microorganisms. Thus, coal liquids may initially eradicate microbial communities that aid the degradation of heavier hydrocarbons and may remain in soils longer than petroleum or shale oils. Lysimeter studies confirmed that coal liquids do not readily degrade. Although germination of barley *(Hordeum vulgare)* occurred during the second growing season following contamination of soils with the SRC-II blend, grain production was still significantly reduced.

Phenol and aniline induced severe phenotypic and toxicity responses in hydroponically grown soybeans. Studies with isotopically labeled compounds showed that the plant absorption rate for $^{14}$C-aniline was substantially lower than that for $^{14}$C-phenol. Unlike phenol, aniline tended to sorb to cell walls. However, absorbed phenol was readily degraded and its carbon metabolized to higher-molecular-weight components; aniline was only partially degraded and persisted as the parent compound or its modified products, or both.

Studies with 1-week-old soybean plants were conducted using $^{14}$C-anthracene (a PAH) in nutrient solution, moist and flooded soil, and the atmosphere. Results showed that $^{14}$C-anthracene was taken up from either roots or foliage, translocated, and catabolized to lower-molecular-weight products.

### Terrestrial Effects

Sulfur-containing gases that are common stack emissions during liquefaction include both reduced [COS, $H_2S$, carbonyl disulfide $(CS_2)$, and methyl mercaptan $(CH_3SH)$] and oxidized [sulfur dioxide $(SO_2)$] forms. Toxicity of liquefaction-emission products to vegetation is a function of deposition rate on foliage and subsequent disruption of metabolic processes. At equivalent ambient concentrations, the principal sulfur gases from liquefaction react with vegetation at rates that vary 10-fold. Reactivity of the gases in descending order is: $SO_2 \geq H_2S > COS > CH_3SH \geq CS_2$. From 0.25 to 0.5 ppm, $SO_2$, $H_2S$, and COS depressed photosynthesis below that of controls, but $CS_2$ and $CH_3SH$ had no effect. Relative toxicity of these gases follows the same order as reactivity. The correlation between reactivity and toxicity suggests that the former may be a screening tool to gauge the potential impact of any coal conversion gas.

Climate also influences plant response to pollutants; relative humidity is a major controlling factor. Uptake of ozone or $SO_2$ by vegetation was 200 to 300% higher at 70% relative humidity than at 35% humidity. Thus, the impact of liquefaction emissions may vary as a function of regional location.

Other atmospheric pollutants also affect plant response to coal liquefaction emissions. Although nitrogen oxides are released from process-fired heaters, boilers, calciners, and controlled combustors during liquefaction, the probability of adverse effects on vegetation is low because emission levels are low. However, when nitrogen oxides occur with $SO_2$ (another liquefaction emission) at concentrations above 262 $\mu g/m^3$ and ozone (a regional pollutant in the eastern United States), growth of vegetation may be depressed.

Studies with barley *(Hordeum vulgare)* exposed to SRC-I solids added to soils in outdoor lysimeters showed little effect on germination, growth, or yield when soil and SRC-I solids were mixed 1:1. When barley was grown on a 3-dm layer of soil placed over a 1-dm layer of SRC-I, growth and yield were reduced, apparently reflecting the inability of roots to penetrate the SRC-I layer. The SRC-II blend added to the soil layer, 10 dm below the surface, resulted in lesions, chlorosis, necrotic tissue, reduced grain yields, and grain with higher nitrogen content. However, yields increased during the second growing season, suggesting a decrease in toxicity due to microbial degradation and/or other processes.

Studies to determine effects of azaarenes on egg production and hatching success of crickets showed an increased frequency of morphologic abnormalities in developing embryos. Several coal liquids were also found to be potent teratogens; eggs developing in soil contaminated with coal-derived materials produced nymphs with extra antennae, eyes, and heads. Standard mammalian assays confirm the teratogenic potential of high-boiling coal liquids (see "Teratogenesis," this chapter). Petroleum products did not cause these developmental abnormalities.

### Aquatic Fate and Transport

Alkyl anilines and pyridines were identified in the SRC-II blend and shown to be significant components (5 to 10%) of the water-soluble fractions (WSFs). The water-soluble components of five synthetic liquids (ranging from a heavy syncrude to LD) were similar, although concentrations varied widely among oils. As expected, major water-soluble components were phenols and cresols with lower levels of xylenols and C3- and C4-substituted phenols. Major neutral components were toluene, xylene, and naphthalene. Basic constituents were aniline and C1- to C3-substituted aniline. Larger multiring compounds (naphthol, alkylnaphthalenes, pyridines, and anilines) were not found at levels above detection limits (~0.1 µg/L). No phenols or bases (except anilines) were detected in water extracts of a petroleum crude.

Studies were also conducted to characterize water-soluble photooxidants produced by sunlight in water underlying coal liquids. Rates of photooxidant formation from four coal liquids were similar and were about one-fourth that from a petroleum diesel oil. Most of the water-soluble photooxidant from coal liquids appeared to be hydrogen peroxide. The remainder appeared to be hydroquinine, a highly toxic nitrogen-containing phenol. Toxicity to *Daphnia magna* of water underlying one coal liquid doubled over 4 d of illumination by sunlight.

Studies were conducted with PAHs to evaluate rate and extent of photolysis (breakdown by sunlight), volatilization, sorption to particles and sediments, and microbial degradation in water and sediments. Volatilization decreased rapidly with increasing molecular size, while photolysis increased for most of the larger potentially carcinogenic PAHs. Microbial transformations in water were extremely slow for PAHs larger than naphthalene (two rings), even in highly polluted environments. Microbial transformation rates in sediments appeared directly related to the amount and size of PAHs entering the water. Transformation rates were sufficiently slow for larger PAHs, like BaP, so that levels in contaminated sediments will likely remain high for several years after release. Sorption of PAHs to particles was rapidly reversible, and resuspension of sediments during high-water periods may result in release of sediment-bound PAH into overlying waters.

### Aquatic Effects

Coal liquids contain relatively high concentrations of phenols, which are highly toxic. The acute toxicities of WSFs of nearly 30 natural and synthetic oils were compared, using aquatic organisms (phytoplankton, invertebrates, fish) representing various trophic levels and habitats. Coal liquids [SRC-I, SRC-II, and H-coal (raw distillate or fuel oil blend)] were all 10 to 1000 times more toxic than petroleum products. Crude and hydrotreated shale oils were more toxic than petroleum equivalents; however, hydrotreated shale oil was less toxic than the crude shale oil.

In chronic-toxicity studies, organisms were exposed to the WSF resulting from an initial contact of coal liquid with water and to a WSF derived from a water-leached coal liquid. Lower-molecular-weight phenols predominated in the initial-contact WSF, while higher-molecular-weight phenols and hydrocarbons characterized the water-leached WSF. Based on percent dilution, the initial-contact WSF was more toxic than the WSF derived from the water-leached material. However, in bioassays of chironomid larvae (*Chironomus tentans* and *Tanytarsus dissimilis*), the water-leached WSF was more toxic than the initial-contact WSF when equal concentrations of total organic carbon (TOC) were present. Although the two WSFs were similar in toxicity to algae *(Selenastrum capricornutum)* over a 5-d exposure period, recovery of algal populations was suppressed to a greater extent in the water-leached WSF.

Sediments were artificially contaminated with the SRC-II blend and subjected to a series of repeated mixing and water replacements to simulate natural river scouring. Adult daphnids and chironomid larvae were used as indicators of toxicity. Readily water-soluble phenolics were rapidly removed from contaminated sediments. Removal rates of total phenolics were linear for both concentrations tested. Rate of removal was dependent on compound class (C1, C2, C3, C4 phenols > C1, C2 indanols > phenol > C3 indanols). Sediment retention of less soluble, high-molecular-weight phenolics affected behavior and survival of the sediment-dwelling chironomids after acutely toxic effects were no longer observed for daphnids in the water column. These studies suggest that, as soluble phenolics are leached from sediments contaminated with coal liquids, pelagic organisms will be exposed to toxic components over relatively short time periods, whereas insoluble components in sediments may result in long-term toxicity to benthic organisms.

### Ecosystem Studies

Stream and pond microcosm experiments were conducted with WSFs of the SRC-II blend and a PDU-derived H-coal oil, respectively. Relatively low doses of coal liquid (0.1 of the 48-h $LC_{50}$ for *Daphnia magna*) caused extensive changes in community structure and function. Many zooplankton species were eliminated, and diatoms were replaced by blue-green algae. Patterns of community metabolism were also affected. That is, detritus (dead algae) replaced diatoms and other algae as a food source for zooplankton. However, eliminating toxic input resulted in partial recovery of the system. Recovery of algal populations was also observed in laboratory bioassays after the coal liquid WSF was removed.

## RISK ASSESSMENT

Risk assessment is an integral part of DOE's coal liquefaction program and integrates the various research and development activities to quantitatively assess potential human health and environmental effects. The assessment incorporates basic information on source terms, exposure mechanisms, dose-risk relationships, and uncertainty and is being conducted on a regional or national scale, concentrating on multiple facilities representing a mature industry.

Preliminary assessments have been performed and results published. Data on regional weather patterns have been used to investigate and evaluate atmospheric dispersion and multiple-facility interactions. A set of generic atmospheric dispersion factors has been employed to evaluate potential health risks associated with airborne pollutants. Many other factors including persistence of pollutants, their solubility in water, pathways of human intake, uptake of synfuel residuals by crops, groundwater movement, toxicity, and epidemiology must also be considered. An iterative process of risk analysis helps guide the direction of health and environmental research programs.

## IMPLICATIONS

Results of DOE's health and environmental research efforts have significant implications for coal liquefaction process designers and developers. High-boiling-range coal-derived materials are mutagenic, teratogenic, and carcinogenic in laboratory test systems. Additionally, coal liquids cause acute and chronic effects in organisms representing various ecological trophic levels. However, knowledge of potential detrimental health and environmental effects and of their causative agents can be used to design environmentally acceptable coal conversion processes.

Studies are in progress to evaluate effects of process modifications, such as reducing extraction severity in the dissolver, on health and environmental effects of coal-derived materials. Additionally, because mutagenic activity is due primarily to PAAs, found only in higher-boiling-range coal liquids, distillation cuts might be adjusted so that the commercial product contains little mutagenic potential. Distillation cuts could also be selected to concentrate mutagenically active compounds in a relatively small process stream, which might receive special treatment (e.g., hydrotreating). In addition to lowering mutagenicity, hydrotreating also lowers carcinogenicity and concentrations of constituents (e.g., phenols) responsible for acute and chronic toxicity and potentially responsible (e.g., nitrogen compounds) for teratogenicity. Although engineering and economic factors must also be considered, the growing biomedical and environmental data base can be incorporated into the decision-making process. Besides adjusting distillation cuts, hydrotreating, or a combination of these, process designers can begin, now, to develop special handling and accident prevention procedures.

Accidental spills of coal liquids and other coal-derived materials are a potential threat to the environment. Aquatic organisms exposed to coal liquid WSFs for long periods will experience a constantly changing spectrum of organic compounds, and different species will experience different toxic effects. Some constituents of coal-derived materials may be taken up and transferred through food chains leading to man. Low-molecular-weight compounds such as phenols, which are responsible for acute effects, degrade rapidly. High-molecular-weight compounds are more persistent and bind to soils and sediments, causing chronic effects at low concentrations. Thus, spill prevention is a major consideration. Assuming that accidental spills of coal liquids will occur, cleanup procedures should be developed to minimize potential chronic effects in aquatic and terrestrial systems. Some aquatic populations (e.g., algae) can recover following exposure to toxic concentrations of coal liquid WSFs after the material is removed.

Potential health and environmental risks associated with developing a large-scale coal liquefaction industry are being assessed during the early design phases of technology development. These efforts are providing guidance for selecting process and product modifications, control technology options, mitigative strategies, accident prevention, spill cleanup, and solid-waste disposal procedures to minimize adverse human health and environmental effects.

## ACKNOWLEDGMENTS

Many individuals were involved in the research and/or made valuable contributions during preparation of the report on which this chapter is based. We are grateful for their support. Authors of the original report included the authors of this chapter and P.J. Mellinger, PNL; and K.E. Cowser, J.L. Epler, R.J. Fry, C.W. Gehrs, J.M. Giddings, M.R. Guerin, J.M. Holland, and H. Inhaber, ORNL. We also wish to thank P. Cho, A.P. Duhamel, G.E. Stapleton, and F.J. Wobber, DOE, Office of Energy Research (OER), who kindly reviewed drafts of the original report and provided critical input to its content. Preparation of the original report was supported by OER under Contract DE-ACO6-76RLO-1830 with Battelle Memorial Institute, Pacific Northwest Laboratory and Contract W-7405-eng-26 with Union Carbide Corporation, Oak Ridge National Laboratory. Financial support for research efforts described was provided by OER and the DOE Office of the Assistant Secretary for Fossil Energy.

## REFERENCES

1. Gray, R.H., and K.E. Cowser, Eds. "Status of Health and Environmental Research Relative to Direct Coal Liquefaction: 1976 to the Present," DOE/NBM-1016, PNL-4176 (Richland, WA: Pacific Northwest Laboratory, 1982).
2. Duhamel, A.P. Chapter 9, this volume.
3. Pelroy, R.A., R.A. Renne, D.D. Mahlum, and M.E. Frazier. "Comparison of In Vivo Carcinogenesis and In Vitro Genotoxicity of Complex Hydrocarbon Mixtures," Chapter 15, this volume.

## DISCUSSION

*C.D. Scott, Oak Ridge National Laboratory:* You mentioned a potential for reducing the problems from such contaminants. One possibility would be distillation. Distillation is a very energy intensive process and conceivably very economically disadvantageous. Do you have an example where that could be used, or have you thought about it from that standpoint?

*R.H. Gray:* Although I am not an engineer, what I was suggesting were a number of potential options that the engineers can begin to consider and take into their data base when they make decisions. There are people in this audience representing the engineering side of the house that might like to comment on that. I do know that some of them are thinking of taking the 700°-plus material and not using it as product material and recycling it in plant.

*C.D. Scott:* The big problem with distillation as I would see it is that you have to remove a large amount of the low-boiling material, water in this case, in order to achieve a separation.

*Carl Mazza, Environmental Protection Agency:* The work that you presented stated that there were no concerns for carcinogenicity or teratogenicity in the middle and light distillates. These appear to be rather definitive statements. Do you mean them as definitive statements or preliminary statements?

*R.H. Gray:* The data just represent results from an SRC-II material using our particular test systems, in which we are looking at potential effects. What I was telling you is that in our test systems we did not get any positive response for those endpoints for those particular distillates. I can also say that some of the additional studies that are now being done with other coal liquids generally support that kind of conclusion. I am not saying anything about carcinogenicity in man. These are laboratory test systems.

*Carl Mazza:* In in vitro type test systems as opposed to animal systems?

*R.H. Gray:* I showed you several endpoints; some of them were in in vitro test systems and some of them were in whole-animal test systems.

*P.H. Buhl:* These tests at PNL, where they are looking at the boiling point ranges and other factors, are not compliance toxicology test systems. They are using limited numbers of animals, and many of the tests are the initiation-promotion tests. We are not saying these materials are any better than petroleum. We are just saying they have significantly reduced activity compared to the heavy distillate studies that we had done before. Until you do a really definitive-type toxicology study, we cannot really say what the end result is going to be.

# CHAPTER 2

## Summary of Health and Environmental Research: Coal Gasification

### K.E. Wilzbach and C.A. Reilly, Jr.
*Argonne National Laboratory*
*Argonne, IL 60439*

This chapter summarizes coal gasification health and environmental research sponsored by the U.S. Department of Energy and conducted by Argonne National Laboratory, the Inhalation Toxicology Research Institute, and Oak Ridge National Laboratory. Following an overview of coal gasification technology and its related health and environmental concerns, the results and conclusions in areas of potential concern are summarized. Emphasis is on chemical and toxicological characterization of materials from a range of process streams in six bench scale, pilot plant, and industrial gasifiers. Ecological effects, industrial hygiene, and environmental control technology performance are also addressed.

### INTRODUCTION

This chapter is based on and in some areas updates a report prepared for the U.S. Department of Energy (DOE) on the status of health and environmental effects associated with coal gasification.[1] It covers studies sponsored by the DOE Offices of Energy Research and Fossil Energy and conducted over the past several years at the Inhalation Toxicology Research Institute (ITRI), Oak Ridge National Laboratory (ORNL), and Argonne National Laboratory (ANL).

Process materials examined in these studies were collected from a number of small coal gasification plants or bench-scale facilities: the 25-tpd (tons per day) slagging fixed-bed gasifier at the Grand Forks Energy Technology Center (GFETC); the 25-tpd pressurized Wellman-Galusha fixed-bed gasifier at Morgantown Energy Technology Center (METC); the 80-tpd HYGAS fluidized-bed pilot plant operated by the Institute of Gas Technology; the

75-tpd two-stage fixed-bed Stoic industrial gasifier at the University of Minnesota in Duluth (UMD); the 75-tpd anthracite-fueled Wellman-Galusha units of the Community Area New Development Organization (CAN-DO) at Hazelton, Pennsylvania, and a bench-scale pyrolysis unit at Carnegie-Mellon Institute of Research (CMIR). Operational objectives at these facilities varied widely, from research (CMIR) and development of advanced processes (GFETC, HYGAS), to investigation of unit operations in gas cleanup (METC) and routine industrial operation (UMD, CAN-DO).

This chapter begins with a brief discussion of coal gasification technology and the potential health and environmental concerns it raises. Emphasis is placed on the toxicological and chemical characterization of organic compounds present in by-product tars, oils, and wastewater or associated with overhead particulates and bottom ash. In addition, ecological effects, industrial hygiene, and environmental control options are addressed.

## COAL GASIFICATION TECHNOLOGY

The health and environmental effects associated with coal gasification are of considerable importance, because the technology can satisfy a variety of our energy needs and eventually will play an important role in our economy. The applications of coal gasification are shown in Table I. The rate of coal consumption varies greatly with plant type, ranging from about 50 tpd of coal for an industrial plant to about 20,000 tpd for a commercial-scale synfuel complex. There is a corresponding variation in the magnitude of potential health and environmental effects.

### Effects Related to Gasification Facility Size

The effects of an individual industrial-scale coal gasifier operating at about 100 tpd are limited to the work force and the local environment. On the

**Table I.** Energy Needs Satisfied by Coal Gasification

| Plant Type | Coal Consumption (tpd) |
|---|---|
| Industrial steam, process heat | 50–200 |
| Combined-cycle power generation | $2–5 \times 10^3$ |
| Regional gaseous fuel | $2–5 \times 10^3$ |
| Substitute natural gas | $15–20 \times 10^3$ |
| Liquid fuels (methanol, gasoline) | $15–20 \times 10^3$ |
| Hydrogen, ammonia, chemicals | $5–20 \times 10^3$ |

other hand, a commercial-scale coal gasification facility can have far-ranging effects. A gasification plant producing 250 million std ft$^3$ of gas per day (equivalent to a liquefaction plant producing 50,000 bbl/d) will process 15,000 to 25,000 tpd of coal. Such a facility could require opening a large new surface mine or two large underground mines. Including coal storage sites and water treatment ponds, the gasification facility may require more than a square mile of land and may employ more than 1500 people. The plant, mine, and associated new dwellings may affect an area of up to 200 sq miles. Additional areas may be affected by new roads, power lines, and pipelines. The total cost of a commercial facility with an equivalent energy production of about 0.4% of current natural gas production can exceed $3 billion.

### Effects Related to Gasifier Design

In addition to facility size, the characteristics of the gasification process and design, as well as the characteristics of the coal, can markedly affect potential health and environmental effects. Coal can be gasified in several ways: by pyrolysis, by flash hydrogenation, or by reaction with steam and oxygen (or air). The last method is by far the most common and was utilized in all of the gasifiers studied thus far. The principal gaseous products of the reaction of steam and oxygen with coal are carbon monoxide, hydrogen, carbon dioxide, and methane. If air is used as the source of oxygen, the nitrogen-containing product gas has a low heat value and must be used locally.

Condensable organic compounds such as oil and tar may be significant components of the raw product gas or virtually absent from it, depending on gasifier design. Likewise, the characteristics of the solid residue (ash or slag) discharged from the gasifier are a function of design and operating conditions. There are many variations in the design of coal gasifiers, but they generally fall into three broad categories: fixed bed, fluidized bed, and entrained flow. The effects of gasifier design on the characteristics of the raw product gas, liquid effluents, and solid wastes will be discussed briefly.

#### Fixed-Bed Gasifiers

In a fixed-bed coal gasifier, such as a Wellman-Galusha or Lurgi gasifier, nut-size coal is introduced periodically from a hopper at the top of the gasifier. As the coal moves downward, it is exposed to progressively higher temperatures and is sequentially dried, devolatilized, gasified, and combusted. Steam and oxygen (or air) are introduced near the bottom of the gasifier and exit at the top, sweeping the products of gasification and the tars and oils formed in devolatilization out of the gasifier. The raw product gas from fixed-bed gasifiers thus contains significant amounts of tar and oil, typically 3 to 5% of the feed-coal weight. When the raw product gas is

cooled by quenching with water, the resulting aqueous phase is highly contaminated (e.g., with ammonia, hydrogen sulfide, phenols, and aromatic
amines) and requires extensive treatment before reuse or discharge. Fixed-
bed gasifiers can be designed and operated to discharge the residual mineral
matter of the coal either as an ash (e.g., the METC gasifier) or as a slag
(e.g., the GFETC gasifier).

### Fluidized-Bed Gasifiers

In fluidized-bed gasifiers, crushed and dried coal (pea-sized) is continuously
introduced, usually near the bottom of the gasifier, and fluidized by air and
steam entering at the bottom. Some caking coals may require mild oxidative
pretreatment. Fine ash entrained in the raw product gas is collected in a
cyclone and recycled. Agglomerated ash, if present, is withdrawn at the
bottom of the reactor.

Because the heat transfer in fluidized beds is rapid, the temperature
throughout the bed is nearly uniform. When the gasifier is operated at high
temperature (near the ash softening point), the coal is gasified very quickly
and little or no condensable organic material appears in the raw product
gas. Consequently, the aqueous phase produced by quenching the product
gas with water is far less contaminated than that from a fixed-bed gasifier.
Furthermore, when the bed temperature is near the ash softening point, the
ash begins to agglomerate, facilitating its separation from the product gas.
Gasifiers in this category, such as the U-gas Process of the Institute of Gas
Technology and the Westinghouse Agglomerating Ash Process, are nearing
commercialization.

### Entrained-Flow Gasifiers

In entrained-flow gasifiers, pulverized coal is entrained by and reacts with
a rapidly flowing stream of steam and oxygen. High temperatures (3000°F)
are required to gasify the coal during the short residence period. The oxygen
required to achieve such temperatures is usually introduced through nozzles
located near the bottom of the gasifier. Char entrained in the product gas
is separated and recycled. Ash is removed from the gasifier as a slag. The
high temperature of operation precludes the survival of significant amounts
of condensable organic matter in the product gas. Gasifiers of this type
require pulverized coal but, in contrast to fixed-bed and fluidized-bed gasifiers, are not sensitive to the caking properties of the feed coal. They are
more suitable for the preparation of synthesis gas than SNG, because the
methane content of the gas is low. The only fully commercial entrained-flow
gasifier is the Koppers-Totzek atmospheric-pressure gasifier. However, the
Texaco gasifier, which has been used extensively for generating synthesis
gas by the partial oxidation of oil residues, has been adapted to the gasification of coal and is nearing commercial status.

## HEALTH AND ENVIRONMENTAL CONCERNS

Discussion of the major areas of environmental concern, applicable to a greater or lesser degree to all coal gasification technologies and individual gasification facilities, and the nature of these concerns, follows.

### Air Quality

The operation of a coal gasification facility generates a large number of potential air pollutants in addition to the conventional coal-combustion pollutants (sulfur dioxide, oxides of nitrogen, carbon monoxide, particulates, and hydrocarbons). These pollutants include toxic or potentially toxic substances such as hydrogen sulfide, carbonyl sulfide, ammonia, hydrogen cyanide, benzene, polynuclear aromatic hydrocarbons and amines, nitrogen- and sulfur-containing heterocyclic compounds, and various trace elements. Carcinogenic chemicals, such as benzo(*a*)pyrene and 2-naphthylamine, have been identified as components of coal gasification tars and particulate-associated organic matter. Although technology is available to control conventional pollutant emissions to mandated levels, protection may be required against fugitive or accidental emission of materials such as polycyclic aromatic hydrocarbons and amines. Such emissions are not expected to affect regional air quality adversely, but are of significant concern in plant areas.

### Water Quality

Overall, water is consumed during coal gasification. However, potential effluents of contaminated water can arise from several sources in a major coal gasification facility. The major water stream (gas liquor) results from gas quenching and scrubbing operations, where sulfur must be removed from the product gas. Contaminated water is also produced during runoff from coal storage piles, ash quenching, desulfurization, impoundment of ash and sludge, raw-water cleanup, boiler blowdown, and cooling tower evaporation. Water from all of these sources can contain high concentrations of dissolved and suspended solids, including toxic trace elements. The gas liquor also can contain ammonia, cyanide, phenols, polynuclear aromatic hydrocarbons, and a range of compounds potentially carcinogenic or otherwise toxic. Conventional industrial wastewater treatment systems may be adequate for most of these streams; but the gas liquor presents unique problems, because of its high phenolic content and the presence of refractory organic compounds.

### Health Effects

The work force in coal gasification plants and the nearby populace may be exposed through inhalation to direct and fugitive emissions of potentially harmful vapors, aerosols, and particulate matter. In addition, the work force can be exposed to tar and oil by-products through ingestion and skin contact during plant operations and maintenance. The nature and extent of these emissions, and hence the risk of exposure, can be expected to vary with gasifier type and operating conditions. For small industrial gasifiers (UMD, CAN-DO), the major health effects are those in the work force. Exposure risks for large-scale commercial facilities are difficult to estimate, because the operating pilot plants do not generate products and emissions completely representative of those expected in commercial operations.

### Ecological Effects

Coal gasification and related mining operations may have significant adverse effects on terrestrial and aquatic ecosystems. The growth and developmental processes of terrestrial vegetation are known to be disturbed by atmospheric pollutants and by deposition of organic and particulate matter. Acute and chronic toxicity to aquatic species can result from the release of untreated liquid effluents. Degradation of surface water and groundwater quality can occur by runoff and leaching at the disposal site of gasifier ash and other solids. An important consequence of these processes is the possibility of biological uptake and bioaccumulation of toxicants in food chains, including those leading to man.

Other potential ecological effects include increased formation of oxidants and acid rain, increased consumption of water resources, disruption of water supply systems (aquifers), and disturbance of ground cover and wildlife populations.

### Industrial Hygiene

The work force in coal gasification plants can be exposed to a variety of toxicants by inhalation of fugitive vapors and particulates and by dermal contact with (or accidental ingestion of) oils, tars, and contaminated water, particularly during maintenance and repair of the facility. Assurance that the work force is adequately protected requires the identification, quantification, and control of exposures capable of producing adverse health effects. These in turn require the development and application of methods for determining area concentrations of and personal exposures to specific or surrogate pollutants; investigation of the effectiveness of various methods for mitigating exposures; and medical surveillance to ensure that gasification-associated health effects are identified at an early stage.

### Adequacy of Environmental Control

Various environmental control technologies may need to be incorporated in commercial coal gasification plants to decrease atmospheric emissions, decontaminate aqueous effluents, and secure solid waste disposal sites. Precautions must also be taken to protect the work force from undue stresses (e.g., heat, noise, and odors) and exposures to toxic vapors or liquids.

Environmental control technologies for dealing with corresponding problems in other industries have been developed and commercialized, but their applicability to coal gasification processes is not well established. In some cases the technologies appear to be applicable with little or no modification. In other cases, however, their applicability is not clear, because the coal gasification process streams have significantly different characteristics. It is not certain, for example, that the wastewater treatment schemes used in oil refineries are suitable for treating the highly contaminated water produced in some coal gasification processes. Similarly, conventional practices may not be suitable for disposal of the solid wastes from some gasifiers such as those in which reducing conditions prevail.

### Socioeconomic Impacts

One of the outstanding features of any future commercial coal gasification facility will be its size. Thus, the construction and operation of a major coal gasification plant may have significant socioeconomic impacts on neighboring communities, especially in less populated regions. These effects can include stresses on worker availability, housing, local tax structure, inflation, and government-provided services such as police protection, schools, and recreational facilities. The magnitude of these stresses and the effectiveness of mitigating measures are at present unknown.

## TOXICOLOGICAL CHARACTERIZATION

A stepwise approach has been used in the toxicological characterization of process samples from the six gasifiers under investigation. First, the process samples were screened for mutagenicity and cytotoxicity with a battery of readily performed cellular bioassays. Then, selected samples with relatively high toxicity and/or potential for exposure were used to determine acute and chronic toxicities in experimental animals.

## Cellular Assays

The mutagenicity of the materials was determined using microbial systems (bacteria and yeasts), with principal reliance on the Ames *Salmonella* microsome assay.[2] Toxicant interaction with mammalian DNA (genotoxicity) was measured by the increase in sister chromatid exchange (SCE) in mouse myeloma cells.[3] A number of mammalian cell systems were used to measure cytotoxicity. Cell viability (lethality or growth inhibition) was determined both in mouse myeloma cells and in dog and rabbit alveolar macrophages. Subcellular damage (release of cellular enzymes[4] or loss of phagocytic ability[5]) was determined in dog and rabbit alveolar macrophages. Generalized results of the cellular assays are presented in Table II.

## Tar

Tars produced in the GFETC, METC, and UMD gasifiers were mutagenic (Ames test, yeast cells) and cytotoxic in various mammalian cell systems. The nonvolatile organic (NVO) components in oil produced in the HYGAS process and a high-temperature raw-gas condensate from the CMIR reactor exhibited similar responses. The mutagenicities of all of these products are generally low relative to mutagenicities of known mutagens (e.g., benzo(a)pyrene) and require metabolic activation to be observed. Although values for the specific mutagenicities of the tars cannot be directly compared, because of inherent day-to-day and laboratory-to-laboratory variations, the values are quite similar. Typical mean mutagenicities of the *Salmonella* histidine revertants induced per microgram of test material (revertants/$\mu$g), with their ranges in parentheses, are: 4 for GFETC tar (1 to 8);[6] 8 for METC tar-trap tar;[7] 3.2 for UMD electrostatic precipitator tar (0 to 41);[8] 7 for the NVO fraction of HYGAS recycle oil (1 to 22);[9] and 19 for CMIR product tar (3 to 80).[10] These levels of activity are approximately 1 to 5% that of benzo(a)pyrene.

   SCE and cytotoxicity (growth inhibition) measurements were made in mouse myeloma cells on GFETC process tar and raw-gas tar condensates, and on the NVO fractions of HYGAS low-temperature reactor condensates. A twofold increase in the induction of sister chromatid exchange (SCE$_{200}$)

**Table II.**  Generalized Results of Cellular Bioassays

|  | Tar | Oil | Ash | Water |
|---|---|---|---|---|
| Mutagenicity | + + | +/− | +/− | − |
| Genotoxicity | + + | + | + | +[a] |
| Cytotoxicity | + | +/− | + | + |

[a]Solvent extracted.

was observed at concentrations of 83 µg/mL for GFETC process tar, 8 µg/mL for GFETC raw-gas tar condensate,[11] and 65 µg/mL for an NVO fraction of HYGAS low-temperature reactor condensate.[12] A 50% reduction in growth ($ED_{50}$) occurred at concentrations of 97, 20, and 96 µg/mL, respectively. A reference toxicant, methyl methanesulfonate, showed an $SCE_{200}$ at a concentration of 3 µg/mL and an $ED_{50}$ of 25 µg/mL. Concentrations that induced a 50% loss ($EC_{50}$) in rabbit alveolar macrophage function ranged from about 80 to 100 µg/mL for these materials. An $EC_{50}$ of 9 µg/mL was found with the reference toxicant vanadium oxide. METC tar-trap tar was cytotoxic to dog alveolar macrophages, as measured by release of the enzyme lactate dehydrogenase, with an $LC_{50}$ (concentration killing 50% of cells) of 45 µg/mL.[7]

## Oil

Mutagenicity of process oil samples from the GFETC gasifier was at the limit of detection (mean specific mutagenicity of < 1 revertant/µg).[11] The samples induced growth inhibition at an average $ED_{50}$ of 90 µg/mL and $SCE_{200}$ at an average concentration of 154 µg/mL. Average $LC_{50}$ and $EC_{50}$ concentrations of 308 µg/mL and 199 µg/mL were observed with rabbit alveolar macrophages. The Venturi condensate at METC had a specific mutagenicity of 3 revertant/µg.[13] No mutagenicity was detectable in the semivolatile organic fractions of HYGAS samples.

## Ash

The chemical composition of the solids discharged from a gasifier (ash, spent char, slag, etc.) varies as a function of coal type, process, and operating conditions. Health concerns center around the leachability of potentially hazardous adsorbed organic compounds and certain trace elements.[11] Bottom ash from the METC gasifier contained very little organic material extractable with dichloromethane (100 µg/g ash), and such extracts were nonmutagenic in the Ames test.[4] Spent char from the HYGAS gasifier contained slightly more extractable organic material (245 µg/g ash), and this extract was essentially nonmutagenic (≤ 0.1 revertant/µg).[12]

Distilled-water leachates of bottom ash from the UMD gasifier were evaluated in a number of bioassays, including the use of amphibian embryos *(Xenopus laevis)*, water fleas *(Daphnia magna)*, freshwater algae *(Selenastrum capricornutum)*, and radish and sorghum seedlings. High concentrations of the leachates were found to be toxic (e.g., the 48-h $LC_{50}$ for *Daphnia magna* was 87%), but in no assay was a toxic effect noted at a 10-fold dilution of the leachate.[14]

Cyclone dust from the METC gasifier contained 0.3 wt % dichloromethane-soluble material. Following metabolic activation, the extracts had specific mutagenic activities ranging from 0.8 to 5.7 revertants per μg of extract, corresponding to 2 to 17 revertants per mg of dust.[7]

At the HYGAS plant, char collected in a cyclone contained 1 to 3 wt % extractable organic material. The nonvolatile organic components of the extracts were shown to be mutagenic in the Ames test (3 to 20 revertants/μg) and genotoxic and cytotoxic to mouse myeloma cells.[12] The doubling of sister chromatid exchanges and the $LC_{50}$ both occur at concentrations of about 60 μg/mL. For these nonvolatile organic fractions, $LC_{50}$ values of cytotoxicity to rabbit alveolar macrophages varied from 100 to 250 μg/mL. Phagocytic capability was reduced 50% by concentrations as low as 30 μg/mL.

Limited information is available on the toxicity of cyclone ash leachates. Neutralized distilled-water leachates of cyclone ash collected at the UMD gasifier were evaluated using the same series of bioassays used with bottom ash leachates.[14] As with the bottom ash leachates, no toxic effects were seen with a 10-fold dilution of the leachate. Some toxic effects were observed at higher concentrations (e.g., the 48-h $LC_{50}$ for *Daphnia magna* was 66%).

## Water

Water quenching of product gas streams is generic to all coal gasification processes where removal of $H_2S$ and $NH_3$ is an objective. In the quenching and scrubbing process, the higher-molecular-weight organic compounds formed during gasification are condensed, and the more polar components (ammonia, phenols, and amines) are concentrated in the aqueous phase. Typically, water used in these process streams is recycled, but it may be eventually released. Water that is actually released must be at least minimally pretreated to remove gross organic contamination. At present, toxicological evaluations have been performed only on raw or minimally treated quench water. The results provide an indication of total toxicity but are not representative of water that could potentially be released after more effective treatment.

Quench water samples from both the gasifier and the pretreater of the HYGAS pilot plant were screened for their toxicological effects. Ames test results indicated that the mutagenicities of both quench water extracts were very low ($\leq$ 1 to 4 revertants/μg), with the concentration of nonvolatile organic compounds being 0.1 and 0.4 wt % in the two extracts, respectively. The toxicity of these samples was also low as measured in the rabbit alveolar macrophage assay: average cytotoxicity, $LC_{50}$ of 166 μg/mL and 179 μg/mL; functional impairment, $ED_{50}$ of 125 μg/mL and 89 μg/mL. However, sister chromatid exchange in mouse myeloma cells indicated that raw quench waters were more toxic ($EC_{50}$ of 13 μg/mL) than the positive control, methyl methanesulfonate.[6]

The toxicity of the crude waste scrubber water at the METC plant was not evaluated, but the concentration of volatilized organic compounds was measured. The inlet water contained 0.003 wt % extractable hydrocarbons, and the outlet water contained 0.17 wt % hydrocarbons. The mutagenicity of the tars extracted from this water was 0.7 revertants/µg.[7]

Untreated process water from the GFETC gasifier, containing 0.6 wt % extractable hydrocarbons, was found to be more cytotoxic in the mouse myeloma and rabbit alveolar macrophage assays than HYGAS quench waters.[11] Solvent extraction of GFETC water eliminated lethal effects to rabbit alveolar macrophages and reduced the functional impairment by 80%.

The teratogenicity and embryotoxicity of aqueous extracts of UMD electrostatic precipitator tar have been determined in vitro for early amphibian embryos *(Xenopus laevis)*.[14] Concentrations of 8 mg/mL caused 50% lethality in 96 h. A 50% induction of abnormalities occurred at a concentration of 0.5%. The high toxicity is not surprising, because these untreated aqueous extracts would be expected to contain large quantities of toxic phenolic compounds.

### Acute Mammalian Toxicity

The acute mammalian toxicity of UMD tar,[15,16] GFETC process tar,[11] and HYGAS recycle oil[12] was evaluated with a number of tests: oral $LD_{50}$ (mouse), intraperitoneal $LD_{50}$ (mouse), dermal toxicity (rat and rabbit), delayed hypersensitivity (guinea pig), and eye irritation (rabbit).

Tar samples from the UMD gasifier were slightly toxic if ingested and moderately toxic following intraperitoneal administration. The oral $LD_{50}$ for mice ranged from 5 to 6.4 g/kg, and the intraperitoneal $LD_{50}$ ranged from 1.1 to 3.2 g/kg. Comparison with data on the acute toxicity of other coal conversion products in mice showed that the UMD samples have about the same acute toxic potential as hydrotreated coal distillates, or crude shale oil and its derivatives. HYGAS recycle oil and GFETC tar were also slightly toxic in mice following oral ingestion, with HYGAS recycle oil having an $LD_{50}$ of 1.3 g/kg and GFETC tar having an $LD_{50}$ of 2.9 g/kg.

UMD tars were essentially nontoxic in contact with rabbit skin; that is, they caused no overt short-term skin damage or sensitization. Exposure of rabbit skin to HYGAS recycle oil resulted in mild to severe inflammatory reactions with some skin necrosis. Only slight dermal toxicities resulted from exposure of rabbit skin to GFETC tar. Marked skin hypersensitivity was detected in guinea pigs with the NVO fraction of HYGAS recycle oil but not with GFETC tar.

UMD tars were irritating to eyes, producing moderate to severe erythematous and edematous conjuctiva in all test animals, with evidence of corneal damage in the majority. However, all lesions were greatly reduced or had disappeared within 7 d after the single exposure. Recycle oil NVO fraction was a severe eye irritant, causing inflammatory reactions, corneal ulcers, and persistent panus (21 d). GFETC tar was a transient eye irritant, producing significant reactions only within the first 24 h after treatment.

### Chronic Mammalian Toxicity

Chronic toxicity studies were focused on carcinogenesis. The carcinogenic potential of UMD tar was evaluated in mice, both in a lung tumor assay and following skin exposure.[14] Multiple (24) intraperitoneal injections (50 to 1000 mg/kg per injection) of the tar resulted in a dose-related increase in lung adenomas. Chronic treatment of skin with this tar (19 mg/week) resulted in a 100% incidence of skin tumors. The tumors were malignant, as evidenced by local invasiveness and their capacity to metastasize. There was an associated chemical dermatitis, but no overt systemic effects resulted.

HYGAS recycle oil was also shown to be a mouse skin carcinogen, inducing tumors in SKH hairless mice following repetitive application of weekly 150-mg doses.[12] The tumorigenic response was considerably less than that produced by benzo(a)pyrene (0.03-mg weekly doses). However, 105 mg weekly of the NVO fraction of the recycle oil approximated the benzo(a)pyrene tumor response. In addition, weekly 75-mg doses of GFETC tar were shown to induce a 100% skin tumor response within 29 weeks.[11]

## CHEMICAL CHARACTERIZATION OF TOXIC COMPOUNDS

Coal-derived liquids are exceedingly complex and contain several hundred components that boil over a wide range of temperatures, from less than 100°C to more than 500°C. Their constituents include weak acids (phenols and other hydroxyaromatics), nitrogen-containing bases (aromatic amines and azaarenes), and a variety of neutral compounds (aliphatics, polycyclic aromatic hydrocarbons, and heterocyclics). Fractionation of such samples into simpler mixtures is necessary, to allow identification and analysis of individual components, by gas chromatography (GC) and gas chromatography/mass spectrometry (GC/MS) and to relate toxicity to specific chemical classes or subclasses. The basis for separation can be physical (volatility, molecular size) or chemical (acidity, polarity).

The separation procedures that have been applied include extraction, distillation, liquid/liquid partitioning, and thin-layer and column chromatography. In almost all cases, the biological activity of the fractions has been monitored with the Ames assay, because of its simplicity. Hence, mutagenicity is the only criterion of toxicity used to date.

Early results established that mutagenicity, if present, was not detectable in the more volatile components (i.e., those boiling below 250°C) nor in the phenolic (acidic) fraction of process oils and tars. The latter point is illustrated in Figure 1, which depicts the distribution of mass and mutagenicity among acidic, basic, and neutral subfractions of a GFETC tar sample. The distribution of mass among the sample fractions, 30% acidic, 4% basic, and 65% neutral, is fairly typical of other gasifier tars. The distribution of mutagenicity between the basic and neutral fractions, 66% basic and 34% neutral, falls within the range observed for other samples and other fractionation procedures. Earlier procedures had led to the conclusion that most (70%) of the mutagenicity appeared in the neutral fractions of coal gasification tars,[17] but more recent results have indicated that the basic fractions are important, and often major, contributors to the mutagenicity of the tar.[8,18]

### Basic Mutagens

Attention was initially focused on the identification of the mutagens in the basic tar fractions, because their specific activity was about 30-fold greater than that of the unfractionated tar. Identification and quantitation of the components by GC/MS and GC indicated that the basic fractions contain polycyclic azaarenes and aromatic amines, with the azaarenes being 4 to 5 times as abundant. The almost complete loss of mutagenicity upon treatment of basic tar fractions with nitrous acid led to the preliminary conclusion that primary aromatic amines are the dominant mutagens and spurred efforts in three laboratories to develop procedures for separating amines from azaarenes. A list of procedures surveyed appears in Table III. One of the more successful is based on the higher basicity of azaarenes and utilizes cation exchange high-performance liquid chromatography (HPLC) with pH-gradient elution. Using this procedure, it is possible to separate not only the two classes of bases but also closely related members of each class

**Figure 1.**   Percent mass and mutagenicity present in acidic, basic, and neutral fractions of a GFETC tar sample.

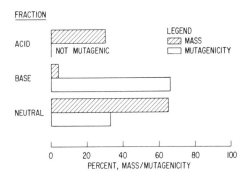

**Table III.**   Fractionation and Analysis of Basic Components of
Coal Gasification Tars

| Sample Type | Facility | Laboratory | Methods |
|---|---|---|---|
| Tar from electrostatic precipitator, holding tank, and cyclone | UMD | ORNL | Aqueous/organic partitioning to separate basic from acidic and neutral components<br>Alumina column chromatography of basic components to separate azaarenes and aromatic amines<br>Sephadex LH-20 chromatography of amine fraction to achieve further enrichment<br>Liquid/liquid partitioning of azaarene fraction to achieve further enrichment<br>GC and GC/MS analysis of derivatized amine fraction |
| Tars and condensates from tar trap, scrubber, and process gas | METC | ITRI | Sephadex LH-20 column chromatography to isolate a more polar fraction<br>Aqueous/organic partitioning of the more polar fraction to separate basic from acidic and neutral components<br>GC and GC/MS analysis |
| Process tar and<br>Condensate from low-temperature reactor; recirculation oil (note that GFETC and HYGAS samples are treated by the same methods) | GFETC<br><br>HYGAS | ANL | Fractional distillation to remove volatile components (both HYGAS and GFETC)<br>Aqueous/organic partitioning to separate basic from acidic and neutral components (both GFETC and HYGAS)<br>Cation exchange HPLC and reverse-phase HPLC of basic components to separate azaarenes and amines (both HYGAS and GFETC)<br>GC and GC/MS analysis of fractions (both HYGAS and GFETC) |

(Figure 2).[18] Ames assays of the HPLC fractions indicated that the mutagenicity was associated predominantly with the amines and, indeed, was concentrated in a rather narrow band within the amine region. Upon

**Figure 2.** Reverse-phase HPLC resolution of the basic fraction of a GFETC tar sample, shown with results of a concurrent determination of the mutagenicity (Ames assay) within each subfraction.

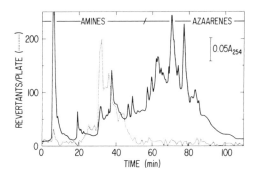

subfractionation of this concentrated mutagenic band by reverse-phase HPLC, it was possible to further purify and characterize the mutagens by GC and GC/MS. Principal mutagenic amines identified in this way include aminophenanthrenes (and anthracenes) and their methyl derivatives.

### Neutral Mutagens

Following the identification of aromatic amines as the dominant mutagens in the basic fractions of coal gasification tars, attention was directed toward the characterization of mutagens in neutral fractions. The procedures used by the various laboratories to separate neutral components of the tars are shown in Table IV. The most definitive results have been obtained by HPLC subfractionation of neutral tar components (isolated by pH fractionation) according to polarity on a silica gel column. Ames assay of the fractions indicated, as shown in Table V, that relatively nonpolar neutral components account for most of the mutagenicity, but that polar neutral components make a significant contribution.[19] Upon subfractionation of the major nonpolar mutagenic band by reverse-phase and normal HPLC it was possible, as in the case of the amines, to obtain mutagenic subfractions that contained, or were very highly enriched in, a single component. The identities of these compounds were established by spectrometric analysis (GC/MS and UV). Compounds conclusively identified included fluoranthene, aceanthrylene/acephenanthrylene, cyclopenta(cd)pyrene, chrysene, and benzo(a)pyrene. The characterization of polar neutral mutagens, many of which are not amenable to identification by GC/MS techniques, is just beginning.

## ECOLOGICAL EFFECTS

Generic studies of the effects of atmospheric pollutants, conducted with volatile hydrocarbons and sulfur-containing gases, have shown that toxicity to vegetation is a function of pollutant reactivity, with sulfur-containing

**Table IV.**   Fractionation and Analysis of Neutral
Components of Coal Gasification Tars

| Sample Type | Facility | Laboratory | Methods |
|---|---|---|---|
| Tar from electrostatic precipitator, holding tank, and cyclone | UMD | ORNL | Aqueous/organic partitioning to separate neutral from acidic and basic components<br>Sephadex LH-20 column chromatography to separate aliphatic, aromatic, and polyaromatic fractions |
| Tars and condensates from tar trap, scrubber, and process gas | METC | ITRI | Sephadex LH-20 column chromatography to separate polycyclic aromatic hydrocarbons from aliphatic, N-heterocyclic, acidic components, and salts<br>Silica column chromatography to separate subfractions of increasing polarity<br>Aqueous/organic partitioning to isolate neutral components of the more polar fraction from LH-20 chromatography |
| Condensate and recirculation oil | HYGAS | ANL | Liquid/liquid partitioning to remove highly polar components; silica column chromatography to obtain fractions of increasing polarity<br>Aqueous/organic partitioning to separate neutral from acidic and basic components |
| Process tar | GFETC | ANL | Aqueous/organic partitioning to separate neutral from acidic and basic components<br>Preparative silica HPLC<br>Semipreparative reverse-phase and normal HPLC |

compounds (e.g., sulfur dioxide) being quite reactive and hydrocarbons having low reactivity. Chemical interactions in pollutants can result in a synergistic magnification of the individual effects.

Ambient air monitoring in the vicinity of small-scale gasification facilities, such as the UMD and GFETC gasifiers, showed no detectable contamination that could be attributed to gasifier operations.[20] Base-line monitoring studies in Pike County, Kentucky, showed that complexity of

**Table V.**   Mass and Mutagenicity of Subfractionated Neutral Tar Components[a]

| Solvent | Fraction No. | Mass g | % | Mutagenicity (revertants/μg) |
|---------|--------------|--------|---|------------------------------|
| | Starting Material | 2.00 | 100 | 2 |
| Hexane | 1 | 0.76 | 38 | <0.1 |
| 5% Benzene in hexane | 2 | 0.32 | 16 | 3.5 |
| 50% Benzene in hexane | 3 | 0.18 | 9 | 2.5 |
| Chloroform | 4 | 0.26 | 13 | <1 |
| Ethyl acetate | 5 | 0.36 | 18 | <1 |
| Methanol | 6 | 0.10 | 5 | 2 |

[a]Neutral components were isolated by pH fractionation and then subfractionated according to polarity on a silica gel column.

terrain and local meteorological conditions can significantly influence the impact of gasifier emissions.[21]

Operation of a commercial coal gasification plant requires large quantities of water, which must be recycled, evaporated, or discharged into surface water systems. The stream of greatest flow and concern is the water used to quench the raw product gas. Analyses of quench water streams from tar-producing gasifiers have shown that they contain phenols, anilines, and a variety of other polyaromatic compounds in considerably higher concentrations than wastewater from oil refineries. Even at high dilution, the untreated quench water was toxic to water fleas and fathead minnows, and significant fractions of the toxicity and chemical oxygen demand remained after extraction with organic solvents.[22] Water-soluble components of the UMD gasifier tar were found to be toxic and teratogenic in frog embryos.[14]

Disposal of solid waste from a commercial gasification facility has been identified as a major ecological concern, because of the large amount of waste generated by the facility and the presence of hazardous and potentially leachable components.[23] Existing data on the leachates of ash and slag from a number of industrial and pilot-plant gasifiers indicate that these leachates would not be classified as toxic or hazardous under current regulations.

## INDUSTRIAL HYGIENE

Industrial hygiene studies at UMD and CAN-DO[14] have indicated that there is a potential for acute carbon monoxide exposure in the gasifier workplace, particularly during initial gasifier startup and during shutdown. Particulate levels at the UMD plant were variable and appeared to be strongly affected by coal quality and handling; however, levels of extractable organic compounds from particulates were low.

Particulate samples collected at four sites in the vicinity of the METC gasifier contained extractable organic compounds in amounts ranging from 11 wt % at a point 0.5 mile upwind of the gasifier to 21 wt % at the top level of the gasifier, just below the flare.[4] The mutagenicity (Ames assay) of the extract from particulates collected near the gasifier was similar to that of process tar, with most of the bioactivity concentrated in the most polar fractions.

Size-fractionated airborne particulates collected at GFETC during operation and shutdown of the gasifier have been analyzed for organic and trace element contents.[24] The bulk (90%) of the organic material consisted of aliphatic and aromatic hydrocarbons and was associated with the smaller respirable particles. Trace elements were bimodally distributed, with modest enrichments of arsenic and lead on submicron particles.

Concentrations of polynuclear aromatics in the ppb range in workplace air have been monitored with the recently developed Duvas spectrophotometer and with passive dosimeter badges. Surface and skin contaminations have been monitored with a fiber-optic luminoscope.[14] Results have shown that coal tar contamination on workers' hands can be a significant problem, not completely alleviated by wearing cotton gloves.

## ENVIRONMENTAL CONTROL TECHNOLOGY

The Environmental Protection Agency has not yet promulgated any New Source Performance Standards for coal gasification or liquefaction plants. However, the provisions of the National Environmental Protection Act and other federal legislation such as the Clean Air and Water Acts, the Resources Conservation and Recovery Act, and the Toxic Substances Control Act will require that commercial-scale coal gasification plants be extensively equipped with environmental control technologies to reduce potentially adverse health and environmental effects. On the other hand, it appears unlikely that industrial-scale coal gasifiers ($\leq$ 100 tpd) will be subject to federal regulation.

Because of the lack of experience in commercial-scale coal gasification, the performance of environmental control technologies in coal gasification plants has not been established. Environmental control technologies have been developed for related applications in coal-fired power plants and oil refineries, but application of these technologies in coal gasification plants is not always straightforward.

Environmental control systems for the larger combustion sources, such as boilers and heaters, generally will be required for compliance with federal and state regulations. The technologies used in the utility industry for control of sulfur dioxide (e.g., wet and spray-dryer scrubbing processes) and for control of particulates (electrostatic precipitators and fabric filters) appear to be applicable without modification in coal gasification plants. However, the applicability of combustion modification methodology for control of oxides of nitrogen in plants burning by-product tars and oils is not as certain. The high nitrogen content of the fuel tends to increase formation of oxides of nitrogen, but decreasing the concentration of excess oxygen to reduce formation of oxides of nitrogen can lead to the formation of potentially toxic polynuclear aromatic compounds, because of the high aromaticity and long burnout time of the tars.

Operation of a commercial-scale coal gasification complex requires large quantities of water (20 to 40 kL/min). Although about 20% of the water is consumed in the gasification process, the remainder must be treated to remove process-derived contaminants before recycling or discharge. A major concern is the highly contaminated, high-volume water stream resulting from quenching the raw product gas in oil- and tar-producing (fixed-bed) coal gasification processes. In the quenching process, tars and heavy oils present in the raw gas are condensed, and their components become distributed between the aqueous phase, a lighter oil layer, and a heavier tar layer. The more polar constituents tend to enter the water, and the resulting solution contains high concentrations of phenols and significant concentrations of other toxic chemicals. The phenolic concentrations must be decreased by dilution or solvent extraction before the water is treatable by conventional bio-oxidation procedures.

Constituents remaining in treated water can be released to the environment in a variety of ways including vaporization from cooling tower water or holding ponds and direct discharge to surface waters. They can also be concentrated to solid or semisolid wastes and potentially enter the environment in this form. The effectiveness of solvent extraction and bio-oxidation in decreasing organic contamination is therefore of considerable importance. The DOE environmental program has included a number of studies in wastewater treatment.

Ammonia stripping and bio-oxidation of the extracted water from the GFETC and HYGAS pilot plants essentially eliminated the biological oxygen demand, but the levels of residual organic carbon and chemical oxygen demand were close to 5% of those in the raw water.[25,26] The identity of the remaining constituents is under investigation.

Gasifier ash (or slag) accounts for most of the solid waste and can amount to 5000 tpd from a commercial-scale coal gasification facility. The gasifier solids contain toxic trace elements and small concentrations of organic compounds that can be mobilized through leaching. The major concern is not the specific toxicity of the leachates, which is low, but rather the possibility that the leaching from the large volumes of ash over long periods of time cannot be accommodated by natural attenuation and dispersion mechanisms and may result in serious contamination of surface waters and groundwaters.

## CONCLUSION

A broad program of health and environmental studies has been carried out under DOE sponsorship, in parallel with the operation of six bench scale, pilot plant, and industrial coal gasifiers. These gasifiers differ in design, but each produces some (2 to 4 wt %) tar and oil as by-products. They are similar in this respect to the Lurgi gasifiers used at Sasol in South Africa and installed in the Great Plains Gasification Project in North Dakota. Cellular bioassays and whole animal tests indicate that the by-product tars and oils contain a variety of toxicants, including carcinogens. It has been shown that these materials contribute to fugitive emissions and can result in work force exposures by inhalation and dermal contact. However, the observed levels of toxicity are low, and the mutagenicity is confined to the less volatile constituents. Because the tars and oils are likely to be used as on-site fuels, potential for general population exposure is limited. Although sufficient data for a firm conclusion are not yet in hand, it appears that potential problems associated with coal gasification tars and oils can be avoided by the use of appropriate control technology and industrial hygiene procedures. There is a clear need to validate this conclusion in studies at larger-scale systems (using advanced as well as Lurgi coal gasification technology) and to investigate other uncertainties (such as ecological effects and environmental control technology performance) that cannot be satisfactorily addressed at pilot-scale facilities.

## ACKNOWLEDGMENTS

The authors wish to acknowledge the research efforts of the scientific staffs involved in generating the information on coal gasification in this chapter and in particular the individual contributors to the DOE report "Status of Health and Environmental Research Relative to Coal Gasification": A.S. Bopari, D.A. Haugen, F.R. Kirchner, M.J. Peak, V.C. Stamoudis, and J.R. Stetter of Argonne National Laboratory; J.M. Benson, R.L. Carpenter, R.L. Hanson, C.E. Mitchell, and G.J. Newton of the Inhalation Toxicology Research Institute; and K.E. Cowser, W.E. Dreibeldis, J.L. Epler, R.B. Gammage, M.R. Guerin, J.M. Holland, F.M. Larimer, J.D. VanHoesen, and C.W. Gehrs of Oak Ridge National Laboratory. The editorial contribution of Marcia Rosenthal and D.A. Haugen, and the secretarial assistance of Terri Vanisko are gratefully appreciated. This work is supported by the U.S. Department of Energy under contract No. W-31-109-ENG-38.

## REFERENCES

1. "Status of Health and Environmental Research Relative to Coal Gasification," DOE/ER-0149 (Washington, DC: U.S. Department of Energy, 1982).

2. Ames, B.N., J. McCann, and E. Yamasaki. "Methods for Detecting Carcinogens and Mutagens with the *Salmonella*/Mammalian-Microsome Mutagenicity Test," *Mutat. Res.* 31:347–364 (1975).

3. Griego, V.M., G.C. Matsushita, and T. Matsushita. "Near-UV Induction of Sister Chromatid Exchanges Under Aerobic and Anaerobic Conditions," *Photochem. Photobiol.* 34:51–55 (1981).

4. Diel, J.H., D.E. Bice, and B.S. Martinez, eds. "Annual Report of the Inhalation Toxicology Research Institute 1979–1980," LMF-84 (Albuquerque, NM: Inhalation Toxicology Research Institute, 1980).

5. Garrett, N.E. "Development and Implementation of Cellular Toxicity Assay for Particulate Matter Using the Alveolar Macrophage and Chinese Hamster Ovary Cell," Report ES-TR-80-06 (Research Triangle Park, NC: Northrup Services, Inc. 1980).

6. Reilly, C., Jr., M.J. Peak, T. Matsushita, F.R. Kirchner, and D.A. Haugen. "Chemical and Biological Characterization of High-Btu Gasification (The HYGAS Process). IV. Biological Activity," in *Coal Conversion and the Environment: Chemical, Biological and Ecological Considerations*, Proceedings of the 20th Annual Hanford Life Sciences Symposium, D.D. Mahlum, R.H. Gray, and W.D. Felix, Eds. (Oak Ridge, TN: Technical Information Center, U.S. Department of Energy, 1981), pp. 310–324.

7. Henderson, R.F., ed. "Low Btu Gasifier Emissions Toxicology," in "Status Report December 1980," LMF-85 (Albuquerque, NM: Inhalation Toxicology Research Institute, 1981), p. 60.

8. Cowser, K.E., ed. "University of Minnesota-Duluth Coal Gasification Project, Semiannual Progress Report for the Period Ending December 31, 1980," ORNL/TM-7730 (Oak Ridge, TN: Oak Ridge National Laboratory, 1981), p. 26.

9. Wilzbach, K.E., and C.A. Reilly, Jr. "Chemical and Toxicological Characterization of HYGAS Pilot Plant Process Streams," in *Proceedings of the 1981 International Gas Research Conference* (Rockville, MD: Government Institute, Inc., 1981), pp. 1550–1561.

10. Stetter, J., V. Stamoudis, S. Vance, M.J. Peak, C.A. Reilly, Jr., and K.E. Wilzbach. "Chemical and Toxicological Characterization of an Experimental Pyrolysis Unit," Argonne National Laboratory (in preparation).

11. Wilzbach, K.E., ed. "Environmental Research Program for Slagging Fixed-Bed Coal Gasification, Final Report," Argonne National Laboratory (in preparation).

12. Reilly, C.A., Jr., ed. "Toxicological Characterization of the HYGAS High-Btu Coal Gasification Process, Final Report," Argonne National Laboratory (in preparation).

13. Benson, J.M., C.E. Mitchell, R.E. Royer, C.R. Clark, R.L. Carpenter, and G.J. Newton. "Mutagenicity of Potential Effluents from an Experimental Low Btu Coal Gasifier," *Arch. Environ. Contam. Toxicol.* (in press).

14. Cowser, K.E., ed. "Life Sciences Synthetic Fuels Semiannual Progress Report for the Period Ending June 30, 1981," ORNL/TM-7926 (Oak Ridge, TN: Oak Ridge National Laboratory, 1981), p. 207.

15. Cowser, K.E., ed. "University of Minnesota-Duluth Coal Gasification Project, Quarterly Progress Report for the Period Ending December 31, 1979," ORNL/TM-7268 (Oak Ridge, TN: Oak Ridge National Laboratory, 1980), p. 39.

16. Cowser, K.E., ed. "University of Minnesota-Duluth Coal Gasification Project,

Quarterly Progress Report for the Period Ending June 30, 1980," ORNL/TM-7466 (Oak Ridge, TN: Oak Ridge National Laboratory, 1980), p. 24.

17. Cowser, K.E., ed. "University of Minnesota-Duluth Coal Gasification Project, Quarterly Report for the Period Ending September 30, 1978," ORNL/TM-7272 (Oak Ridge, TN: Oak Ridge National Laboratory, 1980), p. 46.

18. Haugen, D.A., M.J. Peak, K.M. Suhrbier, and V.C. Stamoudis. "Isolation of Mutagenic Aromatic Amines from a Coal-Conversion Oil by Cation-Exchange Chromatography," *Anal. Chem.* 54:32–37 (1982).

19. Haugen, D.A., and M.J. Peak. "Inhibition of Mutagenesis in the *Salmonella/ Microsome* Assay Caused by Inhibition of Metabolic Activation by Mixtures of Polynuclear Aromatic Hydrocarbons," *Mutat. Res.* 116:257–269 (1983).

20. Suter, G.W., II, and R.M. Cushman. "Preliminary Environmental Assessment of the University of Minnesota-Duluth Coal Gasifier - FY 1980," ORNL/TM-7728 (Oak Ridge, TN: Oak Ridge National Laboratory, 1981), p. 34.

21. Cushman, R.M., D.K. Brown, N.T. Edwards, J.M. Giddings, and B.R. Parkhurst. "Ecotoxicity of Coal Gasifier Solid Wastes," *Bull. Environ. Contam. Toxicol.* 28:39–45 (1982).

22. Singer, P.C., and E. Miller. "Treatment of Wastewater from a Fixed Bed Atmospheric Coal Gasifier," Proceedings of the EPA Environmental Aspects of Fuel Conversion Technology-VI. A Symposium on Coal-Based Synfuels (in press).

23. Francis, C.W., and F.J. Wobber, eds. "Status of Health and Environmental Research Relative to Solid Wastes from Coal Conversion," DOE/NBB-0008 (Washington, DC: U.S. Department of Energy, 1982).

24. Wilzbach, K.E., J.R. Stetter, C.A. Reilly, Jr., and W.G. Willson. "Environmental Research Program for Slagging Fixed-Bed Coal Gasification, Status Report November 1981," ANL/SER-1 (Argonne, IL: Argonne National Laboratory, 1981), p. 34.

25. Stamoudis, V.C., and R.G. Luthy. "Biological Removal of Organic Constituents in Quench Water from a Slagging, Fixed-Bed Coal-Gasification Pilot Plant," ANL/PAG-2 (Argonne, IL: Argonne National Laboratory, 1980), p. 22.

26. Stamoudis, V.C., and R.G. Luthy. "Determination of Biological Removal of Organic Constituents in Quench Waters from High-Btu Coal-Gasification Pilot Plants," *Water Res.* 14:1143–1156 (1980).

## DISCUSSION

*J.A. Klein, Oak Ridge National Laboratory:* You made several comments that I would like to get you to relate together. One, raw wastewaters had the strongest genotoxicity. Do you know what chemicals would cause that? And second, you said that solvent extraction reduces ecotoxicity. Is genotoxicity and ecotoxicity the same thing and what types of compounds do you suspect causes these two?

*C.A. Reilly:* The genotoxicity I specified is the sister chromatid exchange test (SCE) as done in our laboratory. Phenols are the predominant species and probably responsible for it. I am not sure which ones, but clearly if we just do a simple solvent extraction, SCE levels become undetectable. I raised the point to emphasize that raw water is going to have to be cleaned up. In terms of ecotoxicity, I was talking about Singer's work where he is looking at *Daphnia* (fathead minnows) and finds that solvent extraction of waters significantly decreases the toxicity.

*C.D. Scott, Oak Ridge National Laboratory:* One's intuition would say that if you had a hot-gas cleanup, you would reduce the amount of adsorption on the particulates and, thus, you would have a reduction in the potential problem from particulates. Are you aware of data that confirm this?

*C.A. Reilly:* No. I do not really have any idea. All I know with certainty is that we get overhead particulates that contain significantly increased organic deposition.

*R.A. Renne, Pacific Northwest Laboratories:* I would like you to comment on the decreased phagocytosis in the pulmonary alveolar macrophage system. Do you have any explanation for that?

*C.A. Reilly:* No. We run the tests routinely and have from the beginning on all our materials. In our laboratory, we culture the rabbit macrophages for 24 hours with constant exposure to the potential toxicants. We measure lethality by a somewhat cruder measurement than ITRI. ITRI uses release of lactic dehydrogenase to say they are actually dead. We use trypan blue exclusion to determine viability and functional impairment on the basis of the ability to phagocytize latex particles. So, we are saying that some form of toxicity much less gross than killing is, in some way, impairing the normal function of the cells.

*M.E. Frazier, Pacific Northwest Laboratories:* I have a lot of trouble with sister chromatid exchange being accepted as genotoxicity, especially standing all by itself. I was wondering if you might comment on that?

*C.A. Reilly:* If you remember, I was careful to define my terms. In fact, there is a sizeable gap in terms of good mammalian cell mutagenesis assays with gasification materials. Clearly, we take a tremendous jump from Ames assay all the way up to the whole animal test. At Argonne we looked at some samples with the Chinese hamster cell system. We could not get it to work for us, probably because of toxicity. This is an area in gasification where we have to get some data. I am not happy with SCEs as our only mammalian genetic assay, because it is clearly not a mutagenesis assay.

*M.E. Frazier:* In fact, it is not a well-understood phenomenon, and there is some concern that it may represent repair rather than toxicity. It may actually measure adequate repair of some sort, and I think it is a misnomer to call it genotoxicity.

*C.A. Reilly:* I was careful to qualify it, and the reason I discussed it at all was the response we see in terms of testing the water. As I stated, I think we know the answer to that, but there is a big hole and we hope to do something about it.

*H. Roffman, Energy Impact Associates:* You were so nice to show us there are three types of gasifiers, yet you lumped your results together and it is difficult to know who is doing what.

*C.A. Reilly:* All the gasifier studies, with the exception of HYGAS, are fixed-bed gasifiers. HYGAS is a fluidized-bed gasifier, and although I do not have an engineering background, I do not think that it should be compared with those that are currently going to be used. HYGAS makes a lot of overhead organics, and I do not think you are going to see that in the advanced fluidized-bed gasifiers. I can lump them together because I think we are talking about the same kinds of problems as those from fixed-bed gasifiers.

*H. Roffman:* Until we test it, we do not know. Have you done any work on bio-sludges?

*C.A. Reilly:* No.

# CHAPTER 3

## Summary of Health and Environmental Research: Oil Shale

### W.R. Chappell

*Department of Physics*
*Center for Environmental Sciences*
*University of Colorado at Denver*
*1100 14th Street*
*Denver, CO 80202*

The production of oil from shale presents a number of potential risks to human health and the environment. These risks are associated with impacts on air and water quality, solid waste disposal, habitat disturbance, and other effects of shale oil production. Research in the United States, Estonia, and Scotland indicates that sulfur oxides are perhaps the most important air pollutants and will require very high removal efficiencies. High concentrations of organics and salts in the oil shale wastewaters present a considerable challenge in treating these waters. Although the important constituents in leachates of raw and spent shales are fairly well known [total dissolved solids (TDS), fluorine, boron, and molybdenum], the ultimate fate of these constituents is not understood. However, the materials under the spent shale piles will not be impermeable, and it is likely that leachate will eventually reach ground and surface waters and result in significant increases in TDS and, perhaps, other constitutents. While the crude shale oils and other materials are carcinogenic and present a risk of increased cancers, recent research results indicate that nonneoplastic pulmonary health effects (pneumoconiosis, bronchitis, and chronic airway obstruction) will be the most important occupational health concern. Ecological risks are very difficult to quantify; however, adverse impacts on agriculture and wildlife will occur, because of land disturbance and increased TDS in waters. Oil and wastewater spills will have adverse impacts on aquatic organisms, and high levels of molybdenum in plants on the spent shale piles and in irrigation water (from leachates) could result in areas where forage contains molybdenum in concentrations toxic to livestock.

## INTRODUCTION

The first sizeable oil shale industry was begun in Scotland around 1860 and owed its origin to a coal oil industry. In 1850,[1] James Young developed a retort to produce oil from cannel coal. He began commercial production in the West Lothian region of Scotland (near Edinburgh) in 1851. By 1860 the throughput was about 10,000 tons of coal per year (about $10^6$ gal of oil per year). However, the supply of coal was running out. Young had foreseen this possibility earlier and had identified outcrops of oil shale within a few miles of his operation. Since his retort worked for oil shale, he began production of oil from shale in the early 1860s. The expiration of Young's patent in 1864 led to a dramatic increase in oil shale companies, and there were at least 30 oil shale companies by 1870.[1]

In 1871 the total throughput was 800,000 tons of shale per year. However, by that time there was a steady flow of cheap oil from the United States and Russia, which caused a number of oil shale companies to go out of business. By 1905 there were only six oil shale companies; nevertheless, the throughput of oil shale continued to rise until it peaked at over 3 million tons per year during World War I. However, the yield was dropping as the rich seams were exhausted. By 1914–1918 the average annual production was just under 2 million bbl of oil; this corresponded to about 25 gal/ton, as opposed to an average yield of 41 gal/ton in 1879.

The financial problems of the industry continued to worsen, because of cheap imports; in 1928, Winston Churchill, then Chancellor of the Exchequer, instituted a tax exemption for domestic oil producers, which slowed the decline of the industry. By 1950 there were 12 mines and 4 retorting facilities in operation. In 1962 the tax exemption was discontinued and the Scottish oil shale industry was closed.[1]

Several countries, notably the United States, Australia, Brazil, Morocco, and Israel, are actively looking at oil shale as a source of liquid fuels, but the only existing commercial operations are in Estonia and Manchuria. The reason for the widespread interest is clear; there are important oil shale deposits throughout the world. In 1965,[2] it was estimated that $190 \times 10^9$ bbl was recoverable (worldwide) under conditions at that time. On the other hand, the reason that production of oil from shale is very limited at the present is also clear. The process is difficult, is expensive, and could not compete with the cheap oil the world had until very recently. Furthermore, the uncertainties in price and supply since 1973, coupled with economic conditions that are not conducive to large capital investments, have led to a situation in which only one commercial-size operation (Union Oil at Parachute Creek, Colorado) is proceeding at this time in the United States.

Those who have been studying the health and environmental aspects of shale oil are in the position where the data base, like those of the other synthetic fuel technologies, relates either to pilot or demonstration facilities in the United States or to commercial facilities in other countries. The first of these suffers from the inevitable criticism that "the results are not representative of what will happen in a commercial facility" and the second is vulnerable to the criticisms that:

- The feedstock (coal or oil shale) is or was mineralogically and/or chemically different from the U.S. feedstock.
- The technologies are or were different from those proposed for the U.S. industry.
- The control technologies, industrial hygiene practices, and other mitigation strategies were either nonexistent or inferior to those being proposed.
- The countries involved (e.g., Soviet Union and China) are not entirely open in sharing data.
- The operations have ceased (as with the Scottish industry) sometime in the past, and information has been lost.

All of these criticisms have some merit and limit the validity and/or generality of the results of our research. Clearly, the "best of all worlds" for the researcher would be to have a fully installed industry, complete access to all relevant samples and data, and sufficient funds and competent scientific personnel to carry out all the research required to understand the environmental and health consequences of the industry.

To date, most of the environmental and health research in this country has related to the deposits in Colorado, Utah, and Wyoming. Although considerable deposits exist in the eastern United States, this discussion is confined to the western deposits.

## THE RESOURCE AND THE TECHNOLOGY

Most of the oil shale resource in the western United States is contained in the Green River Formation shales, which underlie about 16,000 sq miles of Colorado, Wyoming, and Utah.[3] The richer shales are located in four depositional basins (see Fig. 1): Piceance Creek Basin in Colorado, Uinta Basin in Utah, and the Green River and Washakie Basins in Wyoming. The thickest and richest deposits are contained in the Piceance Creek Basin, which covers an area of about 2000 sq miles.

The origin of the oil shale involved the deposition of organic remains in large (mostly freshwater) lakes under reducing conditions. There are, however, wide variations in mineralogy and in kerogen properties from one deposit to another and even within deposits. We will point out later that these variations can have a significant effect on some environmental parameters.

The Green River Formation oil shales were deposited in the Eocene period in two large lakes. Within each lake complex there were individual

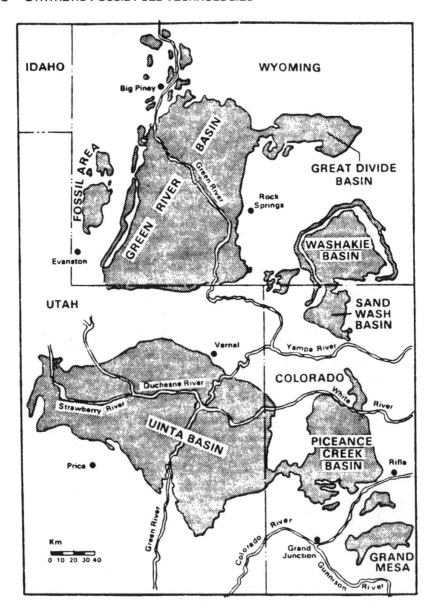

**Figure 1.**   Oil shale resources in the western United States.

depositional basins. Oil shale is "not a lithologic name but an economic name referring to the rock's ability to yield oil."[4] Indeed, the Green River Formation oil shales are a marlstone, with the average mineral composition shown in Table I.

The processes that presently appear to be commercially acceptable

**Table I.** Average Mineral Composition of Mahogany Zone Shale

| Mineral | Wt % |
|---|---|
| Dolomite | 32 |
| Calcite | 16 |
| Quartz | 15 |
| Illite | 19 |
| Albite | 10 |
| Potassium-feldspar | 6 |
| Pyrite | 1 |
| Analcime | 1 |

involve heating the rock to about 900°F or higher. At these temperatures, the kerogen pyrolyzes to yield vapors (which condense to shale oil), gases, and carbonaceous residue. The carbonaceous residue is burned in some processes as a source of heat for the pyrolysis of kerogen. The ideal retorting process has been described as follows: "(a) a preheat zone for the raw shale feed, (b) a pyrolysis zone for shale oil production, (c) a combustion zone for heat production, and (d) a cooling zone for heat recovery from the spent shale."[5] Numerous designs have been proposed to satisfy these criteria, with various options, including supplementing the heat in the combustion zone with a portion of the retort gases.

The technologies for extracting oil from shale can be divided into three broad classes, with many variations within the classes. The three broad classes are surface processes, modified in situ processes, and true in situ processes.

## Surface Processes

In surface processing the oil shale is mined by conventional means (underground, strip, open pit, etc.), crushed, and then retorted in vessels. The various technologies differ in the methods of heating and movement of shale through the retorts. In the United States, three basic methods for heating the shale have dominated.[5,6] These involve the use of (1) recycled hot solids; (2) a combustion zone within the retort; and (3) retorts with an external, fuel-fired furnace. The first method achieves heat transfer by mixing hot solid particles (e.g., hot spent shale or ceramic balls) with the oil shale; this is used in the TOSCO II and Lurgi-Ruhrgas retorts. The second method uses a combustion zone inside the retort to furnish heat, which is transferred to the pyrolysis zone by flowing gases generated in the combustion zone; this is used in the Union A, USBM gas combustion, NTU, and Paraho direct retorts. The third method involves the transfer of heat by gases which are heated outside the retort; this is used in the Union B, Paraho indirect, and Superior retorts.

The foreign industries have primarily involved surface retorting. In Estonia, the retorts have been of either the recycled hot solids (Galoter) or externally heated (Kiviter) variety. In Scotland, many of the retorts were of still another type, involving transfer of heat by conduction through the retort wall (Pumpherston). The Brazilian Petrosix process is very similar to the Paraho indirect retort.

These retorts present a considerable engineering challenge.[5] Large quantities of rock must be heated to 900 to 1000°F; subsequently, the spent shale must be cooled, requiring efficient heat recovery with minimal water consumption. Because of the presence of carbonates which decompose above 1000°F, there must be good temperature control to avoid energy-consuming reactions. In spite of these difficulties, the surface processes are by far the most advanced. However, even these have only been tested at capacities of 500 to 1000 bbl/d, which are five to ten times less than contemplated for commercial-scale retorts.

### Modified In Situ Processes

The problems associated with the handling and disposal of large volumes of solids have encouraged several companies to investigate the potential for in place processing of oil shale. The in situ processes considered have consisted of two general types, which are classed as "modified" and "true" in situ. The modified in situ (MIS) processes involve removing a portion of the material and leaving the remaining material in a rubbled state underground. The rubbled pile is then heated by fuel burners or by the injection of hot gases to ignite the pile.

The purpose of removing some of the material is to increase the permeability and promote uniform rubbling, both of which contribute to greater recovery. Two major field demonstrations have been performed. Occidental Oil Shale Company has blasted and ignited several retorts at its experimental facility at Logan Wash, Colorado. The other major field exercise was by the Rio Blanco Oil Shale Company at Lease Tract C-a in Colorado.

Both the Occidental and the Rio Blanco techniques[6] use a configuration whereby a combustion zone progresses vertically through the rubbled zone. They differ mainly in the way the shale is rubbled and the portion of shale mined out. The latter difference is particularly significant, because Rio Blanco proposes to mine out twice (40%) as much as Occidental (20%).

Multi Mineral Corporation has proposed an MIS method which differs from those of Occidental and Rio Blanco. This method[6] is proposed for extracting both oil and saline minerals containing sodium and aluminum from the saline zone. In this method, a significant fraction of the material is removed after rubbling, crushing, and screening are used to remove the nahcolite (sodium bicarbonate), which is taken to the surface. The remaining oil shale is pyrolyzed by injecting gases, after which the retorts are cooled and leached to obtain aluminum (originally contained in dawsonite) and soda ash from the remaining nahcolite.

Because of the very low thermal conductivity of the surrounding rock, the diminished heat loss to external surroundings, compared with that in surface processes, can lead to substantially higher temperatures in the retorts than encountered in surface retorts. Indeed, the maximum temperatures encountered in MIS retorts could be as high as 2200°F (1200°C),[7] compared with maximum temperatures of 1300 to 1400°F (~750°C) in surface retorts. Moreover, the spent shale in MIS retorts will remain at above-ambient temperatures for long periods of time. It has been suggested[7] that these very high temperatures could initiate solid state reactions that might have a significant effect on the environmental consequences of these processes.

### True In Situ Processes

Clearly, MIS processes still involve a significant amount of materials handling (about 10,000 to 40,000 tons/d). There are zones in the Green River Formation where oil can be extracted without any initial mining out of material. Such processes are called true in situ (TIS) processes and essentially involve access only through wells to the surface. The steps involved in TIS processes are (1) dewatering, if groundwater is present; (2) fracturing or rubbling, if greater permeability is required; (3) injection of a hot fluid or ignition to provide heat; and (4) recovery of oil and gas through wells.[6]

A particularly suitable portion of the Green River Formation for TIS processing is the leached zone of the Piceance Creek Basin, where groundwater has dissolved saline mineral deposits. Some experiments have been conducted in the leached zone using the injection of hot gas or superheated steam.

Another approach involves the exploitation of slightly fractured zones, where various techniques such as hydraulic fracturing, the detonation of explosives in well bores, and the injection of high-pressure water have been used in attempts to increase the permeability of the formations.

One of the most successful TIS methods to date is the Geokinetics process. In this technique, explosives are used to simultaneously lift the overburden (to create a void) and fracture the shale to make it permeable. The shale is ignited by the injection of air and hot gases, a burn zone proceeds horizontally through the rubbled zone, and oil and gas are extracted by perimeter wells. Almost 30 such retorts have been blasted and ignited at the Geokinetics property in Utah. This method may be particularly useful for shallow, thin beds of oil shale.

## Discussion

At present, the technological development of surface-retorting processes is far ahead of that of MIS processes, which, in turn, is ahead of that of TIS processes. Recent uncertainties in future energy demand, coupled with high interest rates and questionable profitability, have led to cancellation or temporary suspension of most development activities, other than the 10,000-bbl/d operation being constructed in Colorado by Union Oil.

In many respects, the single most important factor influencing the environmental impact (and technical and economic feasibility) is the large amount of material that must be processed. For a relatively rich shale, approximately 1.5 tons of oil shale must be processed to obtain 1 bbl of oil. Since most commercial-scale operations proposed to date are at least 50,000 bbl/d, the size of the individual facilities will be very large. Indeed, a 50,000-bbl/d operation would involve the processing of about 75,000 tons of oil shale (either above or below ground) per day with the production of about 60,000 tons of spent shale per day. A million barrel per day industry would process about 500 million tons of shale per year and would "be the world's largest industry processing low-grade minerals."[5]

For surface processing, the underground mines or open-pit operations needed to support some of the projects that have been proposed would be among the largest in the world. In addition to the large size of the mines, some aspects of mining differ from other mines. As presently contemplated, most oil shale mines will operate with large openings and high extraction rates, and many will involve gassy conditions. Other than some salt mines,[8] no other U.S. mines operate under all three of these conditions. The MIS operations are even more unique, since they involve mining and retorting at the same time. This is an unprecedented set of circumstances.

## AIR QUALITY

The oil shale region of Colorado, Utah, and Wyoming is topographically complex. River valleys and basins can be expected to function as corridors for air pollutants, while high plateau areas may be above much of the pollution. The region is located on the western slopes of the Rockies and the eastern end of a 300-km-wide basin between the Wasatch Mountains and the Colorado Rockies. Both mountain groups are massive and influence meteorological structure in the lower troposphere. Thus, the setting for the oil shale industry is very complex and, to date, poorly understood. The primary air quality issues involved revolve around two concerns:

1.  Will air quality regulations, specifically Prevention of Significant Deterioration (PSD) requirements, limit the size of the potential industry and, if so, what is the limit?
2.  What will be the impacts on the health of the people in the region and on the environment?

The first concern has received a great deal of attention, because it has appeared that PSD regulations may be the primary limitation to the size of an oil shale industry. Several years ago, starting in 1976, the U.S. Environmental Protection Agency (EPA)[9] made very conservative estimates of the maximum size of the oil shale industry, using the PSD limits on sulfur dioxide ($SO_2$) and total suspended particulates (TSP) in nearby class I areas such as the Dinosaur National Monument and the Flat Tops Wilderness Area. These early estimates gave figures of 200,000 and later 400,000 bbl/d for the *conservative* maximum level of production.[9] Since most scenarios for a mature industry are in the range of 1 to 2 million bbl/d, these projections, although involving very conservative assumptions, have caused considerable concern. More-recent studies[10] have indicated that the maximum level is probably at least 800,000 bbl/d. Clearly, air quality regulations will impose a limit at some level of production. It is not clear what level that is or whether it is the primary limit (as opposed, for example, to water availability). However, this potential for placing such a limit on the industry has been a strong motivating force for finding ways to reduce emissions, particularly sulfur oxides ($SO_x$) and TSP, and for refining the models with the hope of increasing the projected maximum size.

Dealing with PSD regulations involves a number of extremely complex technical issues. Although the issue of health and environmental effects is not entirely separate from the regulatory issue, it is certainly not the same and adds some complicating factors while simplifying others. Both acute and chronic exposure possibilities need to be addressed. Acute incidents, for example, might arise in connection with nocturnal drainage winds, a condition in which there is no significant large-scale gradient wind, and drainage of cold air into the Colorado River Valley could transport pollutants from several oil shale operations to the area including Grand Junction. On a smaller scale, local stagnation might cause acute effects in the immediate vicinity of a single operation, particularly when coupled with the unlikely, but not impossible, event of an upset condition involving the process or control equipment. On a chronic level, there are several "standard" (e.g., $SO_x$) and "other" (e.g., polycyclic organics) pollutants that might increase the health and environmental risk to humans and their environment. Estimates of some of these risks have recently been made, but much remains to be done because of the extreme complexity of these issues. Whereas the regulatory issues have focused attention primarily on $SO_x$, TSP, and, more recently, visibility, the "effects" issues involve a broader spectrum of inorganic and organic constituents as well as dose-response relationships. However, at least for chronic effects, the transport modeling may be much simpler, since we are not interested in transient effects that might be related to complex terrain (indeed, a simple Gaussian, flat-terrain model may well suffice for many calculations).

The concern with the PSD regulations and with the health and environmental effects of $SO_x$ has focused a great deal of attention on the pres-

**Table II.**   Sulfur Distribution in Mahogany Zone Oil Shale Samples

|  | Stanfield et al.[a] | Smith et al.[b] | Young and Smith[c] |
|---|---|---|---|
| Total sulfur, wt % | 0.63 | 0.72 | 0.45–0.74 |
| Fraction of total, % | | | |
| Pyritic | 68 | 73 | 77 |
| Sulfate | 2 | 3 | 1 |
| Organic | 30 | 24 | 22 |

[a]Reference 10, this chapter.
[b]Reference 11, this chapter.
[c]Reference 12, this chapter.

ence and fate of sulfur compounds in retort off-gases. This has led, in turn, to an interest in the occurrence of sulfur in the initial raw shale and the fate of this sulfur.

Several authors[11,12] have reported the results of studies on the sulfur content of oil shale. As seen in Table II, the sulfur is mostly in the form of pyrite. Most of the remainder is associated with organic material.

Most of the sulfur in the off-gas is in the form of hydrogen sulfide ($H_2S$). The principal reaction believed to be involved[13] is

$$FeS_2 + 2H^+ \rightarrow FeS + H_2S .$$

However, the rate of $H_2S$ emission depends on temperature and gas composition.[14] The uncontrolled emission rates from several processes are given in Table III.

In addition to $H_2S$, minor sulfur species have recently been identified

**Table III.**   Hydrogen Sulfide Emissions from In Situ and Surface Oil Shale Retorts[a]

| | | Sulfur Emissions (as $H_2S$) | |
|---|---|---|---|
| Retort | Type[b] | kg/d | kg/bbl |
| Occidental retort 6 | IS | 936 | 5.5 |
| Rio Blanco retort 1 | IS | 3,414 | 15.9 |
| Geokinetics retort 25 | IS | 377 | 3.8 |
| Paraho semiworks | S | 159 | 1.0 |
| Union B proposed | S | 14,180 | 1.4 |
| TOSCO II | S | 175,000 | 3.2 |

[a]Modified from Fruchter et al., *1982 Potential Air Emissions from Oil Shale Retorting* (Vail).
[b]IS = in situ; S = surface.

in the raw retort gases by researchers at Pacific Northwest Laboratories (PNL) and Lawrence Livermore National Laboratory (LLNL) involved in the U.S. Department of Energy (DOE) research program. These sulfur compounds and their concentrations in off-gases are given in Table IV.[4,14–16]

Although there are no federal New Source Performances Standards (NSPS) for oil shale $SO_2$ emissions, Colorado has enacted an NSPS for $SO_2$. For facilities producing 1000 or more barrels of oil per day, $SO_2$ emissions must be curtailed by BACT (best-available control technology) and are not to exceed 0.14 kg $SO_2$ per barrel of oil. Facilities producing 1000 or more barrels of oil from surface and in situ retorts, however, are exempted from the strict limitation until July 1, 1992. Instead, they may not exceed a daily emission equal to 0.14 kg/bbl multiplied by the rated-design capacity. However, after 1986 no source can emit more than 900 kg $SO_2$/d and all vented

**Table IV.** Trace Sulfur Species and their Concentrations in Off-gases from Different Retorts (adapted from Reference 15, this chapter)

|  | Occidental[a] | Paraho[b] | Rio Blanco Retort 1[c] |
|---|---|---|---|
| Trace species, ppm |  |  | 7/81[c] |
| COS | 50 | 108 | 100 |
| CH$_3$SH | 20 | 18 | 45 |
| C$_2$H$_6$S | NA[d] | ND[e] | ND |
| CS$_2$ | 10 | 10 | 9 |
| Thiophene | NA | ~70[f] | 35 |
| Methylthiophene | NA | NA | 65[g] |
| SO$_2$ | NA | <20 | <10 |
| H$_2$S, % | 0.14 | 0.2–0.3 | 0.9 |
| Non-H$_2$S sulfur species, vol % of total sulfur species measured | 5 | 6.4–9.3 | 2.8 |
| Sulfur in non-H$_2$S species, % total sulfur in sulfur species measured | 4 | 2.7–4.0 | 1.6 |

[a]From Reference 4, this chapter.
[b]Averages during September 17–18, 1980; from Reference 14, this chapter.
[c]Averages during several days of sampling in July 1981; from Reference 16, this chapter.
[d]NA = not available.
[e]ND = not detected.
[f]Original thiophene data were based on a CH$_3$SH standard (thiophene was not available on site at that time). Value was corrected by later comparing the gas chromatography responses of CH$_3$SH and thiophene.
[g]Based on thiophene standard.

gases must contain less than 500 ppm $SO_2$. Calculated[15] sulfur removal efficiencies necessary to meet the Colorado NSPS range from 93.5 to 99.7%.

Two options are available for sulfur removal from raw retort gas: (1) remove the reduced species before oxidation, using technologies such as Stretford; or (2) remove $SO_2$ by scrubbing after oxidation.[15,16] The Stretford approach is economically attractive; however, it will not remove some of the minor sulfur constituents, such as carbonyl sulfide (COS; also called carbon oxysulfide) and carbon disulfide ($CS_2$). The rather high (98.8 to 99.7%) efficiencies required by MIS processes to meet the Colorado NSPS standard may present a considerable challenge,[15] because the non-$H_2S$ species may be several percent of the total sulfur in retort gas.

One promising approach to controlling the sulfur emissions is a change in the retorting conditions, as indicated by work being done at LLNL.[17] This work indicates that steam injection in combustion retorts has the effect of increasing $H_2S$, because of iron sulfide reactions with steam, but at the same time decreases COS production and also decreases the oil pour point. The LLNL work also shows that processes that use retorted shale for heat in a vessel separate from pyrolysis can lead to a significant reduction in $SO_2$ emission (perhaps an order of magnitude) because of reactions of carbonate minerals or resulting oxides with $SO_2$ and $O_2$ to form sulfates.

Nitrogen oxides ($NO_x$) are pollutants of interest associated with retorting. They arise in part from the oxidation of atmospheric nitrogen and in part from the combustion of nitrogen-containing organic compounds and ammonia.[15] Since a portion of the ammonia will be recovered in commercial operations for sale in fertilizer, it is difficult to estimate the actual emissions. The uncontrolled emission from Retort O at Rio Blanco has been estimated[15] to be in the range of 5.5 to 7.3 lb/bbl (mostly as NO).

Studies of the redistribution of trace elements[18–20] show that the major redistribution of elements after C, H, N, and S is of Cd, Hg, and As. The data[19] indicate the possible appearance of significant quantities of Br, Cl, Se, Cr, and F in the off-gas, but it is possible that these were contained in oil mist that was only partially removed before measurement.[15] The high organic content of the gas streams has made speciation of the As and Hg difficult, although there is preliminary evidence of $As_2O_3$ in retort gases. Some laboratories report evidence[15,19] that the Hg may be present as $Hg^0$.

It has been estimated[19] that a 50,000-bbl/d in situ operation could release 8 kg Hg/d. This is about four times the emission rate from a 1000-MW coal-fired power plant and three times the allowable mercury emission rate from chlor-alkali plants. This suggests that Hg may have to be removed from oil shale off-gases.

Over 75 organic compounds have been identified[21,22] in 10 class groups (polyaromatic hydrocarbons, N-heterocyclics, phenols, etc.) in extracts of aerosols. Twenty polyaromatic hydrocarbons were identified (Table V) and their emission rates from Rio Blanco Retort 1 were measured (after scrubbing and incineration).[15] The total emission rate for these 20 compounds

**Table V.** Polyaromatic Hydrocarbon (PAH) Components and Concentrations from Rio Blanco Retort 1 (adapted from Reference 15, this chapter)

| | Concentration ($\mu g/m^3$) | |
| --- | --- | --- |
| PAH Component | In Raw Gas[a] | After Scrubbing and Incineration |
| Naphthalene | $1.82 \times 10^{-2}$ | $1.22 \times 10^{-2}$ |
| Acenaphthylene | | $1.22 \times 10^{-2}$ |
| Acenapthene | $1.66 \times 10^{0}$ | $3.68 \times 10^{-2}$ |
| Fluorene | | |
| 9,10-Dihydroanthracene | $1.64 \times 10^{-1}$ | $6.12 \times 10^{-2}$ |
| Phenanthrene | $8.21 \times 10^{-3}$ | $1.02 \times 10^{-1}$ |
| Anthracene | $2.74 \times 10^{-2}$ | $2.86 \times 10^{-2}$ |
| 2-Methylanthracene | $2.52 \times 10^{-1}$ | $1.76 \times 10^{-1}$ |
| 9-Methylanthracene | $2.34 \times 10^{0}$ | $1.91 \times 10^{0}$ |
| Fluoranthene | $3.13 \times 10^{-1}$ | $3.23 \times 10^{-1}$ |
| Pyrene | $5.03 \times 10^{-1}$ | $5.73 \times 10^{-1}$ |
| Benzo($e$)anthracene | $1.19 \times 10^{-1}$ | $9.42 \times 10^{-2}$ |
| Chrysene | $4.60 \times 10^{-1}$ | $4.00 \times 10^{-1}$ |
| Benzo($k$)fluoranthene | $4.81 \times 10^{-1}$ | $1.67 \times 10^{-1}$ |
| Benzo($b$)fluoranthene | $1.10 \times 10^{-1}$ | $1.64 \times 10^{-2}$ |
| Benzo($e$)pyrene | $2.15 \times 10^{0}$ | $3.75 \times 10^{-1}$ |
| Benzo($a$)pyrene[b] | $8.53 \times 10^{-2}$ | $1.31 \times 10^{-1}$ |
| Indeno(1,2,3-$cd$)pyrene | $4.57 \times 10^{-2}$ | |
| Dibenzo($a,h$)anthracene | | |
| Benzo($g,h,i$)perylene | | |
| Total weight of PAH fraction | 13.2 | 4.7 |

[a]Stack conditions: 600-mm Hg, 71°C.
[b]A large and broad peak obscured the peak for benzo($a$)pyrene.

was 760 $\mu$g/s, which extrapolates to 0.25 g/s for a 50,000-bbl/d operation (without controls).[15] This emission rate is about $10^4$ times that for a 1000-MW coal-fired power plant. Preliminary studies[15] indicate a 50-fold reduction in mutagenicity of the off-gas aerosols from an MIS retort after incineration and scrubbing.

It is important to note that most air emissions measurements have been made on raw retort gases or gases with relatively simple treatment. Moreover, no measurements have been made on a retort of commercial size (5,000 to 10,000 bbl/d for a surface retort), because none yet exists.

Not much information is available on air quality impacts from the use of shale oil. Chemical and biological characterizations of upgraded shale oils

indicate these upgraded oils are very similar to their natural petroleum counterparts. Shale oils before upgrading (which includes arsenic removal) contain more As, Se, Co, and N and less V and Ni than ordinary crudes. Since
arsenic concentrations are 20 to 30 ppm in shale oils, direct burning for
electricity production could cause significant arsenic emissions and controls
may be necessary. However, this particular use may not occur because of
the value of the oil for producing premium fuel.

The health risks associated with these emissions are discussed in detail
in the Health and Environmental Effects Document for 1982[23] and are summarized in a later section of this chapter. The public health risks were
calculated by the application of the sulfate-surrogate model[24] for complex
mixtures of pollutants.

There will also, of course, be fugitive emissions from the mining, retorting, and upgrading facilities, the spent-shale disposal pile, evaporation
ponds, and other related activities. Much less is known about these contributions. Of particular interest is the codisposing of the wastewaters (retort
water, gas condensation, etc. produced by the retorting operation) with the
spent shale. Because of the high organic and ammonia content of these
waters, some pretreatment (e.g., steam stripping) may be necessary. Even
with such pretreatment, it is possible that pollutants in the wastewaters will
be volatilized. Preliminary results from the analysis of static-head-space samples from several retort waters have indicated the presence of several organics, including alkyl benzenes and nitrogen-containing heterocyclics.

Although models of various degrees of sophistication have been run
for the oil shale area and limited field studies have taken place, the studies
of the effects of the complex terrain and meteorology of the area on pollutant transport are still in an early stage of development. Plans are being
developed to move the ASCOT program from the Geysers area to the oil
shale area. However, the limited work to date has given some important
clues to transport in this complex region.[25] Studies of the temperature in-
versions that form in deep western Colorado valleys just before sunset describe the stages involved in the growth and decay of this phenomenon.[26]
Studies of the development of convective boundary layers over the complex
terrain in the region have shown that these layers represent an important
means for dilution of pollutants introduced into the atmosphere.[27] However,
further work is needed to determine seasonal and topographical influences.

Tracer experiments[28] have improved our understanding of drainage
flows, indicating frequent cross-gulch winds, which interrupt these flows, and
significant vertical mixing. Moreover, these experiments indicate a considerably greater (about an order of magnitude) plume depletion at respirable
height than would be expected from transport models with dry deposition
for particle removal. The regional soils have been shown to be very efficient
adsorbers of gaseous mercury, and the controlling parameters are amorphous
oxides, reducible iron and manganese, and surface area.[29] Exposure of this
soil to mercury vapor from oil shale operations could eventually lead to a

significant increase in soil mercury. More work is needed to understand the ultimate fate and effect of this increase. Finally, acid deposition has been an issue receiving more and more publicity in the Rocky Mountain area. Very little work has been done in this area, and whether this is a significant problem is not known.

## WATER QUALITY

Although there are no simple research areas associated with oil shale, the issue of water quality (and quantity) is one of the most complicated. To simplify this problem somewhat, the issue of leachates is treated in the section "Solid Waste," which follows this section, and the questions of water availability and consumption are largely ignored in this chapter.

Because water is scarce and therefore precious in a semi-arid area, almost anything that affects it may be significant. The issue of water availability has been a source of numerous conflicts, both political and technical. These conflicts will probably continue regardless of research results because of the complex institutional problems involved. It would seem possible, however, to estimate the physical resource itself and the likely consumptive requirements for oil shale processing and other uses. Such an estimate was performed by the Colorado Department of Natural Resources with funding provided by the U.S. Water Resources Council.[30] With numerous caveats, the conclusion was that the water demand of an emerging energy technology industry (specifically oil shale and coal gasification) in the Upper Colorado River Basin of about 1.5 million bbl/d (equivalent) (9.6 trillion Btu/d) could be satisfied from surface supplies. Furthermore, this could be done without having to significantly reduce consumption by other projected users in the Upper Basin. Some of the qualifiers include:

1.  Water not under contract would be purchased, and reservoirs, pipelines, and other facilities would be developed as needed.
2.  Only projected consumptive uses were accounted for, and such issues as instream recreational uses were not.
3.  Only those institutional factors such as each state's water rights system and the "law of the river" were considered, and factors such as environmental regulations were not.
4.  Constraints by interstate compact considerations among Upper Basin states could affect availability in any one state.

Another potential source of water for the industry is groundwater. However, the size of this resource in the Piceance Creek Basin is highly uncertain, with estimates ranging from 2.5 to 25 million acre-ft. This range indicates a need for some creative new ways of establishing the storage capacity of large and complex systems.

The important wastewater streams associated with shale oil production are given in Table VI, along with rough estimates of their flow rates.[31]

Most of the wastewater research has focused on the gas condensates and retort water. This research has involved characterization, treatment, and health and ecological effects studies. The last will be described in subsequent sections.

The wastewater studies, particularly the treatment research, have been a source of continuing controversy, partly because of the proprietary nature of much of the industrial research. It is typical for a researcher from a university or national laboratory to deliver a paper in which the researcher states, "We have a problem with constituent x; process Z doesn't remove it," only to have an industrial representative in the audience say, "The consulting firm we hired has no problem with constituent x at all." When the researcher asks how the problem was solved, the industrial person says the information is proprietary. This exchange occurs almost exclusively in this research area and causes considerable consternation to both sides. I

**Table VI.**   Quantities and Flow Rates of the Major Wastewater Streams at Oil Shale Plants Selected as a Basis for Risk Analysis (adapted from Reference 31, this chapter)

| | Quantity per Quantity of Product Oil (lb/lb) | Flow Rate for 50,000-bbl/d Plant (gal/min) |
|---|---|---|
| Process condensates | | |
| Gas condensate[a] | 0.3/1.6 | 400/2200 |
| Retort water (MIS plant, average) | 0.7 | 900 |
| Sour water (based on TOSCO II upgrading) | 0.4 | 520 |
| Utility effluents | | |
| Cooling tower blowdown[b] | 0.7/1.3 | 950/1750 |
| Boiler blowdown[c] | 0.50–1.7 | 70–2250 |
| Regenerant wastes[c] | 0.01–0.4 | 15–500 |
| Service/sanitary wastes | | |
| Service and fire water | 0.01 | 16 |
| Potable and sanitary[a] | 0.01 | 14/11 |
| Runoffs | | |
| Runoff from plant[a] | 0.09/0.04 | 120/60 |
| Runoff from spent shale piles[a] | 0.04/0.01 | 50/10 |
| Excess minewater | 0–8 | 0–15,000 |

[a]Surface/MIS.
[b]Excluding/including upgrading requirements.
[c]Depending on retort steam rate.

mention this issue because I cannot give the status of proprietary research to which I do not have access.

To date, all of the developers have proposed a "zero discharge" water management policy. There are good reasons for adopting this approach. One reason is that much of the water requirement for the operation can be satisfied by water of low to medium quality, which facilitates reuse. This reuse not only reduces the requirement for importing fresh water, but also can save money by eliminating the treatment otherwise required to produce wastewater of discharge quality. Table VII[31] gives a summary of estimates of major water requirements for both surface and MIS facilities (for a 50,000-bbl/d facility). For surface processes, the spent shale moisturization requirements clearly exceed the total process condensate produced. Thus, all the process condensate and some of the blowdown could be consumed by co-disposal with the spent shale. The remaining blowdown might be used for other purposes such as revegetation. Indeed, additional fresh water would be required.

For MIS facilities, much more process wastewater is produced than can be consumed by spent shale moisturization. As a result, other uses such as boiler feedwater must be found for the excess wastewater. Thus, for the "zero discharge" scenario under normal operation, the issue is to what ex-

**Table VII.** Summary of Estimates of Major Water Requirements (gal/min) for a 50,000-bbl/d Plant
(from Reference 31, this chapter)

|  | Surface | MIS |
| --- | --- | --- |
| Water needs |  |  |
| Spent shale |  |  |
| Moisturization | 600–1350 | 370 |
| Revegetation | 260–670 | 250 |
| Dust control |  |  |
| At mine | 380 | 140 |
| Other | 120–280 | 115 |
| Cooling water makeup[a] | 1600 | 2200 |
| Boiler feedwater[a] | 150–1600 | 5000[b] |
| Total | 3110–5880 | 8075 |
| Wastewater produced |  |  |
| Gas condensate | 400 | 2200 |
| Retort water | — | 900 |
| Blowdowns[a] | 1000–1800 | 3850 |
| Total | 1400–2200 | 6950 |

[a]Excluding upgrading requirements.
[b]2200 gal/min consumed in retort.

tent, if any, the wastewaters must be treated to be reused for moisturization, revegetation, dust control, steam raising, etc. Researchers in academe, the national laboratories, and industry have looked at the effectiveness of numerous conventional and some advanced technologies, with varying results.

There is, of course, the possibility of an upset condition leading to a discharge of partially treated or untreated wastewaters. The result of such a discharge could be the contamination of soils, stream sediments, groundwaters, and surface waters. The risk of such an event could be estimated as the probability of occurrence times the consequence. While some information exists about the consequence, little information exists about the probability of occurrence.

The compositions of the gas condensates and retort waters vary with the process design.[32] Because retort waters are in contact with oil and shale (for in situ processes), the contact time could be an important parameter. The ranges of compositions of the retort waters and gas condensates are given in Table VIII.

The organic constituents are largely polar, with the major components consisting of carboxylic acids. The organic nitrogen compounds identified include pyridines, quinolines, anilines, and acridine.[33,34] The environmentally significant trace elements are As, Se, B, F, Zn, Ni, and Mo.[19,32] Retort waters produced by surface processes are typically more concentrated than those produced by in situ processes because of lower water production.

An additional source of potentially large quantities of water is mine dewatering. These waters can have high total dissolved solids (TDS) (400–

**Table VIII.**  Compositions of Retort Waters and Gas Condensates (mg/L except pH and minor elements)

| Parameter | Retort Waters | Gas Condensate |
|---|---|---|
| Alkalinity | 18,000–110,000 | 15,000–25,000 |
| Biochemical oxygen demand | 350–85,500 | 500 |
| Total organic carbon | 1,000–20,000 | 1,100 |
| Total inorganic carbon | 2,000–20,000 | |
| Bicarbonate | 4,200–74,000 | |
| Carbonate | 0–15,000 | |
| Total dissolved solids | 5,000–30,000 | <1,000 |
| Ammonia nitrogen (as $NH_3$) | 2,000–13,000 | 7,600 |
| Organic nitrogen (as N) | 73–1,500 | 190 |
| Suspended solids | 200–2,000 | 200–2,000 |
| Sulfate | 40–2,000 | 0–200 |
| pH | 8–9.4 | 8.6–8.8 |
| Minor elements (Al, As, Ca, Cl, Fe, K, Na, Ni, Zn, B, F), ppm | 1–1,000 | |

60,000 mg/L)[32] and boron and fluorine. Because these waters are not particularly special to oil shale processing, I will not discuss them further.

The codisposal of process waters is a potential problem because of high concentrations of organics and ammonia and the presence of toxic substances. The areas of concern include the exposure of workers to the waters or fugitive emissions, the mobilization of constituents in the spent shale, and the contribution of the constituents in the process waters to leaching of the spent shale. Because of these concerns, there may have to be some level of treatment (e.g., steam stripping) of these waters before codisposal. If codisposal is not feasible, various reuse options will require some degree of treatment. Finally, evaporation or incineration may be feasible options.[33]

Thus, research on oil shale wastewaters has involved:

chemical characterization of the untreated wastewaters, to aid in identifying toxics which require treatment and to assist in the design of treatment technology;

control technology research, to investigate the removal efficiencies of various conventional and advanced technologies;

biological characterization of both treated and untreated wastewaters, to determine the potential hazards due to accidental releases; and

studies of the mixtures of process waters and spent shales, to determine the potential for release of toxic compounds by leaching and volatilization.

Extensive characterizations of various oil shale process waters have been done.[32,33,35–37] The waters are extraordinarily complex, and their compositions are dependent on the retorting process and retorting conditions such as shale grade. Many problems are related to sampling and preservation of samples; for example, numerous reduced species of sulfur are present and are subject to oxidation. The heavy loadings of organics and salts cause difficulties in the analysis for specific compounds, and many "standard" methods do not work. Thus, a considerable amount of analytical research has been performed, and more is required. This includes work on determining inorganic species such as arsenic. One of the principal uncertainties in this work is the relationship of these wastewaters to those that will be produced in a commercial-scale operation. Thus, the Union retort will provide important information when it comes on line in 1984.

Some generalizations can be made about the process wastewater composition.[38] Most of the mobilized organic nitrogen and sulfur not transferred to the oil are reduced to ammonia ($NH_3$) and $H_2S$ gases. There is also formation of gases such as hydrogen cyanide (HCN) and COS. Carbon dioxide is formed from organic carbon and calcination of inorganic carbonates. The $NH_3$ is dissolved in the scrubber water, which then dissolves the acid gases with a preference for $CO_2$. Thus, most of the ammonia in gas condensate is present as ammonium bicarbonate with small amounts of dissolved $H_2S$.

In retort waters, inorganic ions leached from the shale such as sulfates and chlorides can "fix" the ammonia. Fixed ammonia cannot be stripped without addition of alkali. Both retort waters and gas condensates also contain organic nitrogen compounds,[39,40] which are not readily removed. Fractionation studies[39,41] have indicated that the organic acids (mainly carboxylic acids) are highest in concentration, followed by the neutrals (cyclic compounds, aromatic hydrocarbons, paraffins, and sulfur-containing compounds) and the bases (nitrogen-containing species). Of particular interest are alkyl pyridines, because they have been shown[42] to be mobile in the environment and perhaps are unique to shale oils and retort waters, making them useful as a diagnostic indicator.

As mentioned previously, the area of control technology research is muddled by the issue of proprietary data. Studies of various control technologies have been reported.[32,33,43] Of course, all of these studies suffer because they have not been done on the scale that would be required by a commercial operation, or for long periods of time, or on waters that are known to be representative of a commercial operation. In general, the high levels of organics and salts seem to present a challenge to the engineer. Biological oxidation processes seem to have a limited success[32] in organic removal and are not effective in salt removal. Reverse osmosis may be effective for salt treatment, and evaporation is an effective, although expensive, process for separation of heavy metals and salts. It is even possible that there could be a market for the sodium salts recovered.

Because of the potential costs, this is a fruitful area for new ideas, but this also means it is a highly competitive and potentially profitable area where much of the work will probably remain in the proprietary regime.

The interactions of process waters and spent shale have been studied from two points of view—water treatment and codisposal. Spent shale has been shown[44] to be usable in water treatment to reduce organic and inorganic carbon, conductivity, color, and odor and to elevate the pH (to convert ammonium ion ($NH_4^+$) to $NH_3$ in advance of steam stripping). Also, arsenic has been shown[34] to be quantitatively removed by the spent shale. Thus, codisposal, or at least the use of spent shale columns for partial treatment, might provide a means for dealing with the management of oil shale wastewaters.


## SOLID WASTE

Although it is difficult and dangerous to single out one area of concern above all others, certainly the most unique aspect of producing oil from shale is the tremendous volume of solid waste that is generated. For each barrel of oil about 1.5 tons of spent shale is generated; this has a volume of 40 cu ft (uncompacted). Thus, a 50,000-bbl/d plant will generate about 60,000 tons or 40 acre-ft of spent shale per day. Estimates of the ultimate size of the industry have varied considerably in recent years. But even a relatively "low" rate of 300,000 bbl/d would generate about 80,000 acre-ft of uncompacted shale per year (assuming that all of the production is from aboveground retorting). This volume would be reduced slightly by compaction.

These large amounts of solid waste will be disposed of by the construction of large waste dumps on a scale of or larger than the largest mining operations in North America. The projected heights of some of these piles are as much as 800 or 900 ft. While some of this material might eventually be backfilled into mines, a 10 to 25% bulking factor due to mining and crushing prevents total replacement. Moreover, the time lag involved for such backfilling would imply a significant surface storage. While these considerations apply to aboveground retorting, in situ operations result in spent shale underground. In addition to spent shale, there is also a significant quantity of raw shale stored aboveground as feedstock, and these storage piles are potential sources of air and water pollution.

One of the major concerns is the pollution of surface waters and groundwaters by leachates and runoff from piles of raw and spent shale. This area has been the subject of considerable research over a number of years.[44–61] A very comprehensive review of this research will be available in the near future.[61]

## Construction of a Spent Shale Pile

To set the stage for the discussion, I will present a scenario for the construction of the oil shale waste pile.[60] The location of the pile will be chosen on a site-specific basis. Some of the considerations will include:

- sufficient area to contain the amounts of waste;
- hydrologic characteristics that can be managed;
- proper slope, aspect, and other factors to assist in reclamation; and
- proper stabilization so that the site requires no maintenance over long periods of time.

Three types of sites likely to be chosen are mesa top, head-of-valley, and canyon. The canyon has some distinct advantages in terms of convenience, remoteness, and ability to contain large volumes with minimum stabilization. However, canyons exist because of geomorphic reasons, and the drainage will need to be controlled.

During construction and start-up, topsoil and minor overburden would be removed and stored. Springs and seeps would be sealed, and diversion ditches would be prepared to divert overland flow. The first spent shale produced would be used to construct a cross-valley dam. The spent shale might be transported by a covered conveyor to a truck loading point. To control dust, a moisturizer would be used at the plant site to cool the shale and bring the moisture content to about 15%. Processed shale at the discharge point of the conveyor is anticipated to have a temperature of 160 to 200°F.

From the conveyor discharge, 150-ton trucks will transport the shale and deposit it at the disposal site. Dozers will spread the waste in 18-ft lifts, and compactors will be used to bring the shale to the desired density. Water trucks will sprinkle the surface for dust control. A higher degree of compaction and quality control will be specified for the dam and valley liner materials. Drainage diversion structures must be constructed before full disposal operations begin. These consist of ditches and culverts to divert surface runoff around the embankment, ditches to carry runoff from the embankment face, and a settling pond to collect the embankment runoff.

At this point the operational phase could begin, with the area behind the dam used to dispose of spent shale. Dust control will be a major concern in active areas, but inactive areas may be allowed to dry and form a crust. In this case, desiccation cracks will develop, water will migrate upward, and evaporation will lead to salt crusts being deposited within the desiccation cracks.

There will be many sources of heterogeneity. Zones of highly compacted material will be present in areas of heavy traffic, and zones of poorly compacted material will exist elsewhere, for example, where compactors have broken down. Localized flooding due to ditch failures, natural precipitation, and rapid melting of snowfall (due to high surface temperatures) will lead to variations in moisture content. Temperatures may remain high for several years. Gullying due to surface runoff, piping along seeps, and differential settlement will also lead to a heterogeneous solid waste pile. In addition to these factors, the variations in shale grade, shale mineralogy, and operating conditions will lead to variations in the chemical and physical properties of the spent shale as it is laid down. Finally, spent shale is not the only waste material that will be put in the pile. The pile may also contain process wastewaters, raw shale dust, coke, spent catalysts, diatomaceous earth, deactivated carbon, and other solid materials. The final pile, then, will be a very large, nonuniform, and complex mixture of materials that is not in thermodynamic equilibrium.

In spite of the addition of other materials, 95% of the wastes placed in the pile will be spent or retorted shale. The characteristics of this material vary from process to process, but its primary characteristics are dark color, high pH, high concentrations of salts, high mobility of some trace elements (F, B, Mo, Li), and fine texture.

The construction life span of the disposal site will be 20 to 40 years.

During this period, the embankment will experience annual wet and dry cycles due to precipitation and evapotranspiration. Although the hydrologic budget for the area shows a net deficit, there is a period of surplus water during the winter. Percolation into the pile from snowfall can occur even without complete saturation.[59] Thus, it is expected[60] that there will be a downward migration of water from November to April and that not all of this input will be available for evapotranspiration during the dry months. However, there is evidence[62,63] that some of the water will be drawn to the surface by capillary action and, upon evaporation, crusts of sodium sulfate salts will be formed. Thus, both upward and downward movement of solutes may occur.

As the embankment is raised in lifts, the additional weight of each lift will cause consolidation of underlying shale.[60] Although the shale will initially be deposited under partially saturated conditions, the weight of the added material will cause compression of the spent material, forcing air out and increasing the degree of saturation. At some value of stress, all of the occluded air will have dissolved and saturated conditions will exist,[60] and a water table will possibly form within the pile.

The annual wet cycle will cause a wetting front to slowly migrate downward under saturated or partially saturated conditions.[60] Because the degree of saturation behind the first wetting front would be higher than that before the wetting front passed through, the time for a second wetting front to cover a given distance would be shorter, and successive wetting fronts may catch up with previous fronts.[60] As the wetting front intersects either the embankment liner or a water table at some depth, the phreatic surface will rise. If the net seepage loss through the liner is less than the inflow during the wet cycle, there will be a net accumulation of water within the dump. The phreatic level and degree of saturation will affect both the shear strength parameters and overall stability of the shale embankment. Thus, the geochemical, hydrological, and geotechnical properties of the pile are coupled together in a complex manner.

### Raw and Spent-Shale Leachates

Leachates from both raw (unretorted) and spent shale are of potential concern. Large quantities of raw shale will be stored on the surface where it will be subjected to both rainfall and snowmelt. Water sprays for dust control will be another source of input. There is a considerable variation in the leachate composition from various raw shales.[51,56,57,64] These variations are assumed to be caused by variations in mineralogy and other characteristics of the material. Ranges of selected parameters are given in Table IX.

The major ions in raw shale leachates from the Colony Mine are $Ca^{2+}$, $Mg^{2+}$, $Na^+$, $HCO_3^-$, and $SO_4^{2-}$.[48,54] The major ions in raw shale leachates

**Table IX.**   Ranges of Selected Parameters in Raw Shale Leachates (mg/L except conductance and pH)

| Parameter | Concentration |
|---|---|
| Al | <10.05–7.5 |
| As | <0.005–0.4 |
| B | <0.025–43 |
| Ca | 3.3–1550 |
| Carbonate | 0.03–346 |
| Cr | 0.025–0.68 |
| Cu | <0.025–0.69 |
| Electrical conductance, µmho/cm | 125–13000 |
| F | <0.5–75 |
| Li | <0.02–3.1 |
| Mo | 0.1–7.4 |
| Na | <25–7700 |
| Sulfate | 5–6100 |
| Total dissolved solids | 70–31000 |
| Total organic carbon | 13–370 |
| pH | 6.8–12 |

from the Anvil Points Mine are $Na^+$, $SO_4^{2-}$, and $HCO_3^-$, with $Ca^{2+}$ and $Mg^{2+}$ considerably reduced.[57] The reduction of $Ca^{2+}$ and $Mg^{2+}$ may be due to the presence of nahcolite and/or Dawsonite in the Anvil Points shale.[57]

Several trace elements are significantly elevated in the raw shale leachates. Among these are As, B, Cu, F, and Mo. The residence of fluorine in raw shale is primarily in the Illite fraction.[55,56] The residence of other trace elements is not known.

In general, much less work has been done on raw shale leachates than on spent shale leachates. The work that has been done, however, contradicts a widely held belief that raw shale piles do not pose a hazard because the natural geologic materials in the region were derived from that material and therefore such piles would be "natural." Clearly, freshly mined material has the ability to release significant quantities of hazardous trace elements such as B, F, and Mo into the environment, and mining and crushing will expose large amounts of fresh shale at a faster than "natural" rate. However, our knowledge of the geochemistry and the hydrology is not sufficient to enable us to quantify the hazard posed, and much more research is required.

As opposed to raw shale leaching, spent shale leaching has been extensively studied. The most thorough review of this work is contained in Reference 61. However, most of the research has involved spent shale generated by either the TOSCO II or the Paraho processes. Only a few studies have been done on Union or Lurgi shales. Thus, we are in the unfortunate position of having little information about the particular shale (Union B) that will be the first to be generated in large quantities.

As with raw shale leachates, wide variations in composition are seen in spent shale leachates as the process, feedstock, and other parameters are changed. Table X compares some key constituents in leachates from three processes.

The differences seen above are generally consistent with the mineralogical changes expected. For example, the very high pH and calcium concentration in Paraho leachates result from the hydrolysis of CaO and dissolution of $CaSO_4$, whereas the high magnesium concentration probably results from the dissolution of $MgSO_4$; the cause of the high lithium concentrations, however, is not known. The reducing atmospheres, lower temperatures, and lack of char combustion in the Union B and TOSCO II processes result in lower concentrations of Ca, Mg, K, and sulfate and lower pH in these leachates.

While plausible explanations exist for the major and minor species, the behavior of the trace elements is less well understood. In general, the

**Table X.**  Compositions of Leachates from Three Retorting Processes (mg/L except water quality parameters)

| Constituent | Union B | TOSCO II | Paraho (Direct) |
|---|---|---|---|
| Major cations | | | |
| $Na^+$ | 110 | 820 | 820 |
| $Ca^{2+}$ | 240 | 2 | 650 |
| $Mg^{2+}$ | 60 | 0.4 | 250 |
| $K^+$ | 7 | 8 | 60 |
| Major anions | | | |
| $SO_4^{2-}$ | 880 | 630 | 4300 |
| $HCO_3^-$ | 170 | 20 | 180 |
| $Cl^-$ | 7 | 20 | 30 |
| $CO_3^{2-}$ | 0 | | 15 |
| Trace elements | | | |
| B | 1 | 5 | 1 |
| F | 6 | 80 | 7 |
| Mo | 0.4 | 3 | 0.8 |
| Li | 0.1 | <0.1 | 6–20 |
| Water quality parameters | | | |
| TDS[b] | 1520 | 2200 | 7100 |
| TOC[c] | 10 | 100 | 2 |
| pH | 8 | 8 | 10 |

[a]From Reference 61, this chapter.
[b]Total dissolved solids.
[c]Total organic carbon.

concentrations of various ions decrease dramatically with pore volume. This is particularly true for total dissolved solids (TDS), boron, and molybdenum, where, apparently, readily soluble salts on the surface of the shale particles are rinsed out quickly. After these are gone, slow dissolution of less soluble minerals becomes the controlling mechanism. On the other hand, the concentration of fluorine remains constant for many pore volumes, indicating a large reservoir of fluorine in the shale that is capable of being replenished at a rate that compensates for movement of water through the column.[58]

Relatively little is known about the chemical speciation of the elements in leachates. The predominant arsenic species found[65] in TOSCO II leachates are the arsenate ion and methyl arsonic acid. Calculations with chemical equilibrium computer models of speciation in leachates[58] indicate that most of the molybdenum exists as the free molybdate ion, $MoO_4^{2-}$, whereas the fluorine exists primarily as the free fluoride ion, $F^-$. These calculations also indicate that the concentrations of molybdenum and fluorine in the leachates studied are controlled by calcium through $CaF_2$ and $CaMoO_4$. Recent results[61] also indicate that dissolved calcium may also exert a control over arsenic in leachates.

In recent years, evidence has been found that indicates a significant role of bacteria in the cycling of trace elements in spent shale. For example, thiosulfate-oxidizing bacteria play an important role in oil shale leachates by increasing the rate of oxidation of reduced sulfur compounds.[66] There is evidence[67] that bacteria are involved in a biological cycling of arsenic in spent shale; the data[67] show that (1) there is a mobilization from spent shale of initially highly insoluble arsenic after several weeks' incubation with soil bacteria under aerobic conditions, and (2) bacteria can increase the rate of volatilization of arsenic in spent shale. PNL researchers[68] have noted a significant increase in soluble chromium and nickel in field lysimeters containing Paraho spent shale. This increase appeared suddenly after several years of observation and was associated with an increase in organic carbon. These researchers suggest that this phenomenon reflects the development of a microbiological community and solubilization of residual organic carbon.

Several studies have involved the characterization of organic compounds in oil shale leachates; however, the data are perhaps more suspect than the inorganic data because of severe problems with sample preservation and analysis. The organic composition of the leachates is clearly important because of the toxicity and carcinogenicity of some of the compounds that have been identified and because of the potential for interactions between organic compounds and metals, which can affect the mobility and/or toxicity of the metals. Much of the research in this area has focused on polycyclic aromatic compounds in benzene extracts of spent shales.[45,60,69]

In 1978, it was suggested[7] that the higher maximum temperatures (up to 1200°C) encountered in in situ processes compared with those in aboveground processes (up to 750°C) could have positive benefits on the leachates of in situ spent shales; it was proposed that high-temperature reactions would create highly insoluble igneous and/or metamorphic minerals from the original oil shale minerals and their decomposition products. The existence of such minerals was demonstrated in laboratory experiments[70,71] and in a core from a field retort.[71] The study of the leaching behavior of in situ spent shales presents many difficult problems, and only limited progress has been made in this area. Great difficulties are encountered in attempting to obtain samples of in situ spent shale that are appropriate for leaching studies.[72] Cores obtained from Retort 3 at Logan Wash indicate a considerable inhomogeneity, reflecting variations in original mineralogy and process variables.[71] These cores indicated that, while the high temperatures encountered in some parts of an in situ retort can lead to the formation of highly insoluble silicate phases such as akermanite, the formation of such minerals does not guarantee the immobilization of many major, minor, and trace elements. The data suggest that K, Li, F, V, B, Mo, Ni, and As are not incorporated in the silicate matrix or that elements that control their solubilities are not incorporated in the silicate matrix. Thus, much work remains to be accomplished in order to understand mechanisms and rates of leaching of in situ spent shales.

### Environmental Transport and Fate of Leachates

The study of the transport of pollutants through a shale pile and surrounding geological materials into groundwaters and surface waters involves many complex and poorly understood mechanisms. The problems involved and a strategy for dealing with these problems are described in Reference 73. Whether this strategy will be successful remains to be seen. However, one of the first steps in this approach involves the application of a one-dimensional unsaturated groundwater flow model, UNSATID. An initial run of this hydrological model for a shale pile 50 m high under conditions similar to those which would be expected for a shale pile in the Piceance Creek Basin showed[73] that a steady state drainage was reached after about 20 years, leading to an annual drainage of about 10 cm from the pile. Thus, initial results indicate that drainage can occur. However, the uncertainty in these numbers is very high and much work remains. In addition, there are many complexities ignored by the model as presently constructed. Among these are the complex geochemistry, which is still not well understood. Mechanisms such as ion exchange, precipitation, and dissolution must be factored in with hydrological transport. These geochemical mechanisms are being studied, and geochemical models are being developed[58] that could be coupled to the hydrological models.

After leaving the pile, the leachates will be in contact with various geological materials (soils, subsoils, etc.), and the interaction with these materials can lead to further changes in the chemistry of the waters. Investigators[62] of this interaction found a dramatic decrease in soil hydraulic conductivity after the passage of leachate. They attribute this to the exchange of sodium in the leachate for calcium and magnesium originally in the soils, leading to a swelling of the clays. This phenomenon, known as peptization or dispersion, could lead to a dramatic increase in runoff and, perhaps, decreased stability in soils over spent shale piles if these soils are contacted by leachate (such as might happen with upward capillary movement). This phenomenon was further demonstrated in elution chromatography experiments involving the passage of leachate through columns of native geological materials from planned disposal sites in the oil shale region. These materials included valley bottom soil from Davis Gulch and weathered and fresh material from the Uinta Formation. A dramatic increase was observed in the calcium and magnesium concentrations in the eluates obtained in the elution chromatography experiments. A very sizable decrease in the permeability was also observed, and subsequent rinsing with water further decreased the permeability. The retardation experiments showed very little removal of molybdenum or boron as leachates passed through soil or bedrock.[62] These materials showed a greater retention for fluorine than for molybdenum or boron, but this retention was reversible and the fluorine readily went back into the solution. There was very little retention of chloride and sulfate, making these constituents good tracers of leachate movement. All of the materials investigated showed a strong retention of arsenic and aluminum, thus providing good protection against those elements, assuming that the strong irreversibility of this retention observed[62] does not change with time, biological activity, or other variables as seen by others.[67]

A recent study[74] has shown that pattern recognition methods such as principal component analysis, factor analysis, and discriminate function analysis could dramatically increase the ability to detect leachate contamination of natural waters in a cost-effective manner. A large data base of water quality data from Logan Wash that had been collected by Occidental Oil Shale, Inc. was given by that corporation to R.R. Meglen of the University of Colorado at Denver.[74] This data base involved 77 chemical parameters for waters from wells and streams in the area. Almost all of the information in this data base that distinguished between the various natural waters and wastewater from Retort 6 was contained in 12 variables. Essentially all of the remaining distinguishing information was contained in 23 additional variables. The study also revealed several variables (e.g., lithium) for which the analytical methods used were inadequate. A similar study recently completed by Meglen and co-workers for Lease Tract C-b shows that these methods can be used to "fingerprint" the numerous aquitards in the area; it also revealed contamination of alluvial groundwaters by leakage from ponds containing water from the dewatering operation. With the large quantity of data now being generated by research and monitoring, these techniques provide a powerful tool for investigating relationships and trends in multidimensional space and a method for devising optimal, cost-effective data sets which will provide better monitoring information at reduced costs.

The Oil Shale Risk Analysis (OSRA),[23] with numerous assumptions, estimated the impact of leaching of spent shale piles for a million-barrel-per-day industry on the water quality of the region.[23] Among the assumptions were that there was no change in concentrations other than by dilution, that the waste pile depths were 200 m, and that equilibrium moisture conditions were reached in 60 to 200 years; leachate concentrations were taken as average concentrations in the first 0.22 to 0.25 pore volume. The results of the calculations are shown in Table XI, and the discussion of these implications follows.

## HEALTH AND SAFETY

Both the occupational workforce and the general public will be exposed to controlled as well as uncontrolled emissions that could lead to adverse health effects. In addition, accidents of various types, (transportation, falls, etc.) that would lead to injury or death could occur. The considerable research in this area, which consists of work in the United States, Scotland, and Estonia, has recently been reviewed.[75,76] Obviously, all the data relating to commercial operations and most of the data relating to human health come from the foreign experience. The U.S. studies have concentrated on the

**Table XI.**  Upper Bound Increases in Concentrations (mg/L) of Selected Leachate Species at Selected Locations in the Colorado River System[a]

| Species | White River[b] (Watson, Utah) | Green River[c] (Green River, Utah) | Colorado River[d] (Colorado-Utah line) | Colorado River[e] (Lees Ferry, Arizona) |
|---|---|---|---|---|
| TDS[f] | 150 | 42 | 25 | 43 |
| TOC[g] | 1.5 | 0.4 | 0.2 | 0.4 |
| F | 0.1 | 0.03 | 0.02 | 0.03 |
| Na | 40 | 10 | 7 | 12 |
| As | $3 \times 10^{-4}$ | $5 \times 10^{-5}$ | $3 \times 10^{-5}$ | $5 \times 10^{-5}$ |
| Mo | 0.2 | 0.03 | 0.02 | 0.03 |
| Se | $3 \times 10^{-4}$ | $8 \times 10^{-5}$ | $5 \times 10^{-5}$ | $8 \times 10^{-5}$ |

[a]From Reference 23, this chapter.
[b]Includes mass flow from Piceance Creek and White River.
[c]Includes mass flow from Piceance Creek, White River, and Green River.
[d]Includes mass flow from Parachute Creek.
[e]Includes mass flow from Parachute Creek, Piceance Creek, White River, and Green River.
[f]Total dissolved solids.
[g]Total organic carbon.

biological characterization (in vivo and in vitro) of the products and effluents from pilot plants and the characterization of the working environment in these pilot operations. A limited amount of epidemiological data exists for U.S. oil shale workers, but these data are ambiguous because these workers have had complicated work and smoking histories.[77] Thus, all useful human health data on occupational health effects come from the foreign experience. With respect to safety, the U.S. oil shale data base is too sparse and the foreign data base has too many gaps to be useful. Thus, safety is evaluated by inspecting risks in similar industries (coal mining, etc.). Safety is discussed later in this chapter.

### Health Effects

There are a variety of ways in which human health could be adversely impacted by shale oil production. These include:

1.   exposure to gaseous, liquid, and solid effluents;
2.   exposure to raw shale oil and various refined products; and
3.   increased stress due to changes in lifestyle (i.e., socioeconomic effects).

We will not discuss the last item here, although it could indeed be significant.

It is possible to construct scenarios for various exposures. It is also possible to chemically characterize the materials to which people would be exposed in these scenarios. It is much more difficult to evaluate the type and frequency of the health effects of such exposure. One approach is to perform in vivo and in vitro bioassays using mice, rats, tissue cultures, bacteria, etc. This approach suffers because of the difficulty of extrapolating to humans. The other approach is to collect data on the health of people who have been exposed to materials related to oil shale (e.g., in Scotland and Estonia). This approach suffers because the exposure data are poor or nonexistent and the materials may not be relevant to their U.S. counterparts.

### Foreign Data

The Estonian oil shale industry is the largest active such industry in the world. While most of the oil shale has been used for direct combustion to generate power, the Estonian industry has been producing shale oil since about 1925. Estonia has been studying the health effects of oil shale for several years. Most of this research is now conducted at the Institute for Experimental and Clinical Medicine in Tallinn. Some work has also been done by the Institute of Chemistry, Estonian Academy of Sciences. Most of the Soviet efforts have been focused on carcinogenicity. This work, which consists of laboratory, medical, and epidemiological studies, has been extensively reviewed.[75,76] Reference 78 is also recommended for further reading.

The principal results of these studies were summarized[75,76] as follows:

**Animal Studies:**
1.  Direct toxicity of the shale oil and various fractions can be estimated from the phenol content and is more pronounced at higher process temperatures.
2.  The intensity of skin reactions is correlated with the degree of inhalation toxicity.
3.  Higher process temperatures also produce more potent carcinogenic products and by-products. Benzo($a$)pyrene is an important carcinogen in many of the products and by-products, but its presence is not a reliable indicator of the carcinogenic potential.
4.  The solid waste (soot) from direct combustion of shale was more carcinogenic than the soot from oil shale fuel oil.

**Human Studies:**
1.  The incidence of stomach and lung cancer is higher in the general population in the Estonian oil shale districts than for Estonia as a whole. However, at least some of this higher incidence is due to immigration of workers from other Soviet republics, where the background level is higher.
2.  Although there is a higher incidence of gastric cancer in the rural populations of the oil shale region, there is no increase in the benzo($a$)pyrene content of waters, soils, or vegetables in these regions compared with controls.
3.  An increased incidence of skin cancer has been observed among female workers in the industry.
4.  Chronic bronchitis, mild forms of pneumoconiosis, and emphysema are observed in miners. The dust levels in the mines are relatively low with a low percentage of free silica, but the dust is highly respirable.
5.  Diseases of the mucous membranes of the nasopharynx, such as chronic hypertrophic rhinitis, are common in miners but are attributed to the high humidity and cold temperatures. However, the more serious atrophic rhinitis commonly found in workers in contact with oil shale ash (soot) is attributed to the ash and to simultaneous exposure to fugitive gases and the ash.

The Scottish oil shale industry was, as mentioned earlier, the longest-running; it was started in the late 1850s and was closed in 1962. The industry was located in a 200-sq-mile area centered about 20 miles from Edinburgh. The most common health effects reported were skin diseases. The first reported health effect was two cases of scrotal cancer.[79] An extensive study[80,81] of skin diseases in oil shale workers, reported in the early 1920s, disclosed several distinct dermatoses and epithelioma (paraffin worker's cancer). Although baths had been erected at Young's Oil Works in Bathgate in 1883, these were never used.[80] The study emphasized the need for good hygiene and noted that some of the skin ailments diminished significantly when good practices were used. The study also recommended the protective application of castor oil, which is insoluble in the paraffin series and provides an impervious coating for the skin. Lubricating oils from shale oil were widely used in the textile industry to lubricate the spindles (mules). As a result of exposure to these oils, hundreds of workers died from cancer of the scrotum or vulva (mule spinnner's cancer). The incidence of these cancers greatly diminished after the substitution of different lubricants and the use of better hygienic practices.[82]

Skin painting studies[83] in mice using Scottish shale oils indicated that the shale oils were more carcinogenic than California and Pennsylvania crudes, but that some coal-derived liquids were far more carcinogenic than shale oils. These studies also indicated that carcinogenic potential was a function of process temperatures.[84] Shale oils were found to contain benzpyrene, but some fractions in which benzpyrene was below detection limits nevertheless induced tumors in mice.[85] Oil shale dusts were not found to be carcinogenic.[86]

The most frequently cited health effects related to the Scottish industry were dermatoses and skin cancers. This distribution is not surprising, because dermatoses generally dominate other occupational diseases. However, this distribution is also likely to be due to a lack of attention to internal problems. Although no reports of pneumoconiosis appear in the older literature, a long-time resident of the area, whose family worked in the oil shale industry for several generations, has said that pneumoconiosis was a frequent health problem in the industry.[87]

The issue of nonneoplastic pulmonary health effects in the Scottish oil shale industry has been highlighted recently by the diagnosis[88] of pneumoconiosis in four patients whose only occupational experience was in that industry. The clinical and histological features of the disease closely resembled the simple pneumoconiosis of coal miners (CWP) and kaolin workers. Indeed, the only significant difference was that the macrophages contained particles which were brown instead of black. Moreover, the mineralogical analysis of the material in the lung tissue closely matched the composition of shale from West Lothian seams.

Two of the men, whose lung tissue was examined after death, had localized peripheral, well-differentiated squamous carcinomas in their lungs, in addition to complicated pneumoconiosis.[88] The site and association with the scars indicate these carcinomas were directly or indirectly related to the dust rather than to smoking.

To gain more information about the health effects of the Scottish oil shale industry, DOE has recently funded a mortality study of workers previously employed by the industry. This research, conducted at the Institute of Occupational Medicine, Edinburgh, has not been under way long enough for results to be available. In addition, a feasibility study[89] has been conducted for an investigation of a community mortality study. Such a study could be very enlightening, because the oil shale workers and their families lived adjacent to the mines, retorts, refineries, and spent shale piles. Moreover, the city of Edinburgh is only a few miles downwind of the industry.

## U.S. Studies

Several U.S. researchers have been active in studying the health effects of materials related to U.S. oil shales. Most of this work has been done at Los Alamos National Laboratory. However, because a commercial industry does not exist in the United States, the research has focused on materials produced by various experimental and pilot retorts.

Studies have been made of U.S. oil shale workers,[77,90–92] but the results are complicated by a complex work history for the subjects of these studies, which includes work in other mining industries, and by the small sample size; therefore, none of these studies show an effect which can clearly be related to oil shale. It is interesting, however, that one of the researchers[77] suggested that "shalosis," a disease resembling silicosis and caused by oil shale dust, might be found in oil shale miners. This suggestion, although widely criticized, is now of interest because of the recent findings of pneumoconiosis in Scottish oil shale workers.

Numerous in vitro and in vivo tests have been carried out on oil-shale-related materials. Certainly the most extensive in vitro studies have been with the Ames *Salmonella* mutagenic system.[93–96] These studies have shown that crude shale oil and the basic and neutral fractions of crude shale oil are mutagenic. These studies also indicate that significant cytotoxic effects are associated with shale oils and their refined products.

Changes and aberrations in chromosomes caused by exposure to shale oils have been studied[97] by measuring sister chromatid exchange (SCE); this study found that both crude and hydrotreated shale oils increased SCE occurrence.

Although the polycyclic aromatic hydrocarbon content, particularly benzo($a$)pyrene, was earlier thought to be the cause of the mutagenic and carcinogenic action of U.S. shale oils,[98,99] upon fractionation, the mutagenicity is found to be primarily determined by the polycyclic aromatic primary amines in the alkaline fraction.[95,100,101]

Near-ultraviolet radiation has been demonstrated[96] to have a stimulating effect on the mutagenicity of shale oil and process waters. Thus, the combined effect of sunlight and exposure to these materials could increase the risks of skin cancer for workers.

Most in vivo testing has focused on skin painting. Results of this research have shown:

1. Crude shale oils have exhibited a carcinogenic potency that is generally somewhat greater than that of crude petroleums and much less than that of coal-derived liquids;[102–104]
2. Hydrotreating of shale oils greatly reduces, but does not eliminate, their carcinogenic potential;[103,105]
3. Exposure to raw or spent shales did not cause tumors in the test animals;[103,105]
4. Shale oils have also been demonstrated to cause skin irritation, with the frequency of exposure being the primary determinant.[106]

Studies of the effects of inhalation of raw and spent shale dusts in rats have shown a potential for chronic inflammatory response of the lung.[107] More-recent inhalation experiments at very high shale dust exposures have produced lung tumors in rats, in addition to fibrosis.[108] Indeed, it has been suggested that the tumors were a sequel to advanced fibrosis, similar to the lung scar cancer seen in Scottish oil shale workers. Scientists at Los Alamos National Laboratory[108] have begun experiments in which animals are exposed to retort off-gas from an experimental retort; no results have been reported as yet.

The biological activity of process waters has been studied by the use of in vivo and in vitro bioassays. Some of these waters are positive on the Ames test,[109] while others are not. One of the waters demonstrating positive mutagenicity was also given to breeding mice in prenatal toxicity studies. While these studies showed no difference in the number of pregnancies, maternal weight, number of live fetuses or average fetal weight, there was an increase in abnormalities of the hard palate and an indication of an increase in preimplantation fetal loss.

### Implications for Public Health

The emission of gaseous and aqueous effluents, the use of the products, and the solid residue associated with an oil shale industry pose potential risks for the general public. However, these risks are exceedingly hard to quantify for several reasons:

1. The emissions involve complex mixtures which will not be well understood in chemistry or magnitude until commercial retorts are operating.
2. Even if the emissions were well characterized, the transport and transformation in the complex system is not well understood.
3. The biological effects of many of the pollutants and mixtures are poorly known.

The OSRA[23] attempted to quantify the risks associated with the steady state air and water emissions from a million-barrel-per-day industry. Emission rates for criteria pollutants and carcinogens were considered. For the air emissions, a Gaussian, flat terrain model was used to estimate chronic exposure. For a million-barrel-per-day industry, the carcinogens in the air emissions were estimated to produce less than 0.01 case of cancer per year. A model[24] that uses sulfate as a surrogate for the health effects of all air pollutants was used, since none of the individual pollutants causing noncarcinogenic effects was above the "no observed effect level." The application of this model led to an increase of 14 premature deaths for the region and 26 nationwide (for which long-range models were used).[23] There are wide uncertainties in this model and its relevance to this situation. The OSRA estimated an uncertainty range of 0 to 300 for this calculation.

Note that shale oil is very low in sulfur (~ 20 ppm); therefore, if shale oil were to replace higher-sulfur petroleum from the Middle East, a benefit could result (if the pollutants responsible for the health effects are decreased in proportion to the sulfates) that might, at least partially, offset the risk from shale oil. In particular, such a benefit could arise because the emission of sulfur by the production of crude shale oil, estimated at 115 metric tons/d for a million-barrel-per-day industry, would occur in a relatively unpopulated area, whereas the refining of higher-sulfur crude petroleum and the consequent sulfur emission of an estimated 167 metric tons/d for a million-barrels-per-day throughput might occur in the more highly populated Midwest.

The situation for water-borne pollutants is even more difficult, because the hydrological transport models are more uncertain than the air models. Table XI gave values for the increase in several pollutants of interest in surface waters downstream of the oil shale area (as estimated by the OSRA).[23] None of these parameters was found to lead to a significant health effect. However, the crudeness of the model required a calculation of the impact at points far downstream of the oil shale area, which allows for considerable dilution. Moreover, none of the toxic organics were included in the risk calculation.

It is much more difficult to estimate the public health risk associated with unplanned releases. Neither the nature nor the frequency of such releases is known. However, it is obvious that accidental releases will occur. The sill-pillar collapse at Retort 6 in Logan Wash was one such example. It is possible to construct scenarios in which an accidental release could lead to a worst-case situation; an example would be the failure of an air pollution control device during a severe inversion or other atmospheric condition, leading to trapping of pollutants and fumigation of a nearby community. While the chemical characterization of raw off-gas gives some idea of the emission characteristics, no modeling has been done which would allow the estimation of the consequences of such an event. Similarly, while there is a considerable amount of data on the chemical and biological characteristics of shale oils and process waters, the frequencies of accidents that would release these liquids into vulnerable waters are unknown.

One area where there may be a need for research is that of chronic responses to acute exposures. Most of the research being conducted involves either acute short-term response to high short-term exposures or chronic long-term response to low long-term exposures. Little, if any, attention has been paid to chronic long-term responses to acute short-term exposures, as might occur with accidental releases. Such effects, if they exist, might be missed by inadequate follow-up of the exposed population. An example of such an effect might be an irreversible disturbance (as has recently been attributed to asbestos) of the immunological system.

### Occupational Health

The occupational health risks are somewhat easier to estimate than the public health risks. Even here, however, the uncertainties are very large, because the exposures will not be well characterized until one or more commercial or near-commercial operations exist. Nevertheless, the data from the foreign experiences and laboratory studies, as well as data from similar industries, allow us to focus on some specific concerns relating to the health of oil shale workers.

Foremost among these effects are dermatoses, skin cancer, internal cancers, and nonneoplastic respiratory diseases such as pneumoconiosis, silicosis, bronchitis, and chronic airway obstruction. In addition, the presence of large diesel equipment in the mines can be expected to cause high noise levels and lead to some increase in hearing impairment. Estimates of these risks have been made by the OSRA[23] and are given in Table XII.

These numbers were derived by comparison with similar industries such as refining and coal mining.[23] Assumptions were made about the relative carcinogenicity and toxicity of oil shale materials and the size of the work force. These assumptions need to be tested by research on commercial-scale retorts.

Clearly, the nonneoplastic respiratory diseases stand out as the greatest human health risk suggested by this analysis. Dermatoses, which are likely to affect a large number of workers, were not estimated. Dermatoses are rarely fatal or totally disabling, but they are painful, disfiguring, and demoralizing and deserve a significant amount of attention from researchers and industrial hygienists. Finally, diesel exhaust could be of concern in the mines.

### Occupational Safety

In addition to disease, the occupational population is exposed to accidents that can cause injury or death. The OSRA[23] estimates that for a million-barrel-per-day industry, some 10 to 20 worker accident-related deaths will occur per year. In addition, an estimated 1800 to 3600 lost-time accidents

Table XII. Summary of Oil Shale Occupational Health: Incidence, Mortality, and Uncertainty[a] (for hypothetical million-barrel-per-day oil shale industry)

| Disease | Excess Incidence per 1000 | Thousands of Workers at Risk | Case Fatality (%) | Cases Per Year | | Deaths Per Year | |
|---|---|---|---|---|---|---|---|
| | | | | Best Estimate | Uncertainty Range | Best Estimate | Uncertainty Range |
| Internal cancers | | | | | | | |
| Lung, hydrocarbons | 0.115 | 15.0 | 91 | 2 | 0–17 | 2 | 0–16 |
| Lung, arsenic | 0.012 | 20.4 | 91 | 0 | 0–1 | 0 | 0–1 |
| Stomach | 0.039 | 15.0 | 88 | 1 | 0–6 | 1 | 0–5 |
| Kidney | 0.022 | 15.0 | 56 | 0 | 0–3 | 0 | 0–2 |
| Brain | 0.069 | 15.0 | 82 | 1 | 0–10 | 1 | 0–9 |
| Skin cancers | | | | | | | |
| Melanoma | 0.029 | 15.0 | 38 | 0 | 0–4 | 0 | 0–2 |
| Basal cell | 1.080 | 15.0 | 1 | 16 | 1–210 | 0 | 0–2 |
| Squamous cell | 0.290 | 15.0 | 1 | 4 | 0–57 | 0 | 0–1 |
| Pneumoconiosis[b] | | | | | | | |
| Method 1: Coal dust surrogate | | | | | | | |
| 0/1+ | 2.9 | 20.4 | 9 | 60 | 17–210 | 4 | 1–14 |
| 2/1+ | 0.65 | 20.4 | 9 | 13 | 4–47 | 1 | 0–3 |
| PMF | 0.95 | 20.4 | 35 | 19 | 5–69 | 7 | 2–24 |
| Combined, 0/1+ and PMF | | | 43 | 79 | 22–280 | 11 | 3–38 |
| Method 2: Silica | 2.5 | 20.4 | | 51 | 15–170 | 22 | 7–74 |
| Chronic bronchitis[b] | 4.5 | 20.4 | 4 | 92 | 26–330 | 4 | 1–14 |
| Airway obstruction[b] | 0.18 | 20.4 | 3 | 4 | 1–13 | 0 | 0–0.4 |
| High-frequency hearing loss | 1.4 | 20.4 | | 29 | 10–82 | | |

[a]From Reference 23, this chapter.
[b]Estimates of pneumoconiosis, chronic bronchitis, and airway obstruction may overlap.

are expected to occur. These estimates are made by inspecting the types of worker activities such as mining and the accident rates associated with these activities. Most of the serious accidents (two-thirds of the fatalities and one-half of the accidents with days lost) are associated with extraction of the oil shale (mining and crushing).

It should be noted that the OSRA assumed a million-barrel-per-day industry with no surface mines. Since the number of serious accidents in surface mining is about half that in underground mining, a significant reduction is possible by choosing surface mining over underground mining.

There are two significant areas where little information exists. One is the risk presented by gassy mines; the other is the risk posed to miners in an MIS operation by a breakthrough of hot, toxic gases from a burning retort to an area containing miners.

## ECOLOGICAL EFFECTS

Although there are numerous concerns[110,111] about ecosystem effects, ranging from loss of water and habitat to acid precipitation, most of the research efforts directly related to oil shale development have focused on spent shale reclamation. I will, consequently, focus most of the discussion on this particular issue.

### Reclamation of Spent Shale

A mature oil shale industry would produce hundreds of millions of cubic yards of spent shale annually. This material should be (and by Colorado law must be) disposed of in a way that creates a land form requiring (on abandonment) zero maintenance and able to function in equilibrium with the surrounding environment. This goal is not trivial, and while considerable progress has been made in solving this challenge, much remains to be done.

A considerable effort has been devoted to the study of revegetation of spent shale, amended spent shale, and spent shale covered with soil. This research is extensively reviewed in References 112 and 113.

As noted previously, the physical and chemical characteristics of spent shale differ from process to process. But most spent shales share a number of characteristics that pose obstacles to successful revegetation. These are high pH, high soluble salt content, low available nitrogen and phosphorous, and, frequently, unfavorable texture and color.[112] Nevertheless, some success has been obtained in revegetating retorted shales. However, the high salt content and low nutrient content of the spent shales require intensive management (e.g., leaching of salts, irrigation, and fertilization) for successful vegetation; even with such techniques, greater success is obtained when the spent shale is mixed with or covered by soil.

Thus, most researchers[113] believe that some type of soil covering is required for successful reclamation. Soil coverings have been shown[113] to ameliorate salt content in leachates, improve vegetative cover and diversity, and reduce erosion.

The most extensive reclamation research has been that carried out by a Colorado State University team at a site near Lease Tract C-a using Paraho spent shale.[112,113] This research has shown that:

1. Paraho spent shale is a poor growth medium.
2. Topsoil coverings of 91 and 61 cm with 30 cm of gravel as a capillary barrier produce more herbage and cover than shallower coverings.
3. Topsoil covering provides a better growth medium than subsoil, but the latter can be markedly improved with fertilizer and water.
4. For arid sites, native shrubs produce better stands than native grasses or introduced grasses. However, the addition of water or fertilizer enhances the biomass of grasses.
5. For more favorable sites, grasses dominate shrubs.
6. Fertilizers increase total yield, and seeded introduced species respond better to fertilizer than seeded native species.
7. The use of supplemental water favors grasses over forbs and shrubs. But a subsequent withdrawal of the water may lead to a decrease of grasses.
8. Mulches serve to conserve moisture and protect against erosion.
9. Microbial processes are adversely affected by spent shale.

Numerous factors need to be considered when selecting the seed mixture, fertilizer applications, irrigation rates, and other parameters. These factors include the climate, morphology, and wildlife. These complex interactions are not well understood. Short-term success has been achieved, but we do not know how these reclamation attempts will fare in the long term (50 to 200 years). Moreover, the experiments have involved very small plots where reasonably good control is possible. On a very large scale, factors such as burrowing animals (marmots, prairie dogs, ground squirrels, pocket mice, badgers, etc.) may come into play.[114]

In 1974, elevated concentrations of molybdenum were found in plants growing on spent shale.[115,116] Subsequent investigations[117–120] have shown:

1. Significantly elevated concentrations of boron and molybdenum have been observed in several species of plants growing on spent shales and spent shales covered with soil. The boron concentrations have been as high as 200 ppm, and the molybdenum concentrations have been as high as 45 ppm compared with background concentrations of 10 and 1 to 2 ppm respectively.
2. In addition to elevated molybdenum concentrations, the ratio of copper/molybdenum concentration is frequently less than 2. This combi-

nation is generally considered to pose a high risk[121] of molybdenum toxicity to grazing livestock.

3.   Although boron concentrations in the range seen in plants growing on spent shale are known to be toxic to agricultural plants, greenhouse experiments indicate[122] that most of the plants (except for Lewis flax) used in reclamation programs are reasonably tolerant of these high B concentrations. However, it is possible that this tolerance might be lowered by stresses such as drought.

4.   Arsenic and selenium were not found to be taken up by plants from the spent shales investigated to date.[118]

5.   Slight, so far insignificant increases in fluorine have been seen in some plants.

6.   In general, the concentrations of boron and molybdenum decrease with increased soil cover over shale. The concentrations of boron increase with decreased precipitation and increased evapotranspiration. Thus periods of drought can be expected to lead to increased boron concentrations in plants.

These results indicate a possible concern with boron, although the levels observed are not acutely toxic and are a definite concern with molybdenum. If the plants (e.g., fourwing saltbush) high in molybdenum constitute an important part of the diet of cattle or sheep, they could lead to chronic or acute molybdenum toxicity. Little is known about the toxicity of molybdenum to wildlife. Limited experiments on deer[116] indicate a much greater tolerance than livestock, and laboratory rats, mice, rabbits, and guinea pigs also show[121] a greater tolerance than cattle and sheep.

### Agricultural Impacts

In addition to impacts on agriculture caused by the withdrawal of land for energy development and associated urban development and by the purchase of water rights, the uptake of molybdenum by plants may pose a significant problem for livestock grazing. As previously mentioned, several plants such as fourwing saltbush and Indian ricegrass take up significant amounts of molybdenum when grown on spent shale or spent shale covered with soil. In addition, Indian ricegrass in the northern part of the Uinta Basin of Utah has been shown[123] to have an average copper/molybdenum ratio of 1.5, which could pose a molybdenosis hazard to livestock.

Besides the high molybdenum levels to be expected in plants growing on spent shale piles and the low copper/molybdenum ratios in plants indigenous to some areas of the oil shale region, the high molybdenum levels in the leachates provide still another source via irrigation. A National Academy of Sciences report[124] recommends a maximum molybdenum concentration of 0.01 mg/L in irrigation water for continuous use on all soils. For short-term use on soils reacting with this element (primarily acidic soils), a maximum concentration of 0.05 mg/L is recommended. Table XI shows that we might expect to exceed the 0.01 mg/L level as far away as the Imperial Valley.

A model[125] of molybdenum contamination indicates that the use of 10 cm of water containing 0.1 mg/L on a clayey soil will increase the concentration of molybdenum in alfalfa by 10 ppm over 25 years. The model also indicates that as little as 0.02 mg/L molybdenum in irrigation water could lead to concentrations of 5 ppm in forage, a level which has been shown[126] in the United Kingdom to cause chronic molybdenum toxicity in cattle. Thus, while the oil shale area, particularly that portion in the Uinta Basin near the White River, is of special concern because of low indigenous copper/molybdenum ratios, high levels of molybdenum and low copper/molybdenum ratios in reclaimed areas, and higher molybdenum in irrigation water, even areas in the lower Colorado River Basin may be affected by molybdenum leached from the spent shale.

In addition to the molybdenum in the leachate, the total salt loading will have an agricultural impact. The salt loading comes not only from the leachate but also from consumptive use by the industry and indirect uses. Using the TDS figure of 43 mg/L from Table XI and a figure of 14 mg/L for consumptive uses and associated wastewater treatment facilities gives an estimated TDS increase of about 60 mg/L at Imperial Dam for a million-barrel-per-day industry. A 1-mg/L increase is estimated to cause annual damages of about $0.5 million.[127] Thus, the total damages from salt loading by a million-barrel-per-day industry would be about $30 million/year. It is interesting to note that this salinity increase is close to estimates made nearly 10 years ago.[128]

Besides the salt loading, sodium in irrigation presents a specific hazard, because it can affect soil structure, infiltration, and permeability unfavorably. Whether such effects will occur depends on the sodium absorption ratio (SAR). At present, the models are not capable of predicting the sodium risk downstream of the oil shale region.

## Terrestrial Ecosystem Effects

While numerous qualitative[6,110,111,128] discussions of the effects of oil shale development on terrestrial ecosystems (excluding agriculture) exist, very little quantitative data, other than baseline studies, are available. There are several sources of impact, including mine dewatering, water pollution, air pollution, habitat disturbance and loss, solid waste piles, subsidence, noise, and indirect effects such as poaching and road kill. But the relationships between the magnitude of impact and the size of effect (the equivalent of relationships between dose and response in toxicology) are poorly understood at this time.

Efforts have been made to estimate effects on selected species such as mule deer by assuming linear relationships between habitat and population.[23,127] These estimates range from loss of a few mule deer to a 10% reduction in mule deer population from habitat loss for a million-barrel-per-day industry. Such an effect would be small compared with the importance of winter range condition and the severity of winter.[129]

The OSRA[23] attempted to estimate the loss of Indian ricegrass due to $SO_2$ emissions, since this species is particularly susceptible to $SO_2$ toxicity. These estimates indicated a loss of less than 1%. There will also be an impact on various plant communities by construction and spent shale disposal. The ultimate impact will depend on the success of revegetation or (if revegetation is unsuccessful) the size and duration of the industry.

An impact that could be very important for terrestrial ecosystems is that of dewatering. For safe and efficient operations, water will have to be pumped out of the areas where mining takes place. This pumping may lower the phreatic surface by as much as 100 m (for an MIS mine) at distances of as much as 3.5 km from the center of the operation.[130] This may have very significant effects on the plant communities and on the availability of water to wildlife via springs, seeps, surface water, but there are inadequate data at present to estimate the magnitude of this effect.

Some research has been done on the toxicity of in situ process waters to terrestrial plants.[131] This research indicates a low to moderate toxicity, with considerable variation among species. Additional studies of the effects of process waters and leachates on plants as well as soil microorganisms are being conducted at the University of Wyoming. These effects would, of course, be important for accidents involving the unplanned release of process waters and leachates.

### Aquatic Ecosystem Effects

Bergman[132] has demonstrated that accidental spills of process waters into streams could have a significant local effect. For short-term exposures, the results indicate that even when diluted by factors of 200 to 2000, such spills could cause fish kills, indicating the necessity for reliable containment. Steam stripping of the process waters led to a reduction of acute toxicity by two orders of magnitude.[132] An even greater reduction was obtained when steam stripping was followed by biological treatment and/or activated carbon filtration.

Some raw shale leachates were found to cause acute toxicity[132] in *Daphnia magna* and fathead minnows, while others were only minimally acutely toxic. However, the *Daphnia* chronic test showed those that did not cause acute toxicity did cause chronic toxicity. As a result, the release of large volumes of raw shale leachates could cause a significant impact on aquatic organisms.

Research on the effects of spent shale leachate on aquatic organisms is under way at the University of Wyoming. While it is clear that accidental releases of process waters, oil, and raw shale leachates could cause localized damage to aquatic organisms, it is not clear what the effects of runoff or leachates from spent shale piles would be, particularly if the leachates did not come from a containment pond, but resulted from leakage through the bottom of the pile into underlying aquifers. The ultimate answer to this question involves all of the difficult issues discussed earlier in the section on solid waste.

## CONCLUSION

The understanding of the health and environmental effects of a U.S. oil shale industry presents a considerable challenge to researchers. Certainly the absence of commercial-scale facilities in the United States represents the largest handicap because of the inability to obtain data which can be extrapolated to an industry of reasonable size.

Because of the absence of any sizeable development, both the foreign experiences (chiefly those in Scotland and Estonia) and the pilot-scale U.S. operations must be used to obtain a qualitative and quantitative description of the significant impacts of a future U.S. oil shale industry. While a considerable amount of research has been and is being conducted, much remains to be done. Many answers will not be obtained until commercial-scale retorts, such as those being constructed by Union, are in operation.

Certain aspects of this complex array of issues and problems stand out as being potentially significant. In the area of air quality, the control of sulfur emissions, which have both potential regulatory (i.e., PSD requirements) and health/environmental importance (e.g., acid rain), appears to present important research challenges. Trace element and trace organic releases in the off-gas also are potentially important. The understanding of transformation (e.g., photochemistry) and transport (e.g., complex terrain effects) of air pollutants is an important area requiring much more effort.

Water quality research presents a considerable challenge because of the proprietary nature of much of the industrial effort. Although much controversy surrounds the question of treatability, it seems safe to assert that the feasibility and economics of various water management systems pose a considerable challenge. Much remains to be done in understanding the problems associated with the codisposal of wastewaters and spent shale. Many of the problems involved with water availability are institutional rather than technical; however, the question of how much water is stored in the aquifers in the oil shale area poses a very interesting research issue.

Perhaps the solid waste problem presents the biggest challenge at this time, simply because we have not had a realistically sized pile to investigate. Because these piles will be as large as or larger than any spoil piles presently in existence, the potential problems could be large. Considerable research has been performed on the chemical and physical characteristics of spent shale, but we do not have the ability yet to integrate this research to give an overall picture. Of particular concern is the extrapolation in time. When it is laid down, the spent shale will be out of equilibrium with its environment. There will be strong forces acting to bring about equilibrium. The nature and strength of these forces are not well understood, nor are the relaxation times known. It is conceivable that significant phenomena could occur which are completely unexpected based on the research over short terms or on small piles.[133,134]

Much health-related research has been directed toward carcinogens in oil shale materials, but recent evidence indicates that the most important human health effect may be the nonneoplastic respiratory illnesses of pneumoconiosis, bronchitis, and chronic airway obstruction. The causes of these diseases in workers exposed to dust are not well understood. Skin painting studies and other data indicate that shale oil is somewhat more carcinogenic than most crude petroleums, but much less potent than many coal-derived liquids. Mining clearly presents the greatest safety hazard. Of particular concern is the poorly understood hazard to MIS miners working in the vicinity of a burning retort.

There are many gaps in our understanding of the ecological impacts of oil shale development, and data exist for reclamation. While it is possible to revegetate some spent shales, many researchers believe that a soil or subsoil cover is required. The ultimate result of revegetation efforts is not understood, but short-term success has been demonstrated.

Uptake of significant quantities of boron and molybdenum has been observed in some plants in the revegetation plots. The high boron levels could affect the viability of the reclamation effort, while the molybdenum levels are high enough to be toxic to livestock if these plants represent a large part of the diet. Because of high indigenous molybdenum concentrations in plants in some areas coupled with high molybdenum concentrations in leachates from spent shale, molybdenum toxicity could be a significant, long-term problem for cattle and sheep. The molybdenum in the leachate may also cause plants outside the region to reach toxic levels if this leachate reaches irrigation waters. The impacts on terrestrial plants and wildlife are not well understood, and additional research is needed. Although acute effects on aquatic organisms from accidental releases of wastewaters and oils can be expected, the result of chronic releases of leachates into streams is not understood.

Many of the questions posed here and elsewhere will not be answered for decades. We are entering a crucial period for oil shale research. With the first commercial-scale retort soon to be in operation and others likely to follow in the latter half of this decade, the opportunity for significant research will be unprecedented. The ability to obtain the important answers will depend on a number of factors, not the least of which is the degree to which the industry cooperates with the researchers in academe and the national laboratories in allowing access to sites and samples. The encouragement of this cooperation is perhaps the best justification for government support of these projects.

## ACKNOWLEDGMENT

This work has been supported in part by contracts DE-AC02-79EV10298 and DE-AC02-81EV10706 from the U.S. Department of Energy.

## REFERENCES

1. Cook, F.M. "The Scottish Oil Shale Industry," in *Oil Shale: The Environmental Challenges,* K.K. Petersen, Ed. (Golden: Colorado School of Mines Press, 1981), pp. 1–17.
2. Duncan, D.C., and V.E. Swanson. "Organic-rich Shale of the United States and World Land Areas," U.S. Geological Survey Circular 523 (U.S. Geological Survey, 1965).
3. Baughman, G.L. *Synthetic Fuels Data Handbook,* 2nd ed. (Denver: Cameron Engineers, Inc., 1978).
4. Smith, J.W. "Geochemistry of Oil-Shale Genesis in the Piceance Creek Basin, Colorado," in *Energy Resources of the Piceance Creek Basin, Colorado,* D.K. Murray, Ed. (Denver: Rocky Mountain Association of Geologists, 1974), p. 73.
5. Prien, C.H. "Current Oil Shale Technology: A Summary," in *Energy Resources of the Piceance Creek Basin, Colorado,* D.K. Murray, Ed. (Denver: Rocky Mountain Association of Geologists, 1974), pp. 141–150.
6. "An Assessment of Oil Shale Technologies" (Washington, DC: Office of Technology Assessment, U.S. Congress, 1980).
7. Smith, J.W., W.A. Robb, and N.B. Young. "High Temperature Reactions of Oil Shale Minerals and their Benefit to Oil Shale Processing in Place," in *Eleventh Oil Shale Symposium Proceedings,* J.H. Gary, Ed. (Golden: Colorado School of Mines Press, 1979), pp. 100–112.
8. "Safety Issues Related to Synthetic Fuels Facilities" (Washington, DC: National Academy Press, 1982).
9. Thoem, T., E. Bates, C. Dral, E. Harris, and F. Princiotta. "Status of EPA Regulatory and Research Activities Affecting Oil Shale Development," in *Thirteenth Oil Shale Symposium Proceedings,* J.H. Gary, Ed. (Golden: Colorado School of Mines Press, 1980), pp. 288–299.
10. Stanfield, K.E., I.C. Frost, W.S. McAuley, and H.N. Smith. "Properties of Colorado Oil Shale," U.S.B.M. Report Inv. 4825 (Washington, DC: U.S. Bureau of Mines, 1951).
11. Smith, J.W., N.B. Young, and D.L. Lawler. "Direct Determination of Sulfur Forms in Green River Oil Shale," *Anal. Chem.* 36:618–622 (1964).
12. Young, N.B., and J.W. Smith. "Dawsonite and Nahcolite Analyses of Green

River Formation Oil-Shale Section, Piceance Creek Basin, Colorado," U.S.B.M. Report Inv. 7445 (Washington, DC: U.S. Bureau of Mines, 1970).

13. Burnham, A.K., N.K. Bey, and G.J. Koskinas. "Hydrogen Sulfide Evolution from Colorado Oil Shale," UCRL-84066 R.1. (Livermore, CA: Lawrence Livermore National Laboratory, 1980).

14. Burnham, A.K., and R.W. Taylor. "Occurrence and Reactions of Oil Shale Sulfur," in *Fifteenth Oil Shale Symposium Proceedings,* J.H. Gary, Ed. (Golden: Colorado School of Mines Press, 1982).

15. Fruchter, J.S., C.L. Wilkerson, D.S. Sklarew, and K.B. Olsen. "Potential Air Emissions from Oil Shale Retorting," in *Oil Shale: The Environmental Challenges III,* K.K. Petersen, Ed. (Golden: Colorado School of Mines Press, 1983).

16. Bates, E.R., and T.L. Thoem, Eds. "Environmental Perspective on the Emerging Oil Shale Industry," EPA-600/2-80-205a (Cincinnati: U.S. Environmental Protection Agency, 1980).

17. Burnham, A.K. "Effect of Steam on $H_2$, $CO_2$, $H_2S$ and COS Concentrations in Combustion-Retort Off-gas," UCID-19093 (Livermore, CA: Lawrence Livermore National Laboratory, 1981).

18. Fruchter, J.S., C.L. Wilkerson, J.C. Evans, and R.W. Sanders. "Elemental Partitioning in an Aboveground Oil Shale Retort Pilot Plant," *Environ. Sci. Tech.* 14:1374–1381 (1980).

19. Fox, P.F. "The Partitioning of Major, Minor, and Trace Elements During Simulated In-Situ Oil Shale Retorting," LBL-9062 (Berkeley, CA: Lawrence Berkeley Laboratory, 1980).

20. Wildeman, T.R., and R.R. Meglen. "The Analysis of Oil-Shale Materials from Element Balance Studies," *Adv. Chem. Ser.: Analytical Chemistry of Oil Shale and Tar Sands,* 170:195–212 (1978).

21. Ondov, J.M., M.L. Stuart, J.S. Johnson, and R.W. Wikkerink. "Report on Preliminary Results of Aerosol Measurements at the Rio Blanco Oil Shale Retort, Burn #1"; UCID-19306 (Livermore, CA: Lawrence Livermore National Laboratory, 1981).

22. Natusch, D.F.S. "Formation and Transformation of Organic Species Emitted from Oil Shale Conversion." Colorado State University Report (Fort Collins: 1981).

23. Gratt, L.B., W.R. Chappell, B.W. Perry, W.M. Marine, D.A. Savitz, and J.L. Feerer. "Health and Environmental Effects Document for Oil Shale - 1982," (San Diego: IWG Corp., 1982).

24. Lave, L.B., and E.P. Seskin. *Air Pollution and Human Health* (Baltimore: Johns Hopkins Press, 1977).

25. Dickerson, M. "Ideas for Implementing Air Quality Studies in the Western Rocky Mountain Region," in *Oil Shale: The Environmental Challenges II,* K.K. Petersen, Ed. (Golden: Colorado School of Mines Press, 1982), pp. 110–121.

26. Whiteman, C.D. "Temperature Inversion Buildup in Valleys of the Rocky Mountains," in *Proceedings of the Second Conference on Mountain Meteorology* (Beacon Hill, MA: American Meteorological Society, 1982).

27. Laulainer, N.S., C.D. Whiteman, W.E. Davis, and J.M. Thorp. "Mixing Layer Growth and Background Air Quality Measurements Over the Colo-

rado Oil Shale Area," in *Proceedings of the Second Conference on Mountain Meteorology* (Beacon Hill, MA: American Meteorological Society, 1982).

28. Sehmel, G.A. "A Dual-Tracer Experiment to Investigate Pollutant Transport, Dispersion, and Particle Dry Deposition at the Rio Blanco Oil Shale Site in Colorado," in *Proceedings of the Second Conference on Mountain Meteorology* (Beacon Hill, MA: American Meteorological Society, 1982).

29. Klusman, R.W., and C.P. Matoske. "Adsorption of Mercury by Soils From Oil Shale Development Areas in the Piceance Creek Basin of Northwestern Colorado," in *Oil Shale Environmental Research and Coordination, Progress Report 1979–1982*, DOE-10298-3, W.R. Chappell, Ed. (Denver: Center for Environmental Sciences, University of Colorado, 1982).

30. McDonald, J.W. "The Availability of Water for Oil Shale and Coal Gasification Development in the Upper Colorado River Basin" (Washington, DC: U.S. Water Resources Council, 1980).

31. Hicks, R.E., and R.F. Probstein. "Water Management: Use and Reuse and the Potential for Environmental Release," in *Oil Shale: The Environmental Challenges III,* K.K. Petersen, Ed. (Golden: Colorado School of Mines Press, 1983).

32. Fox, J.P., and T.E. Phillips. "Wastewater Treatment in the Oil Shale Industry," in *Oil Shale: The Environmental Challenges,* K.K. Petersen, Ed. (Golden: Colorado School of Mines Press, 1981), pp. 253–293.

33. Mercer, B.W., W. Wakamiya, N.E. Bell, and C.J. English. "Treatment of Retort Water for Co-Disposal with Spent Shale," in *Oil Shale: The Environmental Challenges II,* K.K. Petersen, Ed. (Golden: Colorado School of Mines Press, 1982), pp. 46–72.

34. Sievers, R.E., J.S. Stanley, M.K. Conditt, S.B. Hawthorne, M.A. Caolo, and R.M. Barkley. "Characterization and Treatment of Organic Compounds in Wastewater from Oil Shale Processing," in *Oil Shale Environmental Research and Coordination, Progress Report 1979–1982*, DOE-10298-3, W.R. Chappell, Ed. (Denver: Center for Environmental Sciences, University of Colorado, 1982).

35. Fruchter, J.S., and C.L. Wilkerson. "Characterization of Oil Shale Retort Effluents," in *Oil Shale: The Environmental Challenges,* K.K. Petersen, Ed. (Golden: Colorado School of Mines Press, 1981), pp. 31–63.

36. Fruchter, J.S. "Source Characterization Studies at the Paraho Semiworks Oil Shale Retort," PNL-2945 (Richland, WA: Battelle Pacific Northwest Laboratory, 1979).

37. Wezner, M.A., S. Singhawangcha, R.M. Barkley, and R.E. Sievers. "Selective Electron-Capture Sensitization of Water, Phenols, Amines and Aromatic and Heterocyclic Compounds," *J. Chrom.* 239:145–157 (1982).

38. Hicks, R.E., and R.F. Probstein, "Unplanned Release of Process Wastewaters at Commercial Oil Shale Plants" (Cambridge, MA: Water Purification Associates, 1982).

39. Raphaelian, L.A., and W. Harrison. "Organic Constituents in Process Water from the In-Situ Retorting of Oil from Oil-Shale Kerogen," ANL/PAG-5 (Argonne, IL: Argonne National Laboratory, 1981).

40. Fish, R.H. "Speciation of Trace Organic Ligands and Inorganic and Organometallic Compounds in Oil Shale Process Wastewaters," in *Thirteenth Oil*

*Shale Symposium Proceedings,* J.H. Gary, Ed. (Golden: Colorado School of Mines Press, 1980), pp. 385–390.

41. Haas, F.C. "Analysis of TOSCO II Oil Shale Retort Water," in *Analysis of Waters Associated with Alternative Fuel Production,* L.P. Jackson and V.C.C. Wright, Eds. (Philadelphia: American Society for Testing and Materials, 1981).

42. Riley, R.G., T.R. Garland, K. Shiosaki, D.C. Mann, and R.E. Wildung. "Alkylpyridines in Surface Waters, Groundwaters, and Subsoils of a Drainage Located Adjacent to an Oil Shale Facility," *Environ. Sci. and Tech.* 15:697–700 (1981).

43. Hicks, R.E., R.F. Probstein, I. Wei, D.S. Farrier, J. Lotwala, and T.E. Phillips. "Wastewater Treatment and Management at Oil Shale Plants," in *Thirteenth Oil Shale Symposium Proceedings,* J.H. Gary, Ed. (Golden: Colorado School of Mines Press, 1980), pp. 321–334.

44. Fox, J.P., D.E. Jackson, and R.H. Sakaji. "Wastewater Treatment and Management at Oil Shale Plants," in *Thirteenth Oil Shale Symposium Proceedings,* J.H. Gary, Ed. (Golden: Colorado School of Mines Press, 1980), pp. 311–320.

45. Amy, G.L. "Contamination of Groundwater by Organic Pollutants Leached from In Situ Spent Shale," Ph.D. Thesis, University of California, Berkeley (1978).

46. Fox, J.P. "Water Quality Effects of Leachates from an In Situ Oil Shale Industry," LBL-8997 (Berkeley, CA: Lawrence Berkeley Laboratory, 1979).

47. Fox, J.P., P. Persoff, P. Wagner, and E.J. Peterson. "Retort Abandonment—Issues and Research Needs," in *Oil Shale: The Environmental Challenges,* K.K. Petersen, Ed. (Golden: Colorado School of Mines Press, 1981), pp. 133–168.

48. McWhorter, D.B. "Reconnaissance Study of Leachate from Raw Mined Oil Shale-Laboratory Columns," EPA 60017-80-181 (Cincinnati: U.S. Environmental Protection Agency, 1980).

49. McWhorter, D.B. "Laboratory Leaching of Bi-Modal Porous Media" in *Fourteenth Annual Oil Shale Proceedings,* J.H. Gary, Ed. (Golden: Colorado School of Mines Press, 1981), pp. 376–387.

50. Parker, H.W., R.M. Bethea, N. Güven, M.N. Gazdar, and J.K. Owusu. "Simulated Groundwater Leaching of In Situ Retorted or Burned Oil Shale," *Am. Chem. Soc. Div. Fuel Chem. Preprints* 21(6):66 (1976).

51. Parker, H.W., R.M. Bethea, N. Güven, M.N. Gazdar, and J.C. Watts. "Interactions Between Groundwater and *In Situ* Retorted Oil Shale," *Proceedings of Second Pacific Chemical Engineering Congress 2,* p. 450 (1977).

52. Peterson, E.J., A. Henicksman, and P. Wagner. "Investigations of Occidental Oil Shale, Inc., Retort 3E Spent Shales," LA-8792-MS (Los Alamos, NM: Los Alamos National Laboratory, 1981).

53. Runnells, D.D., M. Glaze, O. Saether, and K. Stollenwerk. "Release Transport and Fate of Some Potential Pollutants in Waters Associated with Oil Shale," in *Trace Elements in Oil Shale: Progress Report 1976–79,* COO-4017-3, W.R. Chappell, Ed. (Denver: Center for Environmental Sciences, University of Colorado, 1979), pp. 134–190.

54. Runnells, D.D., and E. Esmaili. "Inorganic Constituents in Oil Shale," in *Trace Elements in Oil Shale: Progress Report 1980–81,* DOE-10298-1, W.R.

Chappell, Ed. (Denver: Center for Environmental Sciences, University of Colorado, 1981), pp. 163–216.

55. Saether, O.M. "The Geochemistry of Fluorine in Green River Oil Shale and Oil Shale Leachates," Ph.D. Thesis, University of Colorado (1980).

56. Saether, O.M., D.D. Runnells, R.A. Ristinen, and W.R. Smythe. "Fluorine: Its Mineralogical Residence in the Oil Shale of the Mahogany Zone of the Green River Formation, Piceance Creek Basin, Colorado, U.S.A.," *Chem. Geol.* 31:169 (1981).

57. Stollenwerk, K.G. "Geochemistry of Leachate from Retorted and Unretorted Colorado Oil Shale," Ph.D. Thesis, University of Colorado, Boulder (1980).

58. Stollenwerk, K.G., and D.D. Runnells. "Composition of Leachates from Surface-Retorted and Unretorted Colorado Oil Shale," *Env. Sci. and Tech.* 15(11):1341 (1981).

59. Ward, J.D., and S.E. Reinecke. "Water Pollution Potential of Snowfall on Spent Oil Shale Residues," Grant 60111280-Progress Report (Laramie, WY: Laramie Energy Research Center, 1972).

60. Nelson, J. "Long Term Stability Aspects of Spent Oil Shale Waste Management," in *Oil Shale Environmental Research and Coordination: Progress Report 1979–1982*, DOE-10298-3, W.R. Chappell, Ed. (Denver: Center for Environmental Sciences, University of Colorado, 1982), Chap. IX.

61. Fox, P. "Leaching of Oil Shale Solid Wastes: A Critical Review" (Denver: Center for Environmental Sciences, University of Colorado, 1983).

62. Runnells, D.D., and E. Esmaili. "Interaction of Oil Shale-Related Leachates and Natural Geologic Materials," in *Oil Shale Environmental Research and Coordination: Progress Report 1979–1982*, DOE-10298-3, W.R. Chappell, Ed. (Denver: Center for Environmental Sciences, University of Colorado, 1982), Chap. X.

63. Runnells, D.D., and E. Esmaili. "The Interaction of Oil Shale-Related Leachates and Natural Geologic Materials," in *Oil Shale Environmental Research and Coordination: Progress Report 1981–1982*, DOE-10298-4, W.R. Chappell, Ed. (Denver: Center for Environmental Sciences, University of Colorado, 1982), Chap. X.

64. Jackson, L.P., R.E. Poulson, T.J. Spedding, T.E. Phillips, and H.B. Jensen, "The Codisposal of Retorted Shale and Process Waters: Effect on Shale Leachate Composition," *Col. Sch. Mines Q.* 70:105 (1975).

65. Fox, J.P. "Arsenic Species in Leachates from Oil Shale Materials," submitted for publication.

66. Brierley, C., and J. Brierley. "Effect of Microbial Oxidation of Thiosulfate on Water Quality in Oil Shale Processing Operations," in *Oil Shale Environmental Research and Coordination: Progress Report 1979–1982*, DOE-10298-3, W.R. Chappell, Ed. (Denver: Center for Environmental Sciences, University of Colorado, 1982), Chap. III.

67. Klein, D.A., R.A. Hassler, R.R. Meglen, and R. Sistko. "Environmental Effects on Microbial Mobilization of Arsenic from Retorted Oil Shale," in *Oil Shale Environmental Research and Coordination: Progress Report 1979–1982*, DOE-10298-3, W.R. Chappell, Ed. (Denver: Center for Environmental Sciences, University of Colorado, 1982), Chap. IV.

68. Wildung, R.E., and J.M. Zachara, "Effects of Oil Shale Solid Waste Disposal on Water Quality: Current Knowledge, Information Requirements, and Research Strategy," in *Oil Shale: The Environmental Challenges,* K.K. Petersen, Ed. (Golden: Colorado School of Mines Press, 1982), p. 158.

69. Carperter, A. "Characterization of carbonaceous spent shale and shale oil derived from the TOSCO II retort of Green River oil shale," Ph.D. Dissertation, University of Massachusetts, Boston (1980).

70. Park, W.C., A.E. Lindemanis, and G.A. Raab. "Mineral Changes During Oil Shale Retorting," *In Situ* 3:353 (1979).

71. Peterson, E.J., and P. Wagner. "Some Chemical and Mineralogical Considerations Important for Understanding Leachate Chemistry," in *Fifteenth Oil Shale Symposium Proceedings,* J.H. Gary, Ed. (Golden: Colorado School of Mines Press, 1982).

72. The Oil Shale Task Force. "Environmental Research on a Modified *In Situ* Oil Shale Process: A Progress Report from the Oil Shale Task Force," DOE/EV-0078, W.R. Chappell, Ed. (Washington, DC: U.S. Department of Energy, 1980).

73. Wildung, R.E., R. Bond, G. Gee, and J.D. Nelson. "Oil Shale Solid Waste Disposal: Estimation of Embankment Physical Stability and the Movement of Water and Solutes," in *Oil Shale: The Environmental Challenges III,* K.K. Petersen, Ed. (Golden: Colorado School of Mines Press, 1983).

74. Meglen, R.R., et al. "Analytical Laboratory," in *Oil Shale Environmental Research and Coordination: Progress Report 1979–1982,* DOE-10298-3, W.R. Chappell, Ed. (Denver: Center for Environmental Sciences, University of Colorado, 1982), Chap. VII.

75. Holland, L.M. "Health Effects of Oil Shale Development," in *Western Oil Shale Development: A Technology Assessment,* PNL-3830, Vol. 8 (Richland, WA: Pacific Northwest Laboratory, 1982).

76. Holland, L.M. "Health Effects of Oil Shale Development," in *Safety Issues Related to Synthetic Fuel Facilities,* Position Paper F (Washington, DC: National Academy of Sciences, 1982), pp. 126–157.

77. Wright, W.E., and W.N. Rom. "A Preliminary Report: Investigation for Shalosis Among Oil Shale Workers," in *Health Implications of New Energy Technologies,* W.N. Rom and V.E. Archer, Eds. (Ann Arbor, MI: Ann Arbor Science Publishers, Inc., 1980), pp. 481–489.

78. Akkerberg, I.I., Ed. *Industrial Hygiene and Occupational Pathology in the Estonian SSR, 10. Health and Safety in Oil Shale Extraction Processing.* NIH Library Translation NIH-80-467 (Washington, DC: National Institute of Health, 1980).

79. Bell, J. "Paraffin Epithelioma of the Scrotum," *Edinburgh Med. J.* 22:135 (1876).

80. Scott, A. "The Occupation Dermatoses of the Paraffin Workers of the Scottish Shale Oil Industry: With a Description of the System Adopted and the Results Obtained at the Periodic Examinations of These Workmen," *Eighth Scientific Report on the Investigations of the Imperial Cancer Research Fund* (London: Taylor and Francis, 1923).

81. Scott, A. "On the Occupation Cancer of the Paraffin and Oil Workers of the Scottish Shale Oil Industry," *Br. Med. J.* (1922).

82. Weaver, N.K., and R.L. Gibson. "The U.S. Oil Shale Industry, A Health Perspective," *Am. Ind. Hyg. Assoc. J.* 40:460–467 (1979).

83. Twort, C.C., and J.M. Twort. "The Relative Potency of Carcinogenic Tars and Oils," *J. Hyg.* 29:373–379 (1930).

84. Twort, C.C., and J.M. Twort. "The Carcinogenic Potency of Mineral Oils," *J. Hyg.* 30:204–226 (1931).

85. Berenblum, I., and R. Schoental. "Carcinogenic Constituents of Shale Oil," *Br. J. Exp. Pathol.* 24:232–238 (1943).

86. Berenblum, I., and R. Schoental. "The Difference in Carcinogenicity Between Shale Oil and Shale," *Br. J. Exp. Pathol.* 25:95–96 (1944).

87. Hyde, E. Lothian Regional Council, Personal Communication (1980).

88. Seaton, A., D. Lamb, W.R. Brown, G. Sclare, and W.G. Middleton. "Pneumoconiosis of Oil Shale Workers," *Thorax* 36:412–418 (1981).

89. Marine, W.M., R. Annis, and S.A. Sklaroff. "Mortality in the Shale Oil Area of Scotland: A Feasibility Study," Report No. TM/82/20, UDC 622.337: 312,2 (Edinburgh: Institute of Occupational Medicine, 1982).

90. Costello, J. "Morbidity and Mortality Study of Shale Oil Workers in the United States," *Environ. Health Perspect.* 30:205–208 (1979).

91. Costello, J. "NIOSH Studies of Oil Shale Workers," Presented at "Health Issues Related to Metal and Non-Metallic Mining," Fourth Annual RMCOEH Occupational and Environmental Health Conference, Park City, Utah, April 1982.

92. Rudnick, J., L.L. Garcia, G.L. Voelz, and H.F. Shulte. "Paraho Oil Shale Workers Occupational Health Study," Informal Report LA-8459-MS (Los Alamos, NM: Los Alamos Scientific Laboratory, 1980).

93. Eplet, J.L., B.R. Clark, C.H. Ho, M.R. Guerin, and T.K. Rao. "Short-term Bioassay of Complex Organic Mixtures: Part II, Mutagenicity Testing," in *Application of Short-Term Bioassay in the Fractionation and Analysis of Complex Environmental Mixtures,* EPA Publ. 600/9-78-027 (Washington, DC: U.S. Environmental Protection Agency, 1978), pp. 269–289.

94. Pelroy, R.A., and M.R. Peterson. "Mutagenicity of Shale Oil Components," in *Application of Short-Term Bioassay in the Fractionation and Analysis of Complex Environmental Mixtures,* EPA Publ. 600/9-78-027 (Washington, DC: U.S. Environmental Protection Agency, 1978), pp. 463–475.

95. Pelroy, R.A., and M.R. Peterson. "Use of Ames Test in Evaluation of Shale Oil Fractions," *Environ. Health Perspect.* 30:191–203 (1979).

96. Okinaka, R.T., and G.F. Strniste. "Exogenous Metabolic Activation of Shale Oils in Mammalian Cell Culture," in *The Los Alamos Integrated Oil Shale Health and Environmental Program Status Report,* LA-8665-SR (Los Alamos, NM: Los Alamos National Laboratory, 1981).

97. Timourian, H., A. Carrano, J. Carver, J.S. Felton, F.T. Hatch, D.S. Stuermer, and L.H. Thompson. "Comparative Mammalian Genetic Toxicology of Shale Oil Products Assayed *In Vitro* and *In Vivo,*" in Griest, W.H., M.R. Guerin, and D.L. Coffin, Eds., *Health Effects Investigation of Oil Shale Development* (Ann Arbor, MI: Ann Arbor Science Publishers, Inc., 1981), pp. 173–188.

98. Guerin, M.R. "Energy sources of polycyclic aromatic hydrocarbons," in Gelboin, H.V., and P.O.P. Tso, Eds., *Polycyclic Hydrocarbons and Cancer.* Vol. I (New York: Academic Press, 1978), pp. 3–42.

99. Schmidt-Collerus, J.J. "The Disposal and Environmental Effects of Carbonaceous Solid Wastes from Commercial Oil Shale Operations, First Annual Report to N.S.F.," NSF GI 3482XI (Denver: Denver Research Institute, 1974).

100. Guerin, M.R., C.H. Ho, T.K. Rao, B.R. Clark, and J.L. Epler. "Polycyclic aromatic primary amines as determinant chemical mutagens in petroleum substitutes," *Environ. Res.* 23:42–53 (1980).

101. Rao, T.K., J.L. Epler, M.R. Guerin, and B.R. Clark. "Short-term microbial testing of shale oil materials," in Griest, W.H., M.R. Guerin, and D.L. Coffin, Eds., *Health Effects Investigation of Oil Shale Development* (Ann Arbor, MI: Ann Arbor Science Publishers, Inc., 1981), pp. 161–172.

102. Holland, L.M., and J.S. Wilson. "Long-term Epidermal Carcinogenicity Studies of Shale Oil," in Holland, L.M., and C.G. Stafford, *The Los Alamos Integrated Oil Shale Health and Environmental Program Status Report,* LA-8665-SR (Los Alamos, NM: Los Alamos National Laboratory, 1981).

103. Coomes, R.M. "Carcinogenicity testing of oil shale materials," 12th Annual Oil Shale Symposium, Colorado School of Mines, Golden, 1979.

104. Lewis, S.C. "Carcinogenic bioassay of shale oil refinery and downstream products," in Griest, W.H., M.R. Guerin, and D.L. Coffin, Eds., *Health Effects Investigation of Oil Shale Development* (Ann Arbor, MI: Ann Arbor Science Publishers, Inc., 1981), pp. 123–128.

105. Coomes, R.M. "Health Effects of Oil Shale Processing," *Col. Sch. Mines Q.* 71:101 (1976).

106. Wilson, J.S., Y. Valdez, and L.M. Holland. "The effect of exposure conditions on dermotoxicity," in Holland, L.M., and C.G. Stafford, *The Los Alamos Integrated Oil Shale Health and Environmental Program Status Report,* LA-8665-SR (Los Alamos, NM: Los Alamos National Laboratory, 1981).

107. Holland, L.M., E.A. Vigil, M. Gonzales, D. Archuleta, and J.S. Wilson. "Inhalation and intratracheal exposures to oil shale dusts." in Holland, L.M., and C.G. Stafford, *The Los Alamos Integrated Oil Shale Health and Environmental Program Status Report.* LA-8665-SR (Los Alamos, NM: Los Alamos National Laboratory, 1981).

108. Holland, L.M., and J.O. Jackson. "The Relationship of Applied Industrial Hygiene Programs and Experimental Toxicology Studies," in *Oil Shale: The Environmental Challenges III,* K.K. Petersen, Ed. (Golden: Colorado School of Mines Press, 1983).

109. Nichols, J., and G.F. Strniste. "Ames/Salmonella Mutagen Assay of Oil Shale Process Water," in *The Los Alamos Integrated Oil Shale Health and Environmental Program Status Report,* LA-8665-SR (Los Alamos, NM: Los Alamos National Laboratory, 1981).

110. Brown, R., Ed. *Health and Environmental Effects of Oil Shale Technology,* DOE/HEW/EPA-02, MTR-79W00136 (McLean, VA: MITRE Corp., 1979), pp. 111–206.

111. Hakonson, T.E., and G.C. White. "Ecological Effects of Oil Shale Development - Problems, Perspectives and Approaches," in *Oil Shale: The Environmental Challenges,* K.K. Petersen, Ed. (Golden: Colorado School of Mines Press, 1981), pp. 105–132.

112. Redente, E.F., W.J. Ruzzo, C.W. Cook, and W.A. Berg. "Retorted Oil Shale Characteristics and Reclamation," in *Oil Shale: The Environmental*

*Challenges,* K.K. Petersen, Ed. (Golden: Colorado School of Mines Press, 1981), pp. 169–200.

113. Redente, E.F., and T.B. Doerr. "Revegetation Research on Retorted Oil Shale Materials," in *Oil Shale: The Environmental Challenges II,* K.K. Petersen, Ed. (Golden: Colorado School of Mines Press, 1982), pp. 215–244.

114. Gano, K.A., and J.B. States. "Habitat Requirements and Burrowing Depths of Rodents in Relation to Shallow Waste Burial Sites," PNL-4140 (Richland, WA: Pacific Northwest Laboratory, 1982).

115. Ward, G.M. "Molybdenosis and Hypocuprosis in Colorado," in *Transport and Biological Effects of Molybdenum in the Environment,* Progress Report to N.S.F. 1/1/74–1/1/75, W.R. Chappell, Ed. (Boulder: University of Colorado, 1975).

116. Ward, G.M., and J.G. Nagy. "Molybdenum and Copper in Colorado Forages, Molybdenum Toxicity in Deer, and Copper Supplementation in Cattle," in *Molybdenum in the Environment,* Vol. I, W.R. Chappell and K.K. Petersen, Eds. (New York: Marcel Dekker, Inc., 1976), pp. 104–105.

117. Kilkelly, M.K. "Levels of B, Mo, As, Se, and F in Plants from Spent Oil Shales," M.S. Thesis, Colorado State University, 1979.

118. McFadden, R.E. "Arsenic Solubility and Arsenic Uptake by Western Wheatgrass from Processed Shale," M.S. Thesis, Colorado State University, 1979.

119. Kilkelly, M.K., and W.L. Lindsay. "Selected Trace Elements in Plants Grown on Retorted Oil Shales," *J. Environ. Qual.* 11:422–427 (1982).

120. Klusman, R.W., and J.A. Rice. "Concentration of Chemical Elements in Plants Growing on Retorted Oil Shale," in *Oil Shale Environmental Research and Coordination, Progress Report 1979–1982,* DOE-10298-3, W.R. Chappell, Ed. (Denver: Center for Environmental Sciences, University of Colorado, 1982).

121. Chappell, W.R. "Transport and Biological Effects of Molybdenum in the Environment," in *Proceedings of the International Conference on Heavy Metals in the Aquatic Environment,* P.A. Krenkel, Ed. (New York: Pergamon Press, 1975), pp. 167–188.

122. Smith, P.J., and W.L. Lindsay. "Boron Toxicity in Range Plants Grown on Retorted Oil Shale," *J. Environ. Qual.* (to be published).

123. Klusman, R.W., J.A. Rice, and D.G. Brown. "Geochemical Baseline Studies in the Uinta Basin, Utah," in *Oil Shale Environmental Research and Coordination, Progress Report 1979–1982,* DOE-10298-3, W.R. Chappell, Ed. (Denver: Center for Environmental Sciences, University of Colorado, 1982).

124. Committee on Water Quality Criteria, *Water Quality Criteria 1972,* EPA-R3-73-003, R.C. Rooney, Ed. (Washington, DC: National Academy of Sciences, 1972), p. 344.

125. Vlek, P.L.G., and W.L. Lindsay. "Molybdenum Contamination in Colorado Pasture Soils," in *Molybdenum in the Environment, Vol. 2,* W.R. Chappell and K.K. Petersen, Eds. (New York: Marcel Dekker, Inc., 1977), pp. 619–650.

126. Thornton, I., G.F. Kershaw, and M.K. Davies. *J. Agric. Sci. Camb.* 78:151–163 (1972).

127. *Uinta Basin Synfuels Development,* Draft EIS (Salt Lake City: Bureau of Land Management, 1972), p. R-4-54.

128. "A Scientific and Policy Review of the Final Environmental Impact Statement

for the Prototype Oil Shale Leasing Programs of the Department of the Interior," K. Fletcher and M.F. Baldwin, Eds. (Institute of Ecology, 1973), p. 67.

129. Cope, O.B. *Colorado Wildlife Research Review 1977–1979,* DOW-R-R-77-79 (Denver: Colorado Division of Wildlife, 1980).

130. Hessel, D., and I. Levy, Eds. "An Investigation of Dewatering for the Modified In Situ Retorting Process, Piceance Creek Basin, Colorado," in *Western Oil Shale Development: A Technology Assessment,* PNL-3830-Vol. 5 (Richland, WA: Pacific Northwest Laboratory, 1982).

131. Farrier, D.S., J.E. Virgona, T.E. Phillips, and R.E. Poulson. "Environmental Research for In Situ Oil Shale Processing," in *Eleventh Oil Shale Symposium Proceedings,* J.H. Gary, Ed. (Golden: Colorado School of Mines Press, 1978), p. 95.

132. Bergman, H.L., and J.S. Meyer. "Aquatic Ecosystem Effects by Process Waters Produced by Synthetic Fuel Technologies, 1981 Annual Report to EPA" (Laramie: University of Wyoming, 1981).

133. Markos, G. "Geochemical Mobility and Transfer of Contaminants in Uranium Mill Tailings," in *Uranium Mill Tailings Management* (Fort Collins: Colorado State University, 1980), pp. 55–70.

134. Markos, G. "Contamination of Ground and Surface Waters by Uranium Mining and Milling," Bureau of Mines Final Report, Vol. II (Denver: Center for Environmental Sciences, University of Colorado at Denver, 1981).

## DISCUSSION

*J. Hinton, Texaco, Inc.:* You alluded to a health risk assessment of 27 deaths from oil shale. Would you explain further?

*W.R. Chappell:* These are premature deaths, using a sulfate surrogate model for the effects of air pollution. There is a study (Lave and Seskin) that was done on the effects of air pollution on health; basically, the study came up with a relationship that involves sulfates as a surrogate for all air pollution. The study found a correlation between sulfate levels and excess premature death, and this is what was used.

*J. Hinton:* Was this the worker community or general population?

*W.R. Chappell:* This is the general population. In order to get sulfates, among other things, you have to give the $SO_2$ time to change to sulfate. So it is going to be a far-field consideration.

*J. Hinton:* Were the data based on an analysis of what the maximum potentials were or on actual measurements such as in the workplace or in the community?

*W.R. Chappell:* These were actual measurements in the community compared with health records as part of a large epidemiological study. We did not do this study.

*C.W. Francis, Oak Ridge National Laboratory:* I am intrigued with those shale piles outside of Edinburgh. Were there any documented effects on the environment from the solid waste leachates from that area? Were leachates from those shales significantly different than, say, the shales from western Colorado, which are rather alkaline? Were they acid leachates or alkaline leachates?

*W.R. Chappell:* The answer to these questions is that we do not know. The first one is because nobody studied the area, and the last one because we do not have any work going on. We are trying to get our hands on material to do leaching studies.

*C.W. Francis:* Do they have any raw shale left?

*W.R. Chappell:* Believe it or not, it is very hard to find. They mined everything within reach, but they do have some in museums that we are able to obtain.

*C.W. Francis:* Those piles are rather close to Edinburgh, if I remember.

*W.R. Chappell:* Yes, in fact you can see one from the Edinburgh airport. They took a large, spent shale pile and used it to camouflage an area where they are storing the oil from the North Sea. With planting, it is a very attractive way of hiding the tanks. One pile was declared a national monument, but there is a limit as to how many you can do that with.

*J.M. Holland, Oak Ridge National Laboratory:* Did you make the statement that hydrotreatment did not reduce the skin tumorigenicity?

*W.R. Chappell:* No. I said that it does reduce it, but it does not necessarily eliminate it altogether.

*C.D. Scott, Oak Ridge National Laboratory:* A limited amount of work has been carried out on hydroretorting—a little bit with western shales, and there is some interest in it with eastern shales. Have you looked at this, and would you speculate on what this would do to sulfur emissions?

*W.R. Chappell:* We have not studied the hydroretorting process.

*K.N. Frye, U.S. Department of Energy:* Do you have access to the Union research plans, either to the state agencies or directly from the company?

*W.R. Chappell:* There is a certain amount of information that is available through DOE, but we do not have access to the detailed research plans.

# CHAPTER 4

## Summary of Health and Environmental Research: Solid Waste Management

### C.W. Francis

*Environmental Sciences Division*
*Oak Ridge National Laboratory*
*Oak Ridge, TN 37831*

### F.J. Wobber

*Office of Energy Research*
*Office of Health and Environmental*
*Research*
*Ecological Research Division*
*U.S. Department of Energy*
*Washington, DC 20545*

Research results pertaining to potential health and environmental consequences of solid wastes produced by operating commercial-sized coal conversion plants were reviewed and evaluated. Some of these wastes contain toxic metals as well as mutagenic and carcinogenic organic compounds. The major problem, however, is not the acute toxicity or carcinogenicity of the wastes, but rather the generation of solid waste leachates from the large volume of wastes, predominantly coal preparation wastes, gasifier ashes, and slags. The most troublesome wastes appear to be those containing reduced forms of sulfur. When disposed of in landfills, these wastes will, with age and oxidation of sulfur, generate acidic leachates. These leachates will likely contain concentrations of toxic contaminants such as copper, lead, cadmium, and nickel that will overtax natural attenuation or dispersal mechanisms, resulting in their harmful accumulation in surface and groundwater as well as in other sensitive areas of the environment. Some of the organic wastes, such as electrostatic precipitator tars and oily sludges from wastewater treatment, are potential health hazards relative to their exposure at the coal conversion facility and to their handling en route to disposal sites.

Further health and environmental research is needed to identify the risks associated with exposure to the work force as well as exposure to the general population because of landfill disposal practices. Health research should concentrate on investigating the effects of inhalation, contact with skin, and ingestion of wastes. Environmental research should address questions regarding long-term disposal. The major research goal should be the prediction of solid waste leachate movement in subsurface environments.

## INTRODUCTION

This chapter summarizes the progress of health and environmental research relevant to solid wastes from coal conversion processes. The objective is to present selected data sets from which the potential health and environmental implications associated with solid wastes from commercialization of a coal synfuels technology can be evaluated. The principal document from which data sets and evaluations are derived, "Status of Health and Environmental Research Relative to Solid Wastes from Coal Conversion,"[1] was prepared by staff members of Battelle Pacific Northwest Laboratory, Los Alamos National Laboratory, Lovelace Inhalation Toxicology Research Institute, and Oak Ridge National Laboratory (ORNL). Recommendations are included for future research needs so that long-term environmental effects from the disposal of coal conversion solid wastes can be elucidated.

## SOLID WASTE MANAGEMENT

Several alternatives are available in the management of solid wastes from coal conversion technologies: (1) reuse/resource recovery, (2) treatment followed by disposal, or (3) direct disposal. In reuse/resource recovery operations, the waste is used in a manufacturing process or construction application. Reuse/resource recovery is generally considered the most environmentally acceptable management alternative, but markets are often limited and economic viability is heavily influenced by distance to the market. Treatment of wastes by fixation and encapsulation (to add stability) or incineration (to reduce volume and toxicity) tends to be applicable only to small waste streams or is energy-intensive. The prevailing management scenario is terrestrial disposal in on-site landfills or return of the wastes "back-to-pit" where mining and conversion operations are nearby.

### Volume and Type of Waste

Coal conversion processes generate several types of solid waste streams. The major process waste stream is gasifier ash or slag. Liquefaction processes generally produce a char-like material (called vacuum bottoms or mineral ash residuals, depending on the process) rather than an ash/slag when the liquid product is separated. This material, usually containing more than 30% carbon, is gasified for production of either hydrogen or a fuel gas for in-plant generation; thus, the char-like material in liquefaction is not considered a solid waste. A major source of waste, though not directly related to the coal conversion process, is from coal preparation. Other wastes include raw water and wastewater treatment sludges, spent catalysts, adsorbents, and by-product sulfur from acid-gas cleanup, as well as fly ash, bottom ash, and flue gas desulfurization sludges from direct combustion of coal or char for on-site power and steam generation. The amounts and physicochemical characteristics of these wastes vary with the process used and with the characteristics of the feed coal. A commercial-scale liquefaction or gasification plant ($7.9 \times 10^6$ L/d or $7 \times 10^6$ m³/d, respectively) will require approximately 30,000 Mgd coal and will generate the estimated quantities of waste shown in Table I.[2]

## PHYSICAL AND CHEMICAL CHARACTERISTICS OF THE WASTES

A cursory description of the wastes will familiarize the reader with the fundamental processes in which the wastes are generated, as well as with the general form and composition of the wastes. For more detailed descriptions, other references are suggested in Table II.[3-29]

**Table I.**   Estimated Quantities of Solid Waste Produced by Commercial-size Coal Conversion Facilities[a]

| Waste Source | Quantity[b] (Mg/d) |
|---|---|
| Coal preparation | 6900 |
| Raw water sludges | 39 |
| Gasifier ash/slags | 4000 |
| Fly and bottom ash | 330 |
| Elemental sulfur | 540 |
| Spent catalysts | 10 |
| Flue gas-desulfurization sludge | 500 |
| Process wastewater treatment sludge | 710 |
| Total | 13,029 |

[a]Adapted from Tables 3–7 and 3–8 in Reference 2, this chapter. Commercial-scale liquefaction or gasification plant (capacity of $7.9 \times 10^6$ L/d or $7 \times 10^6$ m³/d) consuming approximately 30,000 Mg/d (30,000 metric tons) of coal.

[b]Moisture content is not the same for all wastes.

**Table II.** Selected Literature Pertaining to Physiochemical Characterization of Coal Conversion Wastes[a]

| Wastes | Physical Properties[a] | Elemental Composition[a] | Leaching Character[a] |
|---|---|---|---|
| Gasifier ash/slag | 3 | 3 | 5 |
| | 8 | 4 | 9 |
| | 9 | 6 | 10 |
| | 10 | 7 | 11 |
| | 11 | 8 | 12 |
| | 12 | 9 | 13 |
| | 13 | 10 | 14 |
| | 14 | 11 | 16 |
| | 15 | 12 | 17 |
| | 16 | 13 | 18 |
| | 17 | 14 | |
| | 18 | 15 | |
| | | 16 | |
| | | 17 | |
| | | 18 | |
| Liquefaction mineral residue | 17 | 17 | 17 |
| | | 19 | 20 |
| | | 21 | |
| | | 22 | |
| | | 23 | |
| | | 24 | |
| Gasification char | 17 | 10 | 10 |
| | 25 | 17 | 17 |
| | | 25 | 25 |
| Wastewater treatment sludge | | 21 | 20 |
| | | 22 | 21 |
| | | 26 | 22 |
| | | 28 | 26 |
| | | | 27 |
| | | | 28 |
| Elemental sulfur | | 10 | 10 |
| | | 21 | |
| | | 22 | |
| | | 29 | |

[a]Numbers refer to references in this chapter.

## Gasification Ash and Slag

The difference in terminology between ash and slag is a matter of temperature in the gasifier. When the temperature in the gasifier is sufficient to fuse the mineral matter of the feed coal, the term slag applies; when the fusion temperature is not exceeded, the term ash applies.

Slag is usually produced by entrained-bed-type gasifiers, whereas fluidized- and fixed-bed gasifiers usually produce ash. The important point is that none of the gasifiers generate ashes or slags that resemble combustion fly ash. Gasifier ash/slag is larger in particle size and is generally more acidic in reactivity than combustion fly ash.[9-11] Gasifier ash/slag, however, does have many properties similar to those of combustion bottom ash/slag.[10]

### Liquefaction Mineral Residual

The solidified material resulting from the liquefaction process is not considered a waste. Most processes use this material (carbon content often in excess of 50%) as feedstock to gasifiers to make hydrogen gas or as fuel in auxiliary combustion facilities. In special cases there might be sufficient accumulation of this material for it to be considered a waste: (1) at liquefaction pilot plants that do not have a gasifier, and (2) at a commercial plant as a result of a breakdown of the gasifier. The reducing conditions of the liquefaction process enhance conversion of pyrite in feed coals to pyrrhotite and troilite sulfur forms.

### Gasification Char

The raw product gas stream of many gasification processes contains devolatilized coal (char) separated by using particulate control equipment similar to that used for fly-ash control in conventional coal power plants. Because of the high carbon content of this material (20 to 60%), it is recycled to the combustion zone of the gasifier or used as feedstock in conventional boilers. Because gasification char is often enriched in volatile elements (arsenic, selenium, and mercury), disposal of the material in landfills may produce leachates containing toxic levels of these elements.

### Wastewater Treatment Sludges

The chemical or biological treatment of wastewater streams emanating from a coal conversion facility results in various types of sludges. The moisture content of these sludges varies, depending on the methodology used for concentrating the solid residual. They generally contain in excess of 50% moisture, making them difficult to manage. The few data available on the physicochemical composition or the leaching character of these sludges indicate the presence of mutagenic organic compounds and toxic inorganic constituents.[20,27]

### Elemental Sulfur

For most coal conversion processes, the removal of sulfur (as hydrogen sulfide) from the tail gas results in the production of elemental sulfur. This technology is currently being used in the petroleum and petrochemical industry. For this material and for the wastewater treatment sludges few data are available that define physicochemical or leaching characteristics. The major problem is that the process design and implementation of recovery of sulfur from the tail-gas streams have not taken place except at a few pilot gasification plants;[10,22] thus, there is a limited supply of the material for analysis.

Most designs for elemental sulfur removal show a sulfur purification step. However, information on samples collected to date indicates the presence of considerable carbon as an impurity[10,22] as well as residual Streford chemicals (sodium, vanadium) and major coal-ash elements. Theoretical studies indicate that sulfur recovery processes will likely concentrate semivolatile toxic elements such as As, B, Pb, Se, and Hg.[29] Leaching studies[10] revealed that the leachate from the elemental sulfur sludge recovered at a pilot coal-gasification unit contained several metals in quantities that exceeded the primary and secondary drinking water standards. For instance, mercury was found at concentrations 20 times its allowable drinking water concentration. When stored, the sludge leachate became more acidic, indicating apparent oxidation of the sulfur. The long-term effects of landfilling this material may be the subsequent release of sulfuric acid and acid-soluble toxic metals such as As, Cd, Pb, Zn, Ni, and Hg.

### Miscellaneous Residues

Coal conversion facilities will also generate miscellaneous small-volume residues such as spent catalysts, wastewater treatment resins, various bed sorbents, still bottoms, and various oily sludges. Many of these residues will contain highly toxic constituents. Some may be regenerated or recycled for their valuable materials; thus, they may not leave the coal conversion facility as a waste. As for wastewater sludges and elemental sulfur, little information is available describing the physicochemical composition of these residues.

### Comparison of Coal Combustion and Coal Conversion Wastes

Considerable information is available on the physicochemical and leaching characteristics of coal combustion wastes (i.e., mine spoils, cleaning wastes, fly ash, bottom ash, scrubber sludge, and other residues resulting from the various environmental control processes). Each waste is a product of the starting materials and the process conditions to which these materials were subjected. Fly ashes vary in composition because of feed coal composition, boiler design and operation, and type of particulate control system used for collection. Wastes from coal conversion processes also depend on the character of the feed material and process.

Data have been published[10,30,31] to indicate that slag from high-temperature gasifiers contains fewer leachable toxic metals than fly ash from direct combustion of coal. Solid waste leachates from fly ash are characteristically neutral to alkaline in pH, whereas leachates from some of the gasifier ash/slags are acidic,[10,11,18] particularly if they result from the use of high-sulfur coals. Leachate from gasifier ash and slags usually resembles bottom ash leachate from direct combustion more closely than it does fly ash leachate. The difference in temperature, pressure, and oxidative conditions between coal combustion and coal conversion, even using the same feed coal, will result in noted differences in the wastes. If similarities and differences in chemical composition and leaching characteristics can be identified between coal conversion and coal combustion wastes, the long-term health and environmental effects resulting from the disposal of conversion wastes could be more easily evaluated, based on current information about coal combustion wastes.

## HEALTH AND ENVIRONMENTAL RESEARCH

Research evaluating the potential health and environmental consequences of solid waste management at future commercial coal conversion facilities has been limited. Health effects research has been confined to testing the toxicity of selected coal conversion wastes using mutagenic and carcinogenic biotesting protocols. Environmental research has concentrated on (1) evaluating the toxicity of solid waste leachates to various aquatic and terrestrial organisms, (2) defining the leaching character of the waste under disposal conditions, and (3) evaluating the general importance of various environmental transport routes to man of toxic constituents in the leachate.

Health research has addressed the potential of these wastes to induce cancer in workers at future coal conversion facilities. Tars formed during certain coal conversion processes have exhibited higher mutagenic activity than bottom ash and cyclone dust.[32] The end point of major interest is the potential for cancers in excess of those caused by background levels. Possible routes of exposure to maintenance workers include dermal contact, oral ingestion, and inhalation exposure to tar-containing dusts, to aerosolized tars released during fugitive emissions, and to vapors of organic compounds off-gassing from warm tar wastes.

Environmental research has centered on two goals: (1) a short-term goal addressing the regulatory status of the wastes under the Resource Conservation and Recovery Act (RCRA) of 1976, largely funded by the U.S.

Department of Energy/Fossil Energy (DOE/FE) through the Coal Gasification Demonstration Project to develop solid waste management plans regarding specific waste streams; and (2) the long-term fate and effects of solid wastes in the environment, funded principally by the U.S. Department of Energy/Office of Health and Environmental Research (DOE/OHER). The objectives of this research were to determine acute and chronic effects of solid wastes and their leachates on specific aquatic and terrestrial organisms and ecosystems, and to evaluate the effect of the disposal of wastes on the quality of surface and groundwaters.

### Toxicity of Solid Wastes

Testing the toxicity of a solid waste can be accomplished by either direct testing of the waste, or testing the aqueous extract of the waste. For example, as a first approximation to the waste's biohazard potential, short-term mutagenicity testing of the organic extract of the wastes was often conducted. Because water extractions of solid wastes do not have the ability to mobilize nonpolar organic compounds that characteristically produce mutagenic activity, health-related research was centered on characterizing the bioactivity of the constituents of the waste rather than that of the aqueous extracts. Direct testing of the waste using the various biotests to evaluate mutagenicity, carcinogenicity, and teratogenicity has stronger implications in the interpretations related to human health effects (e.g., worker exposure) than those related to environmental effects. The major difference is in exposure pathway. Environmental effects are those impacts on all organisms, including man, and often result because of exposure via subtle pathways. Health effects, however, tend to be pictured as a consequence of direct exposure. Environmental research has taken the approach of testing the toxicity of the waste's aqueous extracts using the Ames *Salmonella* mutagenicity test[33] as well as various aquatic toxicity and phytotoxicity testing protocols.

### Health Research

Short-term bioassays have been used as indicators of long-term effects such as carcinogenesis.[34] The important feature of these tests is that they are rapid and relatively inexpensive as compared with testing protocol for carcinogenesis. The short-term bioassays are based on testing damage to deoxyribonucleic acid (DNA). Specific cellular and bodily functions are controlled by the DNA code which is also passed on to the next generation through germ cells, thus having a dominant role in heredity. The reliability of these short-term bioassays to predict the incidence of carcinogenesis on existing and future generations is subject to debate, but there appears to be a general agreement that their use can serve as valuable prescreens for setting priorities for further testing. The most prevalent short-term bioassay used on solid wastes was the Ames *Salmonella* mutagenicity test.[33]

Samples of bottom ash, cyclone dust, and electrostatic precipitator (ESP) tar at two low-Btu pilot plant gasifiers [the Morgantown Energy Technology Center (METC) at Morgantown, West Virginia, and the University of Minnesota at Duluth (UMD)] revealed that the ESP tars were by far the most mutagenic of the wastes tested.[32] These tests were carried out on the organic extracts of the wastes. Neither the cyclone dust nor the bottom ash at the UMD gasifier displayed genotoxic activity using the Ames test. Bottom ash sampled at the METC gasifier was not found to be mutagenic with or without metabolic activation. However, the cyclone dust showed specific mutagenic activity upon metabolic activation. The activity of these extracts ranged from 0.8 to 5.7 revertants/μg of cyclone dust. This study and others[20,27] have indicated that selected solid wastes from coal conversion processes do possess mutagenic activity. Data to date indicate that the wastes containing organic compounds resulting from the sorption or precipitation of organic materials are those most likely to show mutagenic activity. For example, wastewater filter cake from the H-Coal direct liquefaction pilot plant[27] showed mutagenic activity in aqueous as well as in organic extracts, indicating the presence of water-soluble mutagenic organic compounds. Further evidence that organic-laden wastes may constitute a health hazard at coal conversion facilities is the observation by researchers at ORNL that a sample of ESP tar from the UMD gasifier was highly carcinogenic in mouse skin over a testing period of 32 weeks.[1] It must be kept in mind that some of these organic-laden materials, such as ESP tars, chars, and cyclone dusts collected in cleanup processes, may not be considered as wastes. For example, these materials may be incinerated or recycled at commercial-scale facilities. However, industrial workers will likely be exposed to fugitive emissions of similar character, and the risk associated with inhalation or contact with these materials during maintenance procedures should not be overlooked.

### Environmental Research

Environmental research pertaining to the toxicity testing of coal-conversion solid wastes has focused on determining the toxicity of the aqueous solid waste extracts rather than on the specific wastes. Three general testing schemes have been used: (1) short-term mutagenicity testing (Ames *Salmonella* test), (2) aquatic toxicity testing (zooplankton, *Daphnia magna,* and fathead minnows, *Pinephales promelas*), and (3) phytotoxicity testing using radish and sorghum seedlings. Because testing is conducted on the aqueous extracts of the waste, the extraction media (pH, ionic strength, and redox potential), procedure (batch or column), liquid-to-solid ratio, and time of extraction will have a profound influence on the chemical character of the extract, and thus on the toxicity. For most studies, the extractions have been RCRA extractions (acetic acid: pH 5, 24 h at a 16:1 liquid-to-solid ratio) or distilled water extractions (24 h at 20:1 liquid-to-solid ratio), although other conditions and procedures have been used.[17,27]

Results of the mutagenicity testing (Ames *Salmonella* test) indicated that only one waste tested positive on the aqueous extract (Table III).[1,27,35-37]

**Table III.**   Short-term Mutagenicity of Coal Conversion Solid Wastes

| | Ref. No. | Salmonella[a] | | Saccharomyces[a] | |
|---|---|---|---|---|---|
| | | Aqueous Extract | Organic Extract | Aqueous Extract | Organic Extract |
| Coal conversion wastes | | | | | |
| Gasifier ash No. 1 | 35 | — | — | — | — |
| Gasifier ash No. 2 | 35 | — | — | — | — |
| Gasifier ash No. 3 | 35 | — | — | — | — |
| UMD bottom ash | 1 | — | nd | — | nd |
| UMD cyclone ash | 1 | — | nd | — | nd |
| UMD tar | 1 | nd | + | nd | + |
| METC bottom ash | 32 | nd | — | nd | nd |
| METC cyclone ash | 32 | nd | + | nd | nd |
| METC tar | 33 | nd | + | nd | nd |
| H-Coal wastewater filter cake | 27 | + | + | nd | nd |
| Direct coal combustion wastes | | | | | |
| Fly ash No. 1 | 35 | — | — | — | — |
| Fly ash No. 2 | 35 | — | — | — | — |
| Fly ash No. 3 | 36 | nd | + | nd | nd |
| Fly ash No. 4 | 37 | nd | + | nd | nd |
| Fly ash No. 5 | 1 | nd | + | nd | nd |
| Bottom ash No. 1 | 35 | — | — | — | — |
| Scrubber sludge No. 1 | 35 | — | — | — | — |
| Treated scrubber sludge No. 1 | 35 | — | — | — | — |
| Other energy-related wastes | | | | | |
| FBC residue | 35 | — | T | — | — |
| Raw oil shale | 35 | — | — | — | — |
| Spent oil shale | 35 | — | — | — | — |

[a]+ = mutagenic; — = nonmutagenic; T = toxic; nd = determined.

This waste, a filter cake from the H-Coal wastewater treatment plant, showed positive toxic and mutagenic responses when several aqueous extractions as well as an organic extraction scheme were used.[27] The major waste stream (gasifier ash) in coal conversion was not observed to be positive in the Ames test when aqueous extracts from any of the wastes were used. The lack of a positive test is due to two factors: (1) the organic content of gasifier ash and slags is generally low, and (2) the organic compounds that are present are nonpolar and difficult to extract by aqueous extractions. In fact, experiments[38] have indicated that these wastes would tend to be accumulators or sorbents for mutagenic organic compounds instead of sources. Thus, the major concern relative to mutagenicity of solid wastes from commercial coal conversion plants would not be the gasifier ash and slags, but rather the organic wastewater sludges and precipitator chars and dusts collected in the off-gas streams.

Considerable data are available that evaluate the toxicity of coal conversion solid waste extracts to aquatic organisms.[17,35,39–45] A comparison was made at ORNL[35,41–45] of the toxicity of gasifier ash from several different gasifiers, cyclone dust from the UMD gasifier, a gasifier tar, and H-Coal vacuum-still bottoms with extracts from industrial, municipal, and other fossil energy solid wastes (ash and flue-gas-desulfurization scrubber sludge from direct-fired coal plants and raw and retorted oil shale) using *Daphnia magna* and seedlings of radish and sorghum. Some toxicities were observed (Table IV), but they were substantially less than solid waste extracts from traditional municipal and industrial wastes. Millemann et al.[42] also compared laboratory-derived extracts using distilled water and well water with pH 5 acetic and sulfuric acid extracts. Acetic acid is used in the RCRA extraction procedure[46] and has been observed to interfere with chronic-toxicity tests using *D. magna* as well as with phytotoxicity tests.[35,41] In the latter study,[42] the effects of acetic acid (measured in terms of enhanced or reduced reproduction of *D. magna*) were not observed in the chronic-toxicity tests. However, the sulfuric acid extracts of the gasifier ash and sulfuric acid controls inhibited *D. magna* reproduction. Because no effects were observed with well water and distilled water controls, it was recommended that distilled water be used as an extracting medium, rather than the pH 5 acid extractions, if toxicity testing were to be implemented.

Similar responses were observed in the toxicity testing of coal conversion solid waste extractions using 1- to 6-d-old fathead minnow fry, *Pimiphales promelas*.[17] The major contributors to toxicity were pH and ionic strength of the solid waste extract. When the pH of the extracts was between 6.2 and 8.0, most wastes were not acutely toxic to the minnows. Acidic extracts neutralized with sodium hydroxide to nontoxic pH ranges (6.2 to 8.0) showed total mortality in all cases. The neutralized extracts had specific conductance values in excess of 7 dS/m, indicating that the toxicities were a result of ionic strength of the extract. It was impossible to determine specifically which chemical constituents were directly responsible for the

**Table IV.**    Summary of Acute Toxicities of Solid Waste Leachates to *Daphnia magna* and Radish and Sorghum Seedlings[a]

| Leachate | *Daphnia magna*[b] (%) | *Radish*[c] (%) | *Sorghum*[c] (%) |
|---|---|---|---|
| **Industrial** | | | |
| Dye waste | 0.0005 | 10 | 5 |
| Plater's waste | 0.005 | 2 | NSE[d] |
| Textile waste | 19.2 | 5 | 5 |
| Metal-processing waste | 28.0 | NSE | 4 |
| Soybean process cake | NSE | NSE | 75 |
| **Municipal** | | | |
| Municipal sewage sludge | 7.5 | NSE | NSE |
| **Coal-fired power plant** | | | |
| Power plant No. 1 fly ash | 90 | 30 | NSE |
| Power plant No. 1 bottom ash | 94 | NSE | 100 |
| Power plant No. 1 scrubber sludge | 85 | 10 | NSE |
| Power plant No. 1 treated scrubber sludge | 81.1 | NSE | 8 |
| Power plant No. 2 fly ash | 15.2 | NSE | NSE |
| Fluidized-bed residue | 12.6 | NSE | NSE |
| **Synthetic fuel** | | | |
| Coal gasification waste No. 1 | <50% mortality | NSE | NSE |
| Coal gasification waste No. 2 | 100 | NSE | NSE |
| Coal gasification waste No. 3 | 70 | 100 | 100 |
| Raw oil shale | 53.9 | NSE | 4 |
| Retorted oil shale | 70 | NSE | 1 |
| UMD bottom ash No. 1 | | | |
|   Distilled-water extract | NSE | 50 | NSE |
|   Acetic acid extract | 85 | 10 | 10 |
|   Sulfuric acid extract | <50% mortality | NSE | NSE |
| UMD bottom ash No. 2 | 82 | NSE | NSE |
| UMD bottom ash No. 3 | <50% mortality | NSE | NSE |
| UMD cyclone-separator char | NSE | NSE | NSE |
| Holston gasifier tar | 9 | Not done | Not done |
| H-Coal vacuum-still bottoms | NSE | NSE | NSE |
| SRC-II oil-contaminated soil | 17 | 1 | 100 |

[a]Adapted from Reference 41, this chapter.
[b]Estimated concentration of the leachate killing or immobilizing 50% of the *D. magna* test organisms in 48 h.
[c]Lowest concentration significantly reducing root growth of radish and sorghum plants after 48 and 72 h respectively. Test concentrations ranged between 0 and 100%.
[d]NSE = no significant effect.

observed toxicities. These and other data[35,41,42] indicate that if aquatic toxicity and phytotoxicity testing are to be used as an indicator of biotoxicity, distilled water should be used as an extracting medium. These testing procedures, when used in conjunction with other biotesting protocols for mutagenicity and cytotoxicity, make it possible to detect detrimental environmental effects of solid waste leachates that would not be detected using inorganic and organic analyses.

### Regulatory Classification under RCRA

Implementation of the regulations[47] under the RCRA has resulted in considerable concern as to the regulatory classification of coal-conversion solid wastes. Classification as a hazardous waste would add significantly to costs of disposal; thus, much of the initial research funded by DOE/FE was directed at assessing the RCRA classification[5,11,13,16,48] of the wastes. Criteria for identifying characteristics of hazardous waste include tests for ignitability, corrosiveness, reactivity, and extraction procedure (EP) toxicity.[47] Certain wastes, such as fly ash, bottom ash, slag, and flue gas emission-control waste from combustion of coal or other fossil fuels, were temporarily excluded as hazardous wastes; however, initial regulations[47] did not exclude solid wastes from emerging energy technologies such as coal conversion. Because of the failure to exclude these wastes in the regulations, considerable interest was focused on the classification of these wastes by the U.S. Environmental Protection Agency (EPA)-EP toxicity test. The data seemed especially important for inclusion in the environmental impact statements required for the DOE Coal Gasification Demonstration Projects.[49-51]

Data available from the EPA-EP toxicity test indicate that all coal-conversion wastes tested would be classified as nonhazardous wastes and thus would be permitted to be disposed of in "nonhazardous" landfills. Nonetheless, certain wastes, such as organic-laden wastewater sludges, various sulfur sludges, and miscellaneous small-volume residues (spent catalysts, still bottoms, etc.), may be listed as hazardous by EPA criteria for listing.[47] Testing of the major waste stream (ash and slags produced on gasification) has shown that concentration of the criteria elements (primary drinking water regulation elements) are factors of 20 to 1000 times below RCRA toxicity limits (Table V).

## FATE AND TRANSPORT OF
## SOLID WASTE LEACHATES

Land disposal of the large quantities of waste to be generated in a commercial coal synfuels industry may lead to contamination of groundwater

**Table V.** RCRA Toxicity Classification of Gasification Ash/Slags Using EPA-EP Toxicity Test Procedure (µg/L)[a]

| | C Ohio No. 9 | T Pittsburgh Seam | E Illinois No. 6 | G Kentucky No. 9 | H[b] Kentucky No. 9 | K Char Kentucky No. 9 | K Slag | I[c] Kentucky No. 9/14 | F Western Coal | RCRA Toxicity Limits[d] |
|---|---|---|---|---|---|---|---|---|---|---|
| As | 0.3 | 0.6 | <0.1 | <1 | <1 | 4 | 4 | 0.5 | 1.4 | 5,000 |
| Ba | <200 | 58 | 500 | 20 | 80 | 73 | 3.3 | <500 | 2000 | 100,000 |
| Cd | <0.1 | <0.1 | 1.0 | <1 | 28 | 45 | 0.1 | 3.4 | 0.47 | 1,000 |
| Cr | 1.6 | 1.4 | 0.4 | <5 | <5 | 8.5 | 0.5 | 0.1 | 0.8 | 5,000 |
| Pb | <0.3 | 0.5 | 0.3 | <10 | <10 | 78 | 1.1 | 1.6 | 2.2 | 5,000 |
| Hg | 0.6 | <0.1 | <0.1 | <1 | 1 | <0.1 | <0.1 | 0.2 | 0.01 | 200 |
| Se | <5 | <1 | 2 | <1 | <1 | <5 | <5 | <1 | 1.8 | 1,000 |
| Ag | <0.1 | <0.1 | <0.1 | <2 | <2 | <0.1 | <0.1 | 0.1 | <0.02 | 5,000 |

[a] Adapted from Reference 11, this chapter.
[b] Fine fraction.
[c] A composite of fine and coarse waste.
[d] RCRA limits for toxicity are 100 times the primary drinking water regulations.

and surface water. The solubilization and transport of inorganic and organic toxic constituents in the waste can potentially render waters unsuitable for drinking and possibly unfit for agricultural and industrial uses. Leachates from solid wastes strongly impact the pH and dissolved-salt content characteristics of groundwater and surface water, thus changing the population patterns of flora and fauna that depend on these waters for existence. The revegetation of disposal areas could result in the biological transport and possible accumulation of toxic constituents in natural and agricultural food chains, some of which lead directly to man. Research evaluating the long-term fate and transport of toxic constituents in coal-conversion solid wastes has been extremely limited compared with research conducted on characterization and short-term leaching. Two experiments are briefly described to illustrate the potential for transport of toxic materials from coal conversion wastes to groundwater and surface water and possible bioaccumulation in food chains.

## Impact on Water Quality

Large columns containing a gasifier ash and a disposal-site soil (sample taken from the B horizon of a Dormont silty clay loam containing 61, 30, and 9% silt, clay, and sand, respectively) were used to evaluate the long-term leaching characteristics of the ash and the attenuating effect of soil on transport of toxic trace metals in the leachate.[52] Fifty kilograms of waste was layered between the disposal site soil (20 kg of soil on top of the waste and 50 kg below the waste, Figure 1) in a plastic drum (56-cm diam). This was replicated twice (columns 3 and 4, Figure 1). Two other treatments were included: a control (column 1, Figure 1, containing only soil), and a treatment to measure the leachate characteristics of the waste (column 2, Figure 1, containing 20 kg of soil over 50 kg of waste). Distilled water was continuously pumped to the columns at a rate slightly less than 1 L/d (equivalent to 135-cm rainfall/year) for 37 weeks. The falling head hydraulic conductivity of the silty clay loam soil was $8.6 \times 10^{-5}$ cm/s, slightly higher than the rate at which distilled water was pumped to the column ($4.3 \times 10^{-6}$ cm/s). Thus, the experiment simulated unsaturated flow.

Leachate collections over the first 12 weeks revealed that the gasifier ash strongly changed the water quality characteristics of the leachates (i.e., lowered the pH and increased the sulfate concentrations). Analyses of the leachate from the columns containing the waste also showed concentrations of sulfate, cadmium, nickel, and boron in excess of drinking water and irrigation criteria in both the waste and the soil leachates (Figure 2). The high concentrations of cadmium and nickel in the leachates were unexpected and revealed that the soil was relatively ineffective in attenuating the hydrologic transport of these toxic metals. Laboratory sorption studies of cadmium and nickel on this soil had indicated that the soil was an effective

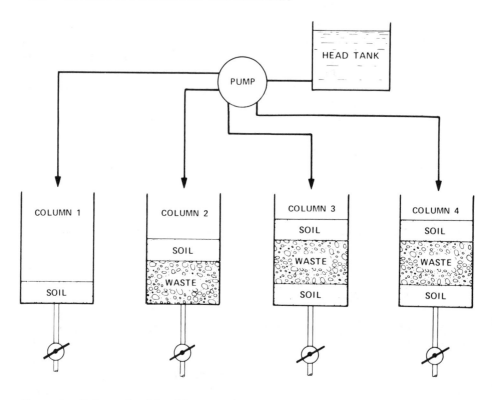

**Figure 1.** Schematic of leaching experiment.

sorbent for these metals. For example, distribution coefficients ($K^d$'s) of 940 and 470 mL/g, respectively, for cadmium and nickel were measured in 5:1 water:soil suspensions. In 0.01 $M$ calcium nitrate:soil suspensions (5:1), the $K_d$ values were 16 and 10 mL/g. These values are appreciably larger than the $K_d$ values of 1.5 and 2.0 mL/g for cadmium and nickel calculated by the one-dimensional FEM/WATER-FEM/WASTE flow model[53] using data from the column-leaching experiment.

The column-leaching experiment indicated that cadmium (concentrations in the gasifier leachate exceeding 10 to 100 times the primary drinking water standard) and nickel transport was not attenuated effectively by the silty clay loam soil. Several factors may have contributed to the ineffectiveness of this soil to sorb these toxic metals: (1) the low pH (~4) and the high ionic strength (2000 to 3000 dS/m) of the leachate may have contributed to the lower sorption on the soil; (2) chemical equilibrium between the aqueous and solid phases may not have been achieved; or (3) soluble inorganic complexes of cadmium and nickel sulfates may have prevailed at these high sulfate concentrations,[54] allowing the movement of neutral or even negatively charged species through the soil. To test this possibility, the comput-

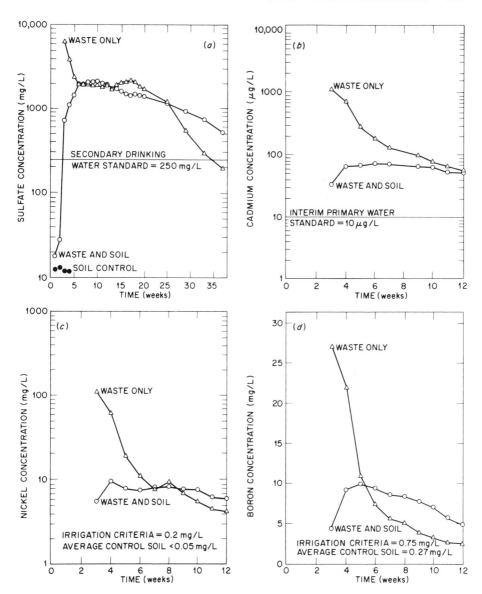

**Figure 2.**    Leachate concentrations from the gasifier waste and underlying soil.

erized thermodynamic model, WATEQ2, was used to partition total analytic concentrations among various aqueous species and to calculate saturation indices.[55] The model indicated that even after 7 weeks of leaching, the leachate was oversaturated relative to gypsum, approximately 40% of the nickel was present as a neutral sulfate complex, and almost 50% of the soluble cadmium was present either as noncharged or negatively charged sulfate species. The presence of such complexes would intensify by major proportions the transport of cadmium and nickel to groundwater aquifers. Thus, gasifier ashes that contain reduced forms of sulfur or high-soluble sulfate will likely impact surface water and groundwater quality adjacent to their disposal areas. The magnitude and duration of impact will depend on sulfur form and content in the waste, the waste loading (quantity disposed over time), oxygen content of the percolating water, characteristics of geologic media underlying the disposal area, chemical characteristics of the groundwater, and general hydrologic conditions.

### Food Chain Transfer

The transport to man of toxic constituents in solid wastes from coal conversion processes is one of the most important environmental and health concerns. The transport and possible bioaccumulation of such materials may result as a consequence of water or soil being contaminated. Bioaccumulation in aquatic food chains may occur as a result of leakage from an ash pond or a shallow land burial site. Transfer along the terrestrial food chain may occur on revegetation of the disposal area. To investigate this possibility, ryegrass was grown on admixtures of soil and gasifier ashes.[1,56] One of the gasifier ashes showed an elevated level of B, Be, Ni, Cd, Zn, and Co in plants growing in the ash/soil mixtures. The concentrations were about 10 to 90 times higher than those measured in control treatments. Dry weight yields from the ash/soil mixture (second harvest) were not significantly different from those from the control, indicating these levels were not phytotoxic; however, yields from later harvests were significantly lower.

These data show that transfer of toxic elements can occur via agricultural food chains (e.g., from animals grazing on revegetated disposal areas or from production of horticultural crops on these areas). The point here is that research is necessary to determine the environmental transport processes associated with long-term management of the disposal area.

## CONCLUSIONS

### Physical and Chemical Characterization

Total elemental analyses and short-term leaching studies have received major attention in solid waste research. Most of the leaching studies have been compliance oriented; that is, the waste has been classified under RCRA. None of the wastes have been classified as hazardous using the EPA-EP toxicity criteria. Short-term leaching research, principally the column-elution studies, has indicated that some gasifier ashes and slags produce leachates that contain high concentrations of sulfate and are generally more acidic than ashes from direct combustion of coal.

## Effects on Health and Environment

Health effects research has centered on testing the organic and aqueous extracts for mutagenicity using the Ames *Salmonella* mutagenesis assay. A few of the ashes and slags from low-Btu gasifiers were found to be mutagenic when an organic extract was used to remove organic compounds. This was principally true for gasifier chars and particulates collected in gas cleanup systems. None of the aqueous extracts from these materials was found to contain mutagenic material. Sludges from wastewater treatment facilities have been observed to contain mutagenic materials in both the aqueous and organic extracts; therefore, these materials and gasifier chars should be handled as carefully as possible by plant personnel to avoid exposure via inhalation or sorption through the skin.

Research identifying environmental effects of solid wastes depended principally on aquatic toxicity and phytotoxicity tests to evaluate exposure to solid waste leachates. Testing of gasifier ashes and slags showed these materials to be considerably less toxic than some industrial and municipal wastes. Interpretations of these tests are constrained because solid waste leaching procedures do not adequately simulate disposal conditions. Most leaching has been conducted with the RCRA-acetic acid extractant (which interferes with biotesting protocols) and distilled water extractants (which is not representative of "real-world" leaching). In many instances, toxicity cannot be identified with any particular solid waste constituent; rather, it is associated with the total ionic strength and pH of the extract. However, these tests give a comparative indication as to the potential toxicity of the wastes. The testing has given little indication of the long-term potential toxicity of the waste that might be expected with disposal in the terrestrial environment.

## Transport and Fate

Few data are available from which long-term transport, fate, and effects of toxic constituents in the wastes can be evaluated. Two experiments, one dealing with uptake of toxic trace elements in ryegrass growing in admixtures of soil and gasifier ash, and the other dealing with a continuous-flow leaching experiment involving overlain waste and soil (both described in the previous section), provide the only data that suggest the potential for long-term effects of these materials in the environment. These data, though limited, clearly demonstrate that potentially damaging effects may occur on disposal of "RCRA-nonhazardous" gasifier ashes and slags. The overriding factor is that the disposal of very large quantities of wastes such as gasifier ashes can overcome the natural ability of soils to attenuate transport via both biotic and abiotic routes, and can pose risks to groundwater.

### Industrial Hygiene and Safety

Research indirectly relating to industrial hygiene and safety is that conducted under "health effects." As mentioned earlier, mutagenic and carcinogenic responses were noted in the testing of electrostatic precipitator tars. Other industrial hygiene work has been aimed at assessing the working environment in coal conversion plants, but no research has been conducted relative to evaluating routes or levels of exposure in handling solid waste after it leaves the plant.

### Environmental Control

Research efforts relating to environmental control of solid wastes have focused on differences in cost of disposal and on variations in operational procedures required for the RCRA's classification of hazardous or nonhazardous waste. These engineering studies generally recommend disposal of the gasifier ashes and slags in clay-lined landfills that have internal and external leachate collection systems. The hazardous wastes would be disposed of in similar landfills, but the clay liner would be thicker and an impermeable synthetic liner would be added. There have been few studies on methods to reduce or contain leachate or to improve the leachate quality.

## NEEDED RESEARCH

Much of the health and environmental research relevant to solid wastes from coal conversion has been process specific and short-term oriented. For example, nearly all leaching studies have involved short-term extraction tests (i.e., RCRA extractions). Some of the ash/slags from certain technologies contain residual reduced forms of sulfur (elemental, pyrite, and pyrrhotite). This sulfur, on oxidation by soil microorganisms in landfill environments, will produce leachates significantly more acidic and containing more acid-soluble toxic metals (e.g., Cd, Cu, Ni, and Zn) than extracts from short-term extraction tests. A major research thrust needs to be made to understand and predict the movement of such leachate through geologic media so that its impact on groundwater quality can be assessed.

Two approaches can be taken to attain this goal. One involves the use of sophisticated mathematical-hydrogeological models to predict transport and fate of the various constituents in the leachate. These models require numerous input parameters. One such input parameter is the sorptivity of the constituents on the geologic media over matrices of pH and ionic strength. Others include rate and pattern of hydrologic flow, dissolution rates of the waste, and influence of redox conditions on dissolution and sorptivity of the waste constituents. In a waste disposal system, physical, chemical, and biological processes operate in a simultaneous and interactive manner; thus, for mathematical models to be applicable, the various processes need to be coupled. No model currently exists to simulate the combined effects of all such processes. However, models do exist that reflect the dominant processes, and these models can be modified and coupled with others in an attempt to simulate the total process.

The alternative approach is empirical. In this approach, the leaching character of the waste is determined under simulated and real-world conditions. This involves medium- to long-term column tests (3 to 10 year) simulating landfill designs, as well as small-scale landfill experiments on terrestrial landscapes. These experiments would require careful and sophisticated instrumentation so that the input parameters to the hydrogeological models mentioned above could be monitored. These values, in turn, could be used to test and modify existing models to simulate transport and fate of leachate constituents. Through a combination of the modeling and empirical approaches, significant knowledge could be attained to estimate the risks of contamination of groundwaters resulting from land disposal of coal conversion waste or any other energy-related solid waste.

### Physical and Chemical Characterization

Future research relative to the physicochemical and leaching characteristics of coal conversion solid wastes should be approached with generic long-term objectives in mind. For instance, elemental composition and leaching characteristics of wastes should be compared among processes (fixed-bed, fluidized-bed, and entrained-flow gasifiers) and wastes generated in direct combustion (coal preparation, fly ash, bottom ash, etc.). Emphasis should be on understanding the chemical, biological, and physical processes responsible for dissolution, and on the potential for transport of the toxic constituents in the wastes. The major concern raised thus far for some of the gasifier ashes and slags (as well as for other wastes) is the oxidation of the reduced sulfur forms present in the wastes, which results in highly acidic leachates, dissolution of toxic metals from the waste, and poor attenuation by surrounding geologic media.

### Health and Environmental Effects

Further health effects research is needed to identify the risks associated with exposure to the work force in the coal conversion facility as well as exposure to the general population as a consequence of disposal practices. The effects of inhalation, skin contact, and ingestion of wastes should be investigated using laboratory animals. Results should be made in a comparative sense so that alternatives relative to possible changes in coal conversion processes as well as energy technologies can be identified.

Future research on environmental effects should address questions regarding the effects of long-term disposal of wastes rather than the short-term effects on aquatic and terrestrial organisms. For instance, research should be conducted to evaluate diversity and resilience of aquatic and terrestrial communities to leachates emanating from disposal areas. In addition, research is needed to evaluate the potential for bioaccumulation of toxic constituents along terrestrial food chains. The latter need is especially relevant with respect to soluble organic compounds observed to be mutagenic in leachates from wastewater sludges.

### Transport and Fate

The prevailing waste management practice involves land disposal in on-site engineered landfills or a "back-to-pit" approach where infiltration by solid waste leachate to groundwater will be common. Thus, the major research goal in the management of solid wastes from a coal conversion technology is the development of the capabilities to predict the movement of solid waste leachate in subsurface environments. To do this, it will be necessary to (1) define the chemical and physical transport mechanisms that control solubilization of the waste under the disposal conditions, (2) characterize the mechanisms controlling leachate attentuation by the surrounding geologic media, and (3) resolve the limits of dispersion for leachates emanating from the disposal area. These boundary conditions then need to be coupled in hydrologic transport models and tested at "real-world" sites.

### ACKNOWLEDGMENTS

Research sponsored by the Office of Health and Environmental Research, Ecological Research Division, U.S. Department of Energy, under contract W-7405-eng-26 with Union Carbide Corporation. Publication No. 2144, Environmental Sciences Division, Oak Ridge National Laboratory.

### REFERENCES

1. "Status of Health and Environmental Research Relative to Solid Wastes from Coal Conversion," DOE/NBB-0008/1 (Washington, DC: U.S. Department of Energy, Office of Energy Research, Office of Health and Environmental Research, 1982).

2. Bern, J., R.D. Neufeld, and M.A. Shapiro. "Solid Waste Management of Coal Conversion Residuals from a Commercial-size Facility: Environmental Engineering Aspects," DOE/ET/20023-5 (Pittsburgh: University of Pittsburgh, 1980).
3. Somerville, M.H., and J.L. Elder. "A Comparison of Trace Element Analyses of North Dakota Lignite Laboratory Ash with Lurgi Gasifier Ash and Their Use in Environmental Analyses," in *Proceedings of the Environmental Aspects of Fuel Conversion Technology-III,* EPA-600/7-78-063 (Washington, DC: U.S. Environmental Protection Agency, 1978), pp. 292–311.
4. Gasior, S.J., et al. "Major, Minor, and Trace Element Balance for the Synthane PDU Gasifier-Illinois No. 6 Coal," *Am. Chem. Soc. Div. Fuel Chem.* 23(2) (1978).
5. Suter, G.W., II, and R.M. Cushman. "Solid Waste Studies," in *Preliminary Environmental Assessment of the University of Minnesota-Duluth Coal Gasifier,* ORNL/TM-7728 (Oak Ridge, TN: Oak Ridge National Laboratory, 1981).
6. Van Meter, W.P., and R.E. Erickson. "Environmental Effects from Leaching of Coal Conversion By-products," Progress Reports FE-2019, (1–7) (Missoula: University of Montana, 1977–1979).
7. Heunisch, G.W., and G.J. Leaman, Jr. "Phase I: The Pipeline Gas Demonstration Plant: Analysis of Coal, By-Products, and Waste Waters for the Technical Support Program," FE-2542-23 (Washington, DC: U.S. Department of Energy, 1979).
8. Lee, S.Y. "Coal Gasification Solid Wastes: Physicochemical Characterization," *Environ. Sci. Technol.* 16:728–731 (1982).
9. Lee, S.Y., and W.J. Boegly, Jr. "Coal Conversion Solid Wastes: Characterization for Environmental Assessment," ORNL/TM-7533 (Oak Ridge, TN: Oak Ridge National Laboratory, 1981).
10. Turner, R.R., and P.D. Lowry. "Comparison of Solid Wastes from Coal Combustion and Coal Gasification Plants," Final Report, Part 1, EPRI EA-2867 (Palo Alto, CA: Electric Power Research Institute, 1983).
11. Francis, C.W., W.J. Boegly, Jr., R.R. Turner, and E.C. Davis. "Coal Conversion Solid Waste Disposal," *ASCE J. Environ. Eng. Div.,* 108:1301–1311 (1982).
12. Martin, E., and G.V. Sullian. "Characterization of Residuals from Selected Coal Conversion Processes," BM-RI-8501 (Washington, DC: Bureau of Mines, 1980).
13. Yu, K.Y., and G.M. Crawford. "Characterization of Coal Gasification Ash Leachate Using RCRA Extraction Procedure," presented at the 5th Symposium on Environmental Aspects of Fuel Conversion Technology, St. Louis, September 16–19, 1980.
14. Keairns, D.L., C.C. Sun, C.H. Peterson, and R.A. Newby. "Fluid-Bed Combustion and Gasification Solids Disposal," *ASCE J. Environ. Eng. Div.* 106:213–228 (1980).
15. Hinckley, C.C., G.V. Smith, H. Twardowska, M. Saporoschenko, R.H. Shiley, and R.A. Griffin. "Mossbauer Studies of Iron in Lurgi Gasification Ashes and Power Plant Fly and Bottom Ash," *Fuel* 59:161–165 (1980).
16. Boegly, W.J., Jr., H.W. Wilson, C.W. Francis, and E.C. Davis. "Land Disposal of Coal Gasification Residue," *ASCE J. Energy Div.* 106(EY2):179–186 (1980).
17. Griffin, R.A., R.M. Schuller, J.J. Suloway, N.F. Shimp, W.F. Childers, and

R.H. Shiley. "Chemical and Biological Characterization of Leachates from Coal Solid Wastes," *Environ. Geol. Notes* 89 (Champaign, IL: State Geological Survey Division, November 1980).

18. Skarlos, L. "Texaco Coal Gasification Process: Leach Characteristics of Slags," presented at the Electric Power Research Institute Workshop on Environmental Control Technology for Coal Gasification, Palo Alto, CA, October 1982.

19. Walker, P.L., Jr., W. Speckman, P.H. Given, A. Davis, R.G. Jenkins, and P.C. Painter. "Characterization of Mineral Matter in Coal and Coal Liquefaction Residuals," final report to Electric Power Research Institute, AP-1634 (University Park: Pennsylvania State University, 1981).

20. Keleti, G., J. Bern, M.A. Shapiro, W.G. Gulledge, and G.T. Moore. "Mutagenicity of SRC-II Coal Liquefaction Wastewater Treatment Residues," *Environ. Sci. Technol.* 16:826–830 (1982).

21. Filby, R.H., K.R. Shah, and C.A. Sautter. "Trace Elements in the Solvent Refined Coal Process," in *Proceedings of the Environmental Aspects of Fuel Conversion Technology-III,* EPA-600/7-78-063 (Washington, DC: U.S. Environmental Protection Agency, 1978), pp. 266–282.

22. Filby, R.H., S.R. Khalil, C.A. Grim, V. Ekabaram, and M.L. Hunt. "The Fate of Trace Elements in SRC Process," in *Pilot Plant Development Work, Solvent Refined Coal (SRC) Process* Vol. 3, Pt. 6, DOE/ET/10104-T11 (Washington, DC: U.S. Department of Energy, 1980).

23. Shiley, R.H., S.J. Russell, D.R. Dickerson, C.C. Hinckley, and G.V. Smith. "Calibration Standard for X-Ray Diffraction Analyses of Coal Liquefaction Residuals: Mossbauer Spectra of Synthetic Pyrrhotites," *Fuel* 58:678–688 (1979).

24. Saporoschenko, M.C., C. Hinckley, G.V. Smith, H. Twardowska, R.H. Shiley, R.A. Griffin, and S.J. Russell. "Mossbauer Spectroscopic Studies of the Mineralogical Changes in Coal as a Function of Cleaning, Pyrolysis, Combustion, and Coal Conversion Processes," *Fuel* 59:567–574 (1980).

25. Leuthy, R.G., P. Vassiliou, and M.J. Carter. "Leach Characteristics of Coal-Gasification Char," *ASCE J. Environ. Div.* 106:81–103 (1980).

26. Maskarinec, M.P., and D.K. Brown. "Determination of Selected Organics in Treated Sludges and Associated Leachates from Coal Conversion Facilities," *Anal. Chim. Acta* 139:257–266 (1982).

27. Brown, D.K., M.P. Maskarinec, F.W. Larimer, and C.W. Francis. "Mobility of Organic Compounds from Hazardous Wastes," in *Annual Progress Report 1981, Toxicity of Leachates Project* (Oak Ridge, TN: Oak Ridge National Laboratory, 1982).

28. Maskarinec, M.P., and R.W. Harvey. "Screening of Sludges and Solid Wastes for Organic Compounds," *Int. J. Environ. Anal. Chem.* 11:53–60 (1982).

29. Anderson, G.L., A.H. Hill, and D.K. Fleming. "Predictions on the Disposition of Selected Trace Constituents in Coal Gasification Processes," in *Proceedings of the Environmental Aspects of Fuel Conversion Technology Symposium,* EPA 600/7-79-217 (Washington, DC: U.S. Environmental Protection Agency, 1979), pp. 302–332.

30. Holt, N.A., J.E. McDaniel, and T.P. O'Shea. "Environmental Test Results from Coal Gasification Pilot Plants," presented at the Fifth Symposium on Environmental Aspects of Fuel Conversion Technology, St. Louis, Sept. 16–19, 1980.

31. Fuch, M.R., D.L. Heenrich, L.J. Holcombe, and K.T. Ajmera. "A Comparison of RCRA Leachates in Solid Wastes from Coal-Fired Utilities and Low-

and Medium-Btu Gasification Processes," presented at *Environmental Aspects of Fuel Conversion Technology-VI,* Denver, Oct. 26–30, 1981.

32. Benson, J.M., C.E. Mitchell, R.E. Royer, C.R. Clark, R.L. Carpenter, and G.J. Newton. "Mutagenicity of Potential Effluents from an Experimental Low Btu Coal Gasifier," *Arch. Environ. Contam. Toxicol.* 11:547–551 (1982).

33. Ames, B.N., J. McCann, and E. Yamasaki. "Methods for Detecting Carcinogens and Mutagens with *Salmonella*/Mammalian Microsome Mutagenicity Test," *Mutat. Res.* 31:347–364 (1975).

34. Kimball, R.F., and N.B. Munro. "A Critical Review of the Mutagenic and Other Genotoxic Effects of Direct Coal Liquefaction," ORNL-5721 (Oak Ridge, TN: Oak Ridge National Laboratory, 1981).

35. Epler, J.L., et al. "Toxicity of Leachates," EPA-600/2-80-057 (Washington, DC: U.S. Environmental Protection Agency, 1980).

36. Fisher, G.L., C.E. Chrisp, and O.G. Reabe, "Physical Factors Affecting the Mutagenicity of Fly Ash from a Coal-fired Power Plant," *Science* 204:879–881 (1979).

37. Kubitschek, H.E., and L. Venta. "Mutagenicity of Coal Fly Ash from Electric Power Plant Precipitators," *Environ. Mutat.* 1:79–82 (1979).

38. Browman, M.G., and M.P. Maskarinec. "Environmental Aspects of Organics in Selected Coal Conversion Solid Wastes," *Environ. Sci. Health* A17(5):736–766 (1982).

39. Griffin, R.A., R.A. Schuller, J.J. Suloway, S.A. Russell, W.F. Childers, and N.F. Shimp. "Solubility and Toxicity of Potential Pollutants in Solid Coal Wastes," in *Proceedings of the Environmental Aspects of Fuel Conversion Technology-III,* EPA-600/7-78-063 (Washington, DC: U.S. Environmental Protection Agency, 1978), pp. 506–518.

40. Schuller, R.M., J.J. Suloway, R.A. Griffin, S.J. Russell, and W.F. Childers. "Identification of Potential Pollutants from Coal Conversion Wastes," Appendix E, FE-0496-176 (Washington, DC: U.S. Department of Energy, 1980).

41. Millemann, R.E., and B.R. Parkhurst. "Comparative Toxicity of Solid Waste Leachates to *Daphnia magna,*" *Environ. Int.* 4:255–260 (1980).

42. Millemann, R.E., B.R. Parkhurst, and N.T. Edwards. "Toxicity to *Daphnia magna* and Terrestrial Plants of Solid Waste Leachates from Coal Conversion Processes," in *Proceedings of the Twentieth Hanford Life Sciences Symposium on Coal Conversion and the Environment* (Richland, WA: Battelle Pacific Northwest Laboratories, 1981), pp. 237–247.

43. Shriner, D.S., H.S. Arora, N.T. Edwards, B.R. Parkhurst, C.W. Gehrs, and T. Tamura. "Physical, Chemical, and Ecological Characterization of Solid Wastes from a Lurgi Gasification Facility," in *Synthetic Fossil Fuel Technology: Potential Health and Environmental Effects,* K.E. Cowser and C.R. Richmond, Eds. (Ann Arbor, MI: Ann Arbor Science, 1980), pp. 181–192.

44. Cushman, R.M., and D.K. Brown. "Composition and Toxicity of Solid Waste Leachates from Industrial Coal Gasifiers," in *Energy Alternatives: International Progress,* T.N. Veziroglu, Ed. (Ann Arbor, MI: Ann Arbor Science, 1982), pp. 425–431.

45. Cushman, R.M., G.W. Suter II, D.K. Brown, N.T. Edwards, W.H. Griest, A.J. Steward, and R.H. Strand. "Environmental Evaluation of the University of Minnesota-Duluth Gasifier," ORNL-8552 (Oak Ridge, TN: Oak Ridge National Laboratory, 1983).

46. "Test Methods for Evaluating Solid Wastes—Physical/Chemical Methods,"

SW-847, Sect. 2.1.4: *Extraction Procedure Toxicity,* 2nd ed. (Washington, DC: U.S. Environmental Protection Agency, July 1982).

47.  "Identification and Listing of Hazardous Waste," Hazardous Waste Management System, U.S. Environmental Protection Agency, 40 CFR Part 261 (1980).

48.  Tamura, T., and W.J. Boegly, Jr. "Leaching Studies of Coal Gasification Solid Wastes to meet RCRA Requirements for Land Disposal," in *Proceedings of the Second DOE Environmental Control Symposium,* CONF-800334/1 (Springfield, VA: National Technical Information Service, 1980).

49.  "Final Environmental Impact Statement for Memphis Light, Gas, and Water Division, Industrial Fuel Gas Demonstration Project," DOE/EIS-0071 (Washington, D.C.: U.S. Department of Energy, 1981).

50.  "Final Environmental Impact Statement, Solvent Refined Coal-I Demonstration Project," Vols. 1 and 2, DOE/EIS-0073 (Washington, DC: U.S. Department of Energy, 1981).

51.  "Final Environmental Impact Statement, Solvent Refined Coal-II Demonstration Project," Vols. 1 and 2, DOE/EIS-0069 (Washington, DC: U.S. Department of Energy, 1981).

52.  Davis, E.C., and C.W. Francis. "Long-Term Leaching of Coal Gasification Ash," (Oak Ridge, TN: Oak Ridge National Laboratory) (to be published).

53.  Yeh, G.T. "Training Course No. 2: The Implementation of FEMWASTE (ORNL-5601) Computer Program," ORNL/TM-8328 (Oak Ridge, TN: Oak Ridge National Laboratory, 1982).

54.  Smith, R.M., and A.E. Martell. *Critical Stability Constants, Vol. 4: Inorganic Complexes* (New York: Plenum Press, 1976), pp. 82–84.

55.  Ball, J.W., D.K. Nordstrom, and E.A. Jenne. "Additional and Revised Thermochemical Data and Computer Code for WATEQ2—A Computerized Chemical Model for Trace and Major Element Speciation and Mineral Equilibrium of Natural Waters," Water-Resources Investigations 78-116 (Menlo Park, CA: U.S. Geological Survey, 1978).

56.  Auerbach, S.I., et al. "Bioaccumulation of Toxic Trace Elements from Coal-Conversion Solid Wastes," in *Environmental Sciences Division Annual Progress Report for Period Ending September 30, 1981,* ORNL-5900 (Oak Ridge, TN: Oak Ridge National Laboratory, 1982), pp. 65–66.

## DISCUSSION

*C.D. Scott, Oak Ridge National Laboratory:* You mentioned that in some of your tests you did get some apparent microbial effects in the leaching experiments. Since, in some cases, this can significantly enhance leaching, would it make sense to structure several experiments in which one introduces a defined microbial population that was sulfur metabolizing and use this to determine the effects of the microbial population on leaching?

*C.W. Francis:* Yes. We are presently conducting such experiments but preliminary data have not been tabulated.

# CHAPTER 5

## Toxicology of Large-Scale Refining of Shale Oil

### C.W. Stallard, Jr., M.D., and G.R. Krautter

*The Standard Oil Co. (SOHIO)*
*Midland Bldg., 805 H.B.*
*Cleveland, OH 44115*

Interest in the development of oil shale deposits in the United States has waxed and waned for several decades even though small-scale operations have taken place for about 100 years. A recent sharp upsurge in activity was followed by a dramatic decline in interest. The future remains uncertain, but the resource is still available. Although the economic aspects of oil shale extraction will undoubtedly determine whether oil is to be produced from shale, the recent activity has established a level of technology that indicates production is feasible and that products derived from extraction are both similar and different from natural petroleum crudes, synthetic crudes, and products derived from other fossil sources. Questions concerning the similarities and differences have instigated research in several disciplines to determine what the nature of the products might be, what toxicological hazard is inherent in the defined materials, and how that hazard is translated into human and environmental risks.

Previously,[1] I presented a methodology to deal with workplace risks and health effects, with the intent that a continuing record could be maintained. Data could then be extracted from this base of information to test hypotheses of causal relationships, that is, whether recorded exposures to defined agents in the workplace could be shown to have statistically significant relationships to the observed health effects, which have also been recorded. This is still a necessary concept, however implemented, and there is a need for a synthetic-fuels worker registry, a subject that has been extensively discussed in oil shale states.

As I pointed out earlier,[1] the proposed methodology lacked an essential element—a toxicological base that could be used in extrapolating biologically specific characteristics into human pathology. This chapter partially deals with our current, admittedly still developing, efforts to correct that deficit.

The Standard Oil Company-Ohio (SOHIO) health organization is dedicated to collecting, validating, analyzing, and evaluating all available toxicologic, workplace, and health-effects data that pertain to agents of concern. These are identified and added to an inventory. Each item is investigated for its intrinsic hazard, and values are assigned for important aspects of its behavior in biological systems, including human systems if data are available. We have attempted to organize these data into a form that allows quick review, and profiles are created for computerization. As applied to shale products, these hazard assessments constitute part of this chapter. Table I summarizes the various current studies in oil shale research.

Identifying the inventory items and testing some of the innumerable fractionations have established certain characteristics. Synthetic liquids derived from shale and coal differ in important aspects from natural petroleum. Petroleum is made up largely of neutral fractions (95 to 100%), whereas shale contains a large percentage of basic components. Coal-derived oils vary widely, some containing even larger quantities of basic plus acid components than shale; others are more nearly neutral, but still contain significant basic constituents. Ames mutagenicity appears to be closely related to this basic fraction, but in coal-derived oils, aromaticity plus the possible

**Table I.** Current Oil Shale Research[a]

| | Cellular Toxicology | Organ/System Toxicology | Teratogenicity/Reproductive Effects | Carcinogenicity and Mutagenicity | Epidemiological Studies | Clinical Studies | Exposure Assessment | Risk Assessment | Total |
|---|---|---|---|---|---|---|---|---|---|
| Raw shale | 1 | 6 | 2 | 4 | 1 | | 2 | 1 | 17 |
| Crude shale oil | 15 | 16 | 7 | 25 | 4 | 2 | 8 | 7 | 84 |
| Hydrotreated shale oil | 9 | 9 | 2 | 17 | 1 | 1 | 2 | 3 | 44 |
| Fuel oil | 1 | 5 | | 2 | | | | | 8 |
| Diesel fuel | | 1 | | | | | | | 1 |
| Diesel marine fuel | 1 | 4 | | 2 | | | | | 7 |
| Jet fuels | | 6 | | 2 | | | 1 | | 9 |
| Retorted shale | 1 | 8 | 2 | 5 | | | | | 16 |
| Process streams | 6 | 4 | 2 | 4 | 1 | | 1 | 1 | 19 |
| Effluents | 12 | 5 | 2 | 11 | 1 | | 14 | 2 | 47 |
| Total | 46 | 64 | 17 | 72 | 8 | 3 | 28 | 14 | 252 |

[a]Adapted by permission from American Petroleum Institute, from Dynamac Corporation Report, API Contract EH 19 ECI (570-1), 1982.

promoting effect of long-chain paraffinics and olefins also produce mutagenic responses. However, a clear gradient of mutagenicity is demonstrated by an ascending scale of biological reactivity, as determined in cellular or animal systems. Petroleum in its natural liquid state is mildly active. Raw shale and solid coal have not proved to be so. The oil must be extracted from shale to exert its biological effect; coal dust has not proved to be carcinogenic unless it is chemically altered.

In 1978, SOHIO's Toledo refinery processed 87,000 bbl of raw shale oil produced by the Paraho process, and samples of the products produced from that refinery run were supplied to Oak Ridge National Laboratory for storage in a depository and for research purposes. The products included jet fuel, J-P 5, to U.S. Navy military specifications; jet fuel, J-P 8; diesel marine fuel; residuum, No. 6 fuel oil; and precursors to the preceding, which were acid treated to produce a "polished" product. All products were tested in sufficiently representative systems to discover their expressed risks, which resulted in a substantial amount of research on these and other products.

The American Petroleum Institute (API) has attempted to correlate these data. Through the efforts of company scientists and the API staff, particularly Group I of the Synthetic Fuels Task Force of the larger API Toxic Substances Task Force, identifiable process streams were classified. The qualification was that conventional petroleum refining processes would produce additional streams that might be defined in the same manner as existing definitions for petroleum streams such as streams resulting from hydrotreating, hydrocracking, catalytic cracking, thermal cracking, solvent refining, and acid treating. The expected products include gasolines, jet fuels, diesel fuel, kerosene, light and heavy fuel oils, lubricating oils, and a variety of light and middle distillates useful for solvents, thinners, and similar products. Table II, which lists the process stream definitions, identifies

**Table II.**  Process Stream Definitions[a]

| Process Stream | Definition | Boiling Range |
|---|---|---|
| Retorting streams | | |
| Shale oil | Complex combination of hydrocarbons from thermal decomposition of kerogen consisting of hydrocarbons and heteroatom compounds containing nitrogen, sulfur, and oxygen[b] | ≥750°F |
| Retorted oil shale | Crushed rock remaining when oil shale, a complex marlstone containing organic material (kerogen), is heated without combustion to substantially remove organic portion; usually contains carbonaceous residue | |

**Table II.** *(continued)*

| Process Stream | Definition | Boiling Range |
|---|---|---|
| Combusted oil shale | Crushed rock remaining when oil shale is heated by process, including combustion of kerogen residues as direct source of retort heat, or when retorted oil shale is subjected to combustion to recover residual fuel value; usually contains virtually no carbonaceous residue | |
| Retort naphtha | Complex combination of hydrocarbons obtained from retorting consisting primarily of hydrocarbons having carbon numbers predominantly in the range $C_4$–$C_{16}$ | ~ −20 to 290°C (−4 to 554°F) |
| Retort gas oil (shale oil) | Complex combination of hydrocarbons obtained from retorting consisting primarily of hydrocarbons having carbon numbers predominantly in the range $C_{11}$–$C_{40}$ | ~200 to 540°C (400 to 1000°F) |
| Retort bottoms (shale oil) | Complex combination of hydrocarbons obtained from retorting consisting primarily of hydrocarbons having carbon numbers predominantly above $C_{25}$ | predominantly >400°C (752°F) |
| Distillation streams | | |
| Light straight-run naphtha (shale oil) | Aliphatic and olefinic hydrocarbons $C_4$–$C_{10}$ | −20 to 180°C (−4 to 356°F) |
| Heavy straight-run naphtha (shale oil) | Hydrocarbons $C_6$–$C_{12}$ | 65 to 230°C (149 to 446°F) |
| Full-range straight-run naphtha (shale oil) | Hydrocarbons $C_4$–$C_{12}$ | −20 to 230°C (−4 to 446°F) |
| Straight-run light distillate (shale oil) | Hydrocarbons $C_9$–$C_{16}$ | 150 to 290°C (320 to 554°F) |
| Straight-run middle distillate (shale oil) | Hydrocarbons $C_{11}$–$C_{20}$ | 205 to 345°C (401 to 653°F) |
| Straight-run gas oil (shale oil) | Hydrocarbons $C_{11}$–$C_{25}$ | 205 to 400°C (401 to 752°F) |
| Atmospheric tower residuum (shale oil) | Hydrocarbons >$C_{20}$ | 350°C (662°F) |

**Table II.**   *(continued)*

| Process Stream | Definition | Boiling Range |
|---|---|---|
| Vacuum tower condensate (shale oil) | Hydrocarbons $C_{11}$–$C_{25}$ | 205 to 400°C (401 to 752°F) |
| Light vacuum gas oil (shale oil) | Hydrocarbons $C_{13}$–$C_{30}$ | 230 to 450°C (446 to 842°F) |
| Heavy vacuum gas oil (shale oil)[c] | Hydrocarbons $C_{20}$–$C_{50}$ | 350 to 600°C (662 to 1112°F) |
| Vacuum residuum (shale oil) | Hydrocarbons $>C_{34}$ | 495°C (923°F) |

Pretreatment streams

| | | |
|---|---|---|
| Pretreated shale oil | Complex combination of hydrocarbons produced from shale oil by pretreatment | |
| Pretreated retort naphtha (shale oil) | Complex combination of hydrocarbons produced from shale oil by pretreatment consisting predominantly of hydrocarbons having carbon numbers predominantly in the range of $C_4$–$C_{16}$ | −20 to 290°C (−4 to 554°F) |
| Pretreated retort gas oil (shale oil) | Hydrocarbons $C_{11}$–$C_{40}$ | 200 to 540°C (400 to 1000°F) |
| Pretreated retort bottoms (shale oil) | Hydrocarbons above $C_{25}$ | above 400°C (752°F) |
| Pretreated light naphtha (shale oil) | Hydrocarbons $C_4$–$C_{10}$ | −20 to 180°C (−4 to 356°F) |
| Pretreated heavy naphtha (shale oil) | Hydrocarbons $C_6$–$C_{12}$ | 65 to 230°C (149 to 446°F) |
| Pretreated full-range naphtha (shale oil) | Hydrocarbons $C_4$–$C_{12}$ | −20 to 230°C (−4 to 446°F) |
| Pretreated light distillate (shale oil) | Hydrocarbons $C_9$–$C_{16}$ | 150 to 290°C (320 to 554°F) |
| Pretreated middle distillate (shale oil) | Hydrocarbons $C_{11}$–$C_{20}$ | 205 to 345°C (401 to 653°F) |
| Pretreated heavy distillate (shale oil) | Hydrocarbons $C_{11}$–$C_{25}$ | 205 to 400°C (401 to 752°F) |
| Pretreated atmospheric tower residuum (shale oil)[d] | Hydrocarbons $>C_{20}$ | 350°C (662°F) |

**Table II.** *(continued)*

| Process Stream | Definition | Boiling Range |
|---|---|---|
| Pretreated vacuum tower condensate (shale oil) | Hydrocarbons $C_{11}$–$C_{25}$ | 205 to 400°C (401 to 752°F) |
| Pretreated light vacuum gas oil (shale oil) | Hydrocarbons $C_{13}$–$C_{30}$ | 230 to 450°C (446 to 842°F) |
| Pretreated heavy vacuum gas oil (shale oil)[c] | Hydrocarbons $C_{20}$–$C_{50}$ | 350 to 600°C (662 to 1112°F) |
| Pretreated vacuum tower residuum (shale oil) | Hydrocarbons $>C_{34}$ | 495°C (923°F) |
| Hydrotreating streams | | |
| Hydrotreated shale oil | Hydrocarbons $C_4$–$C_{50}$ distillation range similar to feed | |
| Hydrotreated retort naphtha (shale oil) | Hydrocarbons $C_4$–$C_{16}$ | −20 to 290°C (−4 to 554°F) |
| Hydrotreated retort gas oil (shale oil) | Hydrocarbons $C_{11}$–$C_{40}$ | 200 to 540°C (400 to 1000°F) |
| Hydrotreated retort bottoms | Hydrocarbons above $C_{25}$ | 400°C (752°F) |
| Hydrocracking streams | | |
| Hydrocracked shale oil | Hydrocarbons $C_4$–$C_{50}$ with higher proportion of lighter components than the feed | |
| Catalytic dewaxing streams | | |
| Catalytically dewaxed shale oil | Hydrocarbons $C_4$–$C_{50}$ with higher proportion of lighter components than the feed; relatively few high-molecular-weight normal paraffins | |
| Catalytically cracked shale oil | Saturated, olefinic, and aromatic hydrocarbons having carbon numbers $C_4$–$C_{50}$ with higher proportion of lighter components than the feed | |
| Thermal cracking streams | | |
| Thermally cracked (coker) distillate (shale oil) | Unsaturated hydrocarbons $C_4$–$C_{50}$ with higher proportion of lighter components than the feed | |

**Table II.** *(continued)*

| Process Stream | Definition | Boiling Range |
|---|---|---|
| Thermally cracked (coker) light naphtha (shale oil) | Unsaturated hydrocarbons $C_4$–$C_8$ | −10 to 130°C (14 to 266°F) |
| Thermally cracked (coker) heavy naphtha (shale oil) | Unsaturated hydrocarbons $C_6$–$C_{12}$ | 65 to 220°C (148 to 428°F) |
| Thermally cracked (coker) light distillate (shale oil) | Unsaturated hydrocarbons $C_{10}$–$C_{22}$ | 160 to 370°C (320 to 698°F) |
| Thermally cracked (coker) heavy distillate (shale oil)[a] | Unsaturated hydrocarbons $C_{15}$–$C_{36}$ | 260 to 480°C (500 to 896°F) |
| Thermally cracked (coker) residuum (shale oil)[c] | Unsaturated hydrocarbons $>C_{20}$ | 350°C (662°F) |
| Coke (shale oil) | Carbonaceous materials and some hydrocarbons having high carbon-to-hydrogen ratio | |

Acid-Treating Streams

| Process Stream | Definition | Boiling Range |
|---|---|---|
| Acid-treated shale oil | Complex combination of hydrocarbons obtained as raffinate when shale oil or pretreated shale oil is treated with sulfuric acid; stream consisting predominantly of saturated hydrocarbons | Above −20°C (−4°F) |
| Acid-treated retort naphtha (shale oil) | Hydrocarbons $C_4$–$C_{16}$ | 20 to 290°C (−4 to 554°F) |
| Acid-treated retort gas oil (shale oil) | Hydrocarbons $C_{11}$–$C_{40}$ | 200 to 540°C (400 to 1000°F) |
| Acid sludge (shale oil) | Complex combination of sulfuric and sulfonic acids, water, esters, amine salts, and high-molecular-weight organic compounds such as polymers of olefinic hydrocarbons, formed during treating of oils with sulfuric acid and usually incinerated to recover the sulfur as sulfuric acid and to dispose of unwanted organic material (CAS Registry No. 64742-24-1) | |

**Table II.** *(continued)*

| Process Stream | Definition | Boiling Range |
|---|---|---|
| Solvent refining streams | | |
| Solvent-refined light paraffinic distillate (shale oil) | Complex combination of hydrocarbons produced as raffinate phase from solvent extraction of shale oil or pretreated shale oil or fraction thereof, consisting predominantly of saturated hydrocarbons having carbon numbers predominantly in the range of $C_{15}$ through $C_{30}$ and producing finished oil with viscosity of <100 SUS at 100°F | 19 cSt at 40°C |
| Solvent-refined heavy paraffinic distillate (shale oil) | Saturated hydrocarbons $C_{20}$ through $C_{50}$; produces finished oil with viscosity of <100 SUS at 100°F | 19 cSt at 40°C |
| Light paraffinic distillate solvent extract (shale oil)[c] | Hydrocarbons $C_{15}$–$C_{30}$ | |
| Heavy paraffinic distillate solvent extract (shale oil)[c] | Hydrocarbons $C_{20}$–$C_{50}$ | |
| Solvent-decarbonized residual oil (shale oil) | Hydrocarbons >$C_{25}$ | 400°C (752°F) |
| Residual oil decarbonized raffinate (shale oil) | Aromatic hydrocarbons <$C_{34}$; high carbon-to-hydrogen ratio | |

[a]Adapted by permission from American Petroleum Institute.
[b]From Chemical Abstracts Registry No. 68308-34-9.
[c]This stream is likely to contain 5 wt % or more of 4- to 6-membered condensed-ring aromatic hydrocarbons.
[d]This stream is likely to contain 5 wt % or more of 4- to 6-membered condensed-ring aromatic compounds.

the complexity of fossil hydrocarbon deposits, man's ingenious treatment of them, their many useful products, and, finally, the compound and interrelated problems of the health scientist in assessing their potential effects on the human populations that will be exposed to them either directly or indirectly.

While like begets like, the differences in raw materials, considering the many kinds of petroleum, the relatively consistent Green River shale, and the different ranks and types of coal, indicate that they do not begin as "likes." Since all are fossil fuel hydrocarbons, treatment will make them resemble each other more closely. As the components that are distinctive to each origin are removed, the likenesses remain, and, if carried to completion, the products will become essentially identical (see Table III for a

**Table III.**  Products Definitions

*Shale oil (CAS 68308-34-9).*    Thick, viscous oil, high in olefins, consisting of hydrocarbons and heteroatoms containing nitrogen, sulfur, and oxygen resulting from heated insoluble kerogen that breaks down into largely soluble nonvolatile material; partial volatilization, cracking, and coking occur at progressively higher temperatures. Arsenic content, about 50 ppm, is typically much higher than in conventional petroleum crudes.

*Retorted oil shale.*    Spent marlstone remaining after heating without combustion. Residual carbonaceous material is present, usually in 4 to 6% range. Alkaline earth carbonates and oxides are present, dependent on retorting method, but product will be alkaline. Free silica is reduced from raw shale values by reacting to form complex silicates. Spontaneous ignition is a concern, and leachates will contain biologically active hydrocarbons.

*Combusted oil shale.*    Spent material remaining after heating by combustion of carbonaceous residues, either during the retorting process (direct retorting, in situ retorting) or combusted to recover fuel values. Little carbonaceous material is present. High temperatures may decompose carbonates, increasing alkalinity. Both retorted and combusted shales can retain significant water content (up to 45 wt %). Compacting and surface drying followed by weathering may result in minimal observed difference between runoff from shale disposal sites and natural loss from nearby scarps and talus slopes in mining region. Efforts to contain and stabilize disposal site are required.

*Hydrotreated shale oil.*    Oil produced by high- and low-pressure hydrogenation of retorted oil, resulting in removal of increasing percentages of sulfur as hydrogen sulfide, nitrogen as ammonia, and oxygen in phenolics and water. Olefinics are saturated, and product is relatively free from heteroatoms and metallic constituents due to coking and removal of adsorptive techniques. Resultant oil is a blend of hydrocarbon distillates (e.g., over boiling range to 950°C) with lowered pour point.

*Treatment residues.*    Residues from hydrotreatment, filtration, adsorptive, or catalytic removal of metallic constituents such as arsenic. Consists of complex hydrocarbons and adsorptive materials such as ceramic balls and filter elements, plus highly viscous, tenacious, oxidized, and polymerized hydrocarbons. Shale oil suitably prepared for refining may serve as sole feedstock or, commingled with petroleum crudes, provide source for conventionally refined petroleum products.

*Major distillate fractions.*    Remaining hydrocarbon mixtures including light and heavy naphthas, carbon numbers $C_4$–$C_{16}$ predominantly and boiling in the range of approximately −20 to 290°C (−4 to 554°F), having lost many of the light-boiling fractions in the retorting process (light naphthas in the boiling range of −259 to 20°F).

definition of the process products). Because treatment is costly, there is an agreeable but not yet discovered configuration that will satisfy the needs of identity, toxic hazard evaluation, and health risk, as well as the need for cost effectiveness. The question is clear: Shall all possible process streams be identified and tested, or can an array of process streams and products be adequately evaluated to provide the necessary level of safety? To make the best use of limited funds and personnel, careful planning is the necessary first step.

Following is an example of shale-derived crude with its toxicological profile, plus an explanation of the profiling system. This is a preliminary treatment of the data only, and is expected to be refined in subsequent use.

**Table IV.** Toxicologic Parameters

| | | | |
|---|---|---|---|
| A | Acute | I | Immunological class |
| S | Subacute | N | Neurological |
| C | Chronic | B | Behavioral |
| O | Ocular | R | Reproductive |
| I | Dermal irritation | M | Mutagenic |
| S | Dermal sensitization | O | Oncogenicity |
| P | Pulmonary | T | Teratogenicity |

**Table V.** Toxicology Rating System

| Level | | Descriptive Terms | |
|---|---|---|---|
| 4 | Extremely toxic (Oral LD$_{50}$ 1 mg/kg) | Irreversible adverse effect, low dose, or short exposure | Severe or extreme effect, low dose toxicant |
| 3 | Highly toxic (Oral LD$_{50}$ 2–49 mg/kg) | Irreversible adverse effect, high dose, or long exposure | Moderate effect, high dose toxicant |
| 2 | Moderately toxic (Oral LD$_{50}$ 50–500 mg/kg) | | Reversible effects after short-term exposure |
| 1 | Slightly toxic (Oral LD$_{50}$ 500–5,000 mg/kg) | | Reversible effects after long-term exposure |
| 0 | Relatively nontoxic (Oral LD$_{50}$ > 5,000 mg/kg) | No effect | Not a toxicant |
| X | No information identified | | |
| Y | Not applicable | | |

## SOHIO HAZARD ASSESSMENT SHEET

Chemical Name: Benzo(a)pyrene                                    Date: 10/11/83

    CAS No.: 5–32–8                                                      Initial: _____

## REGULATORY STATUS

| OSHA STD. (PEL) | ACGIH (TLV) | NIOSH REC'D STD |
|---|---|---|
| (1) | (2)    (2) | (3) |
| TWA = ___ppm; 0.2 mg/m³ | TWA = __ppm;__mg/m³ | TWA = ___ppm; 0.1 mg/m³ |
| CL = ___ppm; ___mg/m³ | STEL = ___ppm; ___mg/m³ | CL = ___ppm; ___mg/m³ |
| PEAK = ___ppm; ___mg/m³ | | |

ODOR THRESHOLD = ___ppm; ___mg/m³

## TOXICOLOGIC PROFILE

### ECOLOGIC PROFILE

| Characterizations | Organ-Systems | Activities |
|---|---|---|
| A  S  C  O  I  S | P  I  N  B  R | M  O  T |
| C  U  H  C  R  E | U  M  E  E  E | U  N  E |
| U  B  R  U  R  N | L  M  U  H  P | T  C  R |
| T  C  O  L  I  S | M  U  R  A  R | A  O  A |
| X  3  3  X  X  X | 3  X  X  X  0 | 1  3  4 |

| Ecologic Profile |
|---|
| P  B  A  B  A |
| E  I  Q  O  T |
| R  O  U  T  M |
| S  A  A  A  O |
| 3 X X X 1 |

## TARGET-ORGAN SPECIFICITY

|      | 0 | 1 | 2 | 3 | 4 | 5 | 6 | 7 | 8 | 9 | X | Y |
|------|---|---|---|---|---|---|---|---|---|---|---|---|
| ACUT | ✓ |   |   |   |   |   |   | ✓ |   |   |   |   |
| CHRO | ✓ | ✓ |   |   | ✓ | ✓ | ✓ |   |   |   |   |   |
| ONCO | ✓ | ✓ |   |   | ✓ | ✓ | ✓ | ✓ |   |   |   |   |

COMMENTS: (1) As coal tar pitch volatiles.

(2) Classified as suspect carcinogenic potential for man. No TLV listed.

(3) Based upon measurements of cyclohexane-extractable fraction of coal tar pitch
products.

## REFERENCE

1. Stallard, C.W., Jr., M.D. "A System for Data Collection and Computer Processing in Occupational Health Programs. The SOHIO Health Information System—Preliminary Report," in *Proceedings of the Symposium on Health Effects Investigation of Oil Shale Development,* W.H. Greist, M.R. Guerin, and D.L. Coffin, Eds. (Ann Arbor, MI: Ann Arbor Science Publishers, Inc., 1981), pp. 73–96.

# CHAPTER 6

## University of Minnesota-Duluth Low-Btu Gasifier Workplace Environment

S.D. Van Hoesen and
W.G. Dreibelbis
*Oak Ridge National Laboratory*
*Oak Ridge, TN 37831*

F.M. Thompson
*University of Minnesota,*
*Minneapolis, MN 55455*

D.B. Hunt
*Radian Corporation*
*Salt Lake City, UT 84115*

Final results are reported for the industrial hygiene evaluation portion of a comprehensive monitoring and testing program focused on a small Foster-Wheeler/Stoic coal gasifier at the University of Minnesota-Duluth. Personnel and plant area measurements for toxic gases, dusts, coal tars, noise, and heat stress are presented. Results of associated toxicology testing and medical monitoring of gasifier employees are discussed. Plant operations and equipment and controls performance are evaluated.

Results of these studies indicate that gasifiers of this size and type can be operated in compliance with current occupational exposure regulations and guidelines. However, it was determined that effective industrial hygiene support during operation was crucial to ensuring that employees were not overexposed. It was noted that plant operation impacted the level of exposure received by employees and that engineering controls were effective in reducing employee exposures.

### INTRODUCTION

Low-Btu gasification offers the potential for increasing coal utilization in industrial, commercial, and institutional applications. The U.S. Department of Energy instituted the Gasifiers in Industry (GII) program to investigate various types and applications of small state-of-the-art gasifiers. Oak Ridge National Laboratory (ORNL) was requested by the Office of Health and Environmental Research to develop an integrated, comprehensive environmental and health program for the GII. Program plans were prepared for two facilities, but the University of Minnesota-Duluth (UMD) gasifier was the only one built; it thus became the major focus of the health and environmental studies conducted in support of the GII program. Although they were not a part of the GII, limited industrial hygiene (IH) studies were also carried out at the Community Area New Development Organization (CANDO) and Morgantown Energy Technology Center (METC) gasifiers.

Because the workers would be so close to the gasifier, it was expected that they would be most likely to receive the highest individual exposures and the most likely to experience health effects, if any occurred. Consequently, evaluation of the occupational exposure and health situation was a major focus of the UMD program.[1] The information on worker exposure and health developed at UMD and presented in this chapter is somewhat site specific. However, information developed by ORNL at the two other low-Btu gasifiers (CANDO and METC) and information developed by Argonne National Laboratory at the Grand Forks Energy Technology Center (GFETC) gasifier and by the Inhalation Toxicology Research Institute at the METC gasifier, as well as the National Institute for Occupational Safety and Health, support the conclusion that the UMD experience can be considered as representative of small size, low-Btu fixed-bed gasifiers.

## INDUSTRIAL HYGIENE PROGRAM

The IH program at UMD has been a truly cooperative effort between University of Minnesota Health Services, Plant Services, and ORNL. The primary goal of the IH effort, protection of plant personnel, has been successfully achieved. Data developed concerning employee exposures and engineering controls have been extremely useful in assessing the employee health impacts that might arise from operation of similar small fixed-bed gasifiers. ORNL efforts at CANDO focused on providing IH support during start-up activities through a subcontract with Radian Corporation. Determination of employee exposures to carbon monoxide (CO) was a major activity. Efforts at METC involved the testing and demonstration of several developmental IH instruments.

The initial step in implementing the IH assessment program at UMD was to develop a plan to (1) identify the potential IH stresses that might be experienced at the gasifier, (2) develop the means for analyzing and monitoring these stresses, and (3) determine the effectiveness of control measures. The original IH plan was developed as part of the overall UMD Health and Environmental Plan.[1]

Through a review of the plant design and available information on coal conversion experience, a number of potential IH stresses were identified. These stresses and the currently recommended limits for worker exposure are presented in Table I. The plan contained provisions for both area and personal monitoring for these stresses. Because it was recognized that some unforeseen stresses might be encountered during UMD operation, the plan was designed to include a broad scoping/screening activity during early gasifier operation and to be flexible enough to respond as needed.

During development of the IH plan, a preoperational health assessment of the UMD gasifier was prepared.[2] The preoperational assessment utilized a general hazard index approach in which exposures to pollutants were compared with limiting values based on human health risk. When the preoperational assessment was conducted, no actual exposure data or UMD process stream composition data were available; therefore, concentrations of potentially hazardous substances that might appear in the UMD work-

**Table I.** Standards for Workroom Air Concentrations

| Contaminant | TLV/TWA[a] | | TLV/STEL[b] |
|---|---|---|---|
| Coal dust, <5% quartz | | | |
| respirable | 2 | mg/m³ | |
| total dust | 4 | mg/m³ | |
| CO | 50 | ppm | 400 ppm |
| NH₃ | 25 | ppm | 35 ppm |
| H₂S | 10 | ppm | 15 ppm |
| HCN | 10 | ppm (ceiling) | |
| Carbon disulfide | 10 | ppm (ceiling) | |
| Coal tar pitch volatiles, CTPV | 0.2 | mg/m³ | |
| Phenol | 5 | ppm | 10 ppm |
| Benzene | 10 | ppm | 25 ppm |
| Toluene | 100 | ppm | 150 ppm |
| Cresol | 5 | ppm | |
| Benzo(a)pyrene, tentative | 0.2 | μg/m³ | |
| Xylene | 100 | ppm | 150 ppm |

[a]The American Conference of Governmental Industrial Hygienists (ACGIH) has developed a threshold limit value—time-weighted average (TLV/TWA), which is a time-weighted average concentration for a normal 8-h workday or 40-h week, to which nearly all workers may be repeatedly exposed, day after day, without adverse effect (1982 ed.).

[b]TLV/STEL is the maximum concentration to which workers can be exposed for a period up to 15 min continuously without suffering from (1) intolerable irritation, (2) chronic or irreversible tissue change, or (3) narcosis of sufficient degree to increase accident proneness, impair self-rescue, or materially reduce work efficiency, provided there are no more than four excursions per day with 60 min between exposure periods and TLV/TWA is not exceeded.

place were estimated based on information available from similar systems. The study concluded that (1) occupational exposures were likely to be more important than public exposures; (2) carbon monoxide and coal tar compounds were likely to pose the most significant health hazard to workers; and (3) carbon monoxide should be a good "indicator compound" for toxic gas exposures at UMD but might not accurately reflect coal tar exposures.

The IH monitoring plan included provisions for evaluating personal exposures to carbon monoxide, other toxic gases, organic materials (coal tar), dust, heat stress, and noise. A toxicology program was undertaken to provide information on important process materials such as electrostatic precipitator (ESP) tar. Newly developed IH instruments were field tested and used as research tools for evaluating exposure to organic materials. A medical surveillance program was also instituted to evaluate worker health. In addition, operational parameters and IH experiences were evaluated to correlate IH monitoring results with plant operating conditions to allow evaluation of exposure controls. The following discussions summarize results of investigations in these areas. A full description of the UMD IH program is available.[3]

## PROCESS DESCRIPTIONS

### UMD Gasifier

An existing gas-fired heating plant at the UMD has been converted to burn low-Btu gas produced by coal gasification. In addition, tar by-product from the gasifier is being collected and used for peak heating requirements in an existing oil-fired boiler. The heating plant is shown schematically in Figure 1.

A Foster-Wheeler/Stoic two-stage gasifier was chosen for this application because (1) it offers a cleaner hot gas (bottom gas) than do single-stage gasifiers, and (2) it can produce a useful tar by-product from its other gas stream (top gas). The term "two-stage gasification" describes the dual offtake of product gases from the lower combustion/gasification zone and from the upper devolatilization zone. Commercially proven in South Africa, the gasifier design was developed by Stoic Combustion (Pty.) United and is licensed through Foster-Wheeler Energy Corporation.

A number of western coals have been used in the UMD gasifier. The coals have been generally low-sulfur low-ash coals that have been screened for size prior to shipment. The majority of gasifier runs during the program were with a Steamboat Springs, Colorado coal. More detail on the operating periods and coals used is presented in Table II.

After tramp iron and fines removal, up to 68 metric tons per day (mtpd) [75 tons per day (tpd)] of coal is dropped through steam-purged lock hoppers into the gasifier. As the coal falls through the 120–590°C (250–

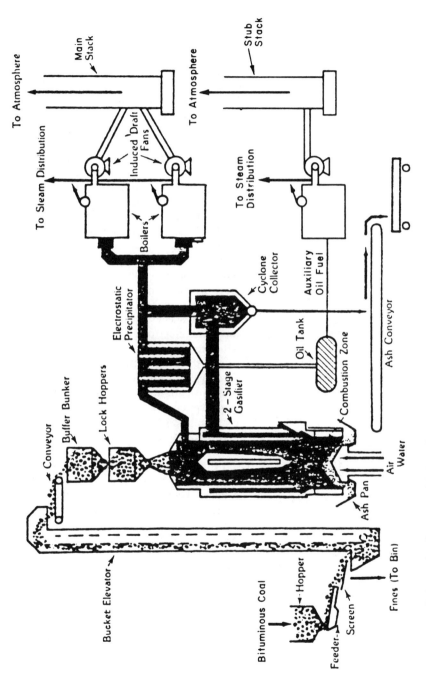

**Figure 1.**   Schematic diagram of UMD heating plant.

**Table II.**  Gasifier Run Data

| Run No. | Start Date | Terminate Date | Comments |
|---|---|---|---|
| 1 | 10/24/78 | 11/16/78 | Short shakedown test using only coke with maximum continuous operation of 20 h. The attempt at operation with a Wyoming Coal was unsuccessful. Numerous leaking flanges were found and the main butterfly gas control valve needed modification. |
| 2 | 2/17/79 | 3/2/79 | Used Wyoming-Big Horn and Indian Freeport Top coals. Maximum continuous operation was for 58 h before a leaking coal hopper and the failure of the ash removal system forced a shutdown. |
| 3 | 5/26/79 | 6/6/79 | Used Wyoming-Grass Creek Coal; terminated with a blowout of the mercury seal on the water pan bearings. Maximum continuous operation was for 105 h. |
| 4 | 9/28/79 | 10/7/79 | Used Colorado-Sun Mine coal; achieved a continuous operation of 170 h. Operation was quite successful until a cracked insulator in the electrostatic precipitator terminated the run. |
| 5 | 11/13/79 | 12/13/79 | This was the longest period of operation to date; used Colorado-Steamboat Springs coal throughout the run. The operation was stopped due to a large crack on the grate holder of the gasifier, which caused a major carbon monoxide leak around the gasifier. |
| 6 | 1/31/80 | 3/2/80 | Used Colorado-Routt County coal for most of the time period. A short ($\sim$1 d) run on a Pennsylvania subanthracite coal was somewhat unsuccessful and discontinued. The run was terminated to modify and repair the coal and ash handling systems. |
| 7 | 4/14/80 | 4/19/80 | Used Colorado-Steamboat Springs coal. The run was terminated due to major cracks appearing in the grate holder. A new grate holder was fabricated. |
| 8 | 1/17/81 | 6/27/81 | The most successful run to date; terminated with the end of the heating season. The main coal used during this time period was Colorado-Steamboat Springs coal, with a short ($\sim$3-d) test on Montana-Colstrip coal at the beginning of April and another test |

**Table II.**  *(continued)*

| Run No. | Start Date | Terminate Date | Comments |
|---|---|---|---|
|  |  |  | with Montana-Decker coal in June. Operation of the gasifier was continuous, except for several hot standby periods (total 135 h) caused by a flange leak, boiler difficulties, and the need to reduce the inventory of accumulated coal tar. |

1100°F) devolatilization zone, gas and tars are produced and exit from the top of the gasifier. Combustion and gasification of the devolatilized coal occur in a 590–980°C (1100–1800°F) zone, fed by air and steam to produce the bottom gas. Ash is removed beneath the gasifier from a water-filled pan, which serves to quench the hot ash and seal the gasifier to operating pressure [<1270 kg/m² (50-in. $H_2O$)].

Top and bottom gases are cleaned of tars and particulates before combination into boiler feed. Since the bottom gas at 980°C is primarily laden with particulates, a hot cyclone removes the dust for disposal. In contrast, the top gas contains tars and some particulates. These are removed in a hot ESP and stored in heated underground tanks for use as boiler feed during the winter months.

Two existing 1300-kg/h (25,000-lb/h) steam Keeler boilers (boilers 1 and 2) have been modified to burn the low-Btu gas rather than natural gas. ESP tar can be burned in either boiler or in a 2700-kg/h (50,000-lb/h) Combustion Engineering boiler (boiler 3). Flue gases from boilers 1 and 2 are fed to the main heating plant stack, while flue gases from the third boiler go to a stub stack.

### CANDO Gasifier

The CANDO gasifier consists of two Wellman-Galusha gasifiers fired with 45–68 mtpd (50–75 tpd) of anthraclite coal. The gas is scrubbed to remove particulate matter and cooled to produce a clean, dry gas that feeds the gas distribution system for a small industrial park. ORNL activities at CANDO primarily involved the provision, through a subcontract with Radian Corporation, of IH support during initial gasifier start-up and shakedown. A major goal was to characterize worker exposures to CO during start-up and user exposures during burning of the gas.

## METC Gasifier

The METC gasifier consists of a 22.7-mtpd (25-tpd) pressurized Wellman-Galusha gasifier. Gas cleanup equipment, including scrubbers and sulfur removal equipment, is provided to produce clean gas that is used in evaluating the potential for low-Btu gas use in industrial applications and in turbines. A variety of coals has been used at METC. ORNL activities primarily involved the testing of several developmental IH instruments.

## OPERATIONAL IMPACTS

Observations at the gasifier facilities during the IH program have indicated that operational parameters and equipment performance can have important effects on worker exposure. In addition, the studies have demonstrated that controls (engineering controls and personal protection) are effective in reducing employee exposures.

The operational parameters found to have the greatest effect on employee exposure for the small, low-temperature fixed-bed gasifiers studied were the type and condition of the coal used, which can directly impact the potential for tar production and consequent exposure. The high volatile content of the subbituminous coals used at UMD and the bituminous coal used at METC resulted in the production of large quantities of coal tar. Tar vapors and aerosols were released as fugitive emissions at many leak points in the process. In addition, processes installed to remove the tars from the gas stream to produce a clean gas also presented the potential for inhalation or skin exposure. Maintenance and cleanup operations were particularly important exposure sources. The low volatile content of the coal used at CANDO resulted in no discernible tar production.

The sulfur content of the coal would be expected to affect the production of hydrogen sulfide and other toxic sulfur compounds. UMD and CANDO both used low sulfur coal. Measurements at UMD indicated that CO levels consistently required more control than hydrogen sulfide levels. Although no gas measurements were made during the ORNL activities at METC, it is expected that with use of high sulfur coal, hydrogen sulfide and other sulfur compounds could be of comparable concern to CO.

The condition of the coal used was noted to strongly impact exposure potential; the fines content and friability of the coal were very important. Due to the nature of the fixed-bed gasification process, accurately sized coal [generally 1.3–6.4 cm (0.5–2.5 in.)] is required for smooth gasifier operation. When coal with a high fines content is used, or if the coal breaks up quickly as it is gasified, the air flow channels in the coal bed become clogged and uneven firebed distribution can occur, causing operational upsets. At UMD, these upsets generally required extensive poking to redistribute the fines material and move it through the gasifier to reestablish normal operation.

As discussed later, the poking operation was associated with higher CO, noise, and heat exposures. Coal of high fines content also resulted in elevated coal dust levels in the plant during coal handling operations.

Gasifier operating temperatures and pressures also had some effects on employee exposure potential. Higher temperature operation at UMD produced a more viscous tar that was difficult to handle, and higher operating pressures generally increased the potential for process gas leaks. At UMD, high pressures tended to cause problems in establishing steam flow to the poke hole injectors and, in a few instances, the pressures were high enough to cause gas to bubble through the main water seal in the ash pan.

Experiences at UMD and CANDO indicated that certain operations and equipment were major sources for emissions that contributed to employee exposures. In most cases, however, these emissions could be reduced or eliminated by using appropriate controls. More detailed discussion of these experiences is provided in the following sections, which summarize employee exposure experiences.

## EMPLOYEE EXPOSURES

### Carbon Monoxide and Other Toxic Gases

The acute toxic air contaminant of most concern generated during the gasification process at UMD is CO. Under design operating conditions, CO levels in the product gas stream can reach 30%. If even a small leak occurs, CO concentrations in the gasifier area can reach levels of concern from an IH viewpoint. This problem is magnified at UMD because the gasifier must be enclosed, because of the extreme weather in northern Minnesota, and any contaminants released in the building can accumulate.

Measurement of CO levels in the gasifier building was accomplished with a number of instruments. Four single-point CO area monitors equipped with visual and audible alarms provided the primary means to detect elevated CO levels. Personal dosimeters were used during the first year of operation to provide daily time-weighted average (TWA) personnel exposures to CO. After the fourth run, two four-point sequential scan CO area monitors were installed and provided data that were logged on the computer system for real-time access and later reference. These data were used to provide plots of CO levels vs time and helped to identify equipment and operations that were release sources. These monitors were also fitted with visual and audible alarms. Two portable, direct reading monitors were used to assist in determining general area CO levels and to locate leaks.

A number of leak points contributed to the CO exposures at UMD. During early runs, the main emission sources were leaky process and equipment flanges and seals. These leaks were usually stopped by tightening flange bolts. In cases where bolt tightening was not effective, either the joints were welded over directly or a U-shaped box was welded over the joint to provide a leak-tight seal. In some cases, additional gasket or packing material was effective. During later runs, leak points were identified with degraded or failed equipment. For example, elevated CO emissions during run No. 5 (see Table III) resulted from the failed grate holder and were eventually severe enough to terminate operation until a new grate could be procured.

Several leak points were also associated with specific pieces of equipment and routine operations. As such, the leaks were highest during early operation and were reduced as equipment was improved or controls such as auxiliary ventilation were added. Major leak sources were associated with initial lighting of the gasifier when the fire was being established under natural draft conditions, cycling of the cyclone lock hoppers to remove char, manual poking operations, and coal-feed lock-hopper cycling.

Carbon monoxide exposures to the plant workers, as determined by personal and area monitoring, were low; in most cases exposures were well below the applicable standard of 50-ppm TWA. As indicated in Table III,

**Table III.**   Summary of UMD Carbon Monoxide Exposures and Measurements

| Personnel dosimetry exposures | | |
|---|---|---|
| *Run* | | *ppm* |
| 1 | Geometric mean | 4.1 |
| | Range | 0.8–18.9 |
| | $\sigma$ | 3.6 |
| 2 | Geometric mean | 12.4 |
| | Range | 2.3–31.2 |
| | $\sigma$ | 1.6 |
| 3 | Geometric mean | 5.5 |
| | Range | 0.3–49.2 |
| | $\sigma$ | 2.7 |
| Area monitoring measurements | | |
| | *Frequency(%)* | |
| 5 | 32.5 | 0–10 |
| | 48.4 | 11–35 |
| | 8.2 | 36–50 |
| | 10.9 | >51 |
| 6 | 66.4 | 0–10 |
| | 30.9 | 11–36 |
| | 2.7 | >36 |
| 8 | 68.1 | 0–10 |
| | 23.4 | 11–35 |
| | 4.2 | 36–50 |
| | 4.3 | >51 |

during run No. 1 a geometric mean TWA exposure of 4.1-ppm CO ($\sigma$ = 3.6 ppm) was measured. During run No. 2, a higher mean TWA exposure of 12.4-ppm CO ($\sigma$ = 1.6 ppm) was determined, while during run No. 3 better control of exposures resulted in a reduced mean TWA of 5.5-ppm CO ($\sigma$ = 2.7 ppm). During run No. 4 difficulties were experienced with the personal dosimeters such as problems with calibration and false alarms. Consequently, data from this run were not considered valid.

For runs 5 through 8, the multipoint recording area CO monitors were operational and TWA exposures at each monitoring station could be calculated. It should be kept in mind that these readings represent potential exposure levels. In most cases, operators spent most of their time at the control panel where CO levels were generally the lowest, and only a small fraction of their time was spent in the areas with higher CO levels. Actual personal exposures would thus be expected to be slightly higher than the TWAs measured at the control panel location.

Analyses of the CO monitoring data identified a number of significant points:

1.  As indicated in Table III, differences in the overall frequency of elevated CO emissions from run to run were noted. The higher frequency of elevated emissions seen during run No. 5 is thought to result from the leaking grate holder assembly. The grate was repaired and emissions were reduced, as indicated by the higher frequency of lower emissions seen during run No. 6. Run No. 8 had a slightly higher emission frequency than No. 6, even though a new grate holder was installed; this grate should have performed at least as well as the repaired grate during run No. 6. It is possible that equipment was degraded somewhat due to the longer run time (5 months for run No. 8 vs 1.5 months for run No. 6). Since some maintenance is generally performed during shutdown, a short run would tend to have slightly better maintained equipment than a long run.

2.  As indicated in Figure 2, no consistent differences in TWAs were noted from shift to shift. This suggests that on an average basis, exposures are independent of shift. Direct observation of specific operators, however, does suggest some difference in exposure from operator to operator.

3.  Differences in TWAs and in frequency of release levels from monitoring point to point are also apparent in Figure 2. In the heating plant, TWA exposures were lowest in the boiler area (locations 225 and 690) and at the gasifier control panel (location 302), with levels measured generally increasing in the following manner:

    basement (location 108) < char hopper (316) < coal scale (802) < poking deck (452) < coal feed level (615).

    In general, exposures measured reflected effects of nearby emission sources and ventilation patterns in the building.

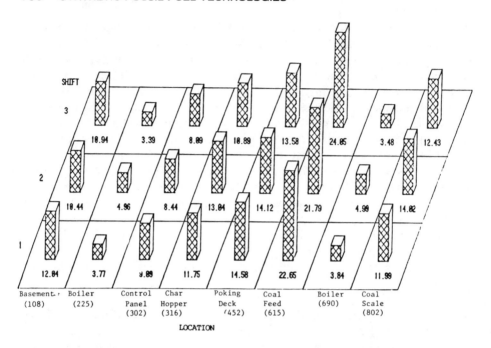

**Figure 2.** Block chart of mean carbon monoxide levels from area monitoring (in parts per million).

Similar CO exposure situations were experienced at CANDO. As with UMD, CO releases were highest during early operations. From Table IV, operator TWAs of 50 to 100-ppm TWA were associated with the start-up of gasifier No. 1 (Phase 1). These relatively high exposures were caused by many leaks in the gasifier body and associated piping, which were located and plugged as operations progressed. Another contributing factor was that the operators were learning how to operate the gasifier and tended to spend a large amount of time at the operator level and the poking level where exposure levels were highest.

Before start-up of gasifier No. 2 (Phase 2), and before start-up of other portions of the system, thorough pressure leak testing was performed to identify leaks so that they could be plugged before operation. Operator exposures during start-up of gasifier No. 2 were reduced significantly to 15-ppm TWA. Once routine operations were established, operator TWAs with one gasifier operating were in the range of 7 to 10 ppm, similar to levels experienced at UMD.

Gas emissions at CANDO were also associated with certain operations. Coal feeding and poking operations were major exposure sources. On the CANDO gasifier, there are no poke hole steam injection mechanisms such as those on the UMD gasifier (described below). Thus, the operator may

**Table IV.**   Summary of Carbon Monoxide Measurements during Startup Operations at CANDO

|  |  | *ppm* |
|---|---|---|
| **Personnel exposures** |  |  |
| Phase 1 | 50–100 ppm TWA |  |
| Phase 2 | 15 ppm TWA |  |
| Routine operation | 7–10 ppm TWA |  |
| **Area levels** |  |  |
| General plant | Average | 5–10 |
|  | Range | <5–>1000 |
| Operator level | Average | 5 |
|  | Range | 5–15 |
| Top of producer | Average | 10 |
|  | Range | 5–10 |
| Coal bin level | Average | 20–50 |
|  | Range | 20–>500 |
| Gas user | Average | 5 |
| **Source emissions** |  |  |
| Poking operation | Average | 100 |
|  | Range | up to 600 |
| Coal bin | Range | 200–>3000 |
| Cyclone flange leaks | Range | 600–2000 |
| Water settling tanks |  |  |
| Leaks |  |  |
| $CO$ |  | >600 |
| $H_2S$ |  | >50 |
| Ambient |  |  |
| $CO$ |  | 10 |
| $H_2S$ |  | 1 |
| Exhaust |  |  |
| $CO$ |  | 1000 |
| $H_2S$ |  | 20 |
| $NH_3$ |  | 20 |

be exposed to CO levels up to 600 ppm (average 100 ppm) for 5 min every 2–4 h, when the poking operation is conducted. Even though operators avoid the major release stream from the poke hole, overall CO levels on the poking deck are elevated.

Elevated levels of CO and other gases were associated with leaks from the scrubbing water settling and surge tanks, which are located under the floor on the ground level. Apparently, fairly substantial amounts of process gas were being entrained or dissolved in the scrubbing water, which resulted in high gas levels in the water tank head space. This gas leaked into the ground floor area through cracks around pump and access hatch openings. Levels associated with these leaks are included in Table IV. To prevent gas leaks into the building and to reduce the possibility of an explosion, the tanks were sealed as tightly as possible and exhausted to the outside through a vent. This effectively eliminated releases into the building.

Carbon monoxide levels associated with use of the product gas by the CANDO industrial customer were in the 5-ppm range, similar to those experienced at UMD.

One of the important questions associated with operation of low-Btu gasifiers is whether CO can be used as an indicator compound to monitor for toxic gases. If it can be shown that when CO levels are kept below threshold limit value (TLV) all other gases are kept below their TLVs, then it would be possible to concentrate monitoring efforts on CO while having confidence that other toxic gas exposures are adequately controlled. Table V presents measured UMD process levels and associated TLVs and short-term exposure limits (STELs). By comparing process levels with the TLVs and STELs, a "reduction factor" can be calculated that reflects the degree of control required to keep the representative gas level below its TLV or STEL. Comparing the reduction factors required for the various gases of interest ($R_{CO}/R_N$) yields a measure of the relative importance of the gases. As can be seen from Table V, the control required for CO is from 41 to 166 times greater than that for other toxic gases ($NH_3$, HCN, $H_2S$, COS) when the TLV is considered. When the STEL is considered, 7 to 20 times better control of CO is required.

At CANDO, no actual process gas measurements are available except for the gases in the water tanks. Because of the uncertainty in the mechanism by which gases are introduced into the tanks (e.g., entrainment or release of dissolved gases), it is possible that the gases in the tanks are not present in the same ratios as in the process streams. A comparison of the gas levels measured in the tanks indicates that better control of CO (as compared to hydrogen sulfide and ammonia) is required by a factor of 10

**Table V.** Comparison of Toxic Gas Exposure Potential at UMD (ppm)

|  | CO | $NH_3$ | HCN | $H_2S$ | COS |
|---|---|---|---|---|---|
| Process | $3 \times 10^5$ | 3660 | 360 | 900 | 370 |
| TLV | 50 | 25 | 10 | 10 | 10 |
| Reduction factor | 6000 | 147 | 36 | 90 | 37 |
| $R_{CO}/R_N$ | 1 | 41 | 166 | 67 | 162 |
| STEL | 400 | 35 | 10 | 15 | 10 |
| Reduction factor | 750 | 104 | 36 | 60 | 37 |
| $R_{CO}/R_N$ | 1 | 7 | 20 | 12 | 20 |
| Actual workplace measurement | 10–20 | <1 | <1 | <1 |  |

to 25 when the TLV is considered and by a factor of 1.9 to 4.4 when the STEL is used as the limiting exposure.

Considering these data, the following conclusions are drawn:

- In all cases encountered, CO required major monitoring attention based on its content in process streams and emissions. Continuous area monitoring for CO, which was supplemented by personal monitoring, is suggested at all low-Btu fixed-bed gasifiers.
- Carbon monoxide appears to be a good candidate for an "indicator compound" with the following qualifications:
    1.  In all instances, a comparison of process stream concentrations and limiting health values should be performed to confirm its appropriateness as an indicator.
    2.  If CO is used as an indicator, a thorough facility-wide survey of all toxic gases should be performed early in operation to confirm that actual workplace measurements are consistent with expectations.
    3.  Both UMD and CANDO use low sulfur (0.5–1%) coal. It is expected that most small, low-Btu gasifiers will use low sulfur coal to comply with air pollution regulations. However, if higher sulfur coals are used, hydrogen sulfide and other sulfur compounds may require expanded monitoring attention. If high-sulfur coal is used and sulfur removal equipment is installed, hydrogen sulfide monitoring will be required in areas containing this equipment and possibly throughout the plant, depending on plant layout and ventilation. The same is true for ammonia recovery systems.
    4.  CANDO experience suggests that water cleanup systems will require careful evaluation because of the potential for mechanisms that could selectively concentrate certain gas (e.g., $H_2S$, $NH_3$).

### Dust

Dust levels at UMD were monitored using high-volume area and lower-volume personal sampling. Experience indicates that dust levels are highly dependent on coal condition and handling operations. During early operations, high levels of dust (to 17.4 mg/m³, as compared with a background of <0.1 mg/m³ and a TLV of 2 mg/m³) were noted. Run No. 5 had the highest levels. The geometric mean for total dust was 3.3 mg/m³ with a range of 1.13–17.4 mg/m³. These excursions resulted from use of coal that had been stored outside over the winter and had become extremely friable and dusty. This was exacerbated by the UMD coal handling system, which was not very "tight" and tended to break the coal up during transport.

Subsequently, more care was used in storing and handling coal, and modifications were made to reduce breakup of the coal during handling and to tighten up the system. During run No. 6, the range of total particulate levels was 0.18–2.97 mg/m$^3$ with a geometric mean of 0.60 mg/m$^3$. During run No. 8, particulate levels were further reduced, with a geometric mean of 0.27 mg/m$^3$ and a range of <0.1–3.32 mg/m$^3$.

A number of the dust samples were evaluated for organic content. As discussed in the section on organic exposure, organic content of the collections was low, as were the coal tar pitch volatile results, suggesting that coal dust was the prime source of particulate matter at UMD. In addition, a concentrated sampling effort was conducted during run No. 6 to evaluate respirable fractions of particulates. An Anderson impactor and a piezo balance were used to develop the total and respirable dust measurements presented in Table VI; respirable levels were quite low.

### Noise

A thorough survey of the UMD facility was conducted to evaluate noise levels. In most parts of the building, noise was associated with specific op-

**Table VI.** Dust Measurements at UMD

| Location | Operating Conditions | Sampling Time | Concentration (mg/m$^3$) |
|---|---|---|---|
| Total dust measurements using Anderson impactor | | | |
| Basement area | Wet coal being conveyed, no visible dust | 3 h 53 min | 0.04 |
| Third level near stairs (coal feed area) | Coal being feed, no visible dust | 7 h 35 min | 1.0 |
| Basement area | Coal being conveyed, no visible dust | 4 h 53 min | 0.4 |
| Basement near coal conveyor | Coal being conveyed | 2 h 9 min | 1.8 |
| Respirable dust measurements using the Piezo balance | | | |
| | | Sample No. | |
| Near coal conveyor | Coal being conveyed | 1 | 0.07 |
| | | 2 | 0.07 |
| | | 3 | 0.05 |
| | | 4 | 0.05 |
| Top of stairs (third level) | Coal buffer bunker being filled | 1 | 0.03 |
| | | 2 | 0.03 |
| | | 3 | 0.03 |
| | | 4 | 0.03 |
| In coal bunker | No coal being conveyed | 1 | 0.05 |
| | | 2 | 0.04 |
| | | 3 | 0.05 |
| | | 4 | 0.02 |

erations, most notably coal handling, coal feeding, and poking. Noise levels in the basement area were of a more general nature.

The highest noise levels at UMD are associated with poking. During poking, a steam venturi injects a curtain of steam into the gasifier poke hole to contain the producer gas while the poke rod is inserted into the gasifier. This high velocity steam creates noise levels from 97 dBA in areas away from the poking to 107 dBA near the poking operation. This noise source is normally active 5–15 min/h. No means have been identified to reduce the noise levels at the source. Consequently, workers wear hearing protection (ear muffs) when poking.

High noise levels were originally associated with cycling of the coal-feed lock-hopper valves. These valves are actuated by compressed air, and noise levels during the exhaust phase of valve operation could reach 105 dBA near the valve. After the fourth run, steel-wool-packed mufflers were installed on the valve operator exhausts, reducing the noise levels to 78 dBA. The effectiveness of the mufflers has degraded over time, and levels have risen to 90 dBA.

Elevated noise levels were measured inside the coal bunker when coal handling equipment was operated. Levels of 91–100 dBA were noted. Personnel who must work in this area when the coal handling equipment is operating wear hearing protection.

Noise levels in the basement are of a more general nature, with vibrations from the coal handling equipment, the hydraulic pump and auger, and the blast air fans. Noise sources varied from 87–95 dBA. Workers wear hearing protection when conducting any extensive activities in the basement.

Noise levels at the gasifier control panel, where workers spend the majority of their time, normally are in the range of 80–86 dBA. Levels can rise to 90 dBA during coal handling and vary from 91–94 dBA during the poking operation. Noise levels in the boiler area range from 85–90 dBA, and in the gasifier area (with the gasifier down) from 73–76 dBA.

### Heat Stress

When the UMD gasifier was operated during warmer months (September and October, May and June), it was observed that worker heat stress could be a problem. The major potential for heat stress was associated with the poking operation. Several factors interacted to cause this situation: (1) poking can require extended vigorous physical activity; (2) workers routinely wear heavy coveralls that limit cooling; (3) the bare metal body of the gasifier at the poking area can reach 130°C; (4) the entire south wall of the gasifier building is glass, which can result in strong solar input; and (5) air movement in the poking area is generally minimal.

Measurements during the poking operation indicated that the potential for heat stress is high when outside temperatures are >4.5°C (>40°F) and the poking operation requires extended activity (longer than the normal 5–

15 min). Avoiding overworking of the gasifier operators during warm periods is the only means currently available to reduce the potential for heat stress at the UMD facility.

### Mercury

As originally designed, the UMD gasifier contained approximately 72.6 kg (160 lb) of mercury in a liquid-column pressure seal. This assembly was located in the undergrate area and maintained gasifier pressure at the seal between the stationary blast air pipe and the rotating ash grate assembly (Figure 3). (A water seal in the ash pan is used to maintain the main pressure seal between the gasifier and the atmosphere.)

Small leaks of elemental mercury and emissions of the vapor were experienced intermittently during early operation. Contributing factors were:

1. The surface of the mercury in the seal was open (i.e., not enclosed), thus providing a means for mercury vapor emission and a path for mercury leaks due to gasifier pressure variations.
2. The seal was not constructed as originally designed, resulting in a

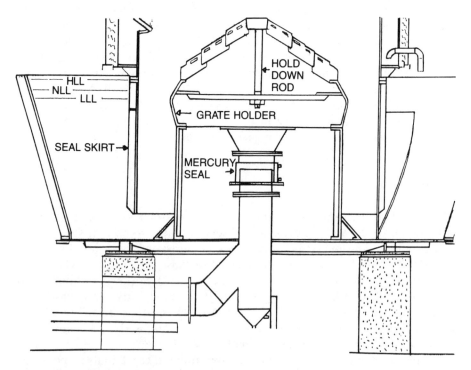

**Figure 3.** UMD mercury seal.

shallower effective seal depth than was needed. This led to fluctuations in the mercury level, causing mercury to leak from the seal.

3.     The seal was apparently overfilled when the gasifier was first started so that mercury leaked down into the blast air pipe and was blown out when the blast air blower was turned on.

As a result of these problems, the gasifier undergrate area and the gasifier building in general experienced mercury contamination. Levels in the undergrate area were highest, with liquid mercury droplets noted on the concrete floor of the access area. General building levels were also elevated, with the basement area and first-floor areas around the gasifier reaching levels high enough to require personnel exclusion.

In March the seal was drained for inspection. During this procedure the mercury levels in the undergrate area rose from 0.01 mg/m$^3$ to 0.6–0.7 mg/m$^3$ 1.5 h later (mercury TLV 0.05 mg/m$^3$, STEL 0.15 mg/m$^3$).

The exposed industrial hygienist and the engineer noted some minor eye irritation after the exposure. No acute symptoms were observed, but a urinalysis was conducted for the hygienist as a precaution. The tests proved negative. Due to recurrent problems, an order was placed for a new mechanical seal to replace the mercury seal, but operations continued pending its arrival. Mercury vapor masks were obtained for employee protection.

Problems with mercury leaks continued throughout the spring of 1979 despite installation of a catch pan and modification of the seal to increase the effective depth. On June 6, 1979, an electrical storm caused a power surge that shut off the gas to the boilers, causing the gasifier to overpressurize. This overpressurization completely blew out the mercury seal, resulting in mercury levels from 0.05–0.7 mg/m$^3$ in the gasifier area and from 0.02–0.03 mg/m$^3$ in the boiler areas. The gasifier area was immediately evacuated. The industrial hygienist wore a self-contained breathing apparatus (SCBA) to inspect the seal area. After the undergrate area was cooled with water, the mercury seal was repoured so that an air-tight pressure seal could be reestablished, allowing workers to gain control of the gasifier and shut it down.

To clean up the undergrate area and remove the mercury seal required 6 weeks. Workers were required to wear SCBA for much of the time until levels were low enough so that vapor masks or no protection was required. The mercury seal was replaced with a Teflon mechanical seal, which has functioned well. The use of a seal containing hazardous material such as mercury should be avoided wherever possible.

### Bottom Ash and Cyclone Char

Two solid wastes are produced at UMD during operation. Significant quantities of bottom ash [~5 mtpd (~5 tpd)], consisting of unconverted coal, ash, and mineral residue, are removed in a wet form from the ash pan. Significant problems were experienced with the ash-handling system and have required many hours of labor for repair and cleanout. During those operations, workers experienced frequent contact with the wet ash. However, based on the chemical composition of the ash and limited toxicity testing results, skin exposure is not expected to be hazardous, and because the ash is wet it produces no dust. Thus, employee hazard from these exposures is negligible. The work involved in cleaning out and repairing the ash-handling system is dirty and difficult and tends to divert attention from other gasifier operations. Improvements to the ash-handling system have reduced the need for these maintenance and repair operations.

Fine particulate matter, consisting primarily of unreacted coal and ash material, is removed from the bottom gas stream in the hot cyclone. A three-valve lock-hopper system is used to discharge the small quantity of char collected into a hopper feeding an auger, which drops the char into a carboy in the basement. Carbon monoxide emissions are associated with the discharge operation, and the very fine nature of the materials can cause elevated dust levels. Although the char does not appear to be a hazardous material, care is used during char handling to keep dust levels controlled.

### Organics and Coal Tars

The use of subbituminous coals at UMD (~35 to 40% volatiles) results in the production of a dense tar aerosol in the top-gas stream. These tar aerosols and associated vapors are emitted at leak points associated with the coal scale and coal-feed lock hoppers. The tar (and associated particulate matter) is removed from the top gas in the ESP and is collected for storage and subsequent burning as a supplemental boiler fuel. Leaks in the tar transfer lines and frequent maintenance and repair associated with tar pump failures present potential for employee skin and inhalation exposure.

Tar produced during gasification is the prime source of exposure to organic materials at UMD. As indicated in Table VII, the tar consists primarily of carbon, hydrogen, and nitrogen.[4] Table VIII shows that (as with other tars produced during gasification processes) the UMD tar is composed primarily of neutral materials, with some acids and generally low levels of base materials. The lower portion of Figure 4 is a chromatogram of a typical UMD tar, which indicates that a major portion of the tar consists of N-paraffins ($C_{15}-C_{36}$). Tar head space vapor analysis identified the presence of alkylated benzenes, naphthalenes, phenol, and m-cresol. More detailed analyses of the tars identified the presence of a number of polycyclic aromatic hydrocarbons, as indicated in Table IX, and a number of aromatic amines, as indicated in Table X. These materials are of particular interest because of their suspected carcinogenic and mutagenic potential.

Worker skin exposures to the tars were evaluated. In general, the

**Table VII.**  ASTM Standard Analyses of ESP Tars[a]

| Gasifier Run | Number of Samples | Tar (wt%)[a] | | | | | | | | |
|---|---|---|---|---|---|---|---|---|---|---|
| | | C | H | N | O | S | Ash | Moisture | Heating Value (Btu/lb) | Pyridine Insolubles (wt %) |
| 2 | 1 | 77.3 | 7.8 | 1.2 | 13.5 | 0.64 | 0 | 0.9 | 16,200 | <0.01 |
| 5 | 5 | 83.0 ± 3.0 | 8.8 ± 1.9 | 1.1 ± 0.2 | | 0.76 ± 0.14 | | 0.99 | 16,200 ± 1,400 | 2.8 |
| 5 | 1[b] | 84.5 | 9.7 | 0.9 | | 0.52 | | <0.06 | 16,500 | 0.04 |
| 6 | 18 | 81.0 ± 3.2 | 8.5 ± 1.1 | 1.3 ± 0.8 | | 0.43 ± 0.13 | | 0.61 ± 0.61 | 16,000 ± 1,100 | |
| 8 | 18 | 84.0 ± 2.3 | 10.4 ± 1.0 | 0.87 ± 0.24 | 3.9 ± 3.2 | 0.34 ± 0.05 | 0.90 ± 0.69 | 2.1 ± 1.2 | 15,800 ± 900 | 1.5 ± 2.3 |
| 8 | 4[c] | 84.6 ± 2.5 | 10.8 ± 1.5 | 0.93 ± 0.41 | 3.1 ± 3.8 | 0.39 ± 0.05 | 0.12 ± 0.06 | 1.8 ± 0.3 | 15,900 ± 500 | 0.02 ± 0.02 |

[a]/Average ± standard deviation listed for sets of more than one sample.
[b]Tar tank tar.
[c]Tar to boiler.

**Table VIII.** Chemical Class Fractionation Results for ESP and Other Tars

| Gasifier Run | Number of Samples | Tar (wt %)[a] | | | | | | | | |
|---|---|---|---|---|---|---|---|---|---|---|
| | | Ether Soluble Bases | Insoluble Bases | Ether Soluble Acids | Insoluble Acids | Neutral Saturates | Neutral Aromatics | Polar Polyaromatics | Total Neutrals | Recovered |
| 2 | 1 | 5.3 | 0.4 | 13.3 | 2.4 | 18.6 | 35.9 | 26.7 | 0.4 | 108[b] |
| 3 | 1 | 1.3 | 0.4 | 13.1 | 2.1 | 14.2 | 33.4 | 26.9 | 3.4 | 104[c] |
| 5 | 5 | 3.8 ± 0.9 | 6.9 ± 9.3 | 12.3 ± 6.2 | 2.0 ± 2.1 | 19.1 ± 9.0 | 30.9 ± 9.9 | 21.0 ± 9.3 | 4.8 ± 1.4 | 97.9 ± 6.3 |
| 5 | 1[d] | 1.8 | <0.1 | 5.1 | 0.6 | 42.0 | 31.3 | 10.9 | 6.6 | 97 |
| 6 | 18 | 4.9 ± 4.5 | 6.7 ± 9.9 | 10.6 ± 5.8 | 1.2 ± 0.7 | 23.8 ± 8.0 | 30.9 ± 6.2 | 16.2 ± 5.0 | 3.2 ± 1.4 | 96.3 ± 6.6 |
| 6 | 1[e] | 1.6 | 12.1 | 4.4 | 0.7 | 23.8 | 20.6 | 7.2 | 3.5 | 70.7 |
| 8 | 4 | 1.9 ± 0.5 | 0.7 ± 0.7 | 9.0 ± 4.1 | 0.6 ± 0.2 | 11.6 ± 13.8 | 35.9 ± 5.1 | 23.7 ± 7.8 | 3.6 ± 2.8 | 97.9 ± 6.1 |
| 8 | 5[f] | 1.3 ± 0.2 | T[g] | 6.3 ± 0.3 | 0.2 ± 0.1 | 24.6 ± 2.9 | 37.9 ± 3.4 | 25.1 ± 4.3 | 2.8 ± 1.0 | 99.7 ± 3.0 |

[a] Average ± standard deviation listed for sets of more than one sample.
[b] Includes 5.1% volatiles.
[c] Includes 2.2% volatiles.
[d] Tar tank tar.
[e] Lock hopper cyclone material.
[f] Composite of 11 tars fractioned 5 times.
[g] T = trace, <0.05%.

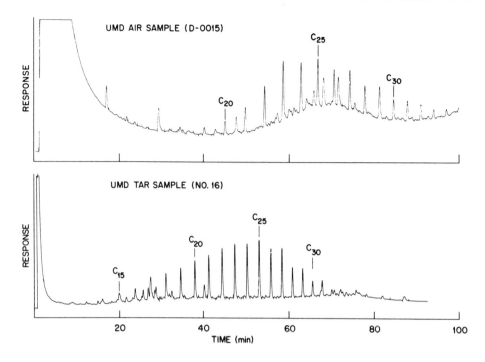

**Figure 4.**  Comparison of UMD tar and air samples.

frequency and extent of skin contamination with tar was found to be low. Routine use of full coveralls and heavy cotton gloves by the gasifier operators was effective in controlling incidental tar contamination. During operations that presented significant potential for tar contamination (e.g., valve

**Table IX.**  Polycyclic Aromatic Hydrocarbons (PAHs) Determined in ESP Tar 16

| PAH | Concentration (µg/g) |
|---|---|
| Fluoranthene | 180 |
| Pyrene | 110 |
| Benzo($a$)fluorene | 150 |
| Benzo($b$)fluorene | 100 |
| 3-Methyl pyrene | 90 |
| Benz($a$)anthracene | 140 |
| Chrysene/triphenylene | 90 |
| Benzo($b + j$)fluoranthenes | 140 |
| Benzo($a$)pyrene | 80 |
| Perylene | 110 |

**Table X.**  Polyaromatic Amines (PAA) Determined in ESP Tar 16

| PAA | Concentration (µg/g) |
|---|---|
| 1-Aminonaphthalene | 9 |
| 2-Aminonaphthalene | 30 |
| $C_1$-Aminonaphthalenes | 4–24[a] |
| $C_2$-Aminonaphthalenes | 7–10[b] |
| $C_3$-Aminonaphthalene | 7 |
| Aminofluorene | 9 |
| 1-Aminoanthracene | 13 |
| 2-Aminoanthracene | 2 |
| $C_1$-Aminoanthracene | 1 |
| Acridine | 26 |

[a]Range of results for five separate isomers.
[b]Range of results for three separate isomers.

maintenance, tar spill cleanup), workers wore rubber gloves and, in some cases, such as when entering the ESP, full-body impervious suits and SCBA. In addition, workers are encouraged to wash if they are aware of any tar contact and to shower at the end of every shift. Measurements with the luminoscope (see the following section) did identify isolated instances of skin contamination on a few workers during one special study. Measurements also indicated that the contamination was fairly easy to remove by washing. Similar measurements at METC indicated that tar produced there was much harder to remove from the skin by washing.

As discussed in later sections, toxicological evaluation indicated that the tar was not acutely toxic to the skin, although contact with the eye could produce temporary irritation. Effective control of acute tar exposures is confirmed by the absence of any worker complaints of skin problems associated with tar contamination.

An inhalation exposure potential also exists from the tar aerosols and vapors emitted from leaks in the top-gas lines, particularly the coal-feed lock hoppers, and from vapors produced by tar contamination on hot surfaces. Coal tar pitch volatiles were determined for a number of air samples; levels were generally low, with none being higher than one-half the 0.2-mg/m³ TLV. Extractable organic levels on high-volume filter pads were quite low and, as indicated in the upper portion of Figure 4 and in Table XI, appeared to reflect quite closely the composition of ESP tar.

Vapor-phase sampling was conducted using charcoal, Tenax, and other absorbants, with Tenax proving to be the most effective collection material. As indicated in Table XII, the vapors detected in the workplace atmosphere are reflective of the tar-headspace vapor analyses conducted. Measurements described in the following section also identified some of these compounds and confirmed the low levels (generally in the parts-per-billion range) of

**Table XI.**  Composite Pad Extract Analysis

| N-Paraffins | Total Identified | Polynuclear Aromatics | Total Identified |
|-------------|------------------|------------------------|------------------|
|             | (%)              |                        | (%)              |
| C-11        | 0.42             | Biphenyl               | 0.06             |
| C-12        | 0.50             | 2,3,5-Trimethylnaphthalene | 0.03         |
| C-13        | 0.82             | Fluorene               | 0.05             |
| C-14        | 1.68             | 1-Methylfluorene       | 0.11             |
| C-15        | 2.00             | Phenanthrene           | 0.62             |
| C-16        | 2.20             | Anthracene             | 0.23             |
| C-17        | 3.67             | 2-Methylphenanthrene   | 0.87             |
| C-18        | 3.67             | 2-Methylanthracene     | 0.13             |
| C-19        | 3.95             | 1-Methylphenanthrene   | 0.43             |
| C-20        | 5.36             | 3,6-Dimethylphenanthrene | 0.19           |
| C-21        | 7.34             | Fluoranthene           | 0.83             |
| C-22        | 7.62             | Pyrene                 | 0.55             |
| C-23        | 7.05             | 3-Methylpyrene         | 0.22             |
| C-24        | 5.36             | Benzo($ghi$)fluoranthene | 0.19           |
| C-25        | 9.03             | Chrysene               | 0.45             |
| C-26        | 5.64             | Benzo($b + j$)fluoranthenes | 0.19        |
| C-27        | 9.88             | Benzo($a$)pyrene       | 0.40             |
| C-28        | 4.51             | Perylene               | 0.15             |
| C-29        | 3.95             | Benz($a$)anthracene    | 0.40             |
| C-30        | 2.26             | Total                  | 6.10             |
| C-31        | 2.26             |                        |                  |
| C-32        | 0.68             |                        |                  |
| C-33        | 3.67             |                        |                  |
| C-34        | 0.87             |                        |                  |
| Total       | 94.39            |                        |                  |

these materials. Some worker complaints of nausea and loss of appetite were associated with early operations when condensed tar leaking from the coal feed valves dripped onto the hot top of the gasifier. The vaporization of this tar contamination was thought to be responsible for the complaints. Drip pans were installed to control the tar contamination, and complaints subsided.

### Developmental Instruments

Four developmental instruments to detect and monitor organic exposure were tested at UMD and METC.[5] The derivative ultraViolet absorption spectrometer (DUVAS) measures the second derivative of absorption of UV light to detect monoaromatic and diaromatic compounds. As indicated in Figure 5, measurements detected benzene, phenol, $p$-cresol, naphthalene,

**Table XII.**  Summary of Tenax Tube Area Sampling

| Location | Sample No. | Concentration (ppm) | | | | | |
|---|---|---|---|---|---|---|---|
| | | Benzene | Toluene | Xylene | Trimethyl Benzene | Acetophenone | Phenol |
| Near tar storage tank in basement | 1 | 0.03 | 0.02 | 0.005 | 0.004 | <0.001 | 0.003 |
| | 2 | 0.01 | 0.01 | 0.003 | 0.002 | <0.001 | 0.006 |
| | 3 | 0.01 | 0.02 | 0.005 | 0.004 | <0.001 | 0.003 |
| 10 ft (3 m) from coal scale (fourth level) | 1 | 0.01 | 0.008 | 0.006 | 0.005 | 0.004 | 0.002 |
| | 2 | 0.001 | 0.003 | 0.005 | <0.001 | 0.001 | 0.003 |
| Operator control panel (level 1) | 1 | 0.003 | 0.004 | 0.005 | <0.001 | <0.001 | <0.001 |
| Manual poking area (second level) | 1 | 0.01 | 0.01 | 0.003 | 0.002 | <0.001 | 0.003 |
| | 2 | 0.02 | 0.02 | 0.005 | 0.006 | 0.002 | 0.003 |
| Near top-gas off-take (third level) | 1 | 0.04 | 0.03 | 0.005 | 0.004 | 0.002 | 0.01 |
| Near ESP (first level) | 1 | 0.003 | 0.01 | 0.005 | 0.006 | 0.002 | 0.02 |
| | 2 | 0.003 | 0.008 | 0.005 | 0.002 | 0.001 | 0.003 |
| Coal feed area, by work-bench (third level) | 1 | 0.003 | 0.005 | <0.001 | <0.001 | <0.001 | 0.002 |
| | 2 | 0.001 | 0.002 | 0.005 | 0.004 | 0.001 | 0.002 |

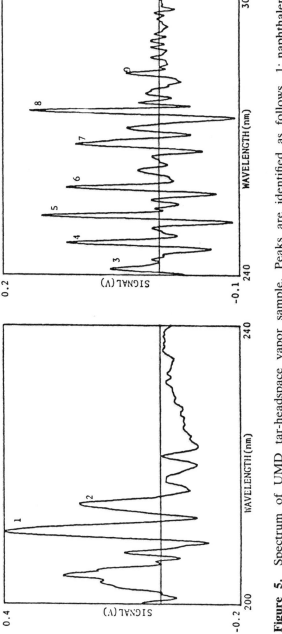

**Figure 5.** Spectrum of UMD tar-headspace vapor sample. Peaks are identified as follows. 1: naphthalene. 2: methyl naphthalene. 3–6: benzene, 7 and 8: phenol. 9: *p*-cresol.

and methyl naphthalene, consistent with tar-headspace analysis and vapor sampling using Tenax. The DUVAS demonstrated its usefulness as a real-time monitoring instrument for these materials during studies at UMD and METC. Measurements for naphthalene were taken during maintenance activities on a packing gland at METC. As indicated in Figure 6, the naphthalene concentrations were reduced significantly as the packing gland was tightened.

The DUVAS is also a very sensitive monitor for several nitrogen compounds such as ammonia and nitric oxide. Figure 7 shows the variation in ammonia concentration near the coal feed system, indicating the varying emissions of product gas as the coal feed system cycles. Figure 8 shows variations in the nitric oxide level produced when a torch was used to heat a tar transfer line to reestablish flow.

A passive dosimeter, sensitive to higher ring polynuclear aromatic compounds, was tested at UMD. Dosimeters were placed at several locations around the gasifier, including a clean area in the computer room. Pyrene vapors were detected at two locations on level 4 near the knife valves and on level 5 near the coal scale. The average concentration of pyrene vapor on level 4 was estimated to be 16 ppb; that on level 5, 100 ppb. These levels were affected to some degree by the nearness of the dosimeters to emission sources. The spectrum of pyrene vapor detected at UMD is shown in Figure 9.

The lightpipe luminoscope for detecting skin contamination by organic materials was tested at UMD and METC. This instrument is a source of UV illumination that collects and detects the ensuing fluorescence. An area of approximately 1 cm$^2$ is illuminated and monitored under a stethoscopic

**Figure 6.** Reduction in naphthalene concentrations with time as packing gland is tightened.

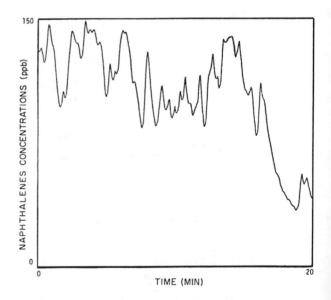

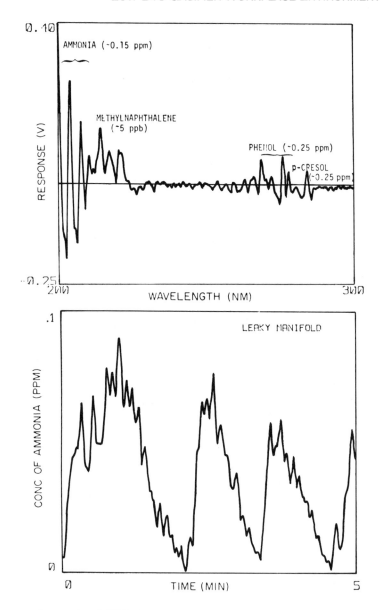

**Figure 7.** DUVAS spectrum of air between 200 and 300 nm, and a plot of ammonia concentration over a 5-min period near a leaky manifold cap.

head pressed against the skin. To minimize the effects of direct toxicity of near-UV light on skin, as well as possible phototoxifying effects of UV light on the PNA compounds, the intensity of the excitation light is reduced to

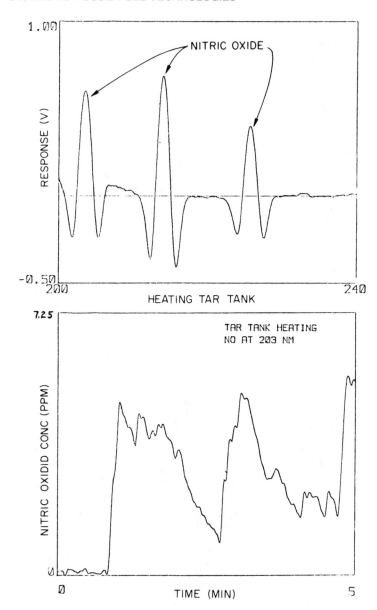

**Figure 8.** DUVAS spectrum of air between 200 and 240 nm, and a plot of nitric oxide concentration over a 5-min period during a tar line heating operation.

0.01 that of directly overhead sunlight in the wavelength region of 320–400 nm.

The luminoscope was most useful in detecting contamination left on the skin after washing (Table XIII). Some tar contamination was visible as

**Figure 9.**  Vapor of pyrene detected at the UMD gasifier by room-temperature phosphorescence spectroscopy.

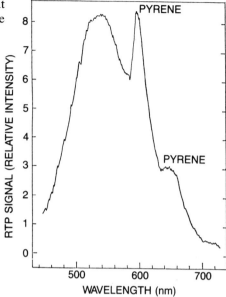

**Table XIII.**  Summary of Results Obtained with the Luminoscope at the UMD Gasifier

| Background Fluorescence of Normal Clean Skin | Fluorescence of Patches of Clean Dried Skin (calluses) | Fluorescence of Contaminated Skin |
|---|---|---|
| The signal intensity varies by 10–15% over the hand and arm area of each worker | Intensity ≥150% of the background level | Intensity >150% of the background level |
| The signal level varies by 10–35% from one worker to another | <1-cm² area | 1–3-cm² area |
| | Signal persists at same level after washing | Signal decreases to normal background level after washing |
| | Detected in 5 of 6 workers | Detected in 2 workers |

brown patches on the skin. Measurements after skin washing indicated that some residue frequently remained, but it could usually be removed by further washing. UMD tar appeared to be easier to remove than METC tar (Table XIV).

The spill spotter for oil and tar spills was designed as a replacement for the hand-held black lamp, and it can be used under almost all lighting

**Table XIV.**  Measurements Obtained by the Lightpipe Luminoscope of Coal Tar Contaminants on Worker Skin Following Repeated Wash Treatments

| Number of Wash Treatments[a] | Fluorescence Signal[b] ($10^3$ photons) | Benzo(a)pyrene Equivalent on Filter Paper[c] ($ng/cm^2$) |
|:---:|:---:|:---:|
| 0 | $1.0 \pm 0.2$[d] | Q[d] |
| 1 | $7.5 \pm 0.2$ | 50 |
| 2 | $6.9 \pm 0.2$ | 42 |
| 3 | $6.5 \pm 0.2$ | 36 |
| 4 | $5.5 \pm 0.2$ | 24 |

[a]Wash treatments used special water skin cleanser for oil removal.
[b]Fluorescence signal includes background of clean skin = $(3.6 \pm 0.4) \times 10^3$ counts.
[c]The net fluorescence signals are compared to that of benzo(a)pyrene spotted on reference paper.
[d]Q = quenching of the fluorescence signal before washing.

conditions. The spotter is a portable UV irradiation source and fluorescence detector. The collimated beam of illuminating UV light is modulated at 1 kH$_z$, while the modulated fluorescence signal is electrically filtered and demodulated to permit discrimination against background illumination from other sources.

The spill spotter is useful for detecting low-level contamination that is not visible to the naked eye. This capability was most useful in evaluating whether clean areas were in fact free of contamination. Many contaminated surfaces and parts of equipment at UMD were detected by the spill spotter, which was also useful in evaluating the effectiveness of cleanup efforts for certain areas and for tools.

## TOXICOLOGY PROGRAM

An extensive program of toxicology testing was conducted on UMD products.[6] Most of the investigations focused on testing UMD tar materials, although aqueous extracts of bottom ash and cyclone fines were also tested. A battery of toxicity tests (Table XV) was applied to these materials. Test results, consistent with investigations conducted by the Inhalation Toxicology Research Institute and Argonne National Laboratory on similar materials from other gasifiers,[7] are summarized below.

1. Distilled water leachates of bottom ash were both embryotoxic and teratogenic in the amphibian system.
2. Electrostatic precipitator tars from the UMD gasifier were mutagenic in the Salmonella/microsome assay. This was confirmed in the yeast assay.

**Table XV.**    UMD Toxicology Testing

Short-term testing
  Microbial mutagenesis
    • Ames - *Salmonella typhimurium*
    • Yeast - *Saccharomyces cerevisiae*
  Amphibian teratogenicity and embryotoxicity
    • FETAX - *Xenopus laevis*
  Mammalian teratogenicity and genotoxicity
    Mouse spot test
    Dominant lethal
    Total reproductive capacity
Mammalian toxicology and carcinogenesis
  Acute toxicity
    Oral and intraperitoneal - mice
    Acute dermal - rats
    Skin irritation - rabbits
    Eye irritation - rabbits
    Delayed skin sensitivity - guinea pigs
  Lung tumor assay
    Intraperitoneal - mice
  Chronic dermal toxicity
    Skin - mice

3. After chemical fractionation of the ESP tars, it was found that the mutagenic activity was contributed principally by the organic constituents of the basic fraction and only secondarily by constituents of the neutral fraction.

4. Mutagenic potential of ESP tars lies between that of the low-activity petroleum crude oils and that of the relatively higher activity coal-derived liquids.

5. Aqueous extracts of ESP tars were embryotoxic and teratogenic in the amphibian system.

6. ESP tars caused decreased postnatal survival, cytotoxicity, and some teratogenicity in the mouse spot test, but there was no evidence of mutation induction.

7. ESP tars caused transient loss of reproductive capacity in mice. There was a detectable increase in dominant-lethal mutations at all stages in spermatogenesis.

8. ESP tars were slightly toxic to mice when given orally. Moderate toxicity was noted following intraperitoneal injection.

9. Tar samples caused moderate, albeit reversible, eye irritation.

10. The data obtained in the lung adenoma bioassay indicate that ESP tar is tumorigenic.

11. ESP tar is carcinogenic in mouse skin.

Results of the acute toxicity testing are consistent with experiences at the gasifier. No worker health effects (skin irritation, etc.) have been noted at UMD to date. However, the chronic skin painting tests, which resulted in a strong carcinogenic response, and the lung adenoma test, which produced positive results, suggest that longer term exposures to the UMD tars may be of concern. Consequently, strong emphasis should continue to be placed on IH procedures designed to limit employee exposures to tar materials, and the medical surveillance program should be continued to ensure that any health impacts that might arise are identified as quickly as possible.

## MEDICAL SURVEILLANCE

A medical surveillance program for the UMD gasifier workers has been established. All gasifier workers must undergo a physical examination before employment at the gasifier, and physicals are conducted every year thereafter. The physical exams include general physical, hearing, and sight evaluations; lung function testing, including x-rays; electrocardiograms; routine blood and urine tests; and a skin examination, including the taking of photographs. To date, no health effects attributable to working at the gasifier have been noted in the employees.

## CONCLUSIONS

A large amount of experience has been developed concerning the IH situations that may be experienced at small, fixed-bed low-Btu gasifiers. The major conclusion is that apparently worker exposures during normal operations can be kept well below *current* regulations and guidelines. It must be strongly emphasized, however, that provision of effective IH support will be an important factor in complying with current exposure regulations. Experiences encountered during the IH program suggest that the potential for employee overexposures is present and may in fact be expected if adequate IH provisions are not implemented.

Carbon monoxide is likely to present the greatest potential for overexposure and, due to its high concentration in process streams, it presents a potential for acute exposures. Hydrogen sulfide and ammonia exposures may occur in certain situations. Experiences have shown that this acute exposure potential is greatest during startup and shakedown operations and that IH support to and interaction with operations is effective in reducing employee exposures.

In contrast, worker exposure to coal-tar-related materials does not appear to present a significant acute exposure hazard. However, it is likely that low level, chronic exposures to these materials through inhalation and skin contact will occur. The hazard potential associated with these chronic exposures is unclear at this time; however, considering the strong activity of these materials in toxicological tests, prudence demands that worker exposures be kept as low as possible. In addition, worker medical surveillance programs should be implemented to ensure that any health effects are detected as soon as possible.

Heat stress, noise, dust, and other toxic material exposures may be important under certain conditions.

Finally, it has been shown that a number of specific operations and pieces of equipment are associated with the major potential for employee exposure. Coal transport and handling, coal feeding, gas scrubbing and cleaning (including tar removal and handling), and poking operations are major sources of emission. Flanges, valves, and seals are generally possible sources of emissions. Proper attention to design and construction and use of appropriate engineering controls should make it possible to reduce and control process emissions and resulting worker exposures. In addition, judicious use of carefully selected personal protection devices can be very helpful in controlling exposures until engineering controls can be applied.

## ACKNOWLEDGMENT

Research sponsored by the Office of Health and Environmental Research, Office of Environmental Programs, and Office of Coal Processing, U.S. Department of Energy, under contract W-7405-eng-26 with the Union Carbide Corporation.

## REFERENCES

1. Cowser, K.E., et al. "Proposed Environmental and Health Program for the University of Minnesota Gasification Facility" (proposal to U.S. Department of Energy, 1978).
2. Walsh, P.J., et al. "Preoperational Assessment of a Foster-Wheeler/STOIC Low BTU Gasifier," Draft (1978).
3. Dreibelbis, W.G., et al. "Personnel and Plant Area Monitoring at the University of Minnesota-Duluth Gasifer," ORNL/TM-8551 (Oak Ridge, TN: Oak Ridge National Laboratory, in press).
4. Griest, W.H., et al. "Sample Management and Chemical/Physical Properties of Products and Effluents From the University of Minnesota-Duluth, Low BTU Gasifier," ORNL/TM-8427 (Oak Ridge, TN: Oak Ridge National Laboratory, 1982).
5. Schuresko, D.D., et al. "Survey of PNA Emissions at the University of Minnesota-Duluth Gasifier," ORNL/TM-8414 (Oak Ridge, TN: Oak Ridge National Laboratory, in press).
6. Epler, J.L., et al. "Biomedical Response to Products and Effluents for the University of Minnesota-Duluth Gasifier," ORNL/TM-8821 (Oak Ridge, TN: Oak Ridge National Laboratory, 1983).

7.  U.S. Department of Energy. "Status of Health and Environmental Research Relative to Coal Gasification, 1976 to Present," DOE/ER-0149 (1982).

## DISCUSSION

*S.L. Morris, Brookhaven National Laboratory:* How long has the worker exposure medical surveillance been going on, and how many workers are involved in it?

*S.D. Van Hoesen:* The medical surveillance program has been in place since the beginning of the gasifier operation in 1978; in fact, there was a requirement that all operators at the gasifier take a preoperational test before they started work. It has only been since 1981 (Run No. 8) that the gasifier has run in what you would call a normal mode with fairly continuous operation. The first five or six runs were of short duration to get the system shaken down. To date (January 1983) a total of 27 workers have had medical data developed as part of the surveillance program. Twenty-two workers are involved currently in the medical surveillance program.

# CHAPTER 7

## Source Discharges and Ambient Air Pollution at the Coal Gasifier at Kosovo

### K.J. Bombaugh
*Radian Corporation*
*Austin, TX 78766*

Emissions from a commercial coal gasification plant were compared with pollutants collected from the air at ground level 1 to 2 km from the plant. A source-receptor relationship was confirmed by identifying profiles of sulfur- and nitrogen-containing hydrocarbons found both in plant discharges and in collected samples. Pollutants collected included polynuclear aromatics, phenols, thiophenes, pyridines, and alkyl aromatics. Quantities collected by each receptor were proportional to the amount of time the receptor site was downwind of the source.

### INTRODUCTION

Coal gasification provides a viable alternative to petroleum as a source of clean fuel. However, the environmental effects associated with long-term production of gas from coal are largely unknown, and the impact of a massive gasification plant is still undetermined. Although significant data have been gathered about the components produced by the gasification process, only limited conclusions can be drawn about the impact of a controlled plant, because information on the composition of effluents from environmental control modules is not available.

Coal gasifiers fit into two broad categories: tar producers or tar nonproducers. The tar producers are generally more energy efficient and therefore are favored for the production of fuel gas. Among the tar-producing processes is the Lurgi-type process, such as is used at Kosovo.

The Kosovo study represented a unique opportunity to evaluate the potential health and environmental problems associated with a commercial Lurgi-type plant lacking modern environmental control devices. The program included a source test, for both regular and fugitive emissions, and an evaluation of the ambient air in the plant vicinity. It is being followed by a prospective/retrospective health effects study. The site was ideal for this purpose because its isolated location is free of other, potentially interfering, pollution sources. The high levels of pollutant discharge made possible an establishable association between pollutants collected and pollutants discharged.

The purpose of this chapter is to show this source-receptor relationship, by comparing profiles of compounds collected at the receptor with those found in the plant's by-products and emissions. Included is a consideration of substances which, although not identified in the collection, are also present in the plant's discharges.

## EXPERIMENTAL

The procedures used in the source-discharge and ambient-air studies were described previously.[1-10] Brief descriptions of the test site, the plant, the gasification and associated processes, and the tests are presented here to facilitate reader understanding.

### Test Site and Gasification Plant

The Kosovo complex is in a large, open valley in southern Yugoslavia where the climate is similar to that in the midwestern United States. The complex is surrounded by farmland interspersed with small villages.

The test facility is an integral part of a large mine-mouth industrial complex, which also includes an ammonia-based fertilizer plant, a Fleissner coal-drying plant, a cryogenic air-separation plant, a steam-generating plant, and a large electric-power generating plant. The gasification plant consists of six pressurized oxygen-blown gas generators with an associated gas-cooling system, a tar and oil separation plant, a Rectisol acid-gas removal plant, a Phenosolvan wastewater extraction plant, and storage facilities for liquid by-products.

### Plant Processes

The gasification plant (Figure 1) consumes dried lignite and produces two primary products: medium-Btu (23–25 MJ/m$^3$ at 25° C) fuel gas and hydrogen for use in ammonia synthesis. It also produces several by-products: tar, medium oil, naphtha, and crude phenol. The lignite fed to the Lurgi gas generators is dried by the Fleissner process (high-temperature steam soak)

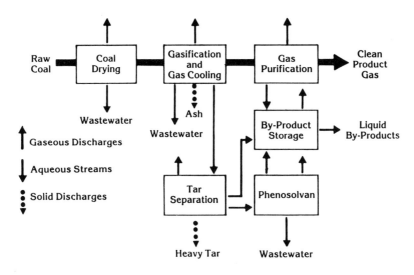

**Figure 1.** Diagram of the Kosovo coal gasification facility, identifying types of discharges from the major process units.[4] (Reprinted with permission of copyright owner.)

and sized to obtain particles between 6 and 60 mm in size. Product gas, generated by the reaction of the lignite with oxygen and steam at 2.3 MPa (23 atm) pressure, is cooled and then cleaned to remove acid gases prior to its transportation by pipeline to the utilization site. In the cooling step, tars, oils, naphtha, and phenolic water are removed from the gas. In the acid-gas removal step, $H_2S$ and $CO_2$ are removed by sorption with cold methanol. The rich methanol is regenerated by depressurization and heating. The $H_2S$-rich waste gas released by the regeneration step is sent to a flare; the $CO_2$-rich waste gas is vented directly to the atmosphere. Tar and oil are separated from the phenolic water by decantation, after which the water-soluble organics (crude phenols) are removed from the wastewater by extraction with diisopropyl ether. Four liquid by-products (tar, medium oil, naphtha, and crude phenol) are collected in storage tanks and used as fuel. Dissolved acid gases and ammonia are removed from the phenolic water by steam stripping and vented to the atmosphere. Each process unit at this plant is a potential source of environmental discharges, as indicated by the ascending arrows in Figure 1, and all operating units in the complex produce gaseous discharges that are a potential source of atmospheric pollution.

### Source Test

Approximately 35 of the plant's gaseous streams were analyzed preliminarily; then 18 were selected for a more detailed study that included:

- stream flow rate measurement,
- particulate measurement via wet impinger, and
- composition analysis.

Composition analyses were made on site by a combination of gas chromatography and wet chemical methods. Stream condensates and by-product analyses were performed off site by a combination of methods including gas chromatography, gas chromatography–mass spectrometry (GC/MS), infrared, and gravimetry.

### Ambient Test

Ambient aerosols and vapors were collected at five sample receptor sites deployed on a perimeter 1 to 2 km from the plant, as identified in Figure 2. Meteorological stations were located at sites 3 and 5. Each site was equipped to collect particles and organic vapors.

Organic analyses of the collected particles and vapors were done by gas chromatography using both universal and element-specific detectors and by GC-MS.

## RESULTS AND DISCUSSION

### Source Results

Mass flows of pollutants from the Kosovo plant are shown in Figure 3. Discharges of hydrocarbons and ammonia are each ten times that of phenol, which is released at a rate of ~11 kg per gasifier hour. Phenol is steam stripped from the phenolic water along with ammonia and is probably transported through the air as an aerosol.

The particulate discharge from the gasifier at Kosovo consists mostly of a water/oil aerosol, which had to be collected in an impinger train that yielded three fractions: tar/oil, filtered solids, and dissolved solids. Discharge rates from the two major sources are shown in Table I. It was assumed that the tar/oil condensate in the gaseous discharge stream is similar in composition to the by-product tar and the by-product oil; therefore, it was informative to determine the concentrations of hazardous polynuclear aromatics (PNAs) in the by-products. The results are shown in Table II. These PNA concentrations were used to estimate PNA concentrations in the discharges from the two major discharge vents, as shown in Table III. On this basis, the level of benzo($a$)pyrene (BaP) in the coal lock discharge can be estimated as between 1700 and 490 $\mu g/m^3$. The determined value was 690 $\mu g/m^3$, as shown in Table IV. The good agreement indicates that the concentrations of all other PNAs can be estimated in the same manner.

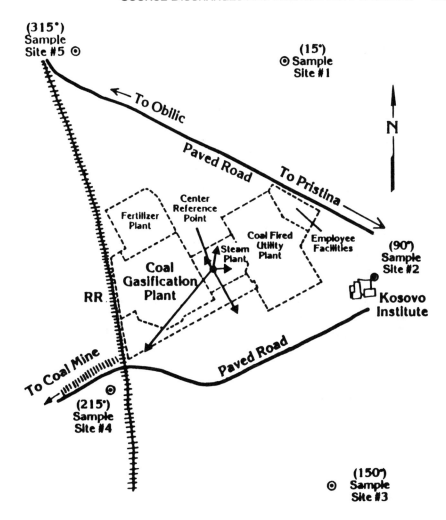

**Figure 2.** . Schematic of the Kosovo complex. Vectors indicate the relative amount of time that each receptor site was downwind.[5] (Reprinted with permission of copyright owner.)

### Ambient Receptor Results

Organics were collected in two overlapping fractions:

- vapors, trapped on Tenax, and
- aerosols, trapped on particles on HiVol filter pads.

Gas chromatograms of the organics thermally desorbed from the Tenax showed a wide range of hydrocarbons, from benzene to perhaps anthracene.

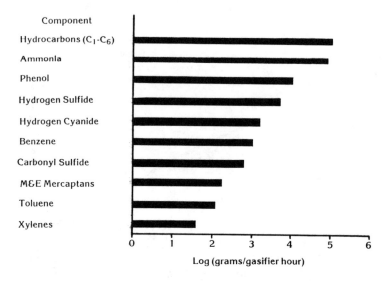

**Figure 3.**   Kosovo mass discharges to the atmosphere, plant wide.[4] The numbers on the abscissa are logarithms to the base 10 of the mass flow rates. (Reprinted with permission of copyright owner.)

**Table I.**   Particulate Concentrations and Flow Rates for Kosovo Gaseous Streams Discharging into the Atmosphere

| | Sampling Point | | |
| --- | --- | --- | --- |
| | Coal Room Vent | Low-Pressure Coal Lock Vent | Gasifier Startup Vent[a] |
| Dry gas flow (m³/gasifier h, 25°C) | 7200 | 21 | 4000 |
| Particulate concentration (mg/m³ at 25°C) | | | |
| Total particulates | 48 | 8100 | 9450 |
| Condensed organics (tars and oils) | – | 7300 | 8980 |
| Dissolved solids | 6 | 650 | 400 |
| Filtered solids | 42 | 220 | 61 |

[a]Stream discharges to atmosphere during startup until a combustible gas is produced.

Isomer groups of alkyl aromatics were recognizable. The pattern was similar to that of by-product medium oil. Element-specific chromatograms for nitrogen compounds and for sulfur compounds showed a striking similarity between the collected vapors and by-product medium oil, as shown in Figures 4 and 5.

The absence of any of these compounds in either the blank or the

**Table II.**    Concentrations of Hazardous Polynuclear Aromatics in Kosovo Tar and Oil (μg/g)

|  | Tar | Oil |
|---|---|---|
| 7,12-Dimethylbenz(a)anthracene | 1090 | 62 |
| Benzo(a)anthracene | 490 | 156 |
| Benzo(b)fluorene | 306 | 115 |
| Benzo(a)pyrene | 210 | 68 |
| Dibenzo(a)anthracene | 23 | 7 |
| 3-Methylcholanthrene | 26 | NF |
| Mass 252 isomer group | 945[a] | 282[a] |

[a]GC/MS analyses show that benzo(a)pyrene comprises 24% of the mass 252 isomer group in both tar and oil.

**Table III.**    Estimated Concentrations of Several Polynuclear Aromatics in Kosovo Atmospheric Discharges[a]

| | Estimated Concentration (mg/m³) | | | |
|---|---|---|---|---|
| | LP Coal Lock Vent | | Startup Vent | |
| Substance | Tar | Oil | Tar | Oil |
| 7,12 Dimethylbenz(a)anthracene | 7.96 | 0.45 | 9.79 | 0.55 |
| Benzo(a)anthracene | 3.58 | 1.14 | 4.40 | 1.40 |
| Benzo(b)fluorene | 2.23 | 0.84 | 2.75 | 1.03 |
| Benzo(a)pyrene | 1.53 | 0.50 | 1.89 | 0.61 |
| Dibenzo(a)anthracene | 0.17 | 0.05 | 0.21 | 0.06 |
| Mass 252 isomer group[a] | 6.90 | 2.06 | 8.49 | 2.53 |

[a]GC/MS analysis shows that benzo(a)pyrene comprises 24% of the mass 252 isomer group in both tar and oil.

**Table IV.**    Concentrations and Mass Flows of Benzo(a)pyrene (BaP) in Kosovo Atmospheric Discharges

| Vent | Stream Flow Rate (m³/h) | BaP Concentration (μg/m³) | BaP Mass Flow (μg/gasifier h) |
|---|---|---|---|
| Startup[a] | 12,500 | 139 | $1.7 \times 10^6$ |
| LP coal lock | 21 | 690 | $1.4 \times 10^4$ |
| Ammonia stopper | 260 | 20 | $5.2 \times 10^3$ |
| Tar tank | 4.5 | 252 | $1.4 \times 10^2$ |
| Naphtha storage tank | 4.5 | 0.085 | $3.8 \times 10^1$ |
| Phenolic water tank | 5.5 | <50 | $<2.8 \times 10^2$ |
| Medium oil tank | 1.7 | <6.5 | $<1.1 \times 10^1$ |
| Total mass flow | | | $1.7 \times 10^6$ |
| Mass flow without startup vent | | | $2.0 \times 10^4$ |

[a]An intermittent stream.

**Figure 4.** Chromatograms of nitrogen species in Kosovo medium oil (bottom) and in downwind samples (top).[2]

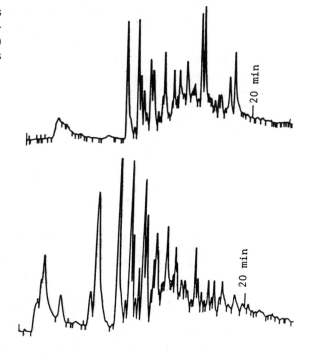

**Figure 5.** Chromatograms of sulfur species in Kosovo medium oil (bottom) and in downwind samples (top).[2]

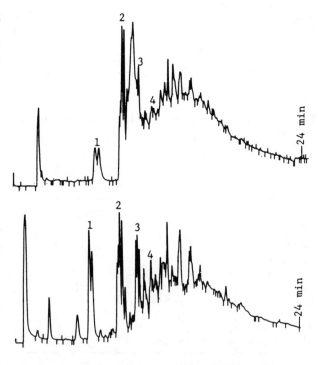

upwind samples (Figure 6) constituted proof that the substances were coming from the plant. These results opened the way to the premise that many other compounds in the Kosovo by-products should be expected at the receptor sites.

Selected nitrogen and sulfur species collected at all five sites were quantified. Concentration values were correlated with the percentage of the time the respective collector site was downwind of the source within $\pm 22.5°$ of the downwind azimuth. The results, presented in Tables V and VI, show correlations greater than 80%.

Analyses by GC/MS showed a range of aromatic compounds, from benzene to anthracene in the vapor and from anthracene to benzopyrene in the particulates. Concentration levels, computed to 100% downwind, are shown in Tables VII and VIII. Benzene and toluene values are not reported here because collection on Tenax was incomplete. The xylenes showed 25% of the collection in the second trap and are therefore considered a complete collection.

The level of benzene at the receptor, as deduced from its ratio with xylene in the plant discharge, is $33 \times 10$ or 330 $\mu g/m^3$. BaP, which is included in the group having a mass ion of 252, is present at a level of 24% of the mixture. On this basis, the level of BaP at a point 1 km from and 100% downwind of the source is 20 $ng/m^3$.

**Figure 6.** Chromatograms of sulfur species in Kosovo upwind samples (top) and in blank (bottom).[2]

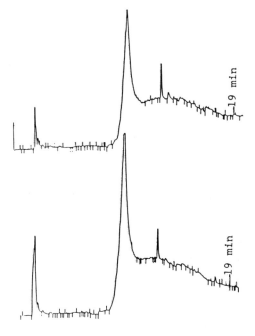

**Table V.**  Correlations of Nitrogen Species
Concentrations with Percent Downwind[a]

| Component | 0% ($\mu g/m^3$) | 45% ($\mu g/m^3$) | Correlation Coefficient | 100%[b] ($\mu g/m^3$) |
|---|---|---|---|---|
| 3-Methylpyridine | <DL[c] | 0.62 | 0.92 | 1.4 |
| C-2 Alkyl pyridine | <DL | 0.55 | 0.83 | 1.2 |
| C-2 Alkyl pyridine | <DL | 0.46 | 0.90 | 1.0 |
| C-2 Alkyl pyridine | <DL | 0.49 | 0.83 | 1.1 |
| C-3 Alkyl pyridine | <DL | 0.56 | 0.84 | 1.2 |
| C-3 Alkyl pyridine | <DL | 0.46 | 0.77 | 1.0 |
| Alkyl pyridine(s) | <DL | 0.74 | 0.76 | 1.6 |
| Quinoline | <DL | 0.94 | 0.91 | 2.1 |
| Alkyl quinoline | <DL | 0.54 | 0.82 | 1.2 |

[a]Values at 19 and 40% downwind are not shown. Percent downwind means the amount of time a receptor site was within ± 22.5° of the downwind azimuth from the source, expressed as a percentage of the total sampling time.
[b]Calculated.
[c]Less than detection limit.

**Table VI.**  Sulfur Species Correlations with Percent Downwind[a]

| Component | 0% ($\mu g/m^3$) | 45% ($\mu g/m^3$) | Correlation Coefficient | 100%[b] ($\mu g/m^3$) |
|---|---|---|---|---|
| C-2 Thiophene | ND[c] | 0.10 | 0.94 | 0.22 |
| C-2 Thiophene | ND | 0.09 | 0.95 | 0.2 |
| C-3 Thiophene | <DL[d] | 0.04 | 0.91 | 0.088 |
| C-3 Thiophene | <DL | 0.08 | 0.78 | 0.18 |

[a]Values at 19 and 40% downwind are not shown. Percent downwind means the amount of time a receptor site was within ± 22.5° of the downwind azimuth from the source, expressed as a percentage of the total sampling time.
[b]Calculated.
[c]Not detected.
[d]Less than detection limit.

## Liquid By-Products and Stream Condensate Compositions

When characterized, the liquid by-products and gas stream condensates showed that these materials contained many types of compounds that could include the following:

- alkyl aromatics
- polynuclear aromatics

**Table VII.**   Aromatics Collected by Tenax at
Receptor Site 1 km Downwind[a]

| Component | Concentration[b] ($\mu g/m^3$) |
|---|---|
| C-2 Benzene | 9.8 |
| C-3 Benzene | 11 |
| C-4 Benzene | 3.0 |
| Naphthalene | 7.5 |
| Biphenyl | 3.8 |
| Acenaphthene | 1.3 |
| Fluorene | 0.60 |
| Anthracene | 1.4 |

[a]Site 4 was 40% downwind.
[b]Values computed to 100% downwind.

**Table VIII.**   Polynuclear Aromatics Collected by HiVol Filters at Receptor Site 1 km Downward

| | Mass | Concentration[a] ($ng/m_3$) |
|---|---|---|
| Anthracene | 178 | 7.5 |
| Fluoranthene | 202 | 17 |
| Pyrene | 202 | 18 |
| Chrysene, benzanthracene, triphenylene | 228 | 90 |
| Benzpyrenes, benzfluoranthenes, perylene | 252 | 82 |

[a]Values calculated to 100% downwind.

- phenols
- nitrogen heterocyclics
    - pyridines
    - diazines
    - pyroles
- sulfur compounds
    - mercaptans
    - thiophenes
    - thiols
- bifunctional compounds
    - oxazoles
    - thiozoles

It is reasonable to conclude that, if these materials are in the condensate of effluent streams, they are also in the air around the plant.

## ACKNOWLEDGMENTS

The author expresses his thanks to the many contributors to this work. The source test was sponsored by the Industrial Environmental Research Laboratory (T. Kelly Janes, Project Officer). The receptor test was sponsored by the Environmental Sciences Research Laboratory (Ronald K. Patterson, Project Officer) of the U.S. Environmental Protection Agency. The study was conducted as a cooperative effort between American and Yugoslav scientists with the cooperation of the plant operator, Elektroprivreda Kosovo.

## REFERENCES

1. Bombaugh, K.J., W.E. Corbett, K.W. Lee, and W.S. Seams. "An Environmentally Based Evaluation of Multimedia Discharges from the Kosovo Lurgi Coal Gasification System," Symposium Proceedings, Environmental Aspects of Fuel Conversion Technology V, September 1980, St. Louis, EPA-600/9-81-006.
2. Bombaugh, K.J., G.C. Page, C.H. Williams, L.O. Edwards, W.D. Balfour, D.S. Lewis, and K.W. Lee. "Aerosol Characterization of Ambient Air Near a Lurgi Coal Gasification Plant, Kosovo Region, Yugoslavia," EPA-600-80-177.
3. Bombaugh, K.J., K.W. Lee, R.G. Oldham, and S. Kapor. "Characterization of Process Liquids and Organic Condensates from the Lurgi Coal Gasification Plant at Kosovo," Symposium Proceedings, Environmental Aspects of Fuel Conversion Technology VI, October 26–30, 1981, Denver, EPA 600/9-82-017.
4. Bombaugh, K.J., K.W. Lee, and T.K. Janes. Chapter 18 in *Energy and Environmental Chemistry, Vol. I,* L.H. Keith, Ed. (Ann Arbor, MI: Ann Arbor Science Publishers, Inc., 1982).
5. Balfour, W.D., K.J. Bombaugh, L.O. Edwards, and R.K. Patterson. Chapter 24 in *Energy and Environmental Chemistry, Vol. I,* L.H. Keith, Ed. (Ann Arbor, MI: Ann Arbor Science Publishers, Inc., 1982).
6. Lee, K.W., K.J. Bombaugh, C.H. Williams, D.S. Lewis, and L.D. Ogle. Chapter 19 in *Energy and Environmental Chemistry, Vol. I,* L.H. Keith, Ed. (Ann Arbor, MI: Ann Arbor Science Publishers, Inc., 1982).
7. Williams, C.H., K.J. Bombaugh, P.H. Lin, K.W. Lee, and C.L. Prescott. Chapter 20 in *Energy and Environmental Chemistry, Vol. I,* L.H. Keith, Ed. (Ann Arbor, MI: Ann Arbor Science Publishers, Inc., 1982).
8. Griest, W.H., C.E. Higgins, R.W. Holmberg, J.H. Moneyhun, J.E. Calon, J.S. Wike, and R.R. Reager. Chapter 21 in *Energy and Environmental Chemistry, Vol. I,* L.H. Keith, Ed. (Ann Arbor, MI: Ann Arbor Science Publishers, Inc., 1982).
9. Huntzicker, J.J., R.L. Johnson, J.J. Shah, and E.K. Heyerdahl. Chapter 22 in *Energy and Environmental Chemistry, Vol. I,* L.H. Keith, Ed. (Ann Arbor, MI: Ann Arbor Science Publishers, Inc., 1982).
10. Boures, L.C.S., J.W. Winchester, and J.W. Nelson. Chapter 23 in *Energy and Environmental Chemistry, Vol. I,* L.H. Keith, Ed. (Ann Arbor, MI: Ann Arbor Science Publishers, Inc., 1982).

## DISCUSSION

*P.H. Buhl, Department of Energy:* The gasification plant seemed to be right next to another utility plant. Was that operating at the same time you were taking these measurements?

*K.J. Bombaugh:* You have reference to the power plant; yes, it was. As a matter of fact, the power plant interfered significantly with our noncarbonaceous particulate measurements, but it did not interfere with our organic measurements.

*P.H. Buhl:* What fuel were they using at the power plant?

*K.J. Bombaugh:* Lignite. The power plant discharges were combustion products and most of the pollutants we collected were from coal devolatilization.

*C.W. Francis, Oak Ridge National Laboratory:* This is one of the first times I have seen where the tars are considered to be a solid waste. I believe it was in your third or fourth slide. Could you tell me what they do with the tar?

*K.J. Bombaugh:* Kosovo has two tar-type products. One is a liquid that they burn; the other, heavy tar, is included with their solid waste in a landfill. Heavy tar was included in our study but not as a part of the air study discussed here.

# CHAPTER 8

## Laboratory-Scale Simulation of Coal Gasification for Biological Studies

F.O. Mixon, J.G. Cleland,
T.J. Hughes, D.A. Green, and
S.K. Gangwal

*Research Triangle Institute*
*P.O. Box 12194*
*Research Triangle Park, NC 27709*

Comparison of operating data from a laboratory-scale coal gasification unit with similar data from large-scale units indicates that the laboratory-scale unit can be a valuable tool in predicting environmental effects of commercial units. A statistical correlation of data on more than 50 operating runs shows that pollutant production in the tar phase is strongly dependent upon coal rank, coal nitrogen content, coal sulfur content, and coal volatile content. Tar base and polynuclear aromatic production as well as the response to Ames testing appear to be related primarily to fuel sulfur content and nitrogen content.

This chapter examines cause-effect relationships that seem to exist among feedstock characteristics, gasifier operating parameters, pollutant production, and bioassay results from gasifier effluents. Mutagenicity of tars and their fractions is emphasized.

### INTRODUCTION

For the past 5 years, the Research Triangle Institute (RTI) has been studying the nature and extent of the production of environmental pollutants in synthetic fuels processes. A laboratory gasifier and associated equipment have been designed, constructed, and operated under various conditions with a number of feedstocks and with extensive sampling and chemical analysis of the effluent streams. Several bioassay studies have been completed including Ames mutagenicity and cytotoxicity tests on samples of the effluent streams as well as of the raw feedstocks.

Figure 1 shows a schematic of the gasifier and sampling train. A steam-generation system and a reactant gas supply and control system are provided to feed the gasifier. Sampling provisions are included for aqueous and organic effluents, product gases, and unreacted reactor contents. Details of the reactor design and sampling system are reported elsewhere.[1]

The reactor system design was intended to provide a flexible research tool, rather than to simulate the performance of large-scale units. Hence, the reactor was designed for operation as follows: (1) in either the fixed-bed or fluidized-bed mode, (2) in either a batch or continuous mode with respect to the coal feed, (3) with either air or oxygen gas feed to cover the conditions of low- and medium-Btu gasification, and (4) with provision for either internal heating by partial combustion of the coal or external heating through electrically heated walls. The primary intent and major emphasis of the program have been to observe the behavior of samples of coal that are subjected to a controlled temperature and controlled gaseous environment to draw conclusions about the fundamental processes (e.g., heat and mass transfer and chemical reaction kinetics), and to apply this fundamental information to understanding the behavior of large-scale units.

In spite of this intention, the program provided considerable experimental evidence that the laboratory reactor is indeed capable of providing a reasonable simulation for many aspects of the performance of full-scale systems and of suggesting the directions for research emphasis in ways to control their environmental effects. Examples of representative data from the RTI unit are compared with literature values for both fixed-bed and fluidized-bed gasifiers in Table I. The overall results that have been achieved with the laboratory gasifier are comparable to those reported for the fixed-bed gasifier of the Morgantown Energy Research Center (MERC) and for the fluidized-bed gasifier of the Synthane process under development at the Pittsburgh Energy Research Center (PERC). The concentrations of hydrogen sulfide, carbonyl sulfide, and ethane from the RTI test runs are of the same order of magnitude as they are from the MERC and PERC results. It can also be noted that the amount of tar produced (0.022 kg/kg coal converted) is the same value for Run 6 at RTI and for the MERC reactor. Finally, the amount of fuel-gas product was 2.7 to 2.9 $Nm^3$/kg coal converted in Runs 6 and 16 at RTI and in the MERC reactor.

The hydrogen-to-carbon monoxide ratio is generally higher from the laboratory reactor than in the other two processes presented. This is directly attributable to lower air-to-steam feed ratios than those typical of commercial or proposed fixed-bed coal gasification reactors.

Another example of the extent to which the RTI laboratory gasifier produces effluents similar to those of larger-scale processes is found in Table II[2-5] and Figure 2, which compare concentrations of selected species in the tar for various gasifiers. The agreement is sufficient to lend credence to the

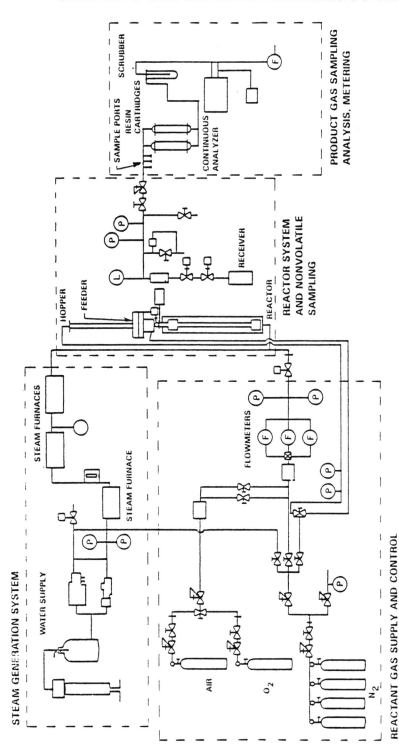

**Figure 1.**   Gasifier and sampling train.

**Table I.**  Coal Gasification: Operating Conditions and Primary Products

| Test Run No: | RTI Data | | | | MERC (airblown) | PERC Synthane (airblown) | PERC Synthane (oxygen-blown) |
|---|---|---|---|---|---|---|---|
| | No. 2 (airblown) | No. 4 (external heat only) | No. 6 (external heat only) | No. 16 (airblown) | | | |
| Feed Material: | FMC Char | FMC Char | Illinois No. 6 | Illinois No. 6 | Illinois No. 6 | Illinois No. 6 | Illinois No. 6 |
| Feed amount, kg | 0.175 | 0.600 | 1.034 | 1.573 | NA[a] | NA[a] | NA[a] |
| Pressure, MPa | 1.5 | 1.5 | 1.5 | 1.5 | 0.22 | 1.9 | 4.2 |
| Temperature (exit) °C | 285 | 353 | 367 | 454 | 650 | NA[a] | 760 |
| Temperature (max) °C | 735 | 833 | 726 | 955 | 1,350 | 987 | 982 |
| Time at sample, min | 77 | 123 | 73 | 78 | NA[a] | NA[a] | NA[a] |
| Component, moisture free | | | | | | | |
| $O_2$, % | 3.0 | | | | | | |
| $N_2$ + Ar, % | 56.9 | 27.7 | 35.2 | 26.6 | 51.5 | 43.4 | |
| CO, % | 2.0 | 3.1 | 4.0 | 17.0 | 21.8 | 10.1 | 13.2 |
| $CO_2$, % | 17.4 | 20.0 | 10.1 | 16.9 | 6.9 | 17.9 | 36.2 |
| $H_2$, % | 9.0 | 38.8 | 29.4 | 36.6 | 17.8 | 21.5 | 32.3 |
| $CH_4$, % | 4.9 | 8.9 | 18.2 | 2.5 | 2.0 | 5.6 | 15.0 |
| $H_2S$, % | 1.3 | 0.6 | 1.2 | 0.5 | 0.2 | 0.7 | 1.6 |
| COS, ppm | 63 | 11 | 83 | 33 | 315 | NA[a] | 150 |
| $C_2H_4$, ppm | 23 | 47 | 1,000 | 8 | | | |
| $C_6H_6$, ppm | 157 | 380 | 4,800 | 37 | 2,000 | 7,000 | 16,000 |
| Tar, kg/kg coal | 12.8 | | 0.022 | 0.035 | 0.022 | 0.047 | 0.047 |
| Gas product, $Nm^3$/kg | | 3.5 | 2.8 | 2.7 | 2.9 | 1.3 | 0.81 |
| Gas product, scf/lb | 220 | 56 | 44.6 | 43.8 | 47 | 20.7 | 13.8 |

[a]NA = Not available.

**Table II.** Comparison of RTI Tar Composition and Production to Those from Other Gasifiers

| | RTI Range 95% Confidence | Synthane[a] Illinois No. 6 | MERC[b] | Chapman[c] Wilputte | GFETC[a,d] | Coal Tar 1 | Coal Tar 2 |
|---|---|---|---|---|---|---|---|
| Total tar, mg/g coal | 15–23 | 37 | 26–34 | 100 | 12–36 | | |
| Cresols | 1.1E4–2.3E4 | | 1.8E4[e] | | | 8.0E3 | |
| Xylenols | 7.1E3–1.7E4 | | | | | 2.0E3 | |
| Dibenzo($a,h$)anthracene | 7.5E2–2.1E3 | | | | | | 2.3E2 |
| Benzo($a$)pyrene | 1.5E3–2.5E3 | | 4.0E3 | 8.0E2 | 7.0E3[f] | | 1.8E3 |
| Perylene | 1.1E3–2.5E3 | | | 8.0E2 | | | 8.0E3 |
| Benzo($a$)anthracene | 2.6E3–5.6E3 | | | | | | 7.0E3 |
| Benzo($g,h,i$)perylene | 3.6E2–1.6E3 | | | | | | 1.9E3 |
| Phenanthrene | 1.9E4–4.1E4 | 1.2E5[g] | | | 4.2E4 | 5.0E4 | 1.8E4 |
| Naphthalene | 3.7E4–1.1E5 | 7.0E4 | 2.1E4 | 2.0E3 | 6.3E4 | 1.0E5 | |
| Acenaphthylene | 1.5E4–2.9E4 | | | | | 2.0E4 | |
| Pyrene | 8.2E3–2.4E4 | 4.2E4 | | | 2.5E4 | 2.1E4 | 1.1E4 |
| Phenol | 4.5E3–1.1E4 | 1.2E4 | 4.0E2 | 2.0E3 | 1.0E5 | 4.0E3 | |
| Biphenyl | 2.6E3–4.0E3 | | | | 1.6E4 | 4.0E3 | |
| Acenaphthene | 3.2E3–5.6E3 | 1.2E5[e] | | | | 3.0E3 | |
| Chrysene | 2.8E3–5.6E3 | 7.6E4[h] | | 3.0E3 | 1.4E4 | 2.0E4 | 2.9E4 |

[a] Reference 4, this chapter.
[b] Reference 5, this chapter.
[c] Reference 2, this chapter.
[d] Reference 3, this chapter.
[e] Analysis of pollutant class.
[f] Includes benzo($e$)pyrene.
[g] Includes anthracene.
[h] Includes benzo($a$)anthracene.

**Figure 2.** Comparisons of
RTI gasifier to other units.

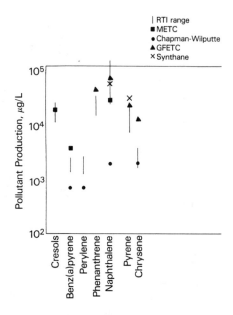

thesis that results of laboratory-scale units are sufficiently representative of those from larger units to be of value in guiding large-scale research and control studies.

Approximately 50 gasification runs have been completed with various coals and various operating conditions. A summary of all the feedstocks used is tabulated in Table III, four of which will be considered in detail in this chapter: Illinois No. 6 bituminous, Wyoming subbituminous, North Dakota lignite, and Western Kentucky No. 9 bituminous. These fuels were used in the runs for which bioassay data were obtained. Operating conditions for these runs are shown in Table IV.

## STATISTICAL ANALYSIS OF DATA

A statistical analysis of the results from all gasifier runs was carried out to identify the most important operating parameters affecting the production of selected potential pollutants. A stepwise linear regression analysis was used to determine the correlation between the operating and production parameters.

A list of the important gasifier operating parameters is shown in Table V. These were used as the independent variables in correlating the pollutant production parameters, which were considered to be the dependent variables in the analysis. The operating parameters were chosen from a more extensive set using engineering judgment and past experience in analyzing gasifier data. Of the 20 variables so chosen, 14 characterize the coal used

**Table III.**  Gasification Feedstocks

| Fuel | Btu/lb (including moisture and ash) | Moisture (%) | Ash (%) | Volatile Matter (%) | Fixed Carbon (%) | Sulfur: Sulfate | Organic | Pyritic | Total | Carbon[a] (%) | Hydrogen[a] (%) | Oxygen (%) | Nitrogen (%) | FSI (%) | Ash Fusion Temp (°F) |
|---|---|---|---|---|---|---|---|---|---|---|---|---|---|---|---|
| Western Kentucky FMC char | 11,090 | 1.90 | 19.70 | 7.80 | 71.50 | | | | 1.80 | 74.02 | 1.48 | 1.70 | 1.3 | <1.0 | 2600[b] |
| Illinois No. 6 bituminous | 11,331 | 6.85 | 13.52 | 32.58 | 47.05 | 0.15 | 1.16 | 1.71 | 3.02 | 63.26 | 5.37 | 13.46 | 1.35 | 3.5 | 2350[b] (2030-2730) |
| Montana Rosebud subbituminous | 9,004 | 21.19 | 8.86 | 31.56 | 38.39 | 0.17 | 0.21 | 0.21 | 0.59 | 53.95 | 6.87 | 28.53 | 1.20 | 0.0 | (2150-2240) |
| North Carolina humus peat | 4,975 | 45.98 | 3.67 | 31.81 | 18.54 | 0.05 | 0.06 | 0.01 | 0.12 | 30.22 | 5.34 | 59.84 | 0.81 | 0.0 | 2270[b] (2060-) |
| Pittsburgh No. 8 | 12,288 | 3.08 | 11.09 | 29.16 | 56.67 | <0.01 | 1.28 | 1.24 | 2.53 | 72.29 | 3.45 | 8.62 | 1.95 | 7 | 2780 |

**Table III.** *(continued)*

| Fuel | Btu/lb (including moisture and ash) | Mois-ture (%) | Ash (%) | Volatile Matter (%) | Fixed Carbon (%) | Sulfur: Sulfate (%) | Organic (%) | Pyritic (%) | Total (%) | Carbon[a] (%) | Hydro-gen[a] (%) | Oxygen (%) | Nitrogen (%) | FSI (%) | Ash Fusion Temp (°F) |
|---|---|---|---|---|---|---|---|---|---|---|---|---|---|---|---|
| Wyoming subbituminous | 7,880 | 15.56 | 6.31 | 38.30 | 39.30 | 0.07 | 0.08 | 0.40 | 0.55 | 56.80 | 5.94 | 30.02 | 0.38 | 0.0 | 2280[b] (2110-2460) |
| North Dakota Lignite | 7,880 | 29.63 | 6.39 | 28.57 | 35.41 | 0.01 | 0.54 | <0.01 | 0.56 | 46.82 | 9.85 | 35.63 | 0.73 | | 2340[b] |
| Western Kentucky No. 9 bituminous | 12,130 | 7.03 | 7.83 | 38.78 | 46.36 | 0.05 | 2.90 | 1.83 | 4.78 | 67.36 | 5.58 | 13.68 | 1.08 | 4 | 2090[b] (1970-2400) |

[a]Includes moisture.
[b]Median fusion temperature.

**Table IV.**   Operating Conditions for Selected Gasification Runs

| | Run 33 Wyoming Subbituminous | Run 35 Wyoming Subbituminous | Run 41 Western Kentucky Bituminous | Run 44 Illinois No. 6 Bituminous | Run 47 Wyoming Subbituminous | Run 51 North Dakota Lignite |
|---|---|---|---|---|---|---|
| Steam, g | 500 | 527 | 1,390 | 1,084 | 528 | 447 |
| Air, g | 2,097 | 2,461 | 3,060 | 4,753 | 2,275 | 1,430 |
| Coal, g | 1,396 | 1,420 | 1,250 | 1,250 | 1,430 | 1,491 |
| Air/coal | 1.5 | 1.7 | 2.5 | | | |
| Steam/coal | 0.36 | 0.37 | 1.1 | 0.87 | 0.37 | 0.30 |
| Air steam | 4.2 | 4.6 | 2.2 | 4.38 | 4.3 | 3.2 |
| $T_{max}$,[a] °C | 1,010 | 790 | 1,034 | 976 | 946 | 939 |
| Carbon conversion, % | 98.9 | 97 | 99.8 | 87.7 | 98.1 | 99.99 |
| Sulfur conversion, % | 91 | 85 | 98 | 91.9 | 94.3 | 74 |
| Tar yield, g/g coal | 0.012 | 0.019 | 0.030 | 0.0210 | 0.0208 | 0.0119 |

[a] Time-averaged maximum bed temperature.

**Table V.** Important Gasifier Operating Parameters (independent variables in the regression analysis)

| Code | Definition |
|---|---|
| PCTVOLMT | Volatile matter in coal, % |
| PCTASH | Ash in coal, % |
| SULFUR | Total sulfur in coal, % |
| HTRT | Heating rate of the coal during pyrolysis phase taken as the slope of the time temperature curve as the coal is heated from 300 to 700°C |
| AC | Air-to-coal ratio, g/g |
| AS | Air-to-steam ratio, g/g |
| PCTMOIST | Moisture in coal, % |
| FBTULB | Higher heating value of coal |
| CLCHRG | Coal charged to the gasifier, g |
| TGAS | Average gas flow rate into gasifier, sLpm |
| TMAXAVG | Mean of the maximum bed temperature averaged over the entire test, °C |
| ORG | Organic sulfur in coal, % |
| SULFATE | Sulfur as sulfate in coal, % |
| SC | Steam-to-coal ratio, g/g |
| FXDCAR | Fixed carbon in coal, % |
| PYR | Sulfur as pyrites in coal, % |
| CARBON | Carbon in coal, % |
| HYDRO | Hydrogen in coal, % |
| OXY | Oxygen in coal, % |
| NITRO | Nitrogen in coal, % |

in the tests and the remainder describe the operation of the gasifier. The heating rate during pyrolysis (HTRT), the air-to-coal (AC) and steam-to-coal (SC) ratios, and the bed temperature (TMAXAVG) are known to affect both the quantity and distribution of products from gasifiers. The amount of coal charged (CLCHRG) and the average gas flow into the gasifier (TGAS) were chosen as independent variables because they are indicative of gas-solid contact and bed height.

Selected pollutant production variables and several other indicators of gasifier performance, which make up the dependent variable set, are shown in Table VI. In general, the pollutant production parameters are yields for a specific compound per unit of carbon gasified or coal loaded. They were chosen because the raw product gas concentration of these compounds typically exceeded published thresholds for adverse health effects.

The stepwise linear regression analysis was carried out using a standard statistical program. Briefly, the stepwise computer program finds the single-variable model that produces the largest $R^2$ statistic (where $R^2$ is the square

**Table VI.** Important Pollution Production Parameters
and Gasifier Performance Variables
(dependent variables in the regression analysis)

| Code | Definition |
|------|------------|
| SCFLB | Total gas produced, scf/lb coal |
| BTUSCF | Higher heating value of gas produced, Btu/scf |
| ORACL | Tar organic acid yield, g × 100/g coal |
| ORBCL | Tar organic base yield, g × 100/g coal |
| NPNCL | Tar nonpolar neutral yield, g × 100/g coal |
| PNACL | Tar polynuclear aromatic yield, g × 100/g coal |
| PCTTARCL | Tar yield from coal, % |
| AR4 | Tar arsenic yield, µg/g carbon converted |
| SU2 | Ash sulfur yield, µg/g carbon converted |
| BEN10 | Benzene production, µg in bulb/g carbon converted |
| BTX | BTX production, µg/g carbon converted |
| PHET | Total phenol production, µg/g carbon converted |
| CRET | Total cresol production, µg/g carbon converted |
| HS10 | $H_2S$ yield in gas, µg/g carbon converted |
| CS10 | COS yield in gas, µg/g carbon converted |
| SRAT10 | Ratio $H_2S$ to COS in gas, g/g |
| MTH10 | $CH_3SH$ yield in gas, µg/g carbon converted |
| NAPT | Total naphthalene yield, µg/g carbon converted |
| PTHT | Total phenanthrene yield, µg/g carbon converted |
| INE8 | Indene yield in gas, µg/g carbon converted |
| BFU8 | Benzofuran yield in gas, µg/g carbon converted |
| FTH4 | Fluoranthene yield in tar, µg/g carbon converted |
| FLU4 | Fluorene yield in tar, µg/g carbon converted |

of the multiple correlation coefficient). After entering the variable with the largest $R^2$, the program uses the partial correlation coefficients to select the next variable to enter the regression. That is, the program enters the variable with the highest partial correlation coefficient (given that the variable with the largest $R^2$ is already in the model). An F-test is performed to determine if the variable to be entered has a probability greater than the specified significance level for entry into the analysis. (For the analysis presented here, this level was 50%.) After the variable is added, the program searches *all* the variables already included in the model and computes a partial-F statistic to determine if these variables should remain in the model. Any variable not producing a partial F significant at the specified significance level of retention (i.e., 0.10) is then deleted from the model. The process then continues by determining if any other variables should be added to the regression. The process terminates when no variable meets the conditions for inclusion or when the next variable to be added to the model is the one previously deleted from it.

## STATISTICAL ANALYSIS RESULTS

The results of the analysis using the independent variables from Table V and the dependent variables in Table VI are summarized in Table VII. Entries in this table correspond to the order of importance of each independent variable in accounting for the variation in each dependent variable. For example, in the row labeled SCFLB (total scf product gas/lb coal), a value of 1+ was entered in column AC (air-to-coal ratio). This means that the air-to-coal ratio was the most important parameter in correlating the total product gas. Also in the same row, the steam-to-coal ratio was the second most important variable in correlating the total product gas with a linear model.

The positive or negative sign following each numerical entry in Table VII is the sign of the coefficient of the corresponding independent variable in the linear model. For example, examination of the first two dependent variables shows that the volume of product gas increases and the heating value of the gas decreases with increase in air-to-coal ratio. This is to be expected due to increased nitrogen concentration in the product gas.

In Figures 3 through 5, the predicted yields for several pollutants are compared to the experimental values obtained from the RTI gasifier. The agreement is reasonable even though the gasifier runs include a variety of coals and operating conditions.

The predicted yield of organic bases (ORBCL) in crude gasifier tar is shown in Figure 3 vs the actual yield. A correlation coefficient of 0.955 was obtained. The amount of scatter in the data is quite low and uniform over the range of the correlation for the 19 values available.

The predicted polynuclear aromatics (PNACL) yield in crude gasifier tar is shown in Figure 4 vs the actual yield. The noticeable degree of scatter seen in this figure is reflected by a correlation coefficient of 0.777. In Table VII, the four independent variables that most successfully represent the yield of polynuclear aromatics are coal sulfur content (SULFUR), coal charge

**Table VII.** Summary of the Statistical Analysis of the RTI Gasifier Screening Run Using All Independent Variables in Table V

| Dependent Variables (from Table VI) | % vol. matter (PCTVOLMT) | % Ash (PCTASH) | % Sulfur (SULFUR) | Heating Rate (HTRT) | Air/Coal (AC) | Air/Steam (AS) | % Moisture (PCTMOIST) | Heating Value (FBTULB) | Coal Charged (CLCHRG) | Inlet Gas Flow (TGAS) | Bed Temperature (TMAXAVG) | % Organic S (ORG) | % Sulfate S (SULFATE) | Steam/Coal (SC) | % Fixed Carbon (FXDCAR) | % Pyritic S (PYR) | % Carbon (CARBON) | % Hydrogen (HYDRO) | % Oxygen (OXY) | % Nitrogen (NITRO) | $R^2$ | Observations (No.) |
|---|---|---|---|---|---|---|---|---|---|---|---|---|---|---|---|---|---|---|---|---|---|---|
| Gas produced (SCFLB) | | | | 4− | 1+ | | | | 3+ | | | | | 2+ | — | | | | | | 0.965 | 34 |
| Gas HHV (BTUSCF) | | | | 3+ | 1− | | | | | | | | | 2+ | 2+ | | | | | | 0.766 | 25 |
| Organic acids (ORACL) | 1+ | | | | | | | | | 2+ | 3− | | | | | | | | | | 0.662 | 19 |
| Organic bases (ORBCL) | 2+ | | 1+ | | 7+ | | | | 3+ | 6− | | | | 5+ | | | | | | 4+ | 0.981 | 19 |
| Nonpolar neutrals (NPNCL) | 2+ | | | | | | | | | | | | | | | 1+ | | | | | 0.338 | 19 |
| PNAs (PNACL) | | 5+ | 2+ | 1+ | | | | | 4+ | 3− | | | | | | | | | | | 0.876 | 18 |
| Tar yield (PCTTARCL) | 2+ | | | | | | | | 3+ | | | | | | | 1+ | | | | | 0.850 | 19 |
| Arsenic in tar (AR4) | | | 1+ | | | | | | 2+ | | | | | | | | | | | | 0.768 | 8 |
| Sulfur in ash (SU2) | | | | | 2+ | | | | | | | 1+ | | | | | | 3+ | | | 0.688 | 18 |

Independent Variables (from Table V)

| Dependent Variables (from Table VI) | % vol. matter (PCTVOLMT) | % Ash (PCTASH) | % Sulfur (SULFUR) | Heating Rate (HTRT) | Air/Coal (AC) | Air/Steam (AS) | % Moisture (PCTMOIST) | Heating Value (FBTULB) | Coal Charged (CLCHRG) | Inlet Gas Flow (TGAS) | Bed Temperature (TMAXAVG) | % Organic S (ORG) | % Sulfate S (SULFATE) | Steam/Coal (SC) | % Fixed Carbon (FXDCAR) | % Pyritic S (PYR) | % Carbon (CARBON) | % Hydrogen (HYDRO) | % Oxygen (OXY) | % Nitrogen (NITRO) | $R^2$ | Observations (No.) |
|---|---|---|---|---|---|---|---|---|---|---|---|---|---|---|---|---|---|---|---|---|---|---|
| Benzene yield (BEN10) | | | | 1+ 4+ | | 3 – | | 2 + | | | | | | | | | | | | | 0.838 | 17 |
| BTX yield (BTX) | | | | 3+ | | | | | | 2 – | 4+ | | | 1+ | | | | | | 5 – | 0.958 | 15 |
| Phenol yield (PHET) | | | | | 2 – | | | | | 3 – | | | 1 + | | | | | | | 1 – | 0.346 | 14 |
| Cresols yield (CRET) | | | | | | | | | 1 – | | | | | | | | | | | | 0.456 | 14 |
| Hydrogen sulfide (HS10) | | | | | | | | | | | 2 – | | | | | 1 + | | | | | 0.715 | 21 |
| Carbonyl sulfide (CS10) | | | | | 1+ | | | | | | | | 3 – | 2+ | 4 – | | | | | | 0.862 | 21 |
| H₂S/COS (SRAT10) | | | | | 2 – | | | | | 3 – | | | 1+ | | | | | | | | 0.731 | 21 |
| Methanethiol (MTH10) | | | | | | | | | | | | | 2 – | 1+ | | | | | | | 0.334 | 19 |

| | | | | | | | | | |
|---|---|---|---|---|---|---|---|---|---|
| Naphthalene (NAPT) | | | | | | | 1+ | | 0.416 | 15 |
| Phenanthrene (PTHT) | | 1+ | | 2+ | | | | | 0.990 | 7 |
| Indene (INE8) | | | | | 1+ | | | 3 − | 0.098 | 16 |
| Benzofuran (BFU8) | | | 1 − | | 2 − | | | | 0.513 | 14 |
| Fluoranthene (FTH4) | 4+ | | | 2+ 3 − | | | 1+ | | 0.871 | 16 |
| Fluorene (FLU4) | | | | | | | 1+ | | 0.261 | 16 |

**Figure 3.** Comparison of the observed and predicted tar organic acid yields for the RTI gasifier screening test.

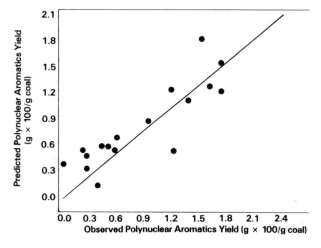

**Figure 4.** Comparison of the observed and predicted tar organic yields for the RTI gasifier screening tests.

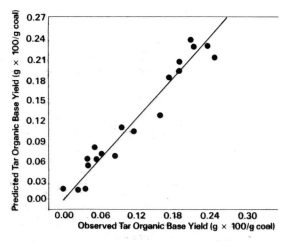

**Figure 5.** Comparison of observed and predicted tar yields for the RTI gasifier screening tests.

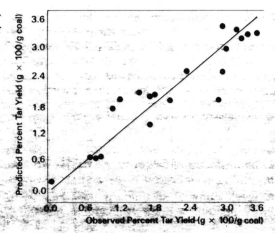

amount (CLCHRG), the gas flow rate (TGAS) to the gasifier, and the air/coal feed ratio (AC).

Figure 5 displays the predicted vs observed yield of crude gasifier tar (PCTTARCL) expressed as percent of the raw coal feed, which appears as tar (i.e., g tar × 100/g coal). A good correlation was obtained; the correlation coefficient was 0.860 based on four significant independent variables: total sulfur (SULFUR), sulfate sulfur (SULFATE), percent volatile matter (PCTVOLMT), and quantity of coal used (CLCHRG).

Relative to the yields of potential pollutants considered in this analysis, the coal characterization parameters of total sulfur, sulfate, and volatile content were the most important parameters. The importance of the volatile matter content of the raw coals undoubtedly reflects the fact that the coal-derived volatiles contain many of the potential pollutants under study here. The three sulfur variables of total sulfur, pyritic sulfur, and organic sulfur exhibited generally the same behavior in the regression analyses. This is explained by the fact that the pyritic sulfur and organic sulfur levels were highly correlated with the total sulfur level, the correlation coefficients being 0.90 and 0.85 respectively.

The importance of sulfur indicated in Table VII may to some extent be a statistical artifact that lacks physical meaning. However, an attempt to further evaluate the possible existence of causative factors has been initiated. The sulfur species (i.e., pyritic, organic, and/or total sulfur content) were intercorrelated as independent variables relative to dependent variables such as hydrogen sulfide yield. Moreover, the iron content of the coal is highly correlated with the pyritic sulfur. Iron is capable of substituting for sulfur in thiophene structures; thus, a higher iron pyrite content for coal can result in a greater potential for the modification of organically bonded sulfur.

Also, sulfur is known to form thioether and dithioether linkages in hydrocarbon media. This process can be a form of "vulcanization" in which the presence of the sulfur promotes the formation and/or maintenance of larger molecular weight hydrocarbons, that is, tars. Clearly, the sulfur, nitrogen, and oxygen content of gasifier tar precursors influences the chemical properties of the tar.

Table VIII gives Ames bioassay results for tars and tar fractions from various coals. Note that in accordance with many other investigations, the primary mutagenic activity appears to lie in the tar base fraction, in the PNA fraction, and occasionally in the polar neutral fraction. We think the exceptionally high specific activity of the polar neutral fraction in Run 44, Illinois No. 6 coal, is an anomaly and results from fractionation errors in the tar base, polar neutral separation. Note that the tar bases for this particular run are abnormally low as well.

Tar and tar fraction yields for the same runs (mg/g coal) are shown in Table IX. Figures 6 through 11 represent a combined plotting of this information in which the tar fractions are plotted along the abscissa and the

**Table VIII.** Mutagenicity for Tars and Fractions from Various Coals, Specific Activity, $\dfrac{\text{Revertants}}{\mu g}$

| Run No. | Tar | Bases | PNA | Polar Neutrals | Acids |
|---|---|---|---|---|---|
| North Dakota lignite, 51 | 1.915 | 17.9 | 0.85 | 1.91 | — |
| Wyoming subbituminous, 33 | 1.189 | 8.5 | 1.56 | 1.42 | — |
| Wyoming subbituminous, 35 | 0.399 | 15.62 | 0.652 | — | — |
| Wyoming subbituminous, 47 | 0.265 | 5.8 | 0.36 | 0.30 | — |
| Western Kentucky No. 9, 41 | 8.69 | 33.79 | 7.72 | 1.77 | — |
| Illinois No. 6, 44 | 11.29 | 6.23 | 1.96 | 37.46 | — |

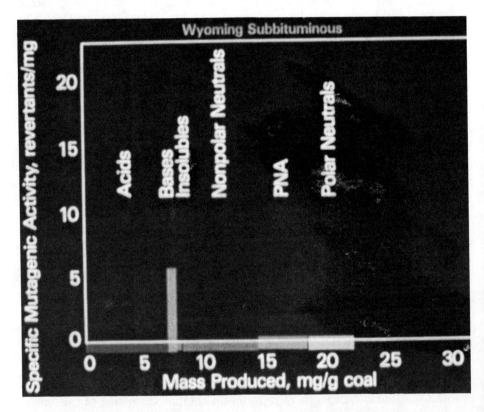

**Figure 6.** Tar fraction productivity and activity, Wyoming subbituminous.

**Table IX.** Tar and Tar Fraction Yields (mg/g coal)

| Run No. | Tar | Acids | Bases | Insolubles | Nonpolar Neutral | PNA | Polar Neutral |
|---|---|---|---|---|---|---|---|
| Wyoming subbituminous, 33 | 12.2 | 3.28 | 0.40 | 0.21 | 2.49 | 4.86 | 0.95 |
| Wyoming subbituminous, 35 | 28.9 | 8.55 | 0.98 | 1.18 | 5.29 | 10.23 | 2.66 |
| Western Kentucky No. 9, 41 | 30.1 | 1.57 | 2.14 | 2.44 | 3.76 | 18.60 | 1.63 |
| Illinois No. 6, 44 | 30.0 | 1.95 | 1.95 | 1.44 | 3.36 | 20.22 | 1.08 |
| Wyoming subbituminous, 47 | 20.8 | 6.76 | 0.57 | 0.44 | 6.06 | 4.03 | 3.95 |
| North Dakota lignite, 51 | 11.9 | 2.80 | 0.54 | 1.31 | 2.03 | 4.31 | 0.92 |

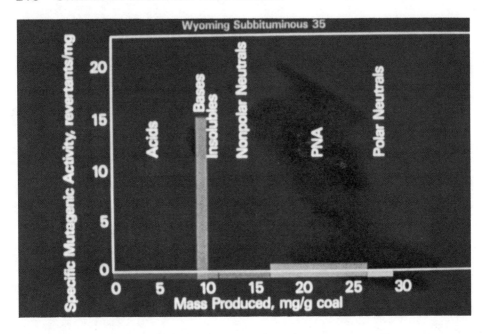

**Figure 7.** Tar fraction productivity and activity, Wyoming subbituminous 35.

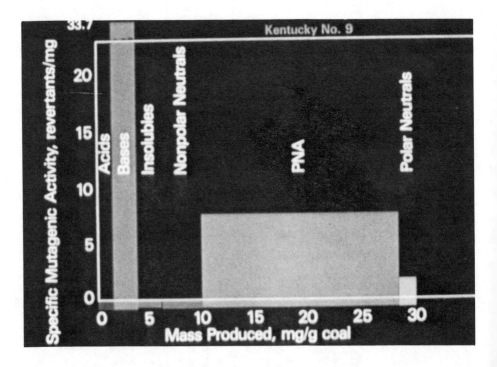

**Figure 8.** Tar fraction productivity and activity, Kentucky No. 9.

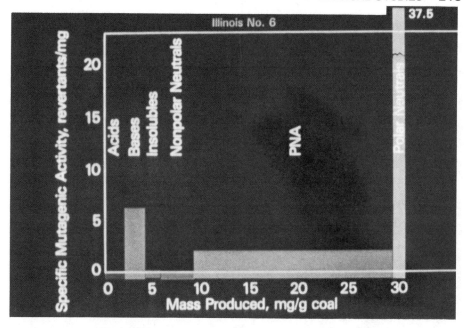

**Figure 9.**    Tar fraction productivity and activity, Illinois No. 6.

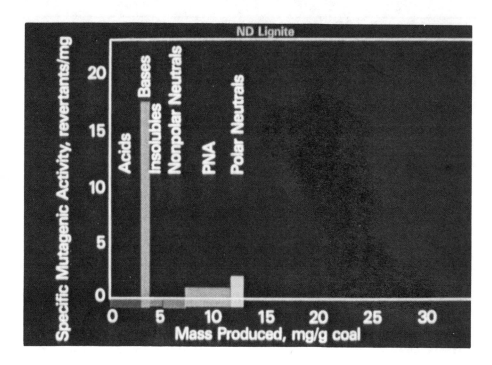

**Figure 10.**    Tar fraction productivity and activity, North Dakota lignite.

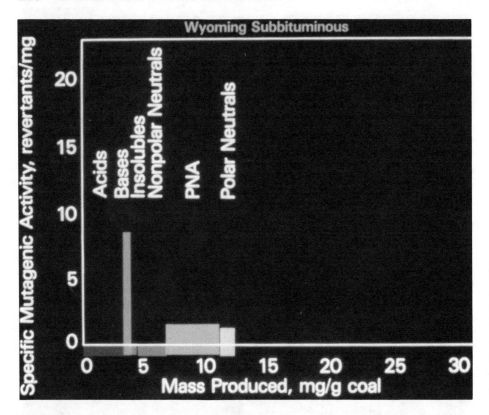

**Figure 11.**   Tar fraction productivity and activity, Wyoming subbituminous.

specific mutagenic activity is plotted along the ordinate. Thus, in some sense at least, the areas as shown represent the product of mutagenic specific activity and quantity of material produced and can be interpreted as an indication of the relative hazard. The similarities from fuel to fuel are evident, as are some notable differences. A discussion of possible reasons for the differences follows.

## DISCUSSION OF FUEL-TO-FUEL DIFFERENCES

Figures 12 and 13, abstracted from the statistical analysis previously discussed, remind us of the major factors influencing the production of tar, tar

**Figure 12.**   Factors influencing tar base production ($R^2 = 0.955$).

| | |
|---|---|
| Volatile matter | Air/steam ratio |
| Sulfur content | Temperature |
| Amount of coal | Air/coal ratio |

**Figure 13.**  Factors influencing PNA production ($R^2 = 0.777$).

| Sulfur content | Amount of coal |
|---|---|
| Heating rate | Inlet gas flow rate |

bases, and polynuclear aromatic hydrocarbons, with factors exhibiting a positive influence in the left column, and those exhibiting a negative influence in the right column.

Figures 14–16 indicate tar yields, tar base yields, and tar acid yields for coals of various ranks. The tar yield increases with rank up through bituminous coals. This could possibly be caused by the development of aromatic structures that are associated with the coalification process that can be envisioned as a long transition from oxygen-containing plant matter to aromatic coal structures.

The coalification process may also account for higher tar base yields

**Figure 14.**  Tar yield for various rank coals.

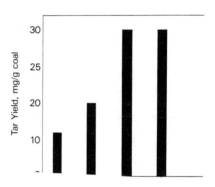

**Figure 15.**  Base yield for various rank coals.

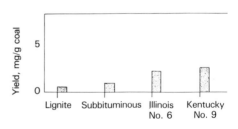

**Figure 16.**  Acid yield for various ranks.

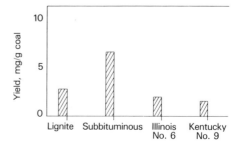

in higher ranked coals; it can be reasonably expected to result in closer association between the nitrogen and the aromatic coal structure. The nitrogen can be either incorporated into the aromatic structure or present in substituents and linkages. The results in gasification processes may well be that the less tightly bound nitrogen is released as ammonia, whereas that which is more closely associated with the coal structure tends to form nitrogen-containing aromatic compounds (e.g., nitrogen heterocycles and aromatic amines) which are the primary constituents of the tar base fraction.

A similar argument applies to the role of oxygen in the coalification process and its contribution to the yield of tar acids, which are primarily phenols.

It is instructive to examine the effect of fuel nitrogen on tar base yield and activity shown in Figures 17 and 18 and Table X. Since the tar bases

**Figure 17.** Effect of fuel nitrogen on tar base yield.

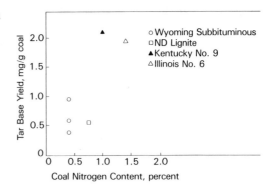

**Figure 18.** Effect of fuel nitrogen on tar base activity.

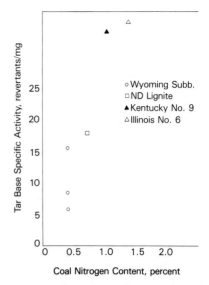

**Table X.**    Tar Base Yields and Specific Activity vs
Fuel Nitrogen and Sulfur Content

| Run No. | Fuel | Tar Base Yield (mg/g coal) | Base Specific Activity (revertants µg) | Nitrogen Content of Coal (%) | Sulfur Content Pyritic (%) | Sulfur Content Total |
|---|---|---|---|---|---|---|
| 33 ⎫ | Wyoming | | 8.5 | | | |
| 35 ⎭ | subbituminous | 0.4 | 15.6 | 0.38 | 0.4 | 0.55 |
| 41 | Western Kentucky No. 9 | 2.1 | 33.8 | 1.08 | 1.8 | 4.8 |
| 44 | Illinois No. 6 | 2.3 | 6.2 | 1.35 | 1.7 | 3.0 |
| 47 | Wyoming subbituminous | 0.4 | 5.8 | 0.38 | 0.4 | 0.55 |
| 51 | North Dakota lignite | 0.5 | 17.9 | 0.73 | — | 0.56 |

are primarily nitrogen compounds, one might reasonably expect fuel nitrogen to be highly correlated with tar base yield. That this is the case is shown by the statistical results as well as the correlation evident in Figure 17. Not only does fuel nitrogen evidently affect the yield of tar bases, but it also appears to affect the mutagenic activity, as shown in Figure 18. We are unaware of the reasons for the evident effects of fuel nitrogen on tar base mutagenic activity.

Is there evidence from the chemical analysis of the tar base fraction that can explain the differences in mutagenic activity from fuel to fuel? Table XI summarizes the results available from our laboratories—no trends are evident to explain such behavior. A number of additional compounds have

**Table XI.**    Tar Base Analyses

| | Tar Base Fraction (%) | | | | | |
|---|---|---|---|---|---|---|
| | 33 | 35 | 41 | 44 | 47 | 51 |
| Fuel Type | Wyoming Subbituminous | | Western Kentucky No. 9 | Illinois No. 6 | Wyoming Subbituminous | North Dakota lignite |
| Aniline | 0.22 | 0.14 | 0.03 | 0.005 | 0.06 | |
| Benzidine | | | | | | |
| Quinoline | 2.52 | 0.35 | 1.55 | 1.23 | 0.92 | 4.67 |
| Acridine | 0.61 | 0.10 | 0.66 | 1.13 | 0.02 | 0.44 |
| Indole | 0.04 | 0.07 | 0.01 | 0.01 | 0.003 | |

been tentatively identified on the basis of boiling-point-retention time plots and the likelihood of their presence. However, any comments on them must await confirmation with more specific instrumentation. Other investigations have pointed out the extreme mutagenicity of compounds such as 2-aminoanthracene. We have quantitated aminonaphthalenes in our tars at concentrations of the same order of magnitude as reported in the SRC-II distillate.[6] Thus, we would expect concentrations of the more mutagenic 2-aminoanthracene and other amino compounds to be similar to those found in the SRC-II distillate. No analytical results are yet available to confirm these expectations.

Is there any information in the chemical characterization of the tars that would account for the higher mutagenic activity of the polynuclear aromatic fraction of the Illinois No. 6 coal? Table XII shows the analytical results available to date for various polynuclear aromatic hydrocarbon compounds in the tar PNA fraction. No trends are evident from these analyses to explain the higher mutagenicity activity of Illinois No. 6 material. We suspect that the higher activity is caused by higher-molecular-weight PNA compounds—those in the 5- and 6-ring range.

The specific mode of operation of the gasifier (whether continuous or batch, with respect to coal addition) appears to exert a strong influence on the mutagenic activities of the tar fractions as indicated in Table XIII. Note that the tar base fractions exhibit much lower specific mutagenic activity for continuous operation than for batch operation. We suspect that the reasons have to do with the severity of conditions encountered during the devolatilization phase of the operation. A lump of coal fed in continuous fashion to the reactor is subjected to a more rapid heating rate during the devolatilization phase and, consequently, can experience a greater opportunity to

**Table XII.** Tar PNA Analyses (mg/g PNA)

| Compound | Run 41 Western Kentucky No. 9 | Run 44 Illinois No. 6 |
|---|---|---|
| Naphthalene | 13.7 | 26.9 |
| 2-Methylnaphthalene | 10.4 | 7.8 |
| Anthracene | 37.2 | 31.5 |
| Phenanthrene | 35.6 | 12.9 |
| 9-Methylanthracene | 7.0 | 2.5 |
| Chrysene | NA[a] | 27.0 |
| Pyrene | 38.8 | 25.5 |
| Perylene | NA[a] | 2.2 |
| Fluorene | 12.1 | 7.6 |
| Fluoranthene | 55.0 | 24.0 |
| Dibenzofuran | 13.1 | 13.7 |

[a]Not available.

**Table XIII.** Effect of Continuous Operation on Mutagenic Activity

| | Tar | Base | PNA | Ratio |
|---|---|---|---|---|
| | Revertants/μg | | | Substituents/Parents |
| Wyoming subbituminous | | | | |
| Batch | 0.3 | 6.6 | 0.80 | 2.5 |
| Continuous | 0.3 | 1.0 | 1.20 | 0.3 |
| North Dakota lignite | | | | |
| Batch | 1.5 | 8.0 | 0.5 | NA[a] |
| Continuous | 1.5 | 0.5 | 1.4 | |

[a]Not available.

undergo cracking and reforming reactions. This hypothesis is partially confirmed by the ratio of substituent compounds to parent compounds for the two runs. In this analysis, parent compounds are aromatic structures with no ring substituents, whereas the substituted compounds have ring substituents of various types.

## SUMMARY

The mutagenic activity that is associated with coal tars appears to be the most strongly associated with tar base fractions, followed by the polynuclear aromatic hydrocarbon fraction. The production of tars and tar bases, as well as their mutagenic activity, appears to be strongly influenced by the sulfur content of raw coal, by the nitrogen content of raw coal, by the coal rank, and by the repetitive heatup during devolatilization.

## ACKNOWLEDGMENT

This work was supported by the U.S. Environmental Protection Agency's Industrial Environmental Research Laboratory in Research Triangle Park, North Carolina, under Cooperative Agreement No. R804979. That assistance is gratefully acknowledged.

## REFERENCES

1. Gangwal, S.K., and D.G. Nichols. "Chemical Characterization of Tars from Fixed-Bed Gasification of Eastern and Western Coals" (Research Triangle Park, NC: Research Triangle Institute, 1980).
2. Page, G.C. "Environmental Assessment: Source Test and Evaluation Report-

Chapman Low-Btu Gasification," EPA-600/7-78-202 (Research Triangle Park, NC: U.S. Environmental Protection Agency, 1978).

3. Ellman, R.C., et al. "Slagging Fixed-Bed Gasification," *Proceedings of the Fourth Annual International Conference on Coal Gasification,* University of Pittsburgh, 1977. (Research Triangle Park, NC: U.S. Environmental Protection Agency).

4. Ghassemi, M., et al. "Environmental Assessment Data Base for High-Btu Gasification," EPA-600/7-78-186a (Research Triangle Park, NC: U.S. Environmental Protection Agency, 1978).

5. Pellizzari, E.D. "Identification of Components of Energy-Related Wastes and Effluents," Final Report (Research Triangle Park, NC: Research Triangle Institute, 1978).

6. Felix, W.D., et al. "Chemical/Biological Characterization of SRC-II Product and By-Products," *EPA Symposium on Environmental Aspects of Fuel Conversion Technology V,* St. Louis, Sept. 16–19, 1980. (Research Triangle Park, NC: U.S. Environmental Protection Agency).

## DISCUSSION

*S.C. Morris, Brookhaven National Laboratory:* Have you looked statistically at the interaction between sulfur and coal rank to see whether the observation that you get of sulfur's predicting PNAs is actually rank instead of sulfur?

*F.O. Mixon:* No. What we did was to define what we thought were appropriate independent and dependent variables for the statistical correlation. The definition produced some 15 or 20 dependent variables and probably another 15 or 20 independent variables that we thought would exhibit some effect on the process. We ran the statistical correlation. Then we took another look at it and asked which of the independent variables were strongly correlated one with the other. Sulfur is a good example—pyritic sulfur, organic sulfur, sulfate sulfur, and total sulfur. All the sulfur forms are indeed strongly correlated. What we did then was to quit looking at pyritic sulfur and organic sulfur as separate independent variables and lumped them into sulfur content. Consequently, we limited the set of independent and dependent variables to a much smaller group than the initial total. So, in a way, we are aware of what you mentioned, but we have not, to my knowledge, looked specifically at the sulfur-versus-rank variables. What I have shown you as sulfur and rank independently could well be the same cause effect.

*S.D. Van Hoesen, Oak Ridge National Laboratory:* What were the maximum temperatures you were able to achieve in the gasifier? Did you see any temperatures where tar productions seem to change drastically?

*F.O. Mixon:* The temperature range we looked at was limited, not so much by the equipment but by the set of runs that we made. We tried to operate the gasifier so that a run would last between 2 h and 10 or 12 h. Consequently, the maximum temperatures obtained were about 1000°C. I believe, as your question suggests, that higher temperatures, notably those characteristic of Koppers-Totzek gasification and some of the slagging gasification units, will burn up the organic materials. We did not have enough temperature variation in our 50 experiments to make that part of the statistical analysis worthwhile.

*S.D. Van Hoesen:* Is the apparatus capable of getting those kinds of temperatures, and do you plan to do anything along those lines?

*F.O. Mixon:* The gasifier is capable of operating at higher temperatures, and we would like to do the studies if we could find the funding. There are no such plans at present.

*M.J. Massey, Environmental Research and Technology:* Do you have any estimate of what the gas residence times were and to what degree they were variable? Similarly, are there correlations of residence time against yield?

*F.O. Mixon:* We have the raw data from which that information can be synthesized, but we have not made the calculations. I will be happy to discuss this with you later.

# CHAPTER 9

## Overview and Findings from Airlie House Retreat: Health and Environmental Research Programs Related to Coal Conversion Technologies and Their Future Directions

### A.P. Duhamel

*Office of Health and Environmental Research*

*U.S. Department of Energy*
*Washington, DC 20545*

The Office of Health and Environmental Research (OHER) formally initiated its coal-conversion research programs in the fall of 1977. The major objective of the programs was, and continues to be, to ensure the environmental acceptability of the emerging energy technologies. The initial phases of the programs were oriented toward short-term issues and the development of an environmental data base that could be used not only to address those issues but also as a building block in assessing longer-term issues. These phases of the program are complete.

To develop strategies for initiation of subsequent phases of the OHER programs related to coal gasification, liquefaction, and combustion, status reports have been prepared by the major laboratories engaged in health and environmental research. They include evaluations of the strengths and weaknesses of the present data bases, conclusions that can be drawn from the data bases, and recommended research.[1–3] Program are summarized in Table I.

In addition, a technical workshop was held at the Airlie House[4] to

**Table I.** Health and Environmental Programs

| Project | Laboratory | Location | Date Initiated | Status |
|---|---|---|---|---|
| *Gasification* | | | | |
| Low-Btu gasification | University of Minnesota/Oak Ridge National Laboratory | Duluth, MN | 1978 | Completed; final report being prepared |
| Low-Btu gasification | Oak Ridge National Laboratory | Pike County, KY | 1979 | Completed; baseline environmental report being prepared |
| Low-Btu gasification | Inhalation Toxicology Research Institute/Morgantown Energy Technology Center | Morgantown, WV | 1977 | Continuing |
| High-Btu gasification | Institute of Gas Technology/Argonne National Laboratory | Hygas, Chicago, IL | 1977 | Completed; final report being prepared |
| High-Btu gasification | Grand Forks Energy Technology Center/Argonne National Laboratory | Grand Forks, IL | 1980 | Continuing |
| In situ gasification | Lawrence Livermore National Laboratory | Hoe Creek, WY | 1978 | Completed; report being prepared |
| *Liquefaction* | | | | |
| H-coal (syncrude) | Oak Ridge National Laboratory | Catlettsburg, KY | 1979 | Continuing |
| SRC-II, SRC-I (boiler fuel) | Pacific Northwest Laboratory | Fort Lewis, WA | 1977 | Continuing |
| Exxon donor | Pacific Northwest Laboratory | Baytown, TX | 1981 | Continuing joint effort with Exxon Corporation |

| | | | |
|---|---|---|---|
| *Combustion* | | | |
| Fluidized-bed combustion | Morgantown Energy Technology Center/Inhalation Toxicology Research Institute | Morgantown, WV | 1977 | Continuing |
| Coal-oil mixtures | Pittsburgh Energy Technology Center/University of California-Davis | Pittsburgh, PA | 1979 | Terminated |
| RDF-coal combustion | Ames Laboratory | Ames, IA | 1978 | Continuing |
| Alcohol fuels combustion | Bartlesville Energy Technology Center | Bartlesville, OK | 1978 | Completed |
| End-use combustion | Pittsburgh Energy Technology Center/University of California-Davis | Pittsburgh, PA | 1979 | Continuing |

facilitate integration of report results across all research areas and to consider future research needs. At this retreat, more than 40 senior scientists responsible for the bulk of the U.S. Department of Energy's (DOE) health and environmental investigations during the past 5 years met and established five panels on health effects, ecological effects, chemical and physical characterization, industrial hygiene, and health and environmental assessment.

Meeting initially in plenary session for an overview of the available data bases in each research area, panelists then conducted separate workshops to discuss strengths and weaknesses of the respective data bases and to address future research needs. Results of these workshops were reported in plenary sessions by the respective panel chairmen. The OHER status reports and the proceedings of the Airlie House workshop are available from the National Technical Information Service.

## SUMMARY OF FINDINGS

### Health Effects

DOE health effects research encompasses the following three areas:

#### Data-Base Management

The health effects program data base has been oriented toward carcinogenesis as the primary health effect, using for the most part a tiered approach of microbial and mammalian in vitro tests and chronic mouse-skin-painting tests.

A substantial data base now exists for short-term test evaluations of available coal-conversion materials. No new methods need development. Recommendations for existing data-base refinement include information on teratogenicity and developmental effects, effects on male fertility, systemic toxicity, inhalation bioassay, correlation of in vitro and in vivo bioassays, further development of in vitro assays, and further biodirected chemical analyses.

#### Development and Deployment of New
#### Methodologies for Toxicological Endpoints

Areas needing investigation include neurotoxicity, respiratory function, hematological effects, cardiovascular effects, reproductive toxicity, liver tumorigenesis, biomedical indices of pathology, pulmonary defense, cytogenetics, mammalian mutagenesis, and carconigenicity other than dermal.

The major problem identified was a lack of standard methods for completing these assays.

*Development and Deployment of*
*Methodologies for Determining Tissue Dose*
*and Metabolism*

Objectives for studies in this research area are to:

1.    establish a correlation between the known effects of coal materials on animals and their potential effects on man,
2.    determine the specific tissues at risk relative to specific compound classes,
3.    provide a basis for worker bioassay programs, and
4.    suggest methods for detoxification or amelioration.

No clear consensus was reached for identifying methods to attain these objectives.

## Environmental Effects

Biomedical research performed to date is most useful for assessing potential effects on workers in coal synfuel industries and has only limited application for addressing potential health effects to the general public resulting from exposure to effluents, emissions, and products. The following analyses were proposed for addressing environmental effects:

1.    analyses of the environmental fate of model compounds considered to be of toxicological concern,
2.    biodirected chemical analyses of materials that might be present or released to the environment and determination of the class of agent causing the biological effects, and
3.    pathological analyses of animal species of ecological concern to determine the cause of death or dominant pathologies.

## Ecological Effects

DOE ecological effects research provides a scientific basis for understanding and predicting pathways by which energy-related materials move through the environment, various physiochemical and biological transport and transformation processes that enhance or reduce levels of energy-related materials, and ultimate environmental effects of the energy-related materials.

### Atmospheric Emissions

Research has centered around a variety of gaseous compounds considered to be of generic importance to (1) determine relative toxicities to plant (vegetation) processes, (2) determine the significance of environmental variables in modifying pollutant toxicity, and (3) identify pathways and fates of polycyclic aromatic hydrocarbons in plant (vegetation) systems. Research has focused on single-pollutant exposures. Future research will be oriented toward multiple-pollutant exposures under a number of approaches including laboratory studies with selected combinations of key pollutant gases and actual field tests around available commercial-scale facilities.

### Coal Liquids and Aqueous Effluents

Research indicates that phenols and anilines contribute significantly to acute toxicities. In addition, higher-molecular-weight organics may persist for longer periods in the environment, particularly when found in association with sediments. Research emphasis for the second-phase studies will include (1) determining the physical, chemical, and biological processes governing dispersal of coal-related materials into aquatic ecosystems (pathways); (2) determining chronic and sublethal effects on representative organisms and communities; (3) evaluating potential for bioaccumulation; and (4) refining transport and effect models to enable predictive evaluation of transport and fate.

Field studies will be needed to test laboratory results and to validate model refinements. These studies could be completed using enclosed portions of natural ecosystems, experimental ecosystems, or areas surrounding operating coal-based synthetic fuels facilities.

### Solid Residues

Research has been oriented toward the physiochemical character of wastes and evaluation of the short-term aquatic toxicity and phytotoxicity of aqueous extracts. Future research, in addition to covering the major areas previously identified under coal liquids and aqueous effluents, will include general toxicological effects of inhaled, sorbed, and ingested solid waste materials and associated contaminants.

## Chemical and Physical Characterization

The present chemical and physical characterization data base has been oriented toward process stream compositions. A considerable data base has been developed for the key chemical materials responsible for the major observed biological responses. Direct chemical and physical characterization support will be required for completion of the long-term research studies being performed for health, ecology, environment, and industrial hygiene. Future research will center around (1) assessing the chemical compounds responsible for toxicity, (2) developing a better understanding of the tests, and (3) improving tests for health and environmental impact measurement.

Substantial activity in characterization, method, and instrument development will be required to complete the research activities. Specific items which should be completed follow.

### Characterization

1. Apply existing methods and techniques to relate new processes and unit operations to the existing data base.
2. Characterize a reference environment (e.g., coke oven, roofing tar, petrochemical/dyes, gas works, asphalt paving) to assist in the extrapolation of epidemiologic and other data for the purpose of providing a comparative risk assessment.
3. Characterize environmental releases: air, water, and solid wastes (source terms).
4. Characterize end-use products of environmental concern (combustion products, chemical feedstocks, end-user wastes, spills), especially emphasizing hazards of products.
5. Improve and expand characterization of volatile compounds.
6. Further identify chemical compounds/classes/properties responsible for biological and ecological effects.
7. Support biotesting and bioassay development (e.g., delivery and dosimetry).

### Method and Instrument Development

1. Develop preparative-scale/high-resolution separations.
2. Develop methods for quantitating marker compounds in complex mixtures.
3. Develop methods for isolating, identifying, and quantifying the intractable constituents in synfuels (especially high-molecular-weight, biologically active material).
4. Develop and deploy new monitoring and surveillance instrumentation in industrial hygiene, safety, and regulatory monitoring activities.
5. Develop and apply methods for classifying inorganics, especially metal/organics.
6. Develop methods for improving isomeric discrimination.
7. Develop instruments for characterizing aerosols for toxicology and industrial hygiene.
8. Develop large-scale air-sampling methods.
9. Synthesize selected standards as required for identifying and quantifying.
10. Develop and apply chemical methods to support research in environmental transport and fate studies.

### Industrial Hygiene

The industrial hygiene data base has grown substantially over the past 5 years. The effort directed toward developing new or improved monitoring tools for dealing with oils and tars and their constituent compounds has produced advances. Worker protection in industry and medicine requires research under workplace conditions. Worker training and acceptance of practices, protective devices, and monitoring requirements are a critical part of any program. Research needs are in applied research oriented toward refinement of existing technologies to the coal-based synthetic fuels industry and in longer-term research primarily oriented toward problems associated with oils and tars and their carcinogenic or potentially carcinogenic constituents.

#### Applied Technology

Laboratory-based studies should assess the efficacy of barriers, creams, soaps, cleaning lotions, and wash treatments. Protective garments should be evaluated for permeation by coal-conversion products and by-products and their service life determined. Efficient cleanup and decontamination options should be evaluated by carrying out spills under controlled conditions. Field tests of recently developed instruments and comparisons of conventional techniques should be conducted. Overall guidelines for workplace practices and exposure limits should be developed from toxicological data and workplace experiences.

#### Long-Term Research

A number of long-term research needs identified include (1) development of measuring and monitoring systems for airborne materials, (2) improved capabilities to deal with skin contamination, (3) development of biological indicators of exposure, (4) development of methods for identifying potential high-risk workers, and (5) epidemiological research at existing synfuel facilities and surrogate industries (e.g., coking facilities).

### Health and Environmental Assessments

The goal of health and environmental assessments (risk assessments) includes consideration of all potentially significant impact sources, transport pathways, and endpoints. Risks associated with the industry must be quantified, compared to reference industries, and bounded by estimates of uncertainty.

### Data Bases

While a substantial data base has been developed over the past 5 years, areas identified as requiring expansion include:

1. Industrial hygiene. Development of uniform systems to monitor work exposures and complete medical surveillance at existing synfuel and related facilities.
2. Chemical and physical characterization. Development of more detailed emission rate estimates for each coal-based technology and development of tracer means to validate transport models.
3. Ecology. Refinement of transport and food-chain models with capabilities of assessing various endpoints.
4. Health. Development of techniques to extrapolate laboratory test results to anticipated human responses.

### Research Needs

Future generic risk assessment research must include consideration of the following items in developing specific risk models:

1. significant exposure pathways defined by sensitivity analyses;
2. employment of surrogate models for synfuels releases;
3. access to more detailed source terms by technology type and release point and scale-up of information (i.e., the most appropriate transformation techniques to move from demonstration plant emissions to full-scale facilities);
4. built-in sensitivity analysis and uncertainty analysis techniques;
5. development of probabilistic risk assessment methods;
6. environmental sampling to validate models;
7. better methods for both human and environmental risk extrapolation (ecosystem);
8. alternatives to the linear, nonthreshold model of dose response at long distances and low doses;
9. acute effects assessment;
10. development of background data for various organics and for trace metals such as As, Cr, Co, Ni, Pb, Be, and Hg;
11. refined risk comparison techniques;
12. access to data on control technology's most probable confinement factors;
13. development of an accident assessment methodology for various pathways;
14. development of region-specific models;
15. development of a conceptual model for ecological risk assessment;
16. definition of a suite of ecological endpoints that is quantifiable and socially relevant;

17.   refined existing methods and new methods of translating effects on environmental test species to ecological endpoints; and
18.   defined and characterized physical, chemical, and biological environments that will be used for ecological risk analyses.

## REFERENCES

1.   Francis, C.W., and F.J. Wobber, Comps. "Status of Health and Environmental Research Relative to Solid Wastes from Coal Conversion," DOE/NBB-0008 (Washington, DC: U.S. Department of Energy, 1982).
2.   Wilzbach, K.E., and C.A. Reilly, Jr., Eds. "Status of Health and Environmental Research Relative to Coal Gasification: 1976 to the Present," DOE/ER-0149 (Washington, DC: U.S. Department of Energy, 1982).
3.   Gray, R.H., and K.E. Cowser, Eds. "Status of Health and Environmental Research Relative to Direct Coal Liquefaction: 1976 to the Present," DOE/NBM-1016 (PNL-4176) (Washington, DC: U.S. Department of Energy, 1982).
4.   "Health and Environmental Research Program Relative to Coal Conversion Technologies and Their Future Directions: Proceedings of the Retreat January 26–28, 1982, Airlie House, Warrenton, VA," CONF-820160 (Washington, DC: U.S. Department of Energy, 1982).

## DISCUSSION

*J.W. Carroll, U.S. Army:* I recognize the spread of your responsibilities primarily focuses on the Department of Energy, and, as you have indicated, the Synthetic Fuels Corporation now has introduced a change in some of these responsibilities. I saw nowhere in the discussion areas relating to research requirements a focus on end-use products, transportation, storage, and combustion products from the fuels that would actually be used commercially. I recognize the Environmental Protection Agency and other people in the regulatory community have that responsibility to some degree, and much of that is being defined for the private sector that would be producing the products. Does the Department of Energy see itself in that picture at all in terms of responsibility? The Department of Defense would be an end-user that would probably be ahead of the civilian community in some areas. We see the user in this case being told that the responsibility is going to be either his or the commercial producer's. It may be a bad analogy, but is this not somewhat remiss in terms of the problems we experienced with the nuclear fission program, where we did not look at the total life cycle issues of the process?

*A.P. Duhamel:* We have been carrying out a program related to end-use for 3 or 4 years where the research involves basically the burning fuels in a dedicated combustor. The problem with synthetic fuels when you say end-use is that very little of it is actually produced at any given time, so we got into the problem of building a combustor that would use fuel at a rate compatible with production. Of course, that gets into the analytical problem of how to obtain very small samples. The answer to that question is yes, we are doing research on end-use and are continuing that program, although with budget restrictions we have had some problems.

Another area involves the oil shale program, and DOE has been working with the Air Force and with 100,000 bbl of oil that existed and was upgraded. So, as you can see, we do have an interest. A lot of people do not know about our program at the Pittsburgh Energy Technology Center and that is kind of bothersome sometimes, because we have done a fair amount of work, specifically, studies in chemical characterization. We have now begun studies in biological characterization of the emissions.

# SECTION II

# TOXICOLOGY

## J.L. Epler
*Oak Ridge National Laboratory*
*Oak Ridge, TN 37831*

## R. Pelroy
*Pacific Northwest Laboratories*
*Richland, WA 99352*

To investigate potential health and environmental hazards associated with the developing synthetic fuel technologies, various laboratories, both academic and governmental, initiated coupled chemical and biological analyses of some existing and proposed energy-generating and energy-conversion systems. In the following chapters, we see that in these studies, "biological" refers to the total picture—specific health effects on man and the environment.

In the initial phase of this parallel approach, now almost complete, investigators sought to identify the specific chemical threats and/or the comparative threat to biological systems. The following chapters deal with the next step, the attempts to begin deciphering the uncertainties and identifying the potential threat by understanding not only the magnitude but the mechanism. The common tie remains the association with energy-related pollutants.

The chapters go beyond illustrating the coupled chemical-biological approach. They bring our attention to the precautions necessary in extrapolating from work with lower organisms to man, not only in the design of new, innovative systems but also in using the existing data base. Our programs have been deficient in monitoring the population potentially affected. We gain a hint of newly developed approaches with skin-in-organ culture and with mammalian cells in both in vitro and in vivo assays. We begin to appreciate a superorganization of data and chemical structure and the possibility of prediction and comparison. We also note the progress in use of parallel environmental and chemical research with real-world materials.

This section opens the door to problem areas that need considerable research and development before we can use the resulting data for accurate predictions.

# CHAPTER 10

## Evaluation of Biohazards Using Skin in Organ Culture

J.Y. Kao, L.R. Shugart, and J.M. Holland

*Oak Ridge National Laboratory
Oak Ridge, TN 37831*

An in vitro short-term organ culture system has been developed for maintaining metabolically viable and structurally intact mouse skin. Using this system, the responses of mouse skin to in vitro chemical insults were assessed by selected biochemical parameters.

Studies with the irritant tributyltin chloride showed that the degree of cellular injury was reflected by inhibition of in vitro incorporation of $^3$H-thymidine and $^{14}$C-leucine into epidermal DNA and protein, respectively. In addition, there was leakage of intracellular enzymes into the culture medium in a dose- and time-related manner. When skin samples were exposed to complex irritant mixtures such as H-coal distillates, leakage of intracellular enzymes was also observed.

This in vitro system is potentially adaptable for use with skin samples from other species, including man. It offers a means whereby species differences may be examined under defined conditions and also allows for a quantitative basis for assessing cutaneous toxicity of chemicals and complex mixtures in vitro.

### INTRODUCTION AND RATIONALE FOR IN VITRO APPROACH TO CUTANEOUS TOXICITY EVALUATION

The skin is the largest and most external organ of the body and has a large surface area for contact exposure. It is often the first organ to be exposed to hazards of the environment, and it is a primary route of exposure to a variety of environmental chemicals. It is sensitive to chemical injuries and is potentially a major target organ for chemical toxicity. In a recent report

243

by the Standard Advisory Committee on Cutaneous Hazards,[1] it was concluded that 45% of all cases of occupational illnesses were skin related. The committee also conceded that this figure is probably low in view of the recognized underreporting of these cases, and it recommended a course of action to the Occupational Safety and Health Administration designed to draw attention to the incidences of occupational skin disorders. Indeed, the National Institute for Occupational Safety and Health (NIOSH)[2] has stated that "skin disorders resulting from exposure to industrial chemicals are the most pervasive current occupational health problem in the U.S."

With the increasing concern over occupational skin disorders, attention has focused on our grossly inadequate understanding of dermatotoxicity and has highlighted the deficiencies of the methods currently in use to study cutaneous toxicity. Cutaneous toxicity can be divided into problems associated with primary irritants and problems related to skin sensitization. While both are important, this chapter is concerned primarily with cutaneous toxicity of the "irritant" variety.

Currently, most methods for evaluating the irritancy of chemicals are based on the early works of Draize et al.[3] and rely on the application of a substance to the shaved back of a laboratory animal (rabbit, guinea pig, or rat), either with or without prior abrasion. The degree of skin irritation is subsequently deduced from the level of nonspecific inflammation induced. There is an effort to make the methods semiquantitative by subjective evaluation of the degree of inflammation. Thus, graded observations of dermal erythema and edema became measures of skin irritation and hence cutaneous toxicity. This approach has proved to be relatively useful in identifying severe irritants and caustic materials. The subjective assessment, however, suffers from considerable variation[4] and is based on the unproven assumption that inflammatory vascular responses of the skin invoked by the chemicals provide an accurate measure of cellular damage. Quantitative evaluation of the degree of injury, particularly with regard to mild irritants, is difficult, and colored materials cannot be visually assessed easily; moreover, the test system provides little if any information regarding the mechanism of toxicity. In general, these test systems will demonstrate that a potential cutaneous toxicant will damage the skin or at least provoke an inflammatory response, but they do not provide any information regarding the kind of damage or its relevance to man. Information of this poor quality would be unacceptable in any other branch of toxicology. Thus it is recognized that a more rational approach to quantitative assessment of cutaneous toxicity should be considered.

A variety of approaches have been considered. Attempts to quantitate cutaneous inflammatory responses have included the measurement of increases in water content and vascular permeability of the skin[5,6] together with increases in the thickness of the epidermis[7] following a toxic insult. Attempts to quantitatively assess some common biochemical manifestations of toxicity in the skin have included the measurement of changes in the incorporation of radiolabeled precursors into cellular macromolecules as an indicator of alterations in cellular proliferation.[7-10] The release of intracellular enzymes from damaged cells as a measure of tissue injury or cellular viability has been used to considerable advantage in clinical biochemistry. It is a technique with extensive diagnostic applications, and increases in certain serum enzymes can often identify a damaged organ and the extent to which it is damaged.[11] Using this approach, attempts have been made to quantitatively assess the degree of cellular damage to skin following exposure to a harmful stimuli.[12-15]

These biochemical changes appear to reflect the degree of cutaneous injuries induced by the harmful stimuli and potentially offer a direct, objective, and quantitative assessment of cellular injuries to skin. Studies of this kind have, by and large, been carried out under in vivo conditions. However, a distinct disadvantage of in vivo methodology is that the animals must be kept alive throughout the duration of the assessment. The attendant difficulties associated with restraint, interindividual variability, and pain induced would indicate that an in vitro approach would be more desirable. A singular advantage of an in vitro approach is that human skin may also be evaluated directly.

## SKIN IN ORGAN CULTURE AND POSSIBLE PARAMETERS FOR IN VITRO CUTANEOUS TOXICITY EVALUATION

Over the past few years our laboratory has been engaged in studying the cutaneous carcinogenic effects of coal-derived fossil liquids. In particular, we are concerned with the interrelationship between the topically applied dose and its carcinogenic and toxic effects on the onset of skin cancer. It has long been recognized that dermatotoxicity can have delaying effects on the expression of epidermal neoplasia.[16,17] An estimate of the influence of dose and cutaneous toxicity should therefore play an important part in the design and interpretation of carcinogenesis bioassay experiments. To better establish a quantitative basis for comparisons and extrapolation of dermal toxicity, we have been developing in vitro systems to study toxicity, translocation, and coupled biotransformation of topically applied chemicals on skin under controlled and defined conditions. The use of skin in organ culture as in vitro models for studying the mechanism of epidermal growth, differentiation, migration, and tumor promotion have been described previously.[18-24] However, its use in dermatotoxicological studies has, to our knowledge, not been previously reported, although Middleton[25] has described biochemical changes in skin slices in vitro following in vivo exposure to irritant chemicals.

For studying dermal toxicity, a short-term (48 h) skin-organ culture for maintaining metabolically viable and structurally intact mouse skin has been developed. Using the culture system, the effects of in vitro topically applied chemicals on the skin may be examined by monitoring some selected biochemical parameters. Details of the methodology are described elsewhere.[26] Briefly, the culture system consists of freshly excised mouse skin discs (1-in. diam) which are maintained in a controlled environment (37°C, 100% humidity in an atmosphere of 5% $CO_2$, 40% $O_2$, and 55% $N_2$), supported on a filter paper in individual organ culture dishes (Figure 1) containing culture media (minimal essential medium containing Earle's salts with L-glutamine, with D-valine in place of L-valine, and contained fetal calf serum and gentamicine). Under these conditions, the mouse skin samples were viable, biochemically functional with active epidermal DNA and protein synthesis, as demonstrated by the incorporation of [3]H-thymidine and [14]C-leucine respectively. Moreover, the overall morphology of the cultured skin was essentially unchanged, and structural integrity was maintained for up to 2 d in culture.[26] An important property of our culture systems is that the skin samples are supported on filter paper over the culture medium so that their epidermal surfaces are not covered. This procedure allows materials to be applied to the skin surface in a manner similar to exposure in vivo. The material reaches the epidermal cells by diffusion through the various strata of the skin and presumably provokes biochemical and cellular responses comparable to in vivo responses.

In vitro cutaneous toxic responses could be assessed by measuring some of the possible common biochemical manifestations of toxicity. Changes in cellular viability could provide a direct measurement in changes in the biological function of the skin. For example, the barrier function properties of the stratum corneum, which ultimately depend on normal cellular proliferation and differentiation, could be assessed directly by measuring, for example, in vitro permeability to water and electrolytes,[27-29] or indirectly by monitoring changes in cellular proliferation and differentiation.

To monitor cellular injury in vitro, the release of intracellular enzymes from damaged skin in organ culture was assessed by examining the culture media for increases in selected intracellular enzyme activities. Changes in the in vitro incorporation of [3]H-thymidine and [14]C-leucine into epidermal DNA and protein, respectively, were also monitored as indicators of the

**Figure 1.** Schematic of skin explants in organ culture.

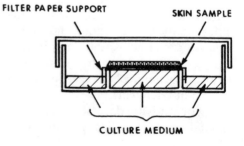

effects on cellular turnover and functional viability of the cultured skins. The methodology for monitoring these changes has been described elsewhere.[26]

## RESULTS OF STUDIES WITH SELECTED AGENTS

### Tributyltin Chloride

Our initial studies with mouse skin in organ culture were to examine the effect of topical application of tributyltin chloride on the selected biochemical parameters. Tributyltin chloride was chosen as the model compound because it is a known skin irritant in both laboratory animals and man.[30–31] It exhibits its toxicity as a potent inhibitor of mitochondrial oxidative phosphorylation,[32] and its effects on in vivo incorporation of $^3$H-thymidine into epidermal DNA and the release of intracellular enzymes into suction-induced blister fluids following topical application to mouse skin[14] have been previously described.

Following a single in vitro topical application of tributyltin chloride, leakage of intracellular enzyme from the skin into the culture medium was apparent. For example, at 50 nmole/cm$^2$, lactate dehydrogenase (LDH) activity was observed to increase with time in the media from both the treated and control cultures, but greater increases were observed in the treated samples, and significant differences were seen towards the latter part of the culture (Figure 2). Similar effects were observed with other intracellular enzyme activities including malate dehydrogenase (MDH), glutamic oxalacetate transaminase (GOT), and glutamic pyrivate transaminase (GPT). At higher doses, the observed increases in the activities of, for example, MDH (Figure 3) were substantially greater than their corresponding controls, and significant increases were apparent during the early part of the incubation. These increases in the relative levels of the enzyme activities in the culture medium were dose related. At 10 h after topical application, detectable increases in MDH activity were observed with an applied dose of 10 nmole/cm$^2$. Increasing the applied dose resulted in increases in the relative level of MDH in the media in a dose-related manner (Figure 4). Maximum release of MDH was apparent at a dose of 500 nmole/cm$^2$, since no differences were observed between samples exposed to 500 nmole/cm$^2$ and 1000 nmole/cm$^2$ of tributyltin chloride. Qualitatively, these results are similar to those previously reported for in vivo exposure to tributyltin chloride[14] and demonstrate that leakage of intracellular enzymes from culture skin samples may provide a quantitative indicator of frank toxicity to skin in vitro.

Exposure to topical tributyltin chloride also has profound effects on the in vitro incorporation of radiolabeled precursors into epidermal cellular

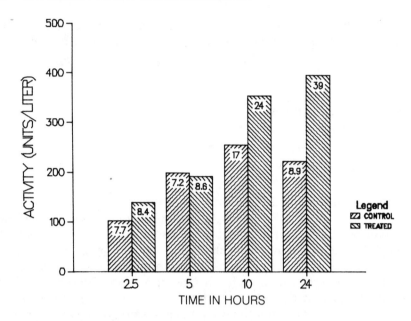

**Figure 2.**    Accumulative LDH activity in culture medium from mouse skin following in vitro topical exposure to tributyltin chloride (TBT). Female mouse skin discs were treated with tributyltin chloride (50 nmole/cm²); controls were treated with acetone. Enzyme activities were determined at the time indicated, and results are expressed as mean ± SE from six individual skin samples (SE are given in the histograms).

macromolecules. At a low dose of 10 nmole/cm², there was significant inhibition in the incorporation of ³H-thymidine and ¹⁴C-leucine into epidermal DNA and protein, and the extent of the inhibition increased with the length of time in culture following exposure (Figures 5 and 6). At higher doses, complete inhibition of incorporation was observed (Table I). Both DNA and protein synthesis are energy-dependent processes; since tributyltins are potent inhibitors of mitochondrial respiration, the inhibition of incorporation of radiolabeled precursors may reflect the effect of tributyltin chloride on energy generation in the cultured skin samples.


### H-coal Distillates and Benzo(a)pyrene

Applying our in vitro approach for examining the dermatotoxicity of some H-coal process distillates, we have examined the effect of topical application of aliquots of the distillates to the mouse skin in organ culture. Preliminary experiments have demonstrated that there was significant release of enzymes

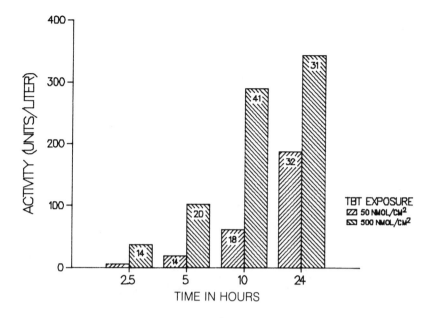

**Figure 3.**    Relative increase in MDH activity in culture media from mouse skin following exposure to tributyltin chloride. Male mouse skin discs were treated. Results are calculated from the difference of the treatment and control mean of six individual skin discs, respectively, and expressed as mean ± SE.

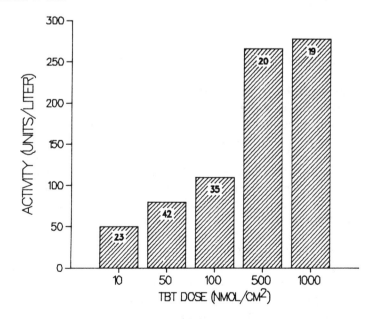

**Figure 4.**    Relative increase in MDH activity in culture medium from female mouse skin 10 h following in vitro topical application of various amounts of tributyltin chloride.

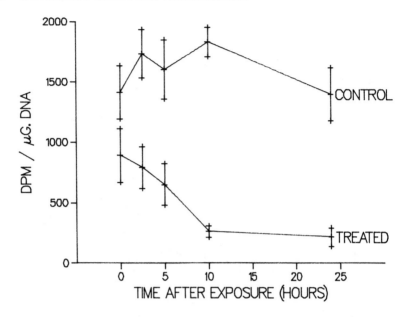

**Figure 5.** In vitro incorporation of ³H-thymidine into epidermal DNA of female mouse skin in organ culture following a single topical application of tributyltin chloride (10 nmole/cm²). At the time, indicated skin samples were "pulse labeled" for 3 h. DNA was isolated and radioactivity incorporation determined. Results are expressed as mean ± SE from six individual skin discs.

into the culture medium following exposure to a number of the distillates (Figure 7).

These same distillates had previously been applied to mouse skin as part of an empirical bioassay to determine their potential skin carcinogenicity. Two were subsequently shown to be potent skin irritants (VOH-S, VOH-F), necessitating discontinuation of exposure of the undiluted materials, while animals tolerated continuous application of materials ASOH-F and ASB-F. This apparent discrepancy between the degree of tissue injury as detected by biochemical criteria in vitro and the actual experience following chronic application to the live animal may, in part, be due to tissue adaptation to toxic insult common in chronic studies. Experiments are planned to compare the response of skin before and after hydrocarbon exposure to evaluate the sensitivity to toxicity.

The significance of these observations in terms of evaluating the relationship between dermatotoxicity and carcinogenicity of these mixtures awaits additional experiments. However, the relative differences in the increase in leakage of enzymes from the mouse skin in culture following cutaneous application of different fossil liquids may offer a simple and direct quanti-

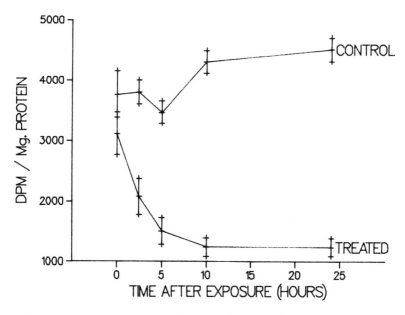

**Figure 6.** In vitro incorporation of $^{14}$C-leucine into epidermal protein of female mouse skin in organ culture following a single topical application of tributyltin chloride (10 nmole/cm$^2$). At times indicated, skin samples were "pulse labeled" for 3 h. Proteins were isolated and radioactivity incorporation determined. Results are expressed as mean ± SE from six skin discs.

**Table I.** In Vitro Incorporation of $^3$H-Thymidine and $^{14}$C-Leucine into Epidermal DNA and Protein of Mouse Skin in Organ Culture Following Exposure to Tributyltin Chloride

|  | Tributyltin Chloride (nmole/cm$^2$) | | |
|  | 10 | 50 | 500 |
|  | % Inhibition of Precursor Incorporation | | |
|---|---|---|---|
| $^3$H-Thymidine | 54.4 | 81.5 | 96.4 |
| $^{14}$C-Leucine | 45.4 | 76.6 | 96.1 |

Conditions: Skin samples were preincubated for 16 h prior to topical application of tributyltin chloride. They were cultured for 2.5 h and "pulse labeled" for 3 h. Epidermal DNA and protein were isolated, radioactivity incorporation was determined, and the results were calculated from the means of four to six skin samples from treated and control cultures.

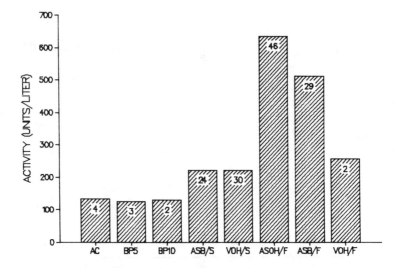

**Figure 7.** LDH activity in culture media from mouse skin treated with various fractions of H-coal distillate. Female mouse skin discs were treated topically with aliquots (50 μl) 50% w/v solution of H-coal distillates in acetone. Enzyme activity in the medium was determined 5 h after treatment. Results are expressed as mean ± SE from four to six individual skin discs. AC = acetone; BP5 = benzo(*a*)pyrene, 5 μg; BP10 = benzo(*a*)pyrene, 10 μg; ASB/s = atmospheric bottom/syncrude; VOH/s = vacuum overhead/syncrude; ASOH/F = atmospheric overhead/fuel oil; ASB/F = atmospheric bottom/fuel oil; VOH/F = vacuum overhead/fuel oil.

tative estimate of their dermatotoxic potential and could provide a measure of their relative dermatotoxic potency.

### Benzo(*a*)pyrene and DNA Binding

The metabolism of benzo(*a*)pyrene to the chemically reactive diolepoxides, which covalently interact with DNA, is believed to be the initiating event responsible for the observed carcinogenic property of benzo(*a*)pyrene.[33] A nonradiometric method has been developed in our laboratory to quantitate femtomole amounts of benzo(*a*)pyrene diolepoxides covalently associated with DNA isolated from mouse skin.[34] The method consists of hydrolyzing the DNA-diolepoxide complex with acid to liberate the benzo(*a*)pyrene adduct in the form of the isomeric tetrols of benzo(*a*)pyrene. These tetrols are fluorescent and can be easily quantitated by high-performance liquid chromatography (HPLC) using a fluorescence detector. Using this fluorometric method and the in vitro culture system, we have examined the interaction of benzo(*a*)pyrene with skin DNA as a function of the amount of in vitro topically applied benzo(*a*)pyrene. Covalent binding to mouse skin DNA was observed (Figure 8). This implies that the enzyme system which metabolically activates benzo(*a*)pyrene is functional in mouse skin in organ culture. Furthermore, the binding to DNA exhibits a dose-response relationship to the amount of benzo(*a*)pyrene applied at doses up to 10 µg. The reduction in binding observed at 20 µg of benzo(*a*)pyrene is probably due to toxicity. Currently, experiments are being conducted to examine the relationship between the applied dose, metabolism, toxicity, and covalent binding.

## SUMMARY

Skin disorders resulting from exposure to industrial chemicals are prevalent, and the accompanying health and economic effects are of serious concern. However, dermatotoxicology, as it relates to the rest of the discipline, is at present an underresearched area of toxicology. In this chapter we have attempted to illustrate an approach for studying cutaneous responses to toxic insults using skin in organ culture by utilizing some selected biochemical parameters as possible quantitative indicators of toxicity. Our results have

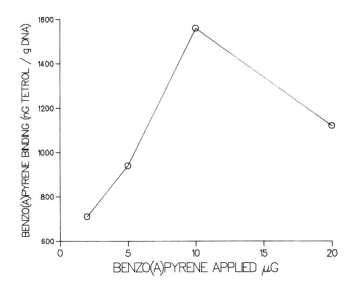

**Figure 8.**  Benzo(*a*)pyrene binding to DNA of female HRS mouse skin in organ culture as a function of the amount of in vitro topically applied benzo(*a*)pyrene. Binding was determined 24 h after the application of benzo(*a*)pyrene and assayed as the amount of tetrol released. Each point represents duplicate determinations.

shown that pieces of mouse skin may be maintained under conditions in which they are metabolically viable and structurally intact, and they respond to toxic chemical insult with biochemical changes that can be quantitatively assessed. Therefore, this approach may be exploited as a tool in the quantitative evaluation of dermatotoxicity of chemicals and complex mixtures from synthetic fossil-fuel technologies. The in vitro approach also allows for a mechanistic approach to the study of dermatotoxicology. Toxicokinetics of penetration, metabolism-coupled translocation, and interaction with important cellular macromolecules at different exposure rates are currently being investigated using biologically viable and intact skin in organ culture. Finally, an important advantage of the culture system is that it is adaptable for use with skin samples from other species, including man. It offers a means whereby the significances of species differences may be examined under defined conditions and also allows for a quantitative basis for the extrapolation of cutaneous toxicity observation from laboratory animals to man. It is in this area that our research effort is being directed, and we hope we can make some contributions to our understanding of dermatotoxicity of chemicals.

## ACKNOWLEDGMENT

This research was sponsored by the Office of Health and Environmental Research, U.S. Department of Energy, under contract W-7405-eng-26 with the Union Carbide Corporation.

## REFERENCES

1. "Standards Advisory Committee on Cutaneous Hazards Findings," *Job Saf. Health Rep.* 9:4 (1979).
2. National Institute for Occupational Safety and Health Notices 4FR 7004. *Chem. Reg. Reporter* 3, 1666 (1980).
3. Draize, J.H., G. Woodard, and H.O. Calvery. "Methods for the Study of Irritation and Toxicity of Substances Applied Topically to the Skin and Mucous Membrane," *J. Pharmacol. Exp. Ther.* 82:377–390 (1944).
4. Weil, C.S., and R.A. Scala. "Study of Intra- and Interlaboratory Variability in the Results of Rabbit Eyes and Skin Irritation Test," *Toxicol. Appl. Pharmacol.* 19:176–260 (1971).
5. Cummings, R., and A.W.J. Lykke. "Increased Vascular Permeability Evoked by Crush Injury in the Skin of the Rat," *Br. J. Exp. Path.* 51:1–27 (1970).
6. Middleton, M.C., and I. Pratt. "Skin Water Content as a Quantitative Index of the Vascular and Histologic Changes Produced in Rat Skin by Di-n-butyltin and Tri-n-butyltin," *J. Invest. Dermatol.* 68:379–384 (1977).
7. Barnes, F.W., W.F. Seip, and C.C. Burch. "Proliferation and Resistance of Epidermis in Response to Harmful Stimuli," *Proc. Soc. Exptl. Biol. Med.* 129:584–593 (1968).

8. Lewis, G.P., J. Peters, and A.M. White. "Intracellular Enzymes and Protein Synthesis in Rabbit Skin after Thermal Injury," *Br. J. Pharmacol.* 42:437–446 (1971).

9. Middleton, M.C., and I. Pratt. "Changes in Incorporation of [3]H-thymidine into DNA of Rat Skin Following Cutaneous Application of Dibutyltin, Tributyltin and 1-Chloro-2:4-Dinitrobenzene and the Relationship of These Changes to a Morphological Assessment of the Cellular Damage," *J. Invest. Dermatol.* 71:305–310 (1978).

10. Peters, R.F., and A.M. White. "The Relationship Between Cyclic Adenosine 3', 5'-Monophosphate and Biochemical Events in Rat Skin After the Induction of Epidermal Hyperplasia Using Hexadecane," *Br. J. Dermatol.* 98:301–314 (1978).

11. Schmidt, E., and F.W. Schmidt. "Clinical Enzymology," *FEBS Lett.* 62: suppl. E62-E79 (1976).

12. Lewis, G.P. "Intracellular Enzymes in Local Lymph as a Measure of Cellular Injury," *J. Physiol.* 191:591–607 (1967).

13. Lewis, G.P. "Changes in the Composition of Rabbit Hind Limb Lymph After Thermal Injury," *J. Physiol.* 205:619–634 (1969).

14. Middleton, M.C. "Evaluation of Cellular Injury in Skin Utilizing Enzyme Activities in Suction Blister Fluid," *J. Invest. Dermatol.* 74:219–223 (1980).

15. Middleton, M.C., and R. Hasmall. "Changes of Enzyme Activities in Suction Blister Fluid from Skin Subjected to Graded Thermal Injury," (abstract) *Br. J. Dermatol.* 102:740 (1980).

16. Holland, J.M., M.S. Whitaker, and J.W. Wesley. "Correlation of Fluorescence Intensity and Carcinogenic Potency of Synthetic and Natural Petroleum in Mouse Skin," *Am. Ind. Hyg. Assoc. J.* 40(6):496–503 (1979).

17. Wilson, J.S., and L.M. Holland. "The Effect of Application Frequency on Epidermal Carcinogenesis Assay," *Toxicol.* 24:45–53 (1982).

18. Reaven, E.P., and A.J. Cox, Jr. "Organ Culture of Human Skin," *J. Invest. Dermatol.* 44:151–156 (1965).

19. Hambrick, G.W., Jr., W.I. Lamberg, and R. Bloomberg. "Observations on Keratinization of Human Skin *in vitro*," *J. Invest. Dermatol.* 47:541–550 (1966).

20. Young, J.M., H.S. Lawrence, and S.L. Cordell. "In Vitro Epidermal Cell Proliferation in Rat Skin Plugs," *J. Invest. Dermatol.* 64:23–29 (1975).

21. Flaxman, B.A., and R.A. Harper. "Organ Culture of Human Skin in Chemically Defined Medium," *J. Invest. Dermatol.* 64:96–99 (1975).

22. Halprin, K.M., M. Leuder, and N.E. Fusenig. "Growth and Differentiation of Postembryonic Mouse Epidermal Cells in Explant Cultures," *J. Invest. Dermatol.* 72:88–98 (1979).

23. Van Der Schueren, B., J.J. Cassiman, and H. Van Den Berghe. "Morphological Characteristics of Epithelial and Fibroblastic Cells Growing out from Biopsies of Human Skin," *J. Invest. Dermatol.* 74:29–35 (1979).

24. Verma, A.K., and R.K. Boutwell. "An Organ Culture of Adult Mouse Skin: An *In Vitro* Model for Studying Molecular Mechanism of Skin Tumor Promotion," *Biochem. Biophys. Res. Comm.* 96:854–862 (1980).

25. Middleton, M.C. "New Approaches to Problems of Dermatotoxicity," in *Testing for Toxicity,* J.W. Gorrod, Ed. (London: Taylor and Francis, 1981), pp. 290–293.

26. Kao, J., J. Hall, and J.M. Holland. "Quantitation of Cutaneous Toxicity: An

In Vitro Approach Using Skin Organ Culture," *Toxicol. Appl. Pharmacol.* 68:206–217 (1983).

27. Schenplein, R.J. "Mechanism of Percutaneous Adsorption. I. Route of Penetration and the Influence of Solubility," *J. Invest. Dermatol.* 45:334–346 (1965).

28. Dugard, P.H., and R.J. Schenplein. "Effect of Ionic Surfactants on the Permeability of Human Epidermis: An Electrometric Study," *J. Invest. Dermatol.* 60:263–269 (1973).

29. Sprut, D., and K.E. Malten. "Epidermal Water Barrier Formation after Stripping of Normal Skin," *J. Invest. Dermatol.* 45:6–14 (1965).

30. Barnes, J.M., and H.B. Stoner. "The Toxic Properties of Some Dialkyl and Trialkyltin Salts," *Br. J. Industr. Med.* 15:15–22 (1958).

31. Lyle, W.H. "Lesions in the Skin of Process Workers Caused by Contact with Butyltin Compounds," *Br. J. Ind. Med.* 15:193–196 (1958).

32. Aldridge, W.N. "The Biochemistry of Organotin Compounds: Trialkyltins and Oxidative Phosphorylation," *Biochem. J.* 69:367–376 (1958).

33. Gelboin, H.V. "Benzo(*a*)pyrene Metabolism, Activation, and Carcinogenesis: Role and Regulation of Mixed-Function Oxidases and Related Enzyme," *Phys. Rev.* 60:1107–1166 (1980).

34. Shugart, L., J.M. Holland, and R.O. Rahn. "Dosimetry of PAH Skin Carcinogenesis: Covalent Binding of Benzo(*a*)pyrene to Mouse Epidermal DNA," (submitted for publication).

## DISCUSSION

*V. Frankos, Clement Associates:* Did you monitor P450 microsomal activity over time in your culture?

*J.Y. Kao:* No, we have not done that yet. That is something I am planning to do.

*V. Frankos:* I think that is an important step.

*J.Y. Kao:* The fact that metabolism and covalent binding occurs indicates that the microsomal P450 enzyme system is active in our skin organ culture.

*V. Frankos:* Can you measure levels of lethal cytotoxicity in the viable portions of the skin in culture?

*J.Y. Kao:* We haven't tried that yet, but I think it is possible.

*A.P. Li, Monsanto Company:* One of the uses of the Draize test, as you mentioned earlier, is to measure irritants. How do you propose to do that in vitro?

*J.Y. Kao:* We are not measuring irritation. Under in vivo conditions, the endpoint for evaluating irritation is an inflammatory response. Under our in vitro conditions we are measuring biochemical changes as endpoints for toxicity resulting from exposure to toxic chemicals. We can define the in vitro biochemical parameters used for toxicity, and we can do this quantitatively and objectively.

# CHAPTER 11

## Use of Gene Locus Mutation Assays in Human Lymphoblastoid Cells to Study the Mutagenicity of Complex Mixtures

H.L. Liber, C.L. Crespi, and W.G. Thilly

*Department of Nutrition and Food Science*
*Massachusetts Institute of Technology*
*Cambridge, Massachusetts 02139*

Gene locus mutation assays have been developed in diploid human lymphoblast cells. In early experiments, which required the addition of an exogenous metabolizing system derived from rat liver, a series of complex mixtures were shown to be mutagenic to human lymphoblasts. These mixtures include a kerosene soot extract, a diesel soot extract, and an air sample standard from St. Louis. This chapter reports the isolation of a line of cells with endogenous oxidative enzymes that permits experiments with polycyclic aromatic hydrocarbons or even whole soot particulates to be done directly. We have found that a carbon-black product containing a variety of polycyclic aromatic hydrocarbons is mutagenic for the cells when provided as a simple dispersed suspension.

### INTRODUCTION

One of the major goals of the Genetic Toxicology Group at the Massachusetts Institute of Technology (MIT) has been to develop human cell systems that measure the mutagenic potential of environmental chemicals. Throughout our efforts we have tried to remain cognizant of the processing steps

257

affecting chemicals in vivo, even while realizing that an in vitro system using single cells can never fully represent a complete human being. Nevertheless, in vitro measurements of genetic change in human cells have developed into a valuable tool in the analysis of complex mixtures.

The toxicological paradigm, shown in Figure 1, diagrams the general fate of environmental compounds that may enter the body. They are absorbed through the skin via inhalation or by ingestion, and chemicals are then distributed throughout the various organ systems. Metabolism may occur in numerous tissues including liver, lung, kidney, and skin. Metabolites will also distribute through the body, depending on their nature. Excretion of the parent compound or its metabolites may occur by various means. Of interest to the genetic toxicologist is that point at which chemicals or their metabolites may interact with target cells to produce genetic changes. Alterations in somatic cells may cause cancer, and changes (mutations) in germ cells may induce heritable disease or birth defects.

A brief outline of the development of human lymphoblast mutation assays and their use in studying the mutagenicity of combustion effluents and air samples is presented in this chapter.

## HUMAN LYMPHOBLAST MUTATION ASSAYS

Human lymphoblast mutation assays have been in use at the Genetic Toxicology Laboratory at MIT since the mid-1970s. The initial cell line used, MIT-2, grew well in suspension but required plating in soft agarose over fibroblast feeder layers in order to form colonies.[1] The availability of fibroblast cultures from Lesch-Nyhan patients deficient in the X chromosome-linked hypoxanthine-guanine phosphoribosyl transferase (HGPRT) activity permitted the measurement of the frequency of HGPRT-deficient, 6-thioguanine (6TG)-resistant human lymphoblasts in a population. Cells deficient in HGPRT activity were resistant to the purine analog 6TG. However, with this system we were limited to mutation measurement at that locus because variant human fibroblasts at other loci were not available. Therefore, we proceeded to isolate a human lymphoblast line derived from WI-L2, designated HH4, which could form colonies efficiently without a feeder layer. This allowed us to score mutations at any locus for which selective conditions could be applied. We were able to isolate a heterozygote of the autosomal

**Figure 1.** Toxicology paradigm.

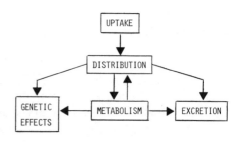

gene coding for thymidine kinase (TK). This TK heterozygote, which was designated TK6, has been used to measure induced mutations to TK deficiency via resistance to the thymidine analog trifluorothymidine.[2,3] We also use other genetic sites such as the ouabain-resistance locus.[4]

The general format of human lymphoblast mutation assays has been described elsewhere.[5] Briefly, lymphoblast cells are treated in suspension culture with a potential mutagen for a defined length of time. After treatment, cells are allowed to grow in nonselective conditions for the appropriate time to permit expression of mutant phenotypes. Cells are then seeded into dishes and incubated for about 2 weeks. Colonies are counted, and the fraction of population capable of forming colonies in the selective agent (the mutant fraction) is calculated.

These human cell systems responded well to a variety of "direct-acting" chemical mutagens. However, they did not contain the capability for xenobiotic metabolism. Therefore, an exogenous metabolizing system was needed if "indirect" mutagens were to be detected. We provided this with a rat liver postmitochondrial supernatant (PMS) and appropriate cofactors and were able to demonstrate that various polycyclic aromatic hydrocarbons (PAH) and mycotoxins were indeed mutagenic.[2,3] However, we have always been somewhat uncomfortable with the use of PMS, because the microsomal particles that form when the liver tissue is disrupted bear little resemblance to the cellular endoplasmic reticulum from which they derive. There is the possibility that they may metabolize foreign compounds differently from intact cells.

Consequently, we set about to isolate a lymphoblast line competent in foreign-compound metabolism. Our initial attempts have recently yielded a cell line, designated AHH-1, capable of activating a variety of PAH to active mutagens. Furthermore, this line is phagocytic and can potentially engulf whole soot particles, and the presence of endogenous metabolic enzymes might activate any compounds that were eluted from the particle. Thus we have developed an in vitro human cell system that can be directly exposed to soot particulates, and in which extraction of mutagens and metabolism are performed by the target cell.

Another advantage of the AHH-1 cell system is that it allows long-term low-dose studies to be performed with compounds requiring metabolic activation. Previous studies with PMS were limited because PMS is toxic to human cells when exposure time is greater than several hours.

## MUTAGENICITY OF COMPLEX MIXTURES AND COMPONENTS IN HUMAN LYMPHOBLAST SYSTEMS

### Mutagenicity of Kerosene Soot

HH4 human lymphoblasts were treated with a methylene chloride extract of a soot obtained by burning kerosene in a continuous-flow combustor.

PMS was used as a metabolizing element. Figure 2 demonstrates that the extract was mutagenic at levels above 6 µg/mL for 3 h.[6]

### Mutagenicity of an Air Sample from St. Louis

TK6 human lymphoblasts were exposed to a methylene chloride extract of an air sample (standard reference material #1648, from the National Bureau of Standards). Figures 3 and 4 show that this extract was mutagenic at two distinct loci only in the presence of PMS, in contrast to what was observed in bacteria (Figure 5). In *Salmonella typhimurium,* the extract was more mutagenic in the absence of PMS. This example is illustrative of the importance of measuring human cell responses in addition to the more rapidly performed bacterial tests.

### Mutagenicity of a Diesel Exhaust Extract and Its Components

In these experiments, we determined that a light-duty diesel engine exhaust extract was mutagenic to TK6 human cells in the presence of PMS. Gas chromatography-mass spectrometry was used to analyze some of the components of this extract, and mutation assays for many of these were performed. We were able to demonstrate that $50\% \pm 20\%$ of the mutagenicity of the extract could be accounted for by summing the mutagenic contribution of components, which totaled less than 1% of the extract (Table I). The major mutagens appeared to be fluoranthene and methylphenan-

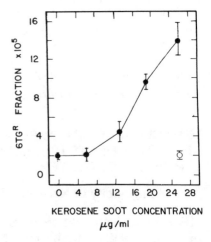

**Figure 2.** Mutagenicity of kerosene soot extract to human cells. HH4 human lymphoblasts in complete growth medium (RPMI 1640 plus 10% fetal calf serum) were treated with an extract of kerosene soot for 3 h in the presence (●) or absence (○) of a 5% (v/v) aroclor-induced rat liver postmitochrondial supernatant. Six days later, cells were seeded in soft-agarose in the presence or absence of 5 µg/mL 6-thioguanine. Error bars are 95% confidence intervals.

**Figure 3.** Mutagenicity of an air sample extract to human cells without metabolic activation. TK6 human lymphoblasts were treated in complete growth medium with an extract of a St. Louis air sample for 2 or 24 h. The mutant fractions were determined 3 d (trifluorothymidine resistance, 1 μg/mL) or 8 d (6-thioguanine resistance, 5 μg/mL) later by seeding cells in microtiter dishes. Error bars are 95% confidence intervals. Dashed line is the upper 95% confidence limit of the background mutant fraction.

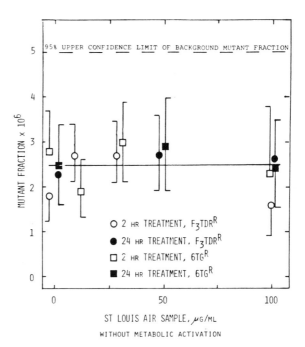

**Figure 4.** Mutagenicity of an air sample extract to human cells with metabolic activation. TK6 human lymphoblasts were treated in complete growth medium with an extract of a St. Louis air sample for 2 h in the presence of 5% (v/v) aroclor-induced rat liver postmitochondrial supernatant. Mutant fractions were determined as in Figure 3.

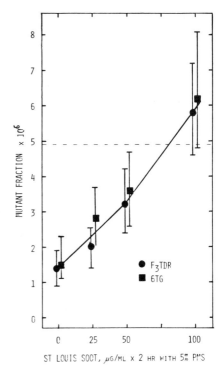

**Figure 5.** Mutagenicity of an air sample extract to bacteria. *Salmonella typhimurium* strain TM677 was treated with the St. Louis air sample in the presence or absence of 10% (v/v) rat liver postmitochondrial supernatant. Additionally, the cells were treated in either the usual minimal bacterial medium or in the more complex human-cell growth medium (RPMI plus 10% fetal calf serum). The 8-azaguanine-resistant (50 µg/mL) fraction was determined immediately after treatment. Error bars are 99% confidence limits. The dashed line is the upper 99% confidence level for *all* measurements of the background mutant fraction.

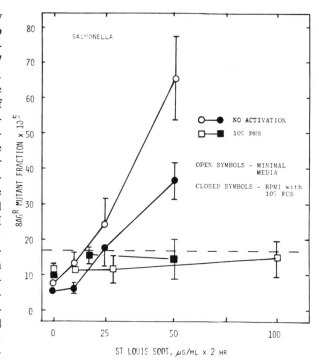

threnes. The identification of other contributing mutagens remains to be accomplished.

### Mutagenicity Assays in Metabolically Competent Cells

A gene locus mutation assay has now been developed in lymphoblast cells partially competent in oxidative xenobiotic metabolism, the AHH-1 line described in the previous section. These cells are mutated by several polycyclic aromatic hydrocarbons in the absence of an exogenous metabolizing element. Their response is compared to TK6 cells (in the presence of PMS) in Table II. The sensitivity of the two cell systems for detecting mutagenesis is about the same except in the case of fluoranthene. AHH-1 cells do not respond to this mutagen, apparently because of a lack of significant levels of microsomal epoxide hydrolase, an enzyme that is necessary for the metabolism of this particular hydrocarbon to a premutagenic DNA-binding intermediate.[7]

**Table I.** Mutagenic Contribution of Individual PAH to Automobile Diesel Exhaust Particulate Extract at 100 μg/mL

| Compound | Wt %[a] | Concentration at 100 μg/mL Extract (μM) | Estimated Contribution to Mutant Fraction[b] (× 10⁶) |
|---|---|---|---|
| Benzo[a]anthracene | 0.007 | 0.03 | 0 |
| Benzo[a]pyrene and benzo[e]pyrene | 0.03[c] | 0.06 | 0.02 |
| Chrysene + triphenylene | 0.01 | 0.04 | 0 |
| Fluoranthene | 0.2 | 1.0 | 1.5 |
| Phenanthrene | 0.2 | 1.1 | 0 |
| 1-Methylphenanthrene | 0.1 | 0.5 | 0.3 |
| 4- and 9-Methylphenanthrene | 0.14[c] | 0.4 | 0.3 |
| Component contribution | 0.6 | | 2.1 |
| Methylene chloride extract | 100 | 100 μg/mL | 4.2 |

[a]Calculations are based on an initial fractionation of the methylene chloride extract of the diesel soot particulate with the PAH-containing subfraction representing 6.5% of the total methylene chloride extract, and the quantitation of the individual PAH in this subfraction is calculated by gas chromatographic-mass spectrometry.

[b]Mutant fractions were determined at the trifluorothymidine-resistant locus (2 μg/mL).

[c]The isomers benzo[a]pyrene and benzo[e]pyrene, as well as 4-methylphenanthrene and 9-methylphenanthrene could not be separated by gas chromatographic-mass spectrometry analysis, and we assumed that both were present in equal amounts for calculation purposes.

**Table II.** Response of AHH-1 and TK6 Cells to PAH Mutagens

| Compound | AHH-1 | TK6 (with PMS) | TK6 (w/o PMS) |
|---|---|---|---|
| Benzo(a)pyrene | (+) $10^{-6}$ M | (+) $10^{-6}$ M | (−) |
| Cyclopenteno-(c, d)pyrene | (+) $3 \times 10^{-8}$ M | (+) $5 \times 10^{-6}$ M | (−) |
| 1-Methylphenathrene | (+) $3 \times 10^{-5}$ M | (+) $6 \times 10^{-6}$ M | (−) |
| Fluoranthene | (−) | (+) $2 \times 10^{-6}$ M | (−) |

Conditions: AHH-1 cells were treated for 24 h, TK6 cells were treated for 3 h, and 6-thioguanine-resistant mutant fractions were determined 7 to 10 d after treatment. (+) means a positive response; (−) indicates a negative response. Numbers listed are the lowest concentrations required to induce a statistically significant response.

## Measuring Mutations by Particle-Bound Components

AHH-1 cells were treated with a carbon black (a gift of R. Hites) to see if chemical compounds could be extracted from particulates, then metabolized directly to mutagens. Treatment of AHH-1 cells with 0.05 to 1.0-mg/mL suspended particulate for 5 d produced a uniform four- to fivefold increase in the 6-thioguanine-resistant mutant fraction. A methylene chloride extract of the carbon black (yield: 7.8-mg/g carbon black) was also assayed for mutagenic activity. Similarly, concentrations of 0.1–1.0 µg/mL for 5 d produced a three- to fivefold increase in the mutant fraction. We feel this procedure represents a significant improvement in methodology for analysis of the biological activity of particulate-borne complex mixtures.

## DISCUSSION

We have developed human lymphoblast assays that can be used to detect mutagenic activity in complex mixtures. We currently hypothesize that the mutagenicity of a mixture can be accounted for by summing the mutagenicities of its components. We expect this relationship to be especially true at low concentrations (which is most relevant to the expected in vivo exposures) where competition for metabolism or reaction with target sites would be minimal or nonexistent. Future work in this area of genetic toxicology will be to further characterize the mutagenicities of complex mixtures. Chemical analyses of these mixtures can be done and the mutagenic potentials of the components measured. It is likely that potent but as yet unidentified mutagens are waiting to be discovered. The further development of mutagenesis tests in human cells will aim toward systems that more and more closely mimic in vivo conditions. Variants of AHH-1 cells may be isolated which contain epoxide hydrolase or other foreign-compound-metabolizing enzymes that increase the spectrum of compounds which can be activated. End points such as chromosome aberrations can be studied in conjunction with gene-locus mutations in order to allow consideration of a wider variety of chemically induced genetic damage. The endocytotic ability of AHH-1 cells appears to allow measurement of mutagenic potential of airborne or combustion-generated compounds in their native form, attached to particulates.

## ACKNOWLEDGMENTS

The work presented in this chapter has been supported by the U.S. Department of Energy grant DE-AC02-EV4267 and by the National Institute of Environmental Health Science grants 5-P01-ES0597 and 1-P30-ES02109. This chapter describes work that has been submitted to referenced journals and is not intended to be original with these proceedings.

# REFERENCES

1. Thilly, W.G., J.G. DeLuca, H. Hoppe IV, and B.W. Penman. "Mutation of Human Lymphoblasts by Methylnitrosourea," *Chem. Biol. Interact.* 15:33–50 (1976).
2. Skopek, T.R., H.L. Liber, B.W. Penman, and W.G. Thilly. "Isolation of a Human Lymphoblastoid Line Heterozygous at the Thymidine Kinase Locus: Possibility for a Rapid Human Cell Mutation Assay," *Biochem. Biophys. Res. Commun.* 84:411–416 (1978).
3. Liber, H.L., and W.G. Thilly. "Mutation Assay at the Thymidine Kinase Locus in Diploid Human Lymphoblasts," *Mutat. Res.* 94:467–485 (1982).
4. Furth, E.E., W.G. Thilly, B.W. Penman, H.L. Liber, and W.M. Rand. "Quantitative Assay for Mutation in Diploid Human Lymphoblasts Using Microtiter Plates," *Anal. Biochem.* 110:1–8 (1981).
5. Thilly, W.G., J.G. DeLuca, E.E. Furth, H. Hoppe IV, D.A. Kaden, J.J. Krolewski, H.L. Liber, T.R. Skopek, S. Slapikoff, R.J. Tizard, and B.W. Penman. "Gene Locus Mutation Assays in Diploid Human Lymphoblast Lines," in *Chemical Mutagens,* F.J. de Serres and A. Hollaender, Eds. (New York: Plenum Press, 1980), pp. 331–361.
6. Skopek, T.R., H.L. Liber, D.A. Kaden, R.A. Hites, and W.G. Thilly. "Mutation of Human Cells by Kerosene Soot," *J. Natl. Cancer Inst.* 63:309–312 (1979).
7. Babson, J., unpublished results.

# DISCUSSION

*V. Frankos, Clement Associates:* Did you possibly combine your AHH-1 line lymphocytes with the PMS fraction to see if you could get increased sensitivity to any given compound?

*H.L. Liber:* No, we have not done that.

# CHAPTER 12

## Comparison of In Vivo Carcinogenesis and In Vitro Genotoxicity of Complex Hydrocarbon Mixtures

R.A. Pelroy, D.D. Mahlum,
M.E. Frazier, R.A. Renne,
D.L. Stewart, and E.K. Chess

*Pacific Northwest Laboratory*
*Richland, WA 99352*

The genetic activity and carcinogenicity of synthetic fuels from several sources were compared. In vitro tests consisted of the standard Ames histidine reversion test with *Salmonella typhimurium* TA-98, the Chinese hamster ovary forward mutation, and the Syrian hamster embryo transformation assays. In vivo carcinogenesis and tumorigenesis tests consisted of the initiation/promotion, mouse skin-painting (initiation phase), and chronic mouse skin-painting assays.

The mammalian in vitro tests appear to be better quantitative indicators of carcinogenicity in mouse skin. However, quantitative correlation between in vitro and in vivo results was not convincingly demonstrated, and the data suggest that relationships are rough, at best. Qualitative correlations appear to be much stronger in relating both genetic and carcinogenic activity to boiling point and to chemical class.

### INTRODUCTION

A number of synfuels have undergone in vitro testing for genotoxicity. Most of the published mutagenicity data have come from the standard plate incorporation version of the histidine reversion or Ames assay with *Salmonella typhimurium*. This test has been systematically used with solvent-refined coal (SRC-I and -II),[1-4] H-coal liquids, coal gasification materials,[5-12] and a number of shale oils.[6-13] A defining characteristic of coal- and shale-derived liquids is the high mutagenic activity of their nitrogen-rich basic fractions in the histidine reversion (Ames) assay with special mutagen-sensitive strains of *S. typhimurium*. A more limited data base for the synfuels is available for mammalian in vitro systems. Mutagenesis induced by basic (i.e., nitrogen rich) fractions from H-coal and both crude liquids and chemical fractions from hydrotreated and nonhydrotreated SRC-II liquids were studied in the Chinese hamster ovary (CHO) forward mutation assay.[14,15] Mammalian cellular transformation in the Syrian hamster embryo (SHE) assay has also been applied to a number of SRC-II coal liquids.[16]

Small-animal skin-painting tests to measure the carcinogenicity of synfuels have also been carried out on a variety of synthetic fuel materials, for example, mouse skin-painting tests on shale oils and coal liquids.[17] Work by Calkins et al.[18] with the initiation/promotion (I/P) mouse skin-painting assay is noteworthy because carcinogenic response appeared to be roughly proportional to mutagenic response in the standard Ames assay. However, the quantitative correlation between Ames test data and carcinogenesis is a controversial subject. Overall, most data do not suggest a strong quantitative relationship between carcinogenic and mutagenic potency in the standard Ames assay.[19-25] However, mutagenic potency in the Ames assay and DNA damage (or mutagenicity) in a mammalian in vitro system taken together may constitute a strong qualitative and quantitative test for carcinogenicity.[26]

Many of the compounds in the high-nitrogen synfuels are reactive (in some cases, highly reactive) as mutagens against the *S. typhimurim* strains used in the Ames test. Examples are from the coal liquids polycyclic aromatic hydrocarbons (PAH), azaarenes, amino polycyclic aromatic hydrocarbons (APAH), hydroxy polycyclic aromatic hydrocarbons (HPAH), polyaromatic carbazoles, and polyaromatic thiophenes.[27-41]

In this chapter we will compare in vitro bioassay data obtained from synfuels with carcinogenesis data from the same materials. Our main objective is to compare mutagenic activity in the standard Ames and CHO assay with tumorigenic activity in mouse skin resulting from exposure to synfuels. Emphasis will be placed on the SRC-II liquids, because there is an extensive chemical and biological data base for these materials. A secondary objective is to relate, both qualitatively and quantitatively, mutagenesis and carcinogenesis to specific chemical classes contained in the synfuels. The performance of the in vitro tests for the complex chemical mixtures represented by the synfuels and, in particular, studies involving coal-derived liquids and their chemical fractions will be emphasized. Since these materials are chemically complex, we will rely heavily on chemical analysis of biologically active fractions to implicate the chemical species that may be responsible for genetic and carcinogenic activity of synfuels.

We anticipate that simple, clear-cut, quantitative relationships between the in vitro and in vivo test results for the synthetic fuel materials are unlikely. However, by analyzing the synfuels in terms of their chemistry and their activity in several bioassay systems, we may be able to draw certain conclusions about the agents responsible for determining these effects and the usefulness of the bioassay systems in screening for such agents in complex mixtures.

## CHEMICAL CLASS FRACTIONATION PROCEDURES

Three methods of separating the major chemical compound classes in synthetic fuels into fractions were employed to produce materials for bioassay. Early bioassay studies were carried out using solvent fractions of basic (acid-soluble), acidic (base-soluble), and neutral PAH components from SRC coal and shale-oil liquids.[6,8,10,13,31] Analysis of the solvent fractions from coal liquids was complicated by the formation of poorly defined tars that contained both polar and PAH components. Formation of tars from the highly aromatic coal liquids during solvent fractionation has been reported for the coal liquids also.[13,42] Various methods have been used to separate solvent fractions into subfractions of greater chemical homogeneity including Sephadex LH20 and alumina-column chromatography[3,4,6,7,9,31,35] and thin-layer chromatography and cation exchange.[32,36,37]

An improved method for separating the SRC coal liquids into well-defined chemical classes was used to prepare chemical class fractions from SRC-II distillate cuts for bioassay.[35] This procedure is based on alumina- and silicic-acid column separations of SRC components into chemical classes for bioassay. It avoids the formation of the poorly defined tar fractions which appear to be characteristic of high-boiling coal liquids.[13,42]

The initial step of the alumina/silicic-acid column fractionation scheme involves separation of the coal liquids into four chemical subclasses: neutral aliphatic hydrocarbons, PAH, NPAC, and HPAH. Three of these classes, the aliphatics, PAH, and NPAC, are well-defined chemically. The HPAH, mainly composed of phenolic and hydroxylated PAH components, also contains other chemically less well-defined polar compounds, including multi-heteroatomic species. The NPAC can be further separated into its major chemical class subfractions (i.e., carbazoles, azaarenes, and APAH) by silicic-acid-column chromatography.[35] Only the bioassay results for the alumina-column fractions will be discussed.

The third method used to generate chemical fractions considered in this chapter was based on separation of components in a coal liquid by high-pressure liquid chromatography (HPLC).[3] In these studies, the SRC-II 850 + °F distillate cut was fractionated by semipreparative HPLC according to polarity and, to a lesser extent, molecular weight. The resulting fractions were analyzed for mutagenesis in both the standard Ames and CHO in vitro assays.

The HPLC procedure employed separates the components in the SRC-II 850 + °F distillate into chemical classes which are similar to those obtained by alumina-column chromatography. A disadvantage of HPLC is its incomplete separation of the aliphatics from PAH in the PAH-rich fractions and incomplete separation of more-polar oxygen and sulfur-containing polycyclics from less-polar NPAC. On the other hand, HPLC yields partial separation of PAH according to molecular weight; in addition, APAH and carbazoles are separated, to a large extent, from azaarenes.

### Composition of PAH and NPAC Fractions from High-Boiling-Point SRC-II Distillate Cuts

Constituents in the PAH and NPAC chemical classes of the high-boiling SRC-II liquids appear to determine most of the in vitro genetic and in vivo carcinogenic or tumorigenic activity of these materials. Following is a summary of some of the more important chemical characteristics associated with these two chemical fractions.

As expected, the average molecular weight of compounds in the various distillate cuts increases with distillation temperature, as illustrated in Tables I and II for selected PAH and NPAC components of the 800–850°F and 850 + °F SRC-II distillate bottoms. These materials were characterized by high concentrations of four-, five-, and six-ring PAH (Table I). The PAH composition of the 850 + °F SRC-II distillate bottoms was surprisingly simple, consisting mainly of five- and six-ring PAH. Comparatively high levels of the potent mouse skin carcinogen benzo(a)pyrene (BaP) were found both in 800–850°F SRC-II distillate cut and the 850 + °F distillate bottoms. Four-ring PAH, including the potent carcinogens for mouse skin 7,12-dimethyl-benzanthracene, 5-methylchrysene, and the less potent benz[a]anthracene, were concentrated mostly in the 800–850°F SRC-II distillate cut. The 800–850°F SRC-II distillate was essentially devoid of six-ring PAH.

With respect to ring number, the composition of the NPAC in these distillate-cut fractions appeared to be similar to that of the PAH (Table II). For example, four-ring azaarenes, APAH, and carbazoles were concentrated in the 800-850°F distillate cut; four- and five-ring compounds were localized in the 850+°F distillate cut. The apparent decrease in APAH concentration in the 850+°F bottoms was dramatic. The five-ring APAH, carbazoles, and five- and six-ring azaarenes appeared to be localized exclusively in the 850+°F distillate cut. In terms of concentration, the APAH were minor constituents of the NPAC compared to the azaarenes and carbazoles. This was also true for the other SRC-II distillate cuts (i.e., < 800°F).

The distribution of PAH and NPAC components in the 800–850°F and 850 + °F SRC-II distillate cuts was also estimated by probe mass spectrometry (MS; Figure 1). Major PAH components in the 800–850°F SRC-II distillate cut were found at m/e 202 (pyrene), 215 (M-1 ion from benzofluorene), and in compounds with molecular weights corresponding to the methyl-,

**Table I.**   Average Molecular Weight of PAH Components

| Compound | Quantity (μg/g) 800–850°F | Quantity (μg/g) 850+°F | Structure |
|---|---|---|---|
| Phenanthrene | 211 (7.4)[a] | 58 (2.7) | |
| Fluoranthene | 732 (8.1) | 30 (1.4) | |
| Pyrene | 2375 (83.1) | 235 (11.0) | |
| Benz(*a*)anthracene | 2997 (104.9) | | |
| Chrysene | 7324 (256.3) | 31 (1.5) | |
| Methylchrysene | 35,201 (1654.4) | 215 (7.4) | |
| 7,12-Dimethylbenzan-thracene | 4532 (213) | | |
| Benzo(*k*)fluoranthene | 3972 (139.0) | 306 (14.4) | |
| Benzo(*e*)pyrene | 6135 (214.7) | 5755 (270.5) | |
| Benzo(*a*)pyrene | 3530 (123.6) | 3637 (170.9) | |
| Benzo(*ghi*)perylene | | 15,311 (719.6) | |

[a]( ) Indicates weight-normalized concentration in the whole-boiling-range SRC-II liquid (800–850+°F).

**Table II.** Average Molecular Weight of NPAC Components

| Compound Type | Quantity (μg/g) | | Representative Structures |
|---|---|---|---|
| | 800°F to 850°F | 850 + °F | |
| Azapyrenes/-fluoranthene | 1381 (48.4)[a] | | |
| Azachrysenes/-benzanthracenes | 2067 (72.3) | 1039 (48.8) | |
| Azabenzopyrenes/-benzofluoranthenes, etc. | | 4431 (208.3) | |
| Azabenzo-(ghi)perylenes | | 2396 (112.6) | |
| Aminophrenanthrene/-anthracene | 154 (5.4) | | |
| Aminopyrenes/-fluoranthenes | 627 (21.9) | 25 (1.2) | |
| Aminochrysenes/-benzanthracenes | | 53 (2.5) | |
| Aminobenzopyrenes/-perylenes, etc. | | 32 (1.5) | |
| Benzocarbazoles | 17,721 (620.2) | 126 (5.9) | , -- |
| Benzocarbazoles | | 2364 (111.1) | , -- |

[a]( ) Indicates weight-normalized concentration of the distillate cuts in the whole-boiling-range SRC-II liquid (800–850 + °F).

dimethylpyrenes, benzofluoranthenes, and benzofluorenes (Figure 1, upper panel). There was also a prominent peak at m/e 252, corresponding to the molecular weight of benzopyrenes, perylenes, etc. These results are generally in accord with the concentrations of individual PAH as determined by gas chromatography (GC) analysis (Table I). However, they also suggest that the "average" compound in the PAH fraction of the 800–850°F distillate cut had four aromatic rings and was alkylated.

Alkylation was especially evident for the NPAC constituents of the 800–850°F SRC-II distillate cut (Figure 1, lower panel). The most intense ions in these mass spectra were obtained at m/e 217 (corresponding to four-ring methylazaarenes) and/or APAH such as the aminopyrenes and/or benzocarbazoles. Intense ions were also observed at m/e 231. From GC and GC/MS analyses, we know these to be mainly dimethylazapyrenes and methylbenzocarbazoles, with smaller concentrations of methylaminopyrenes and other alkylated APAH. The molecular-weight distribution appeared to be skewed toward high mass, with the mass centered near m/e 231. The NPAC fraction mass spectra were characterized by a series of peaks at intervals of 14 amu, suggesting that the mixture was comprised of a homologous series of alkylated aromatic species.

Major PAH components of the 850°F SRC-II distillate bottoms are shown by the mass spectra in Figure 2. The same general pattern observed for the 800–850°F SRC-II distillate cut was repeated: distribution skewed to high mass, with evidence of substantial alkylation. Intense molecular ions were obtained at m/e 252 (mainly benzopyrenes and perylenes), at m/e 266 molecular ions (methylbenzopyrenes and benzofluoranthenes), and m/e 280 (dimethylbenzopyrenes). Molecular ions were also observed at m/e 276 (mainly anthanthrene and benzo[*ghi*]perylene) and, from a series of alkylated homologs, at m/e 290, 304, 318, etc. (Figure 2, upper panel). The data agree with those in Table I in showing a substantial contribution of five- and six-ring PAH components in 850 + °F SRC-II distillate bottoms.

Mass spectra of the NPAC components from the 850 + °F SRC-II distillate bottoms also show a picture consistent with substantial alkylation of the azaarenes, APAH, and carbazoles (Figure 2, bottom panel). For example, the base peak of the NPAC mass spectrum was m/e 267, corresponding to dibenzocarbazole. GC data showed that compounds such as methylazabenanthracene and traces of aminobenzopyrenes contributed to this ion current. Clusters of relatively intense ions at 14-amu increments were again prominent. The average NPAC constituent in the SRC-II 850 + °F bottoms appears to have five aromatic rings and one or more alkyl substituents.

The mass spectra for PAH and NPAC were obtained using electron impact (EI) ionization at 70 eV. This relatively high electron energy gives rise to fragments which, in general, would cause the contributions of alkyl polycyclics in any given complex mixture to be underestimated. Thus, the alkylated compounds were probably more concentrated in the PAH and

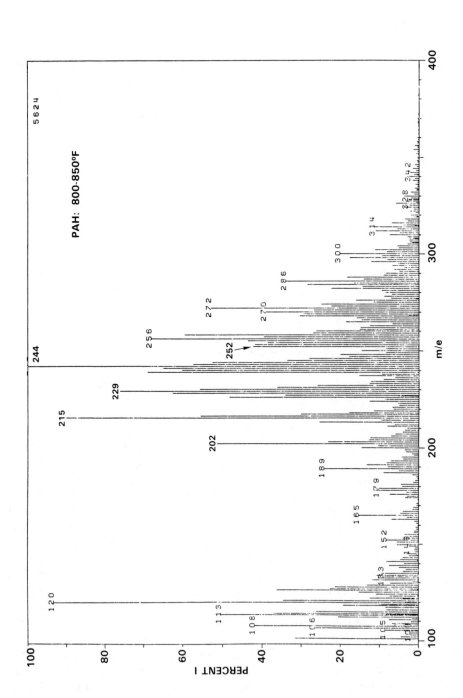

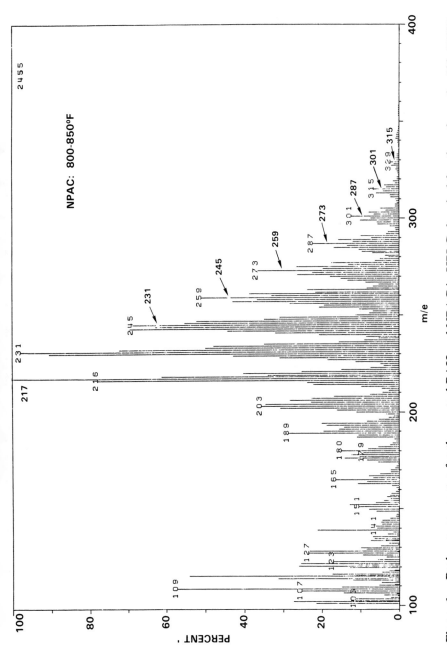

**Figure 1.** Probe mass spectra for the neutral PAH and NPAC in HPLC chemical fractions from the 800–850°F SRC-II distillate cut. The upper panel indicates the PAH fraction and the lower panel indicates the NPAC fraction.

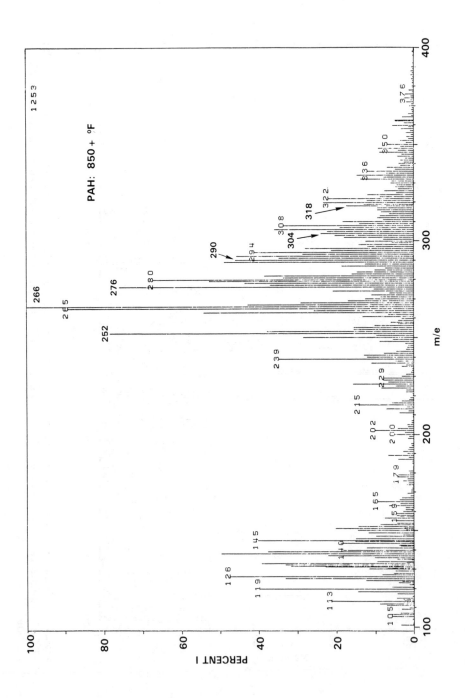

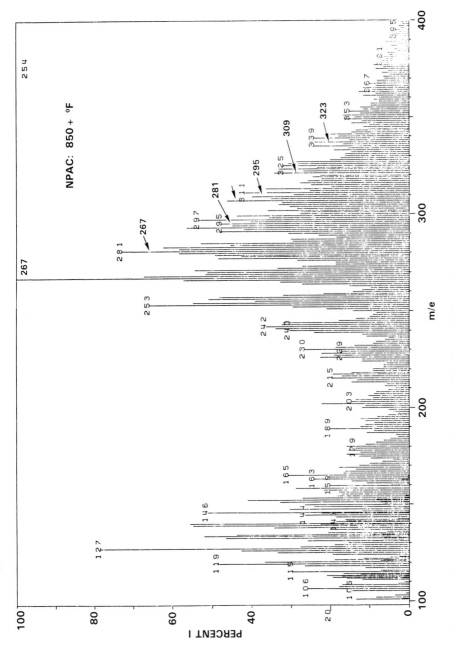

**Figure 2.**   Probe mass spectra for the neutral PAH and NPAC in 850 + °F SRC-II distillate bottoms. The upper panel indicates the PAH fraction and the lower panel indicates the NPAC fraction.

NPAC fractions of the 800 + °F SRC-II distillate cut and bottoms than is suggested by the intensities of their molecular ions in the MS data in Figures 1 and 2.

The data presented for the PAH and NPAC constituents in the SRC-II 800–850°F distillate cut and in the 850 + °F bottoms can be generalized to the other cuts from SRC-II whole-boiling-range liquid. Average molecular weight expressed as the number of aromatic rings for these two chemical classes is shown schematically in Figure 3. There is a progressive increase in the average number of aromatic rings equivalent to approximately one ring for each 50°F increase of distillation temperature. For a given number of aromatic rings, the maximum concentrations of the more-polar APAH were displaced approximately 50°F higher in the SRC-II distillate cuts. Thus, as a function of distillation temperature, three-ring APAH overlap with four-ring PAH, four-ring APAH with five-ring PAH, etc. As a point of reference for later discussion, the most mutagenic/carcinogenic five-ring PAH appear to be localized in the 800 + °F distillate cuts, but the most mutagenically active APAH (those having three and four aromatic rings) were localized in the 750–850°F distillate cuts.

## PARAMETERS FOR COMPARISONS OF IN VITRO AND IN VIVO DATA

We compared in vitro mutagenesis (both microbial and mammalian) and mammalian-cell transformation with in vivo carcinogenesis induced by synfuel materials. The in vitro systems used to generate mutagenesis data are the standard Ames histidine reversion assay with *S. typhimurium* TA-98 and the CHO forward mutation assay at the hypoxanthine-guanine phosphoribosyl transferase (HGPRT) locus. The in vivo assays consist of the complete (chronic) and initiation/promotion (I/P) mouse skin tumorigenesis tests. Particular emphasis will be placed on comparison of mutagenesis data with I/P data.

The endpoints for these assay systems are illustrated by the data in Figures 4 and 5. For the mutagenesis in vitro test systems, potency was estimated by simple linear regression analysis of dose-response data (Figure 4). Where dose response was nonlinear (e.g., PAH fraction enriched in four- and five-ring compounds, Figure 4), mutagenic potency was estimated by subtracting background from response and dividing by dose at the lowest concentration of chemical yielding a statistically significant response, that is, by single-point estimations. For most synfuels or synfuel fractions showing mutagenic activity in these systems, dose response was approximately linear over at least a portion of the dose-response curve.

Figure 4 also shows that, characteristically, variation of the response in duplicate assays was generally less than 10% of the mean.

Response in the I/P mouse skin-carcinogenesis assay was defined as

CARCINOGENIC POTENCY

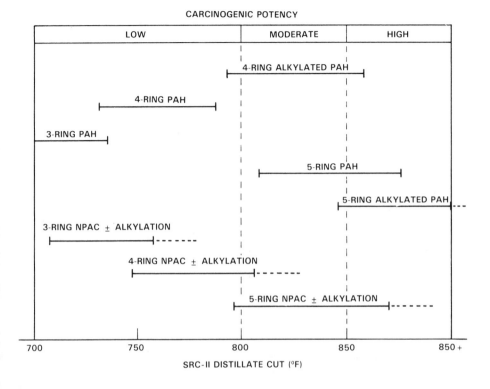

**Figure 3.** Approximate distribution of neutral PAH and NPAC in SRC-II distillate cuts.

either total number of skin tumors or tumor incidence at 120 d after exposure (Figure 5). Response in the chronic mouse skin-painting assay, determined at different concentrations of synthetic fuel materials, was expressed as maximum latency before tumor formation. Response in the I/P mouse skin-carcinogenesis tests was approximately a linear function of the concentration of initiator applied during the exposure step.

## GENETIC, CARCINOGENIC, AND TUMORIGENIC ACTIVITY OF CRUDE MATERIALS FROM VARIOUS SYNTHETIC FUEL PROCESSES

Fifty-degree distillate cuts and/or bottoms from the wide-boiling-range SRC-I and -II liquids were characterized for in vitro genetic, carcinogenic, and tumorigenic activity.

The objective of these studies was to relate in vitro genetic activity and

AMES vs CHO:  850 + °F

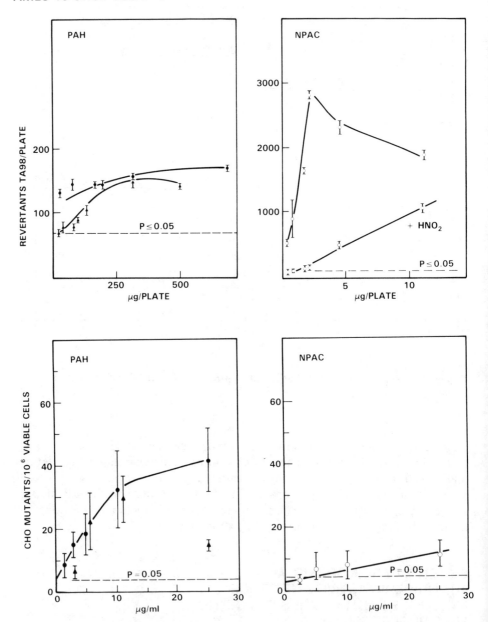

**Figure 4.** Dose-response data for the standard Ames (histidine reversion) test with *S. typhimurium* TA-98 (top panels) and the forward mutation assay with CHO cells (bottom panels) for the neutral PAH and NPAC from the 850 + °F SRC-II distillate bottoms. Symbols: HPLC fractions enriched in four- and five-ring PAH (●), five- and six-ring PAH (▲), the carbazoles and APAH constituents (0).

INITIATION PROMOTION:  SRC-II 850 + °F

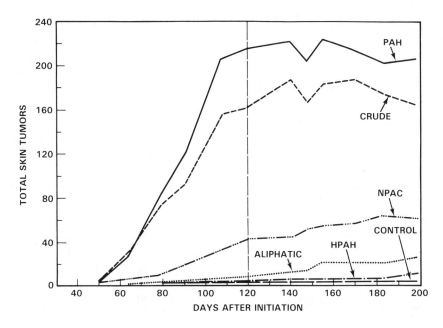

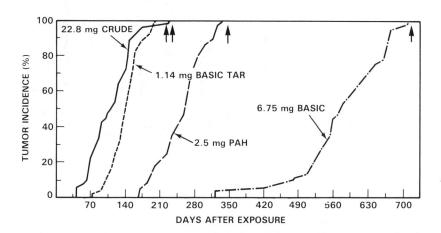

**Figure 5.** Total number of skin tumors in the I/P tests (top panel) and tumor incidence in the chronic mouse skin-painting assays (bottom panel) for chemical fractions of the 850+°F SRC-II distillate bottoms and the 550 to 850°F SRC-II HD. Abbreviations for the alumina-column fractions (top panel): neutral PAH, NPAC, HPAH. The dashed line (upper panel) and vertical arrows (lower panel) indicate I/P response at 120 d after exposure and maximum latency in chronic skin-painting bioassays, respectively.

in vivo carcinogenic activity to specific boiling-point ranges and, thus, to definable molecular-weight species within the distillate cuts. Figures 6 and 7 show that the most active distillate cuts were those that boiled above 700°F. Carcinogenic activity increased monotonically with temperature and reached maximum levels in the high-boiling distillate cuts and/or distillate bottoms (Figures 6 and 7). The dividing line between carcinogenically active and inactive distillate cuts was fairly well defined at approximately 700°F for both the SRC-I and SRC-II distillate cuts. The SRC-II distillate cuts were more active than their SRC-I counterparts over comparable temperature ranges. Responses in the in vitro and in vivo bioassays increased monotonically for the SRC-II materials, reaching the highest levels for the SRC-II 850 + °F distillate bottoms (Figure 6).

Figure 7 summarizes our comparative data base for the SRC-I distillate cuts but does not include data for the ongoing CHO studies. Since chronic

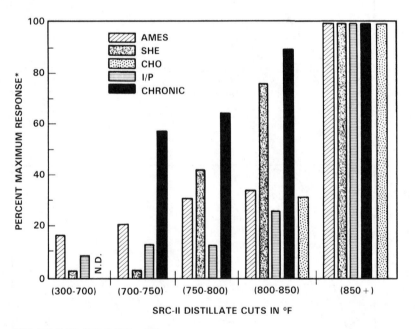

*RELATIVE TO SRC-II 850 + °F

**Figure 6.** Comparison of mutagenesis and mammalian cell transformation results with I/P and chronic skin-painting carcinogenesis results for the SRC-II distillate cuts. To compare these materials on the same scale, bioassay responses were normalized against the most active material. The bioassays included standard Ames test with *S. typhimurium* TA-98, SHE mammalian-cell transformation, CHO mammalian-cell forward-mutation assay, I/P mouse skin-painting carcinogenesis assay (initiation phase; total number of tumors), and chronic mouse skin-painting assay. N.D. = assay not carried out.

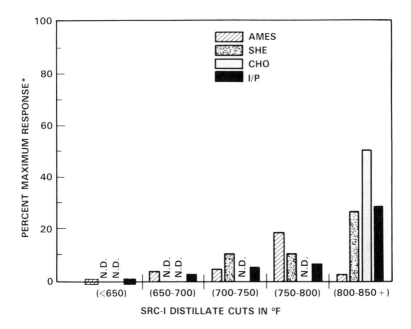

*RELATIVE TO SRC-II 850 + °F

**Figure 7.**   Comparison of mutagenesis and mammalian cell transformation results with I/P skin-painting carcinogenesis results for the SRC-I distillate cuts. N.D. = assay not carried out.

skin-painting assays were not carried out for the SRC-I distillates, comparisons of carcinogenesis to genetic endpoints are based solely on the I/P skin-painting assay system. Nevertheless, it is possible to draw some conclusions about potential relationships between in vivo and in vitro test results and about the relative genetic and carcinogenic activities of the SRC-I vs SRC-II distillate cuts.

The level of assay response for these crude SRC-I distillate cuts increased monotonically for the SHE transformation and I/P initiation tests. However, specific mutagenic activity in the Ames assay systems attained a maximum value for the 750–800°F distillate cut and dropped sharply for the 800–850 + °F distillate cut (Figure 7). Thus, in contrast to the near proportionality among Ames, SHE, and I/P data for the SRC-II distillate cuts, specific mutagenic activity in the Ames assay did not appear to be quantitatively related to results from either transformation or I/P assays with the crude SRC-I distillate cuts. CHO mutagenesis data, available only for the SRC-I 800–850°F distillate, showed less activity than the comparable SRC-II distillates. Moreover, the genetic and carcinogenic activity of the SRC-I distillate cuts, as a whole, was lower than that of comparable SRC-II distillate cuts.

SRC-II heavy distillate (HD), SRC-I process solvent (PS), Paraho shale oil, and Wilmington crude petroleum are compared as genotoxins and skin carcinogens in Figure 8. The boiling points for these two SRC liquids ranged from about 550–850 + °F, thus encompassing the boiling points of the distillate cuts and bottoms. The HD and PS induced strong responses in all five bioassays. In quantitative terms, the potency of HD was approximately two to three times greater than that of PS for both mutagenesis and I/P carcinogenesis tests. Thus, in order of potency, the in vitro and in vivo assay results for the two wide-boiling-range coal liquids were in agreement. The comparative data base for Paraho shale oil and Wilmington crude petroleum was less complete, lacking I/P data for the former and CHO for the latter. Nevertheless, the results suggest important differences between in vitro mutagenesis, mammalian transformation, and mouse skin-carcinogenesis assays.

According to the carcinogenesis assay results, SRC-I and Paraho shale oil are roughly equipotent to mouse skin. Likewise, the CHO assay (mutation) and SHE assay (transformation) suggest near-equivalent potency of these materials for the mammalian in vitro bioassays and I/P assay. However, potency based on Ames data was unexpectedly low, suggesting that

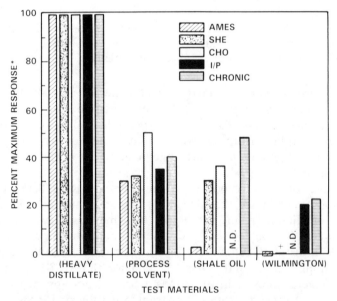

*RELATIVE TO HD

**Figure 8.** Comparison of in vitro and in vivo bioassay results of SRC-II HD, SRC-I PS (coal liquid), Paraho shale oil and Wilmington crude petroleum. N.D. = assay not carried out; + indicates a positive, but weak, response in a given bioassay system.

Ames data from the crude shale oil were not good quantitative indicators of carcinogenic potency for this material.

For the Wilmington crude, no mutagenic activity was detected in the standard Ames test, confirming previous results for crude petroleums.[6,8,13] On the other hand, both carcinogenesis skin-painting tests were positive, indicating that Wilmington crude was capable of initiating tumor formation and inducing carcinogenesis in mouse skin. The CHO system was not used to analyze Wilmington crude; however, low-level, but statistically significant, response to Wilmington crude was demonstrated with the SHE transformation assay. This suggests that, for low-nitrogen-containing petroleum crudes, mammalian-cell transformation assays may be more sensitive to genotoxicants than the Ames test. This possibility should be explored with further comparative studies.

## BIOLOGICAL ACTIVITY VS CHEMICAL FRACTION

### Solvent Fractions

Initial studies on the relationship of genetic and carcinogenic activity of SRC-II liquids to the chemical classes were carried out using fractions prepared from SRC-II HD (550–850 + °F) by acid-base solvent extraction methods.[13]

Nearly all the biological activity associated with the SRC-II HD was in the basic, neutral tar, basic tar, and PAH fractions (Figure 9). Some of these chemical fractions were poorly defined, especially compared to the fraction now employed for bioassays (see below). The tars, which are readily formed from high-boiling coal liquids in the presence of various neutral solvents,[13,42] contained both neutral PAH and basic components. However, the soluble basic and PAH fractions were chemically homogeneous and thus were suitable materials for bioassay studies directed toward relating activity to chemical class. As shown in Figure 9, mutagenicity-specific activities of the tar fractions in the Ames and SHE transformation assays both agreed fairly well with the level of carcinogenic response in the chronic and I/P skin-painting tests. The tars and PAH fractions were, roughly, of equal potency in the mouse skin-carcinogenesis assays. The basic fraction was less carcinogenic than either the tar or PAH fractions. The striking quantitative disparity between the in vivo and in vitro results was caused by the Ames test results. In relative terms, this test showed preferential responses to the basic fraction and very low response to the PAH fraction. As shown elsewhere,[43] most of the genetic activity of the SRC-II basic fractions (and also of the SRC-II basic and neutral tar fractions) is due to one general class of compound, the primary aromatic amines (PAA). Moreover, APAH, a subclass of the PAA, are the determinant Ames test mutagens in these and similar coal liquids.[32,36,37,39,40,42–47]

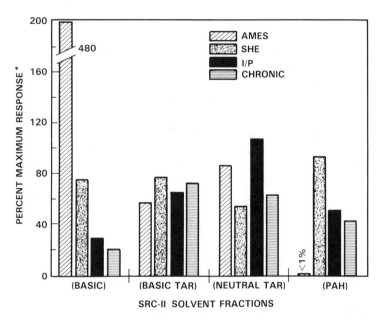

**Figure 9.** Comparison of in vitro mutagenesis and mammalian cell transformation results with I/P and chronic skin-painting carcinogenesis data for solvent fractions from SRC-II HD, bp range of 550 to 850°F.

### Alumina-Column Fractions

Alumina-column chemical-class fractions from the SRC-II 850+°F distillate bottoms, the most carcinogenic of these cuts, were analyzed in detail for genetic and carcinogenic activity. Figure 10 shows that PAH and NPAC from the 850°F distillate were the most active of the alumina-column fractions in the SHE transformation, CHO mutagenesis, and I/P mouse skin-carcinogenesis tests (initiation phase), again showing relatively good agreement between the mammalian in vitro and in vivo test results. Chronic mouse skin-painting tests have not yet been carried out with alumina-column chemical-class fractions.

Differences were observed in the sensitivity of I/P, CHO, and SHE assays to the alumina-column aliphatic and HPAH fractions. Both chemical fractions were negative in the I/P tests but induced low, though significant, responses in both the CHO and SHE test systems. For the HPAH, the disagreement was slight, and responses in CHO and SHE were very weak. For the aliphatic fraction, the disparity, particularly between the CHO and I/P test results, was much greater. At least a partial explanation may be that PAH compounds, which were later shown to be low-concentration contam-

SRC II (850 + °F)

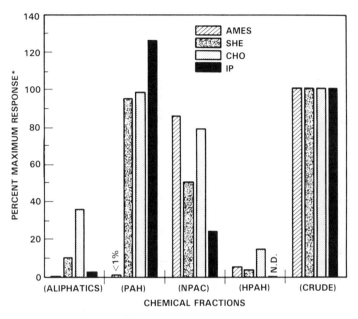

*RELATIVE TO 850 + °F SRC II

**Figure 10.**  Comparison of in vitro mutagenesis and mammalian cell transformation results with I/P skin-painting carcinogenesis data for alumina-column fractions of the 850 + °F SRC-II distillate bottoms. N.D. = assay not carried out.

inants of the aliphatic fraction, were capable of inducing mutation in the CHO assay but were ineffective as carcinogens in mouse skin. This is plausible since, as will be discussed, the forward mutation in the CHO assay appears to be particularly sensitive to PAH in complex mixtures.

Both NPAC and PAH induced mutation in the Ames test, as did HPAH. However, NPAC contained much stronger mutagens in this microbial bioassay system than did PAH, confirming the observations made with solvent fractions (Figure 9). The NPAC, essentially equivalent to the basic solvent fractions, contain APAH, which are particularly potent Ames mutagens. The HPAH were more potent than the PAH fraction in the Ames test. To compare the potency of the four alumina-column chemical-class fractions in the standard Ames test, the relative activities of the HPAH and PAH fractions would be 1 and 0.1%, respectively, if the activity of NPAC is normalized to 100%.

Comparisons of genetic and carcinogenic activity in chemical fractions from the SRC-II distillate cuts are not yet complete. However, the standard Ames test has been carried out for each alumina-column fraction from each distillate cut. These data were compared with tumor incidence for the corresponding unfractionated distillate cut (Figure 11). Ames response for both the PAH and HPAH fractions from different distillate cuts appeared to be highly correlated with tumor incidence induced by the unfractionated distillate cuts. The mutagenicity-specific activity or potency of HPAH was about 10 times greater than that of the PAH in the standard Ames test. The relative Ames mutagenic activity of both these chemical fractions was roughly proportional to tumor incidence in the I/P tests. On the other hand, the specific mutagenic activity of the NPAC fractions from the SRC-II distillate

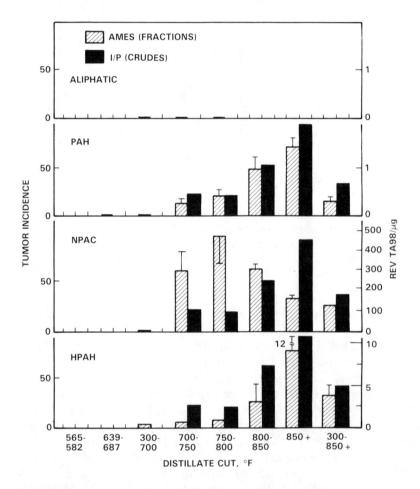

**Figure 11.** In vitro mutagenesis in the standard Ames test with *S. typhimurium* TA-98 induced by alumina-column fractions of the SRC-II distillate cuts. The Ames test response for the fractions is compared with tumor incidence in the I/P skin-painting assay. For definition of abbreviations, see Figure 5.

cuts and distillate bottoms was a poor indicator of mouse skin tumorigenesis in the I/P assays.

## FURTHER COMPARISON OF AMES VS CHO

The strongest CHO mutagens were found in the PAH-rich LC fractions LC 1 and 2. The azaarene-rich fraction, LC 3, was also active in the CHO assay (Figure 12). By comparison, the CHO assay responded weakly to the APAH-rich fraction, LC 4. The activity of LC 1 and 2 was comparatively weak in the standard Ames test. LC 3 showed increasing Ames test activity, and LC

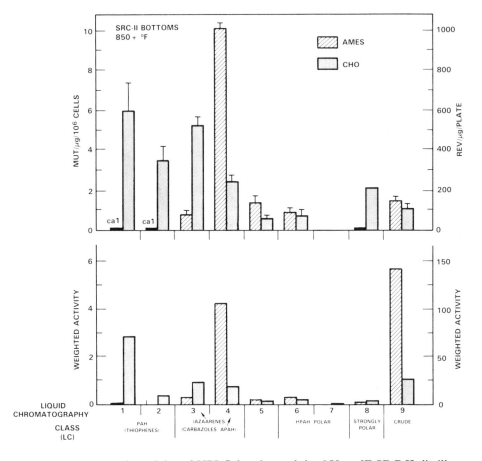

**Figure 12.**   Mutagenic activity of HPLC fractions of the 850 + °F SRC-II distillate bottoms. The top panel indicates specific mutagenic activity. The bottom panel indicates mutagenicity of the LC fractions weighed for composition, that is, expressed as amount of unfractionated, crude distillate cut/mg.

4 was strongly mutagenic in the Ames test, accounting for more than 90% of the total response for all the LC fractions.

Concentrations for selected compounds in LC 1 and 4 fractions are shown in Table III. LC 1 and 2 fractions appeared to contain relatively high concentrations of PAH but were virtually devoid of NPAC. LC 3 contained azaarenes, trace levels of APAH, and carbazoles but was essentially free of PAH. LC 4 appeared to contain essentially only APAH and carbazoles.

If the responses of the Ames and CHO assay to these LC fractions are compared to the main chemical species that are present (Table III), it can be seen that nearly all CHO activity was associated with PAH- or azaarene-rich fractions, while nearly all Ames response was induced by the APAH-rich LC 4. It was determined that LC 4 also contained carbazoles at concentrations much higher than those for the amines. As shown by the dose-response data for this fraction (Figure 4), nearly all Ames mutagenic activity in LC 4 was lost after treatment with nitrous acid. Such losses of activity are diagnostic for APAH.[43,46,47] Since the four- and five-ring APAH were the only PAA present in any significant concentration in LC 4, it is

**Table III.**   Concentration ($\mu$g/g) of Selected Neutral PAH and NPAC in LC Cuts 1 through 4 of the 850 + °F SRC-II Distillate Bottoms

| Compound | LC 1 | LC 2 | LC 3 | LC 4 |
|---|---|---|---|---|
| Azabenzo[*ghi*]perylenes/ azaananthrenes | 2,929 | 10,699 | 2,396 | t[b] |
| Pyrene | 385 | 253 | ND[a] | ND |
| Benzo[*a*]anthracene | 308 | 120 | ND | ND |
| Dimethylbenzanthracene (isomers) | 394 | 269 | ND | ND |
| Benzo[*a*]pyrene | 3,037 | 3,861 | ND | ND |
| Benzo[*ghi*]perylene/ananthrene | 2,929 | 10,688 | ND | ND |
| Azachrysenes/azabenzanthracene | ND | ND | 1,039 | t |
| Azabenzopyrenes/azabenzofluoranthenes | ND | ND | 4,431 | t |
| Azabenzo[*ghi*]perylenes/ azaananthrenes | ND | ND | 2,396 | t |
| Aminopyrene/aminofluoranthenes | ND | ND | t | 25 |
| Aminochrysene/aminobenzoanthracene | ND | ND | t | 53 |
| Aminobenzopyrenes/aminoperylenes | ND | ND | t | 32 |
| Benzocarbazoles | ND | ND | 257 | t |

[a]ND = Not detectable.
[b]t = Trace amounts (<1 ppm).

likely that these compounds were the determinant Ames test mutagens in the 850 + °F SRC-II distillate cut. The other LC fractions (LC 5 through 8) were not particularly active in either the Ames or CHO assays.

The weight-normalized specific mutagenic activity of the LC fractions for the two in vitro assay systems is shown by the bottom panel of Figure 12. Weight-normalized activities (i.e., specific mutagenic activity times the percent weight of a given fraction) give a more accurate picture of the total contribution of a chemical fraction to the genetic activity of the crude material. As can be seen, only the PAH- and azaarene-rich fractions of the 850 + °F SRC-II distillates contributed significantly to the genetic activity of the crude in the CHO assay. The APAH-rich fraction LC 4 appeared to determine nearly all of the genetic activity of the crude 850 + °F SRC-II distillate in the Ames assay with *S. typhimurium* TA-98.

## Determinant Mutagens and Carcinogens in Coal-Derived Synfuels

For clarity we will define a determinant mutagen (or carcinogen) as a compound or type of compound that is quantitatively the most important source of the response under consideration.

For the PAH or NPAC, determinant mutagens are also determinant carcinogens. In previous sections of this chapter, we have shown that PAH fractions most carcinogenically active in mouse skin were also most mutagenically active in the *S. typhimurium* (Ames) and CHO bioassays. These PAH fractions contained comparatively high concentrations of four- and five-ring PAH, that is, 5-methylchrysene, 7,12-dimethylbenzanthracene, and BaP. Each of these compounds is a strong carcinogen in mouse skin, and each shows activity in the mammalian and in vitro mutagenesis assays. The fact that mutagenic response for these PAH fractions in *S. typhimurium* and the mammalian CHO assays was essentially proportional to carcinogenic response measured in terms of initiation suggests that the same compounds are being measured in all three assay systems.

The total concentration of mutagenicity of these known carcinogenic compounds was not related to either mutagenic or carcinogenic activity for their fractions. For example, the PAH fraction from the 800–850°F distillate cut contained higher concentrations of the mutagenically and carcinogenically active four-ring PAH than did the PAH fraction from the 850 + °F distillate cut. Both fractions contained approximately equal concentrations of BaP. Thus, on the basis of known mutagens/carcinogens, the PAH fraction from the 800–850°F distillate should have been more active than its 850 + °F counterpart. However, the PAH fraction from the 850 + °F distillate was several times more mutagenically and tumorigenically active than the 800–850°F distillate. These observations suggest that the expression of both carcinogenicity and mutagenicity in these PAH fractions is strongly dependent on overall composition.

The NPAC fractions were composed of several major subfractions, making it impossible to determine which fraction was responsible for tumorigenesis in the I/P assay. Previous work with a number of coal liquids demonstrated that the APAH component of the NPAC determined virtually all of the mutagenic response in the Ames test with *S. typhimurium*.[42-47] One method used to show this took advantage of the reactivity of APAH with nitrous acid that results in the chemical conversion of the aromatic amine to a phenol or diazonium salt, with subsequent loss of mutagenic activity.[48] The strength of this method is that it can be applied to complex mixtures.[43,46,47] The reaction of polycyclics with nitrous acid can also form direct-acting mutagens such as nitrosamines and oxidation products of PAH.[46,47]

A loss in carcinogenic activity after treatment of NPAC with nitrous acid would be expected if APAH determine the tumorigenicity of the total NPAC from the 850+°F SRC-II distillate cut. As shown in Figure 13, NPAC from the 850°F distillate cut were essentially abolished by nitrous acid at 120 d after initiation; at longer times, the reduction in carcinogenic response in the I/P system was 60 to 80%. It is not clear whether the carcinogenic potency after nitrous acid treatment of the NPAC was due to by-products formed by nitrous acid or to the other compounds originally present in the NPAC (mainly azaarenes and carbazoles of four- and five-ring aromatics). However, the decrease in the potential for the initiation of carcinogenesis in mouse skin after nitrous acid treatment is strong evidence that APAH

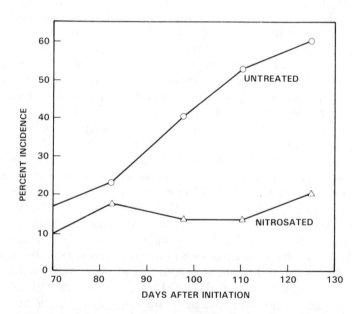

**Figure 13.** Effect of nitrous acid treatment on the tumorigenicity of total NPAC from the 850+°F SRC-II distillate cut.

are quantitatively more important than other subclasses in the 850+°F NPAC as initiators of mouse skin tumorigenesis.

Although APAH in this distillate cut may be important as initiators, it is not clear that these compounds show the same level of activity as chronic carcinogens in mouse skin. As shown in Figure 14, nitrous acid did not reduce the carcinogenic potency of a complex basic tar fraction from the SRC-II HD, bp 550–850 + °F, in chronic skin-painting tests, although nitrous acid treatment of similar basic tar fractions essentially eliminated its mutagenicity in the standard Ames test with *Salmonella typhimurium* TA-98. Thus, a treatment resulting in the chemical destruction of the APAH in the tars did not lead to a loss in their potency in the chronic carcinogenesis skin-painting tests. However, these data are subject to the following reservation. The basic tar fraction contained fairly high concentrations of PAH, including BaP. Thus, the contribution of the aromatic amines to the carcinogenic response may have been overshadowed by that of the PAH. The direct mutagens formed as by-products from the nitrous acid may have been carcinogens. These might include oxidation products of PAH[46,47] or nitrosamines formed from carbazoles, which are major components of the NPAC from the HD.

## SUMMARY

The in vitro genotoxicity and in vivo carcinogenesis and tumorigenesis assay results were in close qualitative agreement for the crude, high-nitrogen synfuels (i.e., the SRC distillate cuts and Paraho shale oil). Particularly important was the observation that all tests indicated 700°F as approximately the temperature boundary between genetically and carcinogenically active and inactive constituents in the coal liquids. In vitro and in vivo test results were not in total qualitative agreement for the chemical fractions bioassayed. For example, all of the alumina-column chemical fracitons from the 800 + °F SRC-II distillate cuts showed some genetic activity in one or more of the in vitro bioassays. However, only the PAH and NPAC chemical fractions induced a tumorigenic response in mouse skin. (None of these fractions were tested as carcinogens in the chronic mouse skin-painting tests.)

The mutagenic activity of the aliphatic fraction in the CHO forward mutation assay may have been due to low concentrations of contaminating PAH. But the contaminating PAH were also present in the aliphatic fractions assayed for tumorigenic activity and failed to elicit tumor formation by 120 d into the assay. However, weak response was observed 185 d after exposure. A possible explanation for this inconsistency is that the CHO assay is much more sensitive to complex PAH fractions than mouse skin in the I/P assay system. Unfortunately, there are no direct data on this point; however, the CHO assay showed many times the sensitivity of the Ames test to the complex PAH fractions from the coal liquids, suggesting that this

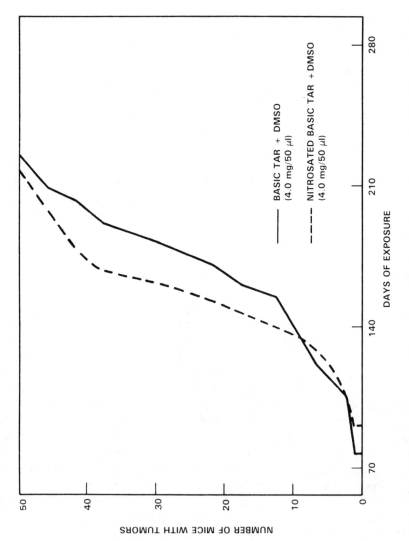

**Figure 14.** Effect of nitrous acid treatment on the carcinogenic potency of basic tar from the SRC-II HD, bp 550–850°F.

mammalian bioassay may possess very high sensitivity for mutagens in complex PAH mixtures compared to the microbial bioassay system.

It is noteworthy that the HPAH chemical fraction of the 850 + °F SRC-II distillate bottoms was mutagenic in the standard Ames assay with *S. typhimurium* TA-98 but very weakly tumorigenic in the I/P assay. This observation is somewhat surprising in view of the exceptional tumorigenicity of various diol epoxides (e.g., BaP)[49] which would be expected as metabolites from HPAH. Moreover, the powerful mouse-skin tumor initiator and complete carcinogen, BaP, and the HPAH (e.g., hydroxy BaP) probably have similar routes of metabolic activation. Preliminary results with the CHO forward mutation assay suggest that HPAH fractions from the SRC-II liquids are strong mutagens in this mammalian bioassay. It is not clear at this time why HPAH failed to elicit a strong response in mouse skin in the I/P assay. Cellular toxicity or inhibition of activating enzyme systems in mouse skin are possible explanations for the apparent weak tumorigenicity of the HPAH fraction. Future studies on the comparative carcinogenicity and tumorigenicity of HPAH versus PAH components of high-boiling coal liquids appear to be called for.

The qualitative correlations between in vivo and in vitro test results on the synfuel materials and the Wilmington crude petroleum can be summarized as follows:

1.  Good agreements were obtained for the synfuel (high-nitrogen) materials but not for Wilmington crude petroleum. Only the SHE mammalian transformation assay results agreed with the mouse skin-painting test results.
2.  Good agreement was obtained for all of the in vitro and in vivo assays in identifying the temperature boundary for biological activity in the SRC-I and -II distillates.
3.  Qualitative agreement was good between initiation activity in mouse skin and mutagenesis induced from chemical fractions of SRC-II liquids. Moreover, there were no "false negative" results; that is, fractions capable of inducing a carcinogenic response in mouse skin were all screened as positive by one or more in vitro tests.
4.  The standard Ames assay system with *S. typhimurium* TA-98 appeared to be reliable for the qualitative assessment of the coal liquids for potentially carcinogenic compounds.

## QUANTITATIVE RELATIONSHIPS

### Crude Oil Fractions

The quantitative relationships between the in vitro and in vivo test results for the synfuels are less clearcut than the qualitative ones just discussed.

There appeared to be a fairly strong quantitative relationship between mammalian in vitro response (mutagenic or transforming activity) to the synfuels and carcinogenic and tumorigenic activity in mouse skin. The high-nitrogen fuels, that is, SRC-I and -II distillate cuts, SRC-I PS and SRC-II HD, and the crude Paraho shale oil, were all ranked in the same order using in vitro mammalian mutagenic and transforming activities or in vivo carcinogenic or tumorigenic activity in mouse skin. On the other hand, the activity of Wilmington crude petroleum in the in vitro bioassays appeared to be a poor indicator of tumorigenic and carcinogenic activity in mouse skin. However, the comparative data base for this and other natural petroleums is much less extensive than for the synfuels. Comparisons of in vitro genetic and in vivo carcinogenic activities for other natural petroleums would be valuable in determining if the results observed for Wilmington crude are generally applicable.

For the crude SRC-II HD, SRC-I PS, and the SRC-II distillate cuts, the mutagenic response of *S. typhimurium* TA-98 in the standard Ames assay was also a good indicator of carcinogenic and tumorigenic response in mouse skin. However, quantitative or semiquantitative relationships between in vitro mutagenic response for *S. typhimurium* TA-98 and tumorigenic response in mouse skin failed to hold true for SRC-I distillate cuts.

In particular, the most tumorigenic of the SRC-I distillate cuts (800–850 + °F) showed much less mutagenicity against *S. typhimurium* TA-98 than the much less tumorigenic 700–750°F and 750–800°F SRC-I distillate cuts. The mutagenicity of crude Paraho shale oil was also much lower than expected, based on its tumorigenic and carcinogenic potency in mouse skin. Moreover, crude Paraho shale oil showed approximately the same carcinogenic potency as SRC-I PS but only about one-tenth as much mutagenic potency against *S. typhimurium* TA-98 of the SRC-I distillate.

### Chemical Types

The fairly strong relationship between mammalian in vitro test results for the synfuels and those observed from in vivo rodent skin-painting tests probably has a straightforward chemical explanation, namely, that carcinogenesis in mouse skin and genetic response in the SHE and CHO bioassays are highly sensitive to PAH components in the synfuels. This was particularly evident in the study showing that the CHO mutagenesis bioassay system was highly responsive to mutagens in the PAH fractions from the high-boiling SRC-II distillates that induced a comparatively weak response in the Ames test. There is no sufficiently large data base for the CHO assay or for other mammalian bioassays to assess the generality of these particular CHO results with the 850+°F SRC-II distillate cut to other synfuel materials. However, studies with pure compounds have provided evidence for a strong quantitative relationship between mammalian-cell mutagenesis and carcinogenesis,[50] suggesting that mutagenic activity in mammalian in vitro systems may be a fairly good general quantitative predictor of carcinogenesis in mouse skin.

The exquisite sensitivity of *S. typhimurium* TA-98 to APAH is well documented[43,45,47,51] and is probably the source of most of the mutagenic response generated in the standard Ames assay by the coal liquids. *S. typhimurium* TA-98 appears to be the most sensitive of the *S. typhimurium* tester strains to mutagens in the coal liquids,[6,13] although *S. typhimurium* TA-100 also responds strongly to mutagens in these materials.[6,13]

Relatively high APAH concentrations in the most carcinogenically and tumorigenically active of the SRC-II liquids (HD and distillate cuts) probably accounted for most of the high mutagenic activity of these materials against *S. typhimurium* TA-98 in the standard Ames test. Thus, for the crudes, the strong quantitative relationship between carcinogenic and tumorigenic activity and mutagenic potency in the standard Ames bioassay with *S. typhimurium* TA-98 was probably coincidental, since PAH are the main determinants of carcinogenicity and APAH are the main determinants of microbial mutagenicity. For example, mutagenically active APAH, especially those of four- and five-rings, are relatively abundant in SRC-II liquids that also contain fairly high levels of the more genetically and carcinogenically active PAH (e.g., four- and five-ring aromatics). The main sources of APAH in the SRC-I distillate cuts (and thus mutagenic activity in the Ames assay with *S. typhimurium* TA-98) were compounds of three-ring aromatics which were concentrated in cuts of low carcinogenic and tumorigenic potency. Very small concentrations of four- and five-ring APAH in the more carcinogenic (tumorigenic) 800 + °F SRC-I distillate cuts were observed. In spite of intrinsic differences in the sensitivity of the various in vitro bioassays to mutagens in the PAH chemical class fractions from the coal liquids, a case can be made that the Ames assay, the CHO assay, and the I/P assay were all responding to the same chemical agents in the individual PAH fractions from the SRC-II distillate. Where comparative measurements were made, the tumorigenic and mutagenic potency appeared to increase proportionately for these chemical-class fractions, with mutagenic potency reaching the highest level in the most carcinogenic of the PAH fractions. In the more active of these PAH fractions, the relative concentrations of known mutagenic/carcinogenic PAH were high. In particular, the concentrations of five-ring PAH, such as BaP, were highest in the most carcinogenic and mutagenic PAH fractions from the SRC-II distillate cuts and distillate bottoms.

The mutagenic activity for the SRC-II NPAC fractions was not closely related to the tumorigenic potency of these materials in mouse skin. For example, the highest specific mutagenic activity in the Ames test was obtained with the NPAC fractions from the 750–800°F and 800–850 + °F distillate cuts, while the NPAC fractions from the 850 + °F distillate bottoms were more active as dermal carcinogens in the mouse. Mutagenic potency of

NPAC fractions in the CHO assay system also appeared to be a poor quantitative indicator of tumorigenic potency in mouse skin.

For SRC-II distillates and distillate bottoms, the NPAC was the only major chemical class other than PAH to show tumorigenic activity. For 800 + °F SRC distillates, APAH, although a minor component of the NPAC, appear to be responsible for most of the tumor-initiating activity. This suggests that PAA, in the chemical milieu of the coal liquids and in particular in APAH or four- or five-ring aromatics, may possess exceptionally high tumor-initiating specific activity in mouse skin.

However, the available data are not sufficient to evaluate these types of compounds as complete carcinogens. As a class, aromatic amines are considered bladder or liver carcinogens rather than skin carcinogens. Most of the large-ring APAH (e.g., four-, five-, and greater-than-five-rings) that are concentrated in the most carcinogenically active NPAC from the SRC-II distillate cuts have not been well studied as dermal carcinogens. In the coal liquids, the possibility of interactions between initiators of carcinogenesis, such as APAH, and promoters of carcinogenesis, such as various carbazoles and PAH, is a virtually unexplored area of research.

## ACKNOWLEDGMENT

This work was supported by the U.S. Department of Energy under Contract No. DE-AC06-76RLO-1830.

## REFERENCES

1. Pelroy, R.A., and M.R. Petersen."Mutagenic Characterization of Synthetic Fuel Materials by the Ames/*Salmonella* Assay System," *Mutat. Res.* 90:309–320 (1981).
2. Pelroy, R.A., D.S. Sklarew, and S.P. Downey. "Comparison of the Mutagenicities of Fossil Fuels," *Mutat. Res.* 90:233–245 (1981).
3. Toste, A.P., D.S. Sklarew, and R.A. Pelroy. "Partition Chromatography/High-Performance Liquid Chromatography Facilitates the Organic Analysis and Biotesting of Synfuels," *J. Chromatogr.* 249:267–282 (1982).
4. Toste, A.P., D.S. Sklarew, and R.A. Pelroy. "Comparison of Chemical and Mutagenic Properties of a Coal Liquid and a Shale Oil," in *Coal Conversion and the Environment,* D.D. Mahlum, R.H. Gray, and W.D. Felix, Eds. (Springfield, VA: Technical Information Center, U.S. Department of Commerce, Symposium Series 54, 1981), pp. 96–114.
5. Rubin, I.B., M.R. Guerin, A.A. Hardigree, and J.L. Epler. "Fractionation of Synthetic Crude Oils from Coal for Biological Testing," *Environ. Res.* 12:358–365 (1976).
6. Epler, J., et al. "Analytical and Biological Analysis of Test Materials from the Synthetic Fuel Technologies. I. Mutagenicity of Crude Oils Determined

by the *Salmonella typhimurium*/Microsomal Activation System," *Mutat. Res.* 57:265–276 (1978).

7.  Jones, A.R., M.R. Guerin, and B.R. Clark. "Preparative-Scale Liquid Chromatographic Fractionation of Crude Oils Derived from Coal and Shale," *Anal. Chem.* 49:1766–1771 (1977).

8.  Epler, J.L., B.R. Clark, C.-H. Ho, M.R. Guerin, and T.K. Rao. "Short-Term Bioassay of Complex Organic Mixtures: Part II, Mutagenicity Testing," in *Application of Short-Term Bioassays in the Fractionation and Analysis of Complex Environmental Mixtures,* M.D. Waters, S. Nesnow, J.L. Huisingh, S.S. Sandhu, and L. Claxton, Eds. (New York: Plenum Press, 1978), pp. 269–289.

9.  Clark, B.R., C.-H. Ho, and A.R. Jones. "Chemical Class Fractionation of Fossil-Derived Materials for Biological Testing," in *Analytical Chemistry of Liquid Fuel Sources,* P.C. Uden, S. Siggia, and H.B. Jensen, Eds. (Washington, DC: American Chemical Society, 1978), pp. 282–294.

10.  Guerin, M.R., I.B. Rubin, T.K. Rao, B.R. Clark, and J.L. Epler. "Distribution of Mutagenic Activity in Petroleum and Petroleum Substitutes," *Fuel* 60:282–288 (1981).

11.  Stamoudis, V.C., S. Bowrne, D.A. Haugen, M.J. Peak, C.A. Reilly, J.R. Stetter, and K. Wilzbach. "Chemical and Biological Characterization of High-BTU Coal Gasification (The Hygas Process). I. Chemical Characterization of Mutagenic Fractions," in *Coal Conversion and the Environment,* D.D. Mahlum, R.H. Gray, and W.D. Felix, Eds. (Springfield, VA: Technical Information Center, U.S. Department of Commerce; *Symp. Ser.* 54, 1981), pp. 67–95.

12.  Schoeny, R., D. Warshawsky, L. Hollingsworth, M. Hand, and G. Moore. "Mutagenicity of Products from Coal Gasification and Liquefaction in the *Salmonella*/Microsome Assay," *Environ. Mutagenesis* 3:181–198 (1981).

13.  Pelroy, R.A., and M.R. Petersen. "Use of Ames Test in Evaluation of Shale Oil Fractions," *Environ. Health Perspect.* 30:191–203 (1979).

14.  Hsie, A.W., P.A. Brimer, J.P. O'Neill, J.L. Epler, M.R. Guerin, and M.H. Hsie. "Mutagenicity of Alkaline Constituents of Coal-Liquified Crude Oil in Mammalian Cells," *Mutat. Res.* 78:79–84 (1980).

15.  Frazier, M.E. "Mutagenic and Carcinogenic Activity of a Hydrotreated Coal Liquid," *J. Toxicol. Environ. Health* (in press).

16.  Frazier, M.E. "Transformation of Syrian Hamster Ovary Cells by Synfuel Mixtures," *J. Toxicol. Environ. Health* (in press).

17.  Holland, J.M., D.A. Wolf, and B.R. Clark. "Relative Potency Estimation for Synthetic Petroleum Skin Carcinogens," *Environ. Health Perspect.* 33:149–155 (1981).

18.  Calkins, W.H., J.F. Deye, R.W. Hartgrove, C.F. King, and D.F. Krahn. "Synthetic Crude Oils from Coal: Mutagenicity and Tumor-Initiation Screening Tests," in *Coal Conversion and the Environment,* D.D. Mahlum, R.H. Gray, and W.D. Felix, Eds. (Springfield, VA: Technical Information Center, U.S. Department of Commerce; *Symp. Ser.* 54, 1981), pp. 462–470.

19.  Coombs, M.M., C. Dixon, and A. Kissonerghis. "Evaluation of the Mutagenicity of Compounds of Known Carcinogenicity, Belonging to the Benz[*a*]anthracene, Chrysene, and Cyclopenta[a]phenanthrene Series, Using Ames's Test," *Cancer Res.* 36:4525–4529 (1976).

20.  Lijinski, W. "Carcinogenic and Mutagenic N-Nitroso Compounds," in *Chem-*

*ical Mutagens,* Vol. 4, A. Hollaender, Ed. (New York: Plenum Press, 1976), pp. 193–217.

21. Lijinski, W., and A.W. Andrews. "The Mutagenicity of Notrosamides in *Salmonella typhimurium,*" *Mutat. Res.* 68:1–8 (1979).

22. Rinkus, S., and M. Legator. "Chemical Characterization of 465 Known or Suspected Carcinogens and Their Correlation with Mutagenic Activity in the *Salmonella typhimurium* System," *Cancer Res.* 39:3289–3318 (1979).

23. Langenbach, R., et al. "Mutagenic Activities of Oxidized Derivatives of N-Nitrosodipropylamine in the Liver Cell-Mediated and *Salmonella typhimurium* Assays," *Cancer Res.* 40:3463–3467 (1980).

24. Parodi, S., S. DeFlora, M. Cavanna, A. Pino, L. Robbiano, C. Bennicelli, and G. Brambilla. "DNA-Damaging Activity In Vivo and Bacterial Mutagenicity of Sixteen Hydrazine Derivatives as Related Quantitatively to Their Carcinogenicity," *Cancer Res.* 41:1469–1482 (1981).

25. Parodi, S., M. Taningher, P. Boero, and L. Santi. "Quantitative Correlations Amongst Alkaline DNA Fragmentation, DNA Covalent Binding, Mutagenicity in the Ames Test and Carcinogenicity for 21 Compounds," *Mutat. Res.* 98:1–24 (1982).

26. Weisburger, J., and G. Williams. "Carcinogen Testing: Current Problems and New Approaches," *Science* 214:401–407 (1981).

27. Schiller, J. "Nitrogen Compounds in Coal-Derived Liquids," *Anal. Chem.* 49:2292–2294 (1977).

28. Schweighardt, F., C. White, S. Friedman, and J. Schultz. "Heteroatomic Species in Coal Liquefaction Products," *ACS Symp.* 71:240–257 (1978).

29. Paudler, W., and M. Chaplen. "Nitrogen Bases in Solvent-Refined Coal," *Fuel* 58:775–778 (1979).

30. Schultz, R., J. Jorganson, M. Maskarinec, M. Novotny, and L. Todd. "Characterization of Polynuclear Aromatic and Aliphatic Fractions of Solvent-Refined Coal by Glass Capillary Gas Chromatography/Mass Spectrometry," *Fuel* 58:783–789 (1979).

31. Ho, C.-H., C.Y. Ma, B.R. Clark, M.R. Guerin, T.K. Rao, and J.L. Epler. "Separation of Neutral Nitrogen Compounds from Synthetic Crude Oils for Biological Testing," *Environ. Res.* 22:412–422 (1980).

32. Wilson, B.W., R.A. Pelroy, and J.T. Cresto. "Identification of Primary Aromatic Amines in Mutagenically Active Subfractions from Coal Liquefaction Materials," *Mutat. Res.* 79:193–202 (1980).

33. Ho, C.-H., B.R. Clark, M.R. Guerin, B.D. Barkenbus, T.K. Rao, and J.L. Epler. "Analytical and Biological Analyses of Test Materials from the Synthetic Fuel Technologies. IV. Studies of Chemical Structure-Mutagenic Activity Relationships of Aromatic Nitrogen Compounds Relevant to Synfuels," *Mutat. Res.* 85:335–345 (1981).

34. Karchar, W., A. Nelson, R. Depaus, J. vanEijk, P. Claude, and J. Jacob. "New Results in Detection, Identification and Mutagenic Testing of Heterocyclic Polycyclic Aromatic Hydrocarbons," in *Proceedings of the Fifth International Symposium on Polycyclic Aromatic Hydrocarbons,* W. Cook and A. Dennis, Eds. (Columbus, OH: Battelle Press, 1981), pp. 59–73.

35. Later, D.W., M.L. Lee, K.D. Bartle, R.C. Kong, and D.L. Vassilaros. "Chemical Class Separation and Characterization of Organic Compounds in Synthetic Fuels," *Anal. Chem.* 53:1612–1620 (1981).

36. Pelroy, R.A., and B.W. Wilson. "Relative Concentrations of Polyaromatic Primary Amines and Azaarenes in Mutagenically Active Nitrogen Fractions from a Coal Liquid," *Mutat. Res.* 90:321–335 (1981).

37. Haugen, D.A., M.J. Peak, K.M. Suhrbler, and V.C. Stamoudis. "Isolation of Mutagenic Aromatic Amines from a Coal Conversion Oil by Cation Exchange Chromatography," *Anal. Chem.* 54:32–37 (1982).

38. Kosuge, T., H. Zenda, H. Nukaya, A. Terada, T. Okamoto, K. Shudo, K. Yamaguchi, Y. Iitaka, T. Sugimura, M. Nagao, K. Wakabayashi, A. Kosuagi, and H. Saito. "Isolation and Structural Determination of Mutagenic Substances in Coal Tar," *Chem. Pharmacol. Bull.* 30:1535–1538 (1982).

39. Later, D.W., M.L. Lee, R.A. Pelroy, and B.W. Wilson. "Identification and Mutagenicity of Nitrogen-Containing Polycyclic Aromatic Compounds in Synthetic Fuels," in *Polynuclear Aromatic Hydrocarbons: Physical and Biological Chemistry*, M. Cooke, A.J. Dennis, and G.L. Fisher, Eds. (Columbus, OH: Battelle Press, 1982), pp. 427–438.

40. Later, D.W., M.L. Lee, and B.W. Wilson. "Selective Detection of Amino Polycyclic Aromatic Compounds in Solvent Refined Coal," *Anal. Chem.* 54:117–123 (1982).

41. Pelroy, R.A., D.L. Stewart, Y. Tominaga, M. Iwao, R.N. Castle, and M.L. Lee. "Microbial Mutagenicity of Three- and Four-Ring Polycyclic Aromatic Sulfur Heterocycles," *Mutat. Res.* (in press).

42. Rao, T., et al. "Analytical and Biological Analyses of Test Materials From the Synthetic Fuel Technologies. II. Extended Genetic and Biochemical Studies with Mutagenic Fractions," *Mutat. Res.* 54:185–191 (1978).

43. Pelroy, R.A., and D.L. Stewart. "The Effects of Nitrous Acid on the Mutagenicity of Two Coal Liquids and Their Genetically Active Chemical Fractions," *Mutat. Res.* 90:297–308 (1981).

44. Guerin, M.R., C.-H. Ho, T.K. Rao, B.R. Clark, and J.L. Epler. "Polycyclic Aromatic Amines as Determinant Chemical Mutagens in Petroleum Substitutes," *Environ. Res.* 23:42–53 (1980).

45. Pelroy, R., and A. Gandolfi. "Use of a Mixed Function Amine Oxidase for Metabolic Activation in the Ames/*Salmonella* Assay System," *Mutat. Res.* 72:329–334 (1980).

46. Haugen, D.A., M.J. Peak, and C.A. Reilly, Jr. "Chemical and Biological Characterization of High-BTU Coal Gasification (The Hygas Process). II. Nitrous Acid Treatment for Detection of Mutagenic Fractions of Mutagenic Primary Aromatic Amines: Nonspecific Reactions," in *Coal Conversion and the Environment*, D.D. Mahlum, R.H. Gray, and W.D. Felix, Eds. (Springfield, VA: Technical Information Center, U.S. Department of Commerce; *Symp. Ser.* 54, 1981), pp. 115–127.

47. Haugen, D.A., M.J. Peak, and C.A. Reilly, Jr. "Use of Nitrous Acid-Dependent Decrease in Mutagenicity as an Indicator of Mutagenic Primary Aromatic Amines: Nonspecific Reactions with Phenols and Benzo[a]pyrene," *Mutat. Res.* 82:59–67 (1981).

48. Yoshida, D., and T. Matsumoto, "Changes in Mutagenicity of Protein Pyrolysates by Reaction with Nitrite," *Mutat. Res.* 58:35–40 (1978).

49. Buening, M.K., P.G. Wislocki, W. Levin, H. Yabi, D.R. Thakker, H. Akagi, M. Koreeda, D.M. Jerina, and A.H. Conney. "Tumorigenicity of the Optical Enantiomers of the Diastereomeric Benzo[a]pyrene 7,8-diol-9,10-epoxides in

Newborn Mice: Exceptional Activity of (+)-7β,8α-dihydroxy-9α,10α-epoxy-7,8,9,10-tetrahydrobenzo[a]pyrene," *Proc. Nat. Acad. Sci. USA* 75:5358–5361 (1978).

50. Clive, D., et al. "Validation and Characterization of the L5178Y/TK + /Mouse Lymphoma Mutagen Assay System," *Mutat. Res.* 59:61–108 (1979).

51. McCann, J., E. Choi, E. Yamasaki, and B. Ames. "Detection of Carcinogens as Mutagens in the *Salmonella*/Microsome Test: Assay of 300 Chemicals," *Proc. Nat. Acad. Sci. USA* 72:5139–5144 (1975).

# CHAPTER 13

## Personnel Monitoring with Cytogenetic and Other Short-Term Bioassays

### M.S. Legator and J.B. Ward, Jr.

*Department of Preventive Medicine and Community Health*
*Division of Environmental Toxicology*
*University of Texas Medical Branch*
*24 Keiller Bldg., F-19*
*Galveston, TX 77550*

## THE PROBLEM

In the regulation of toxic agents, only in recent years (since the establishment of the National Institute for Occupational Safety and Health, the Occupational Safety and Health Administration, and the passing of the Toxic Substance Control Act) have industrial chemicals come under systematic regulatory surveillance. It is an inescapable fact that the hundreds of thousands of chemicals in the workplace have not been evaluated, or evaluated in sufficient depth in mammalian systems, to determine chronic hazards of these materials, specifically the potential to induce cancer or adverse genetic effects. The exact number of hazardous chemicals found in the American workplace is unknown. There may be as many as 55,000 different chemicals in commerce. In 1980, an estimated 8.9 million workers in the manufacturing sector were exposed to hazardous chemicals; moreover, the hazard of working with chemicals is compounded by the likelihood of exposure to more than one chemical which may result in synergistic effects.[1] If one considers only cancer risk associated with occupations and assumes that the annual number of cancer deaths attributed to occupation is $10 \pm 5\%$ (a highly conservative estimate), this would translate to 20,000 to 60,000 avoidable cancer deaths per year.[2] It is anticipated that in the future new chemicals will be tested by relevant assays to preclude the introduction of hazardous elements into the workplace. The almost overwhelming problem facing those of us concerned with chronic toxic effects of industrial chemicals is how to detect hazardous chemicals already present in the industrial environment.

We may consider well-designed classical epidemiological studies as the primary tool for identifying hazardous chemicals in the workplace. The advantages of human epidemiology studies are that

1. the data are directly relevant to man;
2. well-conducted studies with statistically significant positive results are the strongest possible evidence of carcinogenic or mutagenic activity in man;
3. they supply the most reliable data for risk assessment;
4. they are most readily accepted by the public and institutions responsible for control.

However, the weaknesses of human epidemiology studies in detecting chronic effects are numerous, and the following factors must be realized:

1. Difficulties in identifying suitable study populations include adequate size, unreliability of death and birth medical records, and lack of good incidence data.
2. The latency period in onset of effects complicates data collection and prevents detection of effects of new exposures, while assessment of current risks is based on much earlier exposures.
3. There is a lack of sensitivity in that the normal incidence of specific diseases can obscure increased rates, and multiple exposures confound attempts to establish cause-effect relationships. It is difficult to detect effects of ubiquitous exposure, and large populations are required to detect carcinogenic and other common effects.
4. There can be substantial population exposure to an agent prior to detection (carcinogen detection by body count) resulting in a dilution of exposed population and a failure to consider power (error) of study.

The frustrations of epidemiological studies as related to reproductive hazards can be perceived from the introduction to a study by Erickson[3] where the following statement appears.

> If we are lucky we may catch some real associations, but most are likely to get away. Further, because of the small numbers involved, this sort of exploration can do virtually nothing to help us in pronouncing an occupation or industry "safe" for reproducing humans. On the other hand, utmost caution in the interpretation of those associations which do appear is in order. Due to the large number of comparisons made, many associations might be expected to result from chance alone. Our approach is less than ideal but does represent a start in a rather barren field.

The acknowledgment of the present and projected limitations of epidemiological studies to detect chemical carcinogens-mutagens by industry can be further perceived from a recent survey conducted by Karstadt and Bobal.[4] Manufacturers of 75 known International Agency for Research on Cancer (IARC) animal carcinogens were asked about the status of epidemiological studies with these chemicals. Of the 75 chemicals, epidemiological data were available for only 8, and studies with 5 other chemicals were reported in progress. With 62 of the 75 chemicals, no epidemiological data were available, nor do the manufacturers contemplate future studies. Of the 75 IARC animal carcinogens, 18 were reported to have volumes greater than $10^6$ lb, and epidemiological data were not available or anticipated for 10 of these 18 high-volume chemicals.

If sufficient animal testing has not been carried out with existing industrial chemicals and epidemiological studies cannot be considered a primary tool for detecting hazardous chemicals, is there a practical approach to this problem? We believe there is. At the present time, a series of noninvasive short-term procedures are available for monitoring high-risk populations, and these procedures should detect in relevant human studies carcinogenic-mutagenic agents. This chapter will describe these procedures and present their advantages and disadvantages.

## RATIONALE FOR SHORT-TERM TESTS
## FOR HUMAN MONITORING

Although fixed heritable mutations occur with a low frequency ($10^{-5}$ to $10^{-6}$ per cell generation) and are technically difficult to demonstrate, even in intact animals, other manifestations of damage to the genetic apparatus occur at much higher frequencies following exposure to genetically toxic agents. The types of damage observed at high frequency may include chromosome damage, physical damage to DNA such as strand breaks or crosslinks, induced abnormalities in sperm morphology and number, and the excretion of mutagenic substances that can be detected by using in vitro mutagenicity tests to analyze urine samples. These endpoints can be evaluated in specimens of human blood, semen, or urine. A growing number of studies have been conducted in human populations exposed to mutagenic agents in which parameters such as chromosome damage or sperm morphology were evaluated and abnormalities were observed. For example, the International Agency for Research on Cancer has categorized 18 chemicals as carcinogenic for humans, 18 as probably carcinogenic for humans, and an additional 18 as suspected but with insufficient data for classification.[5] Among these compounds, four in the first group, arsenic,[6,7] benzene,[8,9] bis (chloromethyl) ether and chloromethyl methyl ether,[10] and vinyl chloride,[11,12] have been tested for their ability to produce chromosome damage in man and found positive. Similarly, 3/3 compounds tested in the second category, cyclophosphamide,[13] epichlorohydrin,[14,15] and thiotepa,[16] have been checked and shown to cause chromosome damage in man.

In the third category, 4/4 compounds tested, chloroprene,[17,18] ethylene oxide,[19] lead,[20,21] and styrene,[22] caused chromosome damage in man. The limited data available suggest that human cytogenetic analysis is an accurate measure to detect exposure to carcinogens.

It must be clearly understood that these types of changes are not adverse health outcomes in themselves. Rather, these are observable changes which we know from controlled animal studies, supported by the limited human data available, to be produced by agents capable of inducing heritable mutations and the diseases which are their sequelae. The presence of increased levels of these types of changes is an indicator of the presence of a process in which exposure of an individual to a mutagenic agent may produce widespread genetic damage, the bulk of which is resolved through repair processes or cell death. Only a small residual of the initial damage results in fixed mutations or other alterations which contribute to the process of neoplasia. Abnormalities such as chromosome aberrations are, in fact, by-products of the initial interaction of mutagenic agents with cellular DNA.

The development of a strategy for human monitoring for exposure to genetically hazardous substances is based on the use of laboratory tests to detect genetic damage. To be useful in detecting environmental hazards, the tests must be used as endpoints in studies based on the design principles of epidemiology. This approach possesses the immediacy and quantitative properties of laboratory methods while preserving the relevance to human health of epidemiological studies.

Several important conditions must be considered in study design. First, results must be interpreted on a group rather than an individual basis. Individual responses to the same exposure can differ substantially for intrinsic biological reasons such as metabolic characteristics and variations in DNA repair or replication processes. In addition, human exposures to specific agents are not isolated events but are components of complex environments that can differ markedly between individuals. Factors such as nutritional status, lifestyle, health status, and use of medications can influence responses.

To make meaningful associations between observed genetic damage and a specific agent or environmental influence, groups must be carefully identified that have a common exposure experience. Whenever possible, environmental measurements should be made to determine both the identity and concentrations of agents in the study environment. Confounding environmental factors and interindividual variations must be controlled by the selection and simultaneous evaluation of a control population matched for as many variables, other than the exposure of interest, as possible. Individual variations over time can be controlled by sampling the exposed and control populations more than once.

Mutagenic agents differ in pharmacokinetic properties and mechanisms of interaction with DNA. As a result, they may differ in tissue specificity and in the types of observable genetic damage produced. In designing a test battery for human genetic monitoring, the characteristics of the principal agent must be considered. As many tissues and endpoints as possible should be examined, but tests inappropriate for the type of exposure should not be included. For example, radiations do not produce metabolites, so tests for excreted mutagens or adduct formation would be inappropriate. Because heritable effects are among the serious possible consequences of mutagen exposure, evaluation of germinal cells should be included whenever possible.

Human genetic monitoring could be particularly appropriate in situations involving complex environmental mixtures. In these circumstances, the reconstruction of environmental conditions in laboratory tests may be difficult or impossible. Furthermore, the effects in man of interactions between agents may not be reproducible in animal or in vitro systems. Only by examining human populations exposed to the specific environment can the presence of a genetic risk be documented.

## AVAILABLE TESTS THAT CAN BE APPLIED TO MAN

### Cytogenetic Test

Since the early 1960s, cytogenetic analysis in animals and humans has played a central role in most programs designed to detect mutagenic agents. Most identified mutagenic or carcinogenic agents can be detected by cytogenetic analysis, as previously discussed. Although the association remains unresolved, numerous observations implicating the relationship between instability in the structure and number of chromosomes and carcinogenesis have been discussed in detail and can be summarized as follows:

1.    Marker chromosomes, which are derived from normal chromosomes through breakage and rearrangement, can be identified in some clones of cancer cells. In fact, the consistency of marker chromosomes in cancer cells of a given host provides one of the main bodies of evidence supporting a clonal origin of cancer. While most marker chromosomes are unique to that one clone of cancer cells, at least two human cancers consistently have the same chromosome abnormality: the Philadelphia chromosome in as many as 90% of the cases of chronic granulocytic leukemia, and an extra band on the long arm of chromosome 14-in. cells from Burkitt's tumors and in cell lines derived from these tumors.

2.    In general, progression from simple chromosomal anomalies to more complex ones is associated with increasing malignancy of a cancer.

3.    Aneuploidy is a common finding in cancer cells. By comparison, certain aneuploid states in man have higher incidences of certain cancers: leukemia in Down's syndrome, breast cancer in Klinefelter's syn-

drome, cancers of neural crest origin in Turner's syndrome, and go-nadoblastoma in the dysgenetic gonad having a Y-chromosome cell line. Furthermore, in vitro irradiation with x-rays induces a greater frequency of chromosomal aberrations in lymphocytes cultured from individuals with Down's syndrome as well as other trisomic (but not monosomic) disorders than in cells cultured from normal diploid donors.

4.  *De novo* chromosomal aberrations are observed in lymphocytes cul-tured from individuals at increased risk of developing cancer because of their inheritance of certain genetic diseases: ataxia telangiectasia, Bloom's syndrome, and Fanconi's anemia. Lymphocytes cultured from these afflicted individuals also show a heightened radiosensitivity as measured by an increased frequency of x-ray-induced chromosomal aberrations. Similarly, fibroblasts cultured from individuals to develop skin cancer are sensitive to the cell-killing and chromosome-breaking effects of uv irradiation and some chemical agents.

5.  *De novo* chromosomal aberrations are observed in cells cultured from individuals at increased risk of developing cancer because of their ex-posure to ionizing radiation and certain chemical carcinogens (e.g., benzene, cyclophosphamide, and vinyl chloride).

Of course, many of these observations can have different interpreta-tions. For example, marker chromosomes and worsening karyotype could be features that are just temporally but not causally associated with cancer induction, or they may, indeed, contribute causally to the progression of a cancer that was initiated by some other preceding event(s). Patients with aneuploidy and rare genes for chromosome instability suffer from many afflictions, including immunological disorders, which could also account for their predisposition to cancer development. However, the argument that some known human carcinogens cause chromosome damage is not as easily rebuked. All carcinogens that have been thoroughly tested have been found to induce some kind of chromosomal rearrangement.[23]

Our current understanding of the neoplastic process indicates that chromosomal rearrangement is a step in the neoplastic process. Current information indicates that carcinogens can act to induce chromosomal rear-rangements by inducing or exposing sites on DNA for recombination or by inducing or activating cellular systems resulting in stimulation of recombi-nation. Chromosomal rearrangement may affect carcinogenesis by altering gene expression, perhaps by allowing the activation of cellular cancer genes.[24] Estimates of the lifespan of human lymphocytes vary widely but are on the order of at least a few years.[25-28] The observation of unstable aberrations in mitogen-stimulated lymphocytes years after radiation exposure[29] suggests that certain types of genetic damage can persist for long periods in non-replicating cells. Because the lymphocyte is long-lived and tolerant of some types of genetic damage, when not proliferating, it is a very suitable target cell in which to look for cumulative damage resulting from long periods of exposure. The techniques for culturing lymphocytes and analyzing for chromosome aberrations are now well established.[30]

From available information and theoretical considerations, the detection of chromosome abnormalities in man induced by chemical exposure indicates that the chemical is in all likelihood a human carcinogen-mutagen, and lymphocytes are suitable cells for analysis.

The development of the BudR/Hoecsht 33258 staining technique for visualizing sister chromatids[31] has facilitated the development of assays for induced DNA damage resulting in sister chromatid exchanges (SCEs). The refinement of the technique using Giemsa staining eliminates the need for observation by fluorescence microscopy and simplifies scoring. A variety of chemical mutagens have been shown to induce SCEs in several types of mammalian cells including human lymphocytes.[32] Several studies of SCEs in human lymphocytes from individuals with environmental exposures to mutagens have been reported.[33-37] An analysis of factors influencing baseline variation has been recently reported.[38]

### Hemoglobin Alkylation

Most mutagenic and carcinogenic chemicals are electrophilic agents or are converted to electrophilic agents in vivo. Alkylating agents react with nucleophilic centers in DNA (guanine-N-7, guanine-0-6, adenine-N-3, etc.) but also react with nucleophilic centers in proteins such as cysteine-S and -N-1 or -N-3 of the imidazole ring of histidine. Ehrenberg and his colleagues[39] have developed techniques and principles for the determination of the degree of alkylation of specific nucleophilic sites in macromolecules and calculation of the tissue-specific dose of an agent in an exposed animal. Techniques using radiolabeled compounds have been used in animals to determine the degree of alkylation of amino acids of hemoglobin in erythrocytes. The dose (time integral of concentration of free agent) in the erythrocyte can be calculated from the degree of alkylation.[40,41] By comparing agents of varying stabilities, it has been possible to estimate the relationships between the dose in the erythrocytes and other tissues including the gonads.[40,42] More recently, nonisotopic techniques have been developed for measuring the degree of hemoglobin alkylation in man.[43] A major value of hemoglobin alkylation as a monitor of human exposure is that the time integral exposure to an agent over a period equal to the life-length of the erythrocyte (four months in man) can be measured.[40,42] In addition, the technique is relatively insensitive to confounding influences of incidental exposures or biological effects not related to the exposure of primary interest. This is because the endpoint measured is the formation of a specific adduct of the target amino acid. Consequently, the determination of hemoglobin alkylation can be a powerful technique for evaluating chronic occupational exposures to specific chemicals.

## Sperm Analysis

A semen sample is an important source of information in any evaluation of the mutagenic impact of a human exposure. Sperm in a semen specimen is the one germinal cell type available in large number and without the use of any invasive procedures. Several different observations can be made on sperm that may reveal the impact of mutagenic activity on their development. The detection of events related to mutation in sperm has direct implications for the reproductive status of the individual and for the transmission of genetic damage to his offspring.

Over the last few years, two assays have been developed which detect abnormalities in human sperm that have been associated with exposure to mutagenic agents.

One procedure detects Y chromosome nondisjunction in sperm.[44] It is based on the observation in quinacrine-banded human chromosomes that the Y chromosome absorbs a substantial amount of dye.[45] In quinacrine HCl-stained human sperm, the Y chromosome is sufficiently bright to be observed through the cell membrane.[46] In good preparations, about 40 to 50% of the sperm heads are observed to contain a Y fluorescent (YF) body as expected on genetic grounds. Sperm containing two fluorescent bodies (YFF) have been observed in about 0.7% of sperm from donors with no known chemical exposures. Furthermore, frequencies of YFF in unexposed individuals are usually quite stable over time.[47] The presence of two YF bodies indicates the occurrence of nondisjunction of the Y chromosome in meiotic anaphase II. The fact that YFF sperm survive and are sometimes capable of fertilization is shown by the existence of XYY individuals (one per-thousand male births). Exposures to several known mutagenic agents including adiramycin, x-irradiation, and the nematocide dibromochloropropane (DBCP) have produced increases in YFF frequency. DBCP, which produced aspermia and oligospermia in exposed males, was shown to produce a mean YFF frequency of 3.8% (range 2.0 to 5.3%) in 18 exposed individuals as compared to a frequency of 1.2% (range 0.8 to 1.8%) in a matched control group.

The second assay detects agents that increase the frequency of sperm with abnormal morphologies.[48] The normal human sperm head shape is distinctive, and changes are easily recognized. In mice, several lines of evidence indicate that sperm-head shaping is under rigorous genetic control. Studies of strains with different head shapes and hybrids among them indicate that about 10 genetic regions on the X and Y chromosomes as well as autosomes control sperm morphology. In addition, sperm head abnormalities are induced in mice by x-rays and several clinical mutagens. Spermatocytes and late spermatogonia are the most sensitive cell types. The $f_1$ generation of treated males also has increased rates of abnormality, suggesting that induced abnormalities are heritable. Sperm abnormalities do not correlate with the presence of chromosome abnormalities such as translocations, indicating that point mutations may be responsible for the occurrences.[49,50]

## Urine Analysis

The analysis of urine for excreted mutagens using various microbial indicator organisms is a widely used technique.[51,52] Numerous studies in humans have also evaluated the urinary excretion of mutagens following exposures to various drugs.[53-55] The appearance of mutagens in urine usually occurs rapidly following exposure to mutagens, and the technique is sensitive provided an indicator organism is chosen that is responsive to the agent to be monitored.[56] Body fluid analysis is a simple and rapid process appropriate for general screening purposes. It can be used to screen for continued or repeated exposures or to evaluate the magnitude of isolated acute exposures.

Although urine has been the most frequently studied body fluid, there may be distinct advantages to evaluating blood. The presence of active chemicals in the circulatory system may be more important than detecting mutagens in an excretory product such as urine.

## DNA Filter Elution

The technique of alkaline elution of DNA from filters was developed originally by Kohn et al.[57] for examining size distribution of strands during DNA replication. It has subsequently been modified by several groups[58,59] and adapted to detection of chemical and radiation damage to DNA. Alkaline filter elution relies on the fact that alkaline denaturing and unwinding of double-stranded DNA and the release of single strands occurs at a rate inversely proportional to single-strand size.[57] In practice, then, DNA from mutagen-damaged cells is eluted through a plycinyl chloride filter under alkaline conditions over a period of many hours. The total eluate of 20–25 mL is collected in 1-mL fractions; the DNA distribution over these fractions compared with control is indicative of the occurrence of a degree of DNA damage resulting in single-stranded breaks.

Alkaline elution has been used successfully to detect carcinogens in whole-animal studies.[59,60] Swenberg et al.[61] have shown that results of such studies in mammalian cells treated with various noncarcinogens, procarcinogens, and direct-acting carcinogens correlate well with the in vivo activity of those compounds. Parodi et al.[59] recently adapted the alkaline elution technique for use with the method of Kissane and Robins[62] for microfluorometric quantitation of extremely small amounts of DNA. The nature of the alkaline elution technique suggests that, from the same sample, it may also be possible to determine the degree of DNA interstrand linkage and

DNA-protein linkage caused by a test agent.[63] Because the alkaline elution technique can now be employed with mammalian cells whose DNA has not been labeled by incorporation of isotopic precursors, the technique appears to be ideally suited to the monitoring of human populations for exposure to genetically active agents.

### Point Mutation in Human Lymphocytes

A promising but new and relatively untried technique determines the frequency of 6-thioguanine-(6-TG-) resistant lymphocytes in peripheral blood.[64] The resistance to 6-thioguanine presumably occurs because of the inactivation of the gene for hypoxanthine-guanine phosphoribosyl transferase (HGPRT) through mutation. The technique for identifying 6-TG-resistant cells has been developed using reconstruction experiments with lymphocytes from Lesch-Nyhan Syndrome patients who are genetically deficient in HGPRT as a result of mutation of the X-chromosome-linked gene. The frequency of 6-TG-resistant cells has been shown to increase in patients on cytotoxic cancer chemotherapy drugs, x-rays, or psoriatic patients treated with 8-methoxypsoral in an ultraviolet light.[64,65] Early studies were plagued with excessively high frequencies of 6-TG-resistant cells in both normal and exposed individuals, suggesting that phenocopies were being observed; however, this technical problem appears to be better controlled in more recent work.[66] The remaining problem with the technique is the direct confirmation that 6-TG-resistant cells are genuine HGPRT-deficient mutants. This is the most promising currently available technique for development into a somatic mutation assay in man.

### RATIONALE FOR COORDINATED TESTING IN MAN AND ANIMALS

By using several of the methods described above, a battery of tests can be developed for the investigation of human exposures to mutagenic environments. Careful test selection would allow the efficient observation of several types of genetic endpoints. Both somatic and germinal cells could be observed, and genetic damage at the chromosome level and at the molecular level could be detected. The sensitivity and interpretability of the human test battery could be further strengthened in many instances by coordinating specific studies in animals with human monitoring.

Unless the chemical nature of the human environment is well described and the principal agents have been previously well studied, it might not be possible to predict which tests are most appropriate for detecting exposure. Preliminary studies of individual agents or environmental samples in animals could greatly improve the selection of tests for human monitoring. Even when the major environmental agents have been identified, human monitoring alone might not identify the component most responsible for mutagenic activity. Animal or in vitro studies could be used to evaluate the activities of individual agents. One of the primary reasons for conducting animal tests in coordination with human monitoring is to establish the dose response for specific endpoints in the animal. The magnitude of effects in human subjects could be related to responses in animals in order to estimate the exposure level when it could not be determined accurately by environmental measurements. In addition, comparison of human and animal effects might provide an indication of degree of risk posed by the human exposure.

For some tests that must be modified to detect the effects of specific agents, animal or in vitro studies might be necessary to establish methods and conditions for conducting human studies. For example, urine testing for the presence of mutagens might require the use of extraction or concentration procedures. Animal or in vivo studies might be needed to optimize or validate these procedures and facilitate the identification of active metabolites. Hemoglobin alkylation monitoring in man requires that a specific adduct be identified and that techniques for its isolation and measurement be established. Preliminary studies in vitro in animals are necessary to accomplish these objectives.

## CRITIQUE AND CONCLUSIONS

One of the most promising areas in the field of genetic toxicology is the use of a series of noninvasive tests to detect hazardous chemicals directly in humans. These procedures form a bridge between animal studies and the classical epidemiological approach.

The ultimate objective of genetic monitoring is to protect individuals from disease. The ideal approach for accomplishing this goal would be to continuously monitor high-risk populations by suitable techniques so corrective measures could be taken soon after a positive response is detected. Currently, however, those studies that have been carried out using short-term procedures were initiated only after the presence of mutagenic-carcinogenic chemical or processes was already suspected. These studies were usually carried out after prolonged exposure had occurred. The use of these tests on a routine basis in a high-risk population should offer the optimum approach to worker protection.

In interpreting results from these tests, several points should be kept in mind. Interindividual and temporal variation as well as confounding environmental factors make interpretation on an individual basis unjustifiable.

These tests are advanced warning procedures which indicate that the individuals are exposed to hazardous substances. The distinct advantage of this monitoring approach is that remedial action can be taken to prevent the final disease outcome. A positive finding, in all likelihood, signifies an early stage in a multistage process, a process that we would like to abort. These techniques should be considered as analogous to a *group* film badge capable of providing an early indication that a particular environment contains a genetically hazardous agent.

Confounding factors including seasonal variation, age, sex, smoking, viral infection, and various medications have been listed as factors that may invalidate the results. The so-called confounding factors, however, are present in many human studies and are not a problem specifically associated with these procedures. Proper experimental design should take into account these factors and neutralize the problems associated with these possible sources of error.

Individual variation may also be a source of error. It should be borne in mind that there is considerable variation in the way individuals metabolize different chemicals, and this variation will be reflected in all human studies measuring a chemically induced response. Table I illustrates differences in individual response to antipyrine half-life and clearance to cytochrome P-450, and benzo(*a*)pyrene binding.[67] Chemical studies will reflect these inherent individual variabilities. Suitable experimental techniques where appropriate numbers of subjects are included should compensate for expected individual variability.

The sensitivities of the various tests of human exposures to mutagens are not well established. In fact, enlarging the base line data bases for these assays and evaluating sensitivities are major objectives of investigations in this area. We do know that some tests such as cytogenetics have been successfully used in several circumstances to detect human exposure to carcinogens. A statistical analysis by Whorton et al. indicates that a 1% increase in chromosome aberration rate over a background rate of 2% could be detected with 80% certainty at an error rate (p value) of 5% in a population

**Table I.**   Variability in Human Studies

| Experimental Systems | Individuals (No.) | Parameter Measured | Variability (Fold) |
|---|---|---|---|
| Unselected patients | 200 | Antipyrine half-life | 25 |
|  |  | Antipyrine clearance | 41 |
| Liver biopsies | 200 | Cytochrome P-450 | 65 |
| Liver biopsies | 27 | Aryl hydroxylase | 30 |
| Bronchus explants | 37 | Benzo(*a*)pyrene binding | 75 |
| Bladder explants | 16 | Benzo(*a*)pyrene binding | 34 |
| Colon explants | 15 | Benzo(*a*)pyrene binding | 31 |
| Esophageal explants | 15 | Benzo(*a*)pyrene binding | 31 |

Modified from Pelkonen, O., E.O. Sotaniemi, and N. T. Karki, "Interindividual Variation in Sensitivity to Mutagens," in *Mutagens in Our Environment*, M. Sorsa and H. Vairo, Eds. (New York: Alan R. Liss, Inc., 1982), pp. 61–74.

of less than 50 exposed and 50 control individuals.[68] The sperm morphology and YFF tests need additional work for validation in man and to define more thoroughly the relationship between observed effect and genetic damage.

Validation may be required for some of the techniques in the battery; other procedures, however, should be viewed as suitable for use. Validation of assays (i.e., an assay as an acceptable means of testing compounds in industrial populations) as opposed to a research technique poses a difficult problem. In a report from the United Kingdom Environmental Mutagen Society,[69] one guide to mutagenicity testing, validation of assays is discussed. It is suggested that the decision as to when a technique is sufficiently validated for routine application depends to a great extent on the nature of the assay, the purpose for which it will be used, and the interpretation placed on the word "validation." If one wishes to validate an in vitro test as indicating a chemical that induces genetic damage in an animal, one would test by an in vitro system a series of chemicals known to be either active or inactive in animals. A positive genetic response in animals would need no further validation to indicate a chemical that induces genetic damage. If a chemical causes chromosome damage in man, then the compound is a human clastogen, and further testing would be superfluous. We have already established that the assay is valid for indicating chromosome damage in the target species, namely man. Given the number of human carcinogens that cause chromosome aberrations and the theoretical basis linking chromosome aberration to cancer, it is logical to conclude that a positive response indicates an exposure to a carcinogenic-mutagenic agent. The other procedures in the battery of tests that can be used for human monitoring should be viewed in a similiar manner.

Although there may be procedural problems that would restrict the use of these procedures for monitoring industrial populations, certainly there is no compelling scientific reasons for not proceeding to monitor high-risk populations. These noninvasive tests are short-term, comparatively inexpensive, and allow remedial action to be taken shortly after exposure. The results obtained with these procedures to date are indeed impressive.

## REFERENCES

1. "The Role of Genetic Testing in the Prevention of Occupational Illness" (Washington, DC: Congress of the United States, Office of Technology Assessment) (in press).
2. Infante, P., R. Hurwitz and P. Marlow, Occupational Safety and Health Administration, personal communications.
3. Erickson, D. "Contribution to Epidemiology in Biostatistic: Prenatal Occupation in Birth Defects Report," *Environ. Mutagens* 1:107–117 (1979).
4. Karstadt, M., and R. Bobal. "Availability of Epidemiological Data on Humans Exposed to Animal Carcinogens," *Teratog. Carcinog. Mutag.* 2:151–167 (1982).

5.  International Agency for Research on Cancer. IARC Monographs on the Evaluation of the Carcinogenic Risk of Chemicals to Humans. *Environ. Res.* 19:131–156 (1979).
6.  Beckman, G., L. Beckman, I. Nordenson, and S. Nordstrom. "Chromosomal Aberrations in Workers Exposed to Arsenic," in *Genetic Damage Caused by Environmental Agents.* (New York: Academic Press, 1979), pp. 205–211.
7.  Nordenson, I., G. Beckman, L. Beckman, and S. Nordstrom. "Occupational and Environmental Risks in and Around Smelter in Northern Sweden, II. Chromosomal Aberrations in Workers Exposed to Arsenic," *Hereditas* 88:47–50 (1978).
8.  Tough, I.M., P.G. Smith, W.M. Court-Brown, and D.G. Hardner. "Chromosome Studies on Workers Exposed to Atmospheric Benzene: The Possible Influence of Age," *Eur. J. Cancer* 6:49 (1970).
9.  Picciano, D.J. "Cytogenetic Study of Workers Exposed to Benzene," *Environ. Res.* 19:33–38 (1979).
10. Zundova, Z., and K. Landa. "Genetic Risk of Occupational Exposures to Haloethers," *Mutation Res.* 46:242–243 (1977).
11. Funes-Cravioto, F., B. Lambert, J. Lindsten, L. Ehrenberg, A.T. Natarajan, and S. Osterman-Golkar. "Chromosome Aberrations in Workers Exposed to Vinyl Chloride," *Lancet* 1:459 (1975).
12. Ducatman, A.K., K. Hirschhorn, and I.V. Selikoff. "Vinyl Chloride Exposure and Human Chromosome Aberrations," *Mutation Res.* 31:163–168 (1975).
13. Etteldorf, J.N., C.D. West, J.A. Pitchock, and D.L. Williams. "Gonadal Function Testicular History and Meiosis Following Cyclophosphamide Therapy in Patients with Nephrotic Syndrome," *J. Pediat.* 88:206–212 (1976).
14. Kucerova, M., V.S. Zhurkor, L. Polivkova, and J.E. Ivanove. "Mutagenic Effect of Epichlorohydrin, II. Analysis of Chromosomal Aberrations in Lymphocytes of Persons Occupationally Exposed to Epichlorohydrin," *Mutation Res.* 48:355–360 (1977).
15. Picciano, D.J. "Cytogenetic Investigation of Occupational Exposure to Epichlorohydrin," *Mutation Res.* 66:169–173 (1979).
16. Silezneva, T.G., and N.P. Korman. "Analysis of Chromosomes of Somatic Cells in Patients Treated with Anti-Tumor Drugs," *Sov. Genet.* 9:1575–1579 (1973).
17. Katosova, L.D. "Cytogenetic Analysis of Peripheral Blood of Workers Engaged in the Production of Chloroprene," *Gigiera. fuda i professional nye Zabolevaniia.* 10:30–32 (1973).
18. Sanotskii, I.V. "Aspects of the Toxicity of Chloroprene: Immediate and Long-Term Effects," *Environ. Health Persp.* 17:85–93 (1976).
19. Garry, V.F., J. Hozier, D. Jacobs, R.L. Wade, and D.G. Gray. "Ethylene Oxide: Evidence of Human Chromosomal Effects," *Environ. Mutagen.* 1:375–382 (1979).
20. Forni, A., and G.C. Secci. "Chromosome Changes in Preclinical and Clinical Lead Poisoning Correlation with Biochemical Findings," *Proceedings of the International Symposium Environmental Health Aspects of Lead,* Amsterdam, Oct. 2–6, 1972.
21. Garza-Chapa, R., C.H. Leal-Garza, and G. Molina-Ballestros. "Analysis Eromosomico en Personas Professionalmente Expuestas a Contaminancion con Plomo," *Arch. Invest. Mexicol* (Mexico) 8:11–20 (1977).

22. Meretoja, T., H. Vainio, M. Sorse, and H. Harkonen. "Occupational Styrene Exposure and Chromosomal Aberrations," *Mutation Res.* 56:193–197 (1977).
23. Legator, M.S., and S.J. Rinkus. "Mutagenicity Testing: Problems in Application," in *Short-Term Tests For Chemical Carcinogens,* H.F. Stich and R.H.C. Sav, Eds. (Springer, Verlag: 1981), pp. 483–504.
24. Radman, M., P. Jeggo, and R. Wagner. "Chromosomal Rearrangement and Carcinogenesis," *Mutation Res.* 98:249–264 (1982).
25. Norman, A., M.S. Sasaki, and R.E. Ohoman. "Elimination of Chromosome Aberrations from Human Lymphocytes," *Blood* 27:706–714 (1966).
26. Buckton, K.E., P.G. Smith, and W.M. Court-Brown. "Estimation of Lifespan from Studies on Males Treated with X-Rays for Ankylosing Spondylitis," in *Human Cytogenetics,* H.J. Evans, W. Court-Brown, and A.S. McLean, Eds. (Amsterdam: North Holland, 1967), pp. 106–114.
27. Dolphin, G.W., D.C. Lloyd, and R.J. Purrot. "Chromosome Aberration Analysis as a Dosimetric Technique in Radiological Protection," *Health Phys.* 25:7–15 (1973).
28. Nowell, P.C. "Unstable Chromosome Changes in Tuberculin-Stimulated Leukocyte Cultures from Irradiated Patients. Evidence for Immunologically Committed, Long-Lived Lymphocytes in Human Blood," *Blood* 26:798–804 (1965).
29. Bloom, A.D., S. Neriishi, N. Kamada, T. Iseki, and R.J. Hehha. "Cytogenetic Investigation of Survivors of the Atomic Bombings of Hiroshima and Nagasaki," *Lancet* ii:672–674 (1966).
30. Evans, H.J., and M.L. O'Riordan. "Human Peripheral Blood Lymphocytes for the Analysis of Chromosome Aberrations in Mutagens Tests," in *Handbook of Mutagenicity Test Procedures,* B.J. Kilby, M.S. Legator, W. Nichols, and C. Ramel, Eds. (Amsterdam, New York: Elsevier Scientific Publishing, 1977), pp. 261–274.
31. Latt, S.A. "Localization of Sister Chromatid Exchanges in Human Chromosomes," *Science* 185:74–76 (1974).
32. Latt, S.A., J.W. Allen, W.E. Rogers, and L.A. Jeurgens. *"In Vitro* and *In Vivo* Analysis of Sister Chromatid Exchange Formation," *Handbook of Mutagenicity Test Procedures,* B.J. Kilbey, M.S. Legator, W. Nichols, and C. Ramel, Eds. (Amsterdam, New York: Elsevier Scientific Publishing, 1977), pp. 275–291.
33. Raposa, T. "Sister Chromatid Exchange Studies for Monitoring DNA Damage and Repair Capacity after Cytostatics In Vitro and in Lymphocytes of Leukemic Patients under Cytostatic Therapy," *Mutation Res.* 57:241–251 (1978).
34. Crossen, P.E., W.F. Morgan, J.J. Horan, and J. Stewart. "Cytogenetic Studies of Pesticide and Herbicide Sprayers," *New Zealand Med. J.* 88:192 (1978).
35. Nevstad, N.P. "Sister Chromatid Exchanges and Chromosomal Aberrations Induced in Human Lymphocytes by the Cytostatic Drug Adriamycin *In Vivo* and *In Vitro,*" *Mutation Res.* 57:253–258 (1978).
36. Lambert, B., U. Ringborg, E. Harper, and A. Lindblad. "Sister Chromatid Exchanges in Lymphocyte Cultures of Patients Receiving Chemotherapy for Malignant Disorders," *Cancer Treatment Reports* 62:1413 (1978).
37. Musilova, J., K. Michalova, and J. Urban. "Sister Chromatid Exchanges and Chromosomal Breakage in Patients Treated with Cytostatics," *Mutation Res.* 67:289 (1979).
38. Carrano, A.V., J.L. Minkler, D.G. Stetka, and D.H. Morre. "II. Variation

in the Baseline Sister Chromatid Exchange Frequency in Human Lymphocytes," *Environ. Mutagenesis* 2:325–337 (1980).

39.  Ehrenberg, L., and S. Osterman-Golkar. "Alkylation of Macromolecules for Detecting Mutagenic Agents," *Teratog. Carcinog. Mutag.* 1:105–127 (1980).

40.  Osterman-Golkar, S., L. Ehrenberg, D. Segerback, and I. Hallstrom. "Evaluation of Genetic Risks of Alkylating Agents II. Hemoglobin as a Dose Monitor," *Mutation Res.* 34:1–10 (1976).

41.  Osterman-Golkar, S., D. Hultmark, D. Segerback., C.J. Calleman, R. Goethe, L. Ehrenberg, and C.A. Wachtmeiser. "Alkylation of DNA and Proteins in Mice Exposed to Vinyl Chloride," *Biochem. Biophys. Res. Commun.* 76:259–266 (1977).

42.  Segerback, D., C.J. Calleman, L. Ehrenberg, G. Lofroth, and S. Osterman-Golkar. "Evaluation of Genetic Risks of Alkylating Agents IV. Quantitative Determination of Alkylated Amino Acids in Hemoglobin as a Measure of the Dose After Treatment of Mice with Methyl Methanesulfonate," *Mutation Res.* 49:71–82 (1978).

43.  Calleman, C.J., L. Ehrenberg, B. Jansson, S. Osterman-Golkar, D. Segerback, K. Svennson, and C.A. Wachtmeister. "Monitoring and Risk Assessment by Means of Alkyl Groups in Hemoglobin in Persons Occupationally Exposed to Ethylene Oxide," *J. Environ. Pathol. Toxicol.* 2:427–442 (1979).

44.  Kapp, R.W., Jr., and C.B. Jacobson. "Analysis of Spermatozoa for Y Chromosome Nondisjunction," *Teratog. Carcinog. Mutag.* 1:193–212 (1980).

45.  Zeck, L. "Investigation of Metaphase Chromosomes with DNA Binding Fluorochromes," *Exp. Cell Res.* 58:463 (1969).

46.  Barlow, P., and D.G. Vosa. "The Y Chromosome in Human Spermatozoa," *Nature* (Condon) 226:961–962 (1970).

47.  Kapp, R.W., Jr., D.J. Picciano, and C.B. Jacobson. "Y Chromosomal Nondisjunction in Dibromochloropropane Exposed Workmen," *Mutation Res.* 64:47–51 (1979).

48.  Wyrobek, A.J., and W.R. Bruce. "The Induction of Spermshape Abnormalities in Mice and Humans," in *Chemical Mutagens Principles and Methods for Their Detection*, Vol. 5., A. Hollaender and F.J. deSerres, Eds. (New York: Plenum Press, 1978), pp. 257–285.

49.  Wyrobek, A.J. "Changes in Mammalian Sperm Morphology After X-Ray and Chemical Exposures," *Genetics* 92:104–119 (1979).

50.  Gabridge, D.A., A. Denuzio, and M.S. Legator. "Microbial Mutagenicity of Streptozotocin in Animal-Mediated Assays," *Nature* 221:68–70 (1969).

51.  Durston, W., and B.N. Ames. "A Simple Method for the Detection of Mutagens in Urine: Studies with the Carcinogen 2-Acetylaminofluorene," *Proc. Natl. Acad. Sci. USA,* 71:737–741 (1974).

52.  Commoner, B.A., A. Vithayathil, and J.L. Henry. "Detection of Metabolic Carcinogen Intermediates in Urine of Carcinogen-Fed Rats by Means of Bacterial Mutagenesis," *Nature* 249:850–852 (1974).

53.  Siebert, D., and A. Simon. "Genetic Activity of Metabolites in the Ascitic Fluid and in the Urine of a Human Patient Treated with Cyclophosphamide: Induction of Mitotic Gene Conversion in Saccharomyces Cerevisiae," *Mutation Res.* 21:257–262 (1973).

54.  Minnich, V., M.E. Smith, D. Thompson, and S. Kornfield. "Detection of

Mutagenic Activity in Human Urine Using Mutant Strains of *Salmonella typhimurium,"* *Cancer* 38:1253–1258 (1976).

55. Legator, M.S., T.J. Conner, and M. Stoeckel. "Detection of Mutagenic Activity of Metronidazole and Niridazole in Body Fluids of Humans and Mice," *Science* 188:1118–1119 (1975).

56. Connor, T.H., M. Stoeckel, J. Evrard, and M.S. Legator. "The Contribution of Metronidazole and Two Metabolites to the Mutagenic Activity Detected in Urine of Treated Humans and Mice," *Cancer Res.* 37:629–633 (1977).

57. Kohn, K.W., L.C. Erickson, R.A.G. Ewig, and C.A. Friedman. "Fractionation of DNA from Mammalian Cells by Alkaline Elution," *Biochem.* 15:4629–4637 (1976).

58. Kohn, K.W., C.A. Friedman, R.A.G. Ewig, and Z. Iqbal. "DNA Chain Growth During Replication of Asynchronous L1210 Cells Alkaline Elution of Large DNA Segments from Cells Lysed on Filters," *Biochem.* 13:4134–4139 (1974).

59. Parodi, S., M. Taningher, L. Santi, M. Cavanna, L. Sciaba, A. Maura, and G. Brambilla. "A Practical Procedure for Testing DNA Damage *In Vivo,* Proposed for a Prescreening of Chemical Carcinogens," *Mutation Res.* 54:39–46 (1978).

60. Petzold, G.L., and J.A. Swenberg. "Detection of DNA Damage Induced *In Vivo* Following Exposure of Rats to Carcinogens," *Cancer Res.* 38:1589–1594.

61. Swenberg, J.A., G.L. Petzold, and P.R. Harback. "*In Vitro* DNA Damage/Elution Assay for Predicting Carcinogenic Potential," *Biochem. Biophys. Res. Commun.* 72:732–738 (1976).

62. Kissane, J.M., and E. Robins. "The Fluorometric Measurement of Deoxyribonucleic Acid in Animal Tissues with Special Reference to the Central Nervous System," *J. Biol. Chem.* 233:184–188 (1958).

63. Ross, W.E., and N. Shipley. "Relationship Between DNA Damage and Survival in Formaldehyde Treated Mouse Cells," *Mutation Res.* 79:277–283 (1980).

64. Strauss, R., and R.J. Albertini. "Enumeration of 6-Thioguanine Resistant Peripheral Blood Lymphocytes in Man as a Potential Test for Somatic Cell Mutations Arising *In Vivo,*" *Mutation Res.* 61:353–379 (1979).

65. Albertini, R.J. "Drug-Resistant Lymphocytes in Man as Indicators of Somatic Cell Mutation," *Teratog. Carcinog. Mutag.* 1:25–48 (1980).

66. Albertini, R.J., E.F. Allen, A.S. Quinn, and M.R. Albertini. "Human Somatic Cell Mutation: *In Vivo* Variant Lymphocyte Frequencies as Determined by 6-Thioguanine Resistance," in *Birth Defects Institute Symposium XI.* E.B. Hood and I.H. Porter, Eds. (New York: Academic Press, 1980), pp. 235–263.

67. Pelkonen, O., E.O. Sotaniemi, and N.T. Karki. "Interindividual variation in sensitivity to Mutagens," in *Mutagens in Our Environment,* M. Sorsa and H. Vairo, Eds. (New York: Alan R. Liss, Inc., 1982), pp. 61–74.

68. Whorton, E.B., Jr., D.B. Bee, and D.J. Kilian. "Variations in the Proportion of Abnormal Cells and Required Sample Sizes for Human Cytogenetic Studies," *Mutation Res.* 64:79–86 (1979).

69. Dean, B., B. Bridges, D. Kirkland, J. Parry, and N. Taylor. "Framework of Supplementary Testing Procedures," in *The United Kingdom Environmental Mutagen Society.* (United Kingdom Environmental Mutagen Society, 1983), pp. 175–176.

## DISCUSSION

*S.V. Kaye, Oak Ridge National Laboratory:* I wish to take issue with your downplay
of the usefulness of epidemiologic studies. I think you said epidemiology is a
limited approach, if I remember your words, and this is where short-term
procedures come into play. The entire strategy of research in the area that
supports health protection and safety is predicated upon not any single science
or any single test or any single methodology. We start at the atomic level, the
molecular level, the cellular system, testing in terms of screening and mechanistic studies. We work up into animal-level studies and then we follow
this up with studies on human populations. We have to do well-planned studies, either prospective or retrospective studies, to look at how a suspected
agent might affect a human population. These are called epidemiological studies, and I think they are absolutely necessary. They have proven to be extremely valuable, and they are really unsubstitutable. Perhaps you consider
that epidemiology can prove something, unequivocally. I don't think it has
been built up to do that, but it does give inferences. Sometimes, through
biostatistics and different statistical tests, we can learn a great deal about some
of our mistakes of the past. Would you like to comment on that?

*M.S. Legator:* First of all, I indicated that epidemiology is an insensitive tool in the
area of chronic toxicity. Secondly, given the number of chemicals, the resources available, and the cost of the study (see the reference to Karstadt and
Bobal), we cannot rely on classical epidemiology to make an immediate significant contribution to detecting those chemicals in our environment that may
be hazardous. The beta error in many reported epidemiological studies is
usually so high that their major value is to determine the upper limits of
concern rather then to confirm a chemical-induced health hazard. Epidemiology is the obvious confirmatory approach, but there are severe limitations to
its use. These short-term procedures are the most effective tools we now have
for detecting carcinogens and mutagens in high-risk populations.

*R. McKee, Exxon Corporation:* I was unclear about one of the points you were
trying to make. You seemed to say that the major thrust of these programs
would be to look at occupational settings where people were exposed to chemicals that had been introduced without prior testing. But then you talked about
the coal liquefaction industry where the chemicals that will be introduced have
already been tested through programs that have been described at this meeting. Do you see a role for cytogenetic monitoring in a situation where the
biological effects of materials are already fairly well understood?

*M.S. Legator:* Let me say two things to clarify what I meant. The first point I was
trying to make is that with new chemicals being introduced into commerce
the testing is far better than in the past, but we have a definite concern for
the majority of materials that are now in the work place that have not been
extensively tested. The second point has to do with our difficulty in finding
industrial populations to study, for a variety of practical reasons. I suggested
that in new areas of technology such as coal liquefaction, where we don't have
the historical exposure of workers which could lead to problems, we're starting
out afresh. These plants may be the best place to initiate these kinds of studies.
Finally, in response to the third part of your question, one of the valuable
attributes of these methods is that we can determine effects of various chemical

interactions or processes. Thus, my answer to your question is yes, I do think that even with new products there may also be a role for cytogenetic monitoring and I also think that new areas of technology may be the place to start.

*R.H. McKee:* Considering the fact that the active materials have already been fairly well established as polycyclic aromatic hydrocarbons and primary aromatic amines, which are not very potent clastogenic agents and would not tend to show up very well in either cytogenetic or SCE assays, the most likely result you would get from this kind of a test would be a negative result. Perhaps the issue of sensitivity of the test system is one that needs to be addressed before any kind of program of this type is implemented.

*M.S. Legator:* In terms of the issue of sensitivity, I quite agree. It is like any other approach and we could possibly miss active materials. I would suggest though, again with our limited data base, that we have seen the cytogenetic technique detect several chemicals in the industrial setting. Now if we detect activity in the industrial setting, the worker exposure is obviously too high. Yes, we could fail to detect a hazardous chemical, but we have already demonstrated that some of the most important chemicals in the industrial setting have been detected by these procedures. In terms of the chemicals that you allude to that may not be picked up by either SCE or chromosome effects, I think we would have to evaluate them on a chemical-by-chemical basis. I have been rather impressed, even though most of my work has not been in the area of chromosome effects, by how the cytogenetic technique has detected chemicals that do not cause, or at least have not been shown to induce point mutations; an example is benzene.

*P. Buhl, U.S. Department of Energy:* Dr. Hunter Montgomery at Exxon has started a limited cytology program with the Exxon coal liquefaction pilot plant (ECLP) workers in which he had taken about 50 plant workers that were going to work at the ECLP plant and have a cohort study of the ones that were going to stay in the petroleum group. He has been monitoring them quite extensively, including medical surveillance and certain cytology tests. I talked with him recently, and he says that they are having a little problem with the control cohorts in that they have lost interest. The participation of the ECLP workers has been very good. They continue to provide samples, but the petroleum workers are losing interest and don't like the sample routine. Thus, the cohort study may not be as good as originally planned.

*M.S. Legator:* If you have workers that perceive they may have a problem, they are going to cooperate, but finding the control group can be difficult. The one technique that we found to be useful is the "buddy system." After we identify the exposed individual, we ask him if he has a friend, a buddy. The exposed individual will usually identify someone in the same socioeconomic group and also an individual of similar age. We have used this system rather effectively for trying to find a nonexposed individual in case-control studies.

*P. Buhl:* There is another point about the Exxon study. The workers involved at ECLP will return to the main refinery, and the study is supposed to continue for about five more years.

# CHAPTER 14

## Extrapolation to Health Risk: Use of Comparative Approaches

S.C. Morris, J.I. Barancik,
H. Fischer, L.D. Hamilton,
S. Jones, P.D. Moskowitz,
J. Nagy, S. Rabinowitz, and
H.C. Thode, Jr.

*Brookhaven*
*National Laboratory*
*Upton, NY*

This is a preliminary report of work in progress to estimate cancer induction in the general population from an indirect coal liquefaction plant at an eastern U.S. site. Emissions are grouped into risk assessment categories to simplify the task of dealing with many different chemical compounds. Effects are estimated from exposures via air, surface water, and terrestrial and aquatic food chains. Dose-response functions for cancer are extrapolated from animal data by techniques previously used for food and pesticide exposures.

This chapter demonstrates the approach for a single health effect, cancer, and for a single risk assessment category, polycyclic aromatic hydrocarbons.

### Risk Analysis

In a symposium principally directed to chemical and biological research, it is appropriate to discuss briefly what risk analysis is. Risk analysis describes and quantifies risk and the uncertainties associated with health effect estimates, thus providing a rational basis for regulatory action and policy as well as for guiding future research and development efforts. Risk analysis consists basically of four steps:

1. Hazard identification and evaluation.

2. Effects evaluation (e.g., the development of dose-response functions).

3. Exposure evaluation (i.e., estimation of the population exposure). The complexity of the exposure estimate depends on the dose-response function to be used. This may be a single number as in man-rem or, for more complex dose-response functions, disaggregated by population and dose categories.

4. The dose-response function and the exposure estimate are combined to estimate the size or probability of harm.

### Objectives

Risk assessment is best done in stages, first screening to identify important sources of risk to guide later, more detailed analysis. This is a screening-level analysis. It is the first part of a comparison of chemical groupings to identify those groups of most importance to health consequences, specifically cancer in this case.

The principal objective at this point is to demonstrate the method using one chemical group. A second objective is to determine if any one pathway dominates the others. Of course, different pathways may dominate for different chemical groups.

### Risk Assessment Categories

A difficulty in assessing health impacts of emissions from a synthetic fuels plant begins with the seemingly endless list of chemical compounds that can be emitted. An adequate chemical-by-chemical health-risk analysis is precluded due to the number of compounds, the inability to fully characterize their distribution and transformation in the environment, and gaps in toxicological literature. Some method of grouping or indexing these emissions is necessary to come to grips with the task.

In response to this problem, the concept of risk assessment categories (RAC) was developed by Moghissi.[1] Table I lists criteria developed by the U.S. Environmental Protection Agency and Oak Ridge National Laboratory (ORNL) for determining these categories. The current listing of 38 RACs is given in Table II. Toxicological data do not come by RACs, however, but by individual compound. Development of dose-response functions by RAC requires that results from multiple studies of single compounds be combined for several compounds in an RAC. Here, the combination was taken by using the full range of possible results. This assumes the RAC

**Table I.**    Criteria for Determining Risk Assessment Categories (RAC)

| Category | Criteria |
|---|---|
| Engineering relevance | A goal of risk assessment is to provide useful guidance to industry. Therefore, process streams must be characterized in terms of their RAC content so that plant designers and operators can apply the results of the risk assessment. |
| Analysis capability | The categories must correspond to practical chemical characterizations of the products and effluents of interest as revealed by biotesting. RACs that are divided more finely than existing chemical and biological analysis schemes will not be useful. |
| Completeness | All constituents of the industry's products and effluents must be included in the system of RACs. |
| Nonoverlap | The RACs should be mutually exclusive; that is, none of the constituents should be assessed twice. Chemicals with multiple functional groups can be handled by assigning them to the RAC which they follow during chemical fractionation. |
| Data compatibility | The correspondence between the RACs and commonly used chemical classes should be clear enough to allow use of existing data and regulatory standards in the risk assessment. |

exposure to be composed entirely of either the most innocuous or the most potent compound; actual exposure is likely to be somewhere between, although it may lie beyond these bounds due to compounds that are unknown or for which no toxicological data exist.

Results presented are examples for RAC 15, polycyclic aromatic hydrocarbons, a grouping containing a number of known and suspected carcinogens. More than 20 of the RACs include one or more known or suspected carcinogens (Table II).

### Overall Scheme

The present work consists primarily of developing dose-response information and applying it to exposure information to estimate public health effects. The overall study involves quantifying (1) emissions to various media by RAC; (2) environmental transport, dispersion, and population exposure; and (3) health impact. The first two steps are being carried out at ORNL.[2] Only cancer has been examined as a health impact to date. The overall

**Table II.** Risk Assessment Categories (RAC)

| RAC No. | Category |
| --- | --- |
| 1 | Carbon monoxide |
| 2[a] | Sulfur oxides |
| 3 | Nitrogen oxides |
| 4 | Acid gases |
| 5 | Alkaline gases |
| 6[a] | Hydrocarbon gases |
| 7[a] | Formaldehyde |
| 8[a] | Volatile organochlorines |
| 9 | Volatile carboxylic acids |
| 10[a] | Volatile O&S heterocyclics |
| 11[a] | Volatile N heterocyclics |
| 12[a] | Benzene |
| 13[a] | Aliphatic/alicyclic hydrocarbons |
| 14[a] | Mono/diaromatic hydrocarbons (excluding benzene) |
| 15[a] | Polycyclic aromatic hydrocarbons |
| 16 | Aliphatic amines (excluding N-heterocyclics) |
| 17[a] | Aromatic amines (excluding N-heterocyclics) |
| 18[a] | Alkaline nitrogen heterocyclics ("azaarenes") |
| 19[a] | Neutral N, O, S, heterocyclics (excluding "volatiles") |
| 20[a] | Carboxylic acids (excluding "volatiles") |
| 21[a] | Phenols |
| 22 | Aldehydes and ketones ("carbonyls") (excluding formaldehyde) |
| 23[a] | Nonheterocyclic organo sulfur |
| 24[a] | Alcohols |
| 25[a] | Nitroaromatics |
| 26[a] | Esters |
| 27[a] | Amides |
| 28[a] | Nitriles |
| 29[a] | Tars |
| 30[a] | Respirable particles |
| 31[a] | Arsenic |
| 32 | Mercury |
| 33[a] | Nickel |
| 34[a] | Cadmium |
| 35[a] | Lead |
| 36[a] | Other trace elements |
| 37[a] | Radioactive materials |
| 38 | Other remaining materials |

[a]Indicates RAC includes known or suspected carcinogens.

scheme for the study is shown in Figure 1. There is a high degree of uncertainty in such analysis, and consideration of uncertainty is an important aspect of the study. Uncertainties stem from experimental error (or even lack of experimental data), biological variation, high-dose to low-dose ex-

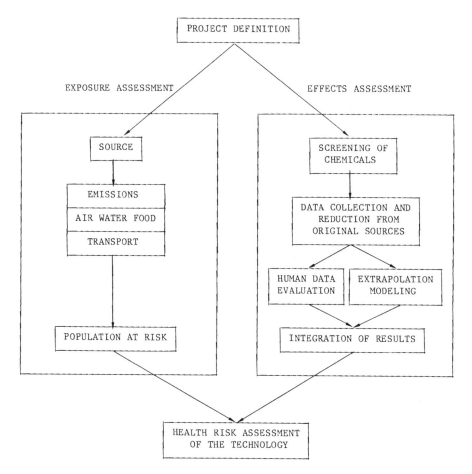

**Figure 1.** Overall scheme of study.

trapolation, animal-to-man extrapolation, and inability to predict the precise nature or magnitude of exposure.

## EXTRAPOLATION METHODS

Ideally, epidemiological data are the best guide for estimation of risk to the public from exposures to chemicals emitted by complex technologies. Use of human data to estimate cancer risks to the public often presents difficulties, however. Most studies are of industrial workers who are not representative of the public at large. Exposures are poorly defined. Moreover, occupational exposures are likely to be to mixtures which may differ from public exposure. Epidemiology cannot provide the controlled experimental conditions of the laboratory; bias from various uncontrolled or unknown factors must be considered. The fact that clinically recognizable cancer does not appear until years after exposure aggravates this problem.

Animal studies offer many advantages over epidemiological studies. Experiments can be better controlled, higher doses given, lifetime studies carried out more easily and quickly, invasive techniques used, and some ethical problems circumvented. Use of animal bioassay data rests upon the commonly accepted premise that effects in animals resemble effects in humans. Susceptibilities often differ, but experimental data show in the main that chemicals that are carcinogenic to animals are likely to be carcinogenic to humans.

Mice, rats, and other commonly used test species have physical and metabolic characteristics and sensitivities different from humans. As a result, models or scaling factors must be used to account for these differences. Furthermore, experimental exposures differ from actual or expected human experiences. These differences must also be accounted for in the conversion.

### Interspecies Extrapolation

Here, interspecies extrapolation is based on an assumption of uniformity of lifetime effect on a milligram dose per kilogram body weight (mg/kg) basis, in which dose is the amount of material consumed (by inhalation, ingestion, injection, etc.) by the animal. This is a simple conversion method; others exist, for example, dose per body surface area. It does not consider metabolic and other factors which may lead to interspecies differences. Crouch and Wilson use a mg/kg base in investigating interspecies differences.[3] These differences are generally less than an order of magnitude, however, compared with the larger differences among studies and among high-dose to low-dose extrapolation models shown below.

### High- to Low-Dose Extrapolation

Because it is not practical to use sufficiently large numbers of animals in laboratory experiments for rigorous determination of effects at low doses, animal doses are usually much higher than equivalent public exposures of interest. Several extrapolation techniques have been developed to estimate low-dose effects. Historically, most have dealt with food safety and aimed at estimating the dose to produce some "acceptable" risk. Krewski and Brown provide a guide to this literature.[4] The methods have been modified to yield dose-response relationships estimating risk at any dose. Extrapolation models used here are detailed in an earlier report.[5]

The models are divided into two groups by the biological concepts of environmental carcinogenesis upon which they are based. Statistical or tolerance-distribution models are based on individual tolerance levels or thresholds of exposure above which cancer occurs. In these models, a statistical distribution of individual susceptibility is assumed. Thus, at any dose level, some fraction of the population will develop cancer. Probit, Logit, and Weibull models are statistical.

Stochastic models form the second group. They are based on the premise that everyone is equally susceptible to cancer, and an event or series of independent events—each with a specific probability dependent on dose— must occur in order to generate a response. Hit models and multistage models are stochastic.

None of the models assumes that a threshold exists. Spontaneous or background risk is an estimated parameter, however.

An extrapolation example is shown in Figure 2. Response is measured as the percentage of animals exhibiting tumors. Response is a nonlinear function of dose, but, since relatively small increments tend to result in linear increases in effect, particularly at low doses, the derivative of the dose-response curve is useful (Figure 3). Using this curve, the percentage response for an incremental dose at any given background level can be

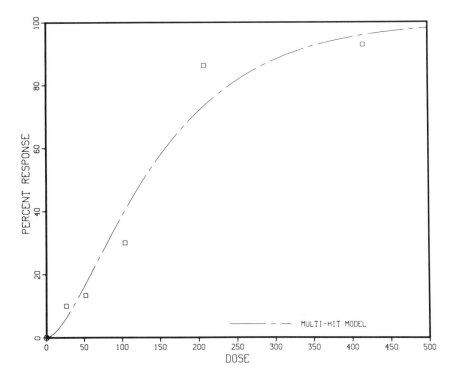

**Figure 2.** Example of cumulative percentage of animals exhibiting tumors over their lifetime vs mg/kg dose with data from an animal experiment. Human backgrounds of 0.5 to 5 mg/kg appear close to zero on this scale.

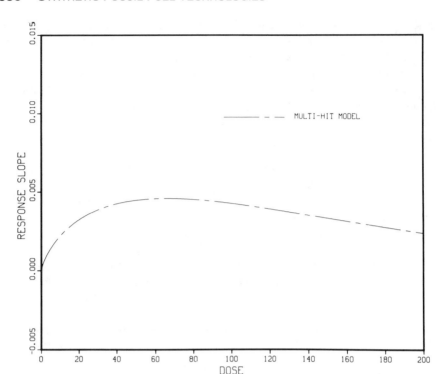

**Figure 3.** Example of lifetime tumor risk per mg/kg dose vs background dose. Derivative of cumulative curve in Figure 2.

determined. Figure 4 shows the differences among the six models used. Figure 5 enlarges the portions of the curves of interest for effects estimates.

## DOSE-RESPONSE COEFFICIENTS

Table III provides the dose-response coefficients derived from four studies of two compounds in RAC 15 using the six extrapolation models (i.e., the derivatives of the dose-response curves at the specified background dose levels). Coefficients are expressed as lifetime tumor risk per individual per milligram dose per kilogram body weight. One study (B) showed evidence of acute toxicity at higher doses and was reanalyzed to avoid incorporating that effect in the results. Background dose is assumed to range from 0.5 mg/kg to 5 mg/kg, and coefficients are calculated at both levels.[6]

As previously noted in exercises of this kind, there are orders of magnitude differences among the individual results.[7] In this case, differences

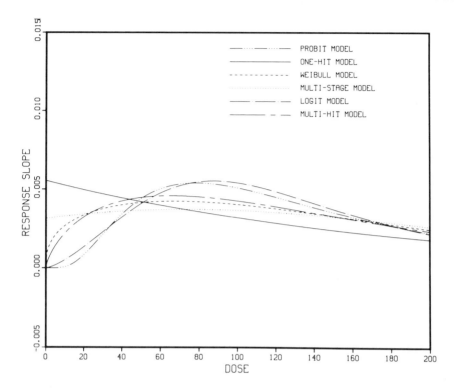

**Figure 4.**    Lifetime tumor risk per mg/kg dose vs background dose level from example study. Results of one-hit, multihit, multistage, Weibull, logit, and probit models are shown. Human background exposure is 0.5–5 mg/kg.

range more than 25 orders of magnitude. In considering this problem, one must realize that all orders of magnitude do not have the same practical significance. The difference between 100 and 1000 predicted cancers per year is much more important than the difference between 0.01 and 0.1 predicted cancers per year. The order of magnitude range in background dose affects only the low estimates. High estimates are quite robust over this range. While the range is >25 orders of magnitude, more than 75% of the estimates cluster in a much narrower range, $10^{-4}$ to $10^{-2}$. This may shed no light on the real answer, but it shows that disagreement among models is not as large as might at first appear.

Although one cannot justify any specific cutoff point in this coefficient, because the resulting cancers depend also on dose, it is reasonable to assume that below some level the coefficient is essentially zero. It will be seen below that, for this case, a coefficient of 0.01 yields ~ 10 tumors/plant-year. Thus a coefficient of $10^{-4}$ yields < 1 tumor/year and one of $10^{-6}$ yields < 1 tumor/ 30 years of plant operation—a reasonable approximation of zero.

Use of zero as a lower bound is appropriate on two additional grounds.

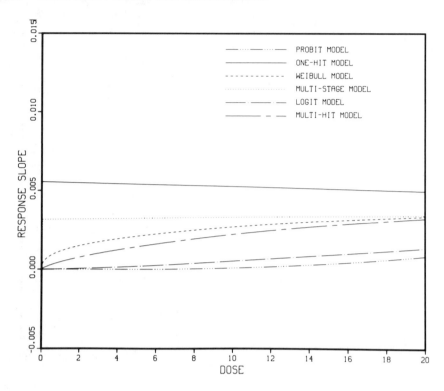

**Figure 5.** Lifetime tumor risk per mg/kg dose vs background dose level from example study. Enlarges the portion of curves in Figure 4 to show rates over range of human background to polycyclic aromatic hydrocarbons (0.5 to 5 mg/kg).

First, experimental data are seldom sufficient to assure there is a carcinogenic effect at low dose, and second, all RACs contain noncarcinogens, and the exposure to any RAC could be made up entirely of noncarcinogens. Use of the highest estimate—the worst combination of compound, study, and model—as the upper bound probably far overstates reality. In this case, however, although the highest slope estimate is 10,000 times the geometric mean of all the values of Table III, it is only 25 times the median and 1.8 times the sixteenth (the value that only 1/16 of the estimates exceed). This brings the upper bound estimate into perspective but does not address the problem of mixing the carcinogenic compounds analyzed with noncarcinogens in the same RAC.

In Table III, the range over studies and the range over models are roughly the same. The range over studies may be improved by considering fraction retained, metabolic models, specific organ dose, or other factors introducing extraneous differences among studies. The range over models can only be improved through better understanding of mechanisms that will lead to better selection of models.

**Table III.**   Lifetime Tumor Risk per mg/kg Dose for Risk Assessment for Four Studies (A–D) Category 15 (polycyclic aromatic hydrocarbons)

| Model/Study | $A^a$ | $B^b$ | C | D |
|---|---|---|---|---|
| *0.5 mg/kg Background* | | | | |
| 1-Hit | $4 \times 10^{-4}$ | $1 \times 10^{-2}$ | $6 \times 10^{-3}$ | $5 \times 10^{-4}$ |
| Multihit | $4 \times 10^{-7}$ | $1 \times 10^{-8}$ | $3 \times 10^{-4}$ | $2 \times 10^{-3}$ |
| Multistage | $2 \times 10^{-4}$ | $1 \times 10^{-4}$ | $3 \times 10^{-3}$ | $5 \times 10^{-4}$ |
| Probit | $2 \times 10^{-28}$ | $2 \times 10^{-25}$ | $4 \times 10^{-14}$ | $1 \times 10^{-3}$ |
| Logit | $5 \times 10^{-9}$ | $2 \times 10^{-7}$ | $8 \times 10^{-6}$ | $2 \times 10^{-3}$ |
| Weibull | $2 \times 10^{-5}$ | $3 \times 10^{-5}$ | $9 \times 10^{-4}$ | $2 \times 10^{-3}$ |
| *5.0 mg/kg Background* | | | | |
| 1-Hit | $4 \times 10^{-4}$ | $1 \times 10^{-2}$ | $5 \times 10^{-3}$ | $5 \times 10^{-4}$ |
| Multihit | $5 \times 10^{-6}$ | $4 \times 10^{-4}$ | $1 \times 10^{-3}$ | $1 \times 10^{-3}$ |
| Multistage | $2 \times 10^{-4}$ | $1 \times 10^{-3}$ | $3 \times 10^{-3}$ | $5 \times 10^{-4}$ |
| Probit | $1 \times 10^{-15}$ | $1 \times 10^{-8}$ | $3 \times 10^{-16}$ | $1 \times 10^{-3}$ |
| Logit | $2 \times 10^{-7}$ | $6 \times 10^{-5}$ | $2 \times 10^{-4}$ | $1 \times 10^{-3}$ |
| Weibull | $6 \times 10^{-5}$ | $6 \times 10^{-4}$ | $2 \times 10^{-3}$ | $1 \times 10^{-3}$ |

[a]Gastric cancers only.
[b]Respiratory tract cancers only.

## ESTIMATING POPULATION EXPOSURE AND HEALTH EFFECTS

Population exposure and health effects have been estimated for several pathways: direct inhalation, terrestrial food chain (local), aquatic food chain, and drinking water. Pathways not yet assessed include long-range atmospheric deposition and resulting exposures via food chain, water, and direct ingestion by children (pica), and groundwater.

The work is at the screening level; thus, simple approaches have been used. Because of the incremental nature of the exposure, the dose-response function is assumed to be linear over the region of interest, as discussed above. Thus, induced tumors can be estimated from the total mass of exposure alone without regard to individual doses. Where this is done, equivalent-population exposed is also estimated so that the average percentage increase in cancer rate can be estimated. Both the total number of cancers and the percentage increase in the cancer rate are useful measures of health impact. For this purpose, predicted tumors are assumed to be indicative of cancer. Calculations are shown and methods, assumptions, and caveats discussed by pathway in the following section on method.

Consistent with the needs of a screening-level analysis, the calculations of effects are kept as straightforward and as simple as possible. Several assumptions are necessary in the analysis (Table IV).[8] The latency period leads to an effective dose smaller than total lifetime dose because some

**Table IV.** Assumptions in Calculations

Steady-state population
70-year Average lifetime
60-kg Average body weight[a]
20-year Latent period
20-m³/d Inhalation rate[a]
2-1/d Water ingestion rate[a]
512-g/d Cereal and produce ingestion rate[a]
26-g/d Aquatic food ingestion rate[a]

[a]Based on Reference 8.

people receiving a dose die before cancer can be manifested. Total cancers induced over the lifetime of the exposed population due to exposure to a single year of plant operation are calculated. These are equivalent to annual effects for a steady state, continuous exposure. For a plant with a 30-year life, the calculated estimates are maximum increases in cancer rate. Under these assumptions, induced cancers will occur over a period of 80 years, that is, during the last 10 years of plant operation (after 20 years of latency following startup) and continuing a full lifetime of 70 years after plant closing. During this 80-year period, average increase in cancer will be 30/80 of the values of the maximum levels.

Table V summarizes the effects estimated above. In comparing results from different pathways, several factors must be considered.

**Table V.** Effects Summary for RAC 15 Indirect Coal Liquefaction—Eastern U.S. Site

| Route | Population Exposed (millions) | Annual Risk[a] | | |
| | | Background[b] | Induced | % Increase |
|---|---|---|---|---|
| Direct inhalation | | | | |
|   Local | 0.35 | 1,200 | 0–6.4 | 0–0.6 |
|   Long range | 166 | 550,000 | 0–5.0 | 0–0.0009 |
| Drinking water | 3 | 9,900 | 0–1.5 | 0–0.02 |
| Aquatic food chain | 0.33 | 1,100 | 0–1.6 | 0–0.1 |
| Terrestrial food chain | | | | |
|   Local | 0.04 | 130 | 0–0.6 | 0–0.5 |
|   Long range[c] | | | | |

[a]Annual cancers induced over all time per plant-year. Percent increase is during peak effects years. Average percentage increase over period cancers expressed is about 40% of stated values for a plant with a 30-year life.

[b]Annual cancer incidence rate 330/10⁵, derived from 1973 to 1976 National Cancer Institute Surveillance, Epidemiology, and End Results Program Data (Reference 9).

[c]Not calculated.

The interface between the short- and long-range air transport models is not smooth since the models are of different form. There may be significant population exposure in the 50 to 100-km range not adequately captured in either model.

The range of effects in Table V reflects only uncertainty in dose response. Exposure values were calculated as point estimates. Both direct inhalation and terrestrial food chain estimates are based on "best-estimate" exposures, whereas drinking water and aquatic food chain exposure estimates are "upper bound." Thus, for purposes of comparison, the latter are overestimated compared to the former.

The local terrestrial food chain appears lowest in total number of cancers induced, but this is largely because the amount of food produced within 50 km of the site is small; production will only support 0.1 of the population. Were sufficient food grown to make the area self-supporting, cancers resulting from food contamination would equal those from local inhalation.

To provide an additional perspective, the percentage increase in cancer rate is calculated as well as the number of cancers induced. For example, the number of cancers produced are about equal from long range and local inhalation, but the percent increase in risk seen by the population exposed differs markedly (0.6% locally compared to 0.0009% at long range). Percent increases for food chains are based on full-time-equivalent population exposed. Since the food will contribute part of the diet of a larger number of people, these percent increases are upper-bound estimates.

## METHOD

### Inhalation—Local

Source rate to air for RAC 15 is $2.5 \times 10^7$ g/year. Local population exposure ($\leq$50 km) was modeled by the Oak Ridge National Laboratory (ORNL) using a Gaussian plume model. Estimated population exposure was 7500 person-$\mu$g/m$^3$ for a plant with a total of 353,000 people exposed. Effects calculations are:

7.5 person-mg/m$^3$ $\times$ 7300 m$^3$/year $\times$ 0.7 effectiveness factor/60 kg
$$= 639\text{-mg/kg effective dose per plant-year}$$

639 mg/kg $\times$ (0 to 0.01) lifetime cancer/(mg/kg)
$$= 0 \text{ to } 6.4 \text{ cancer/plant-year.}$$

Uncertainties in the Gaussian plume model for annual average exposure would contribute an additional uncertainty factor of 2 in the result.

### Inhalation—Long Range

Again, source strength is $2.5 \times 10^7$ g/year. Air concentrations at long range were calculated by ORNL on a $13 \times 15$ grid covering the eastern United States. County populations were mapped into this grid to obtain population exposure of 5.83 person-mg/m$^3$ over 166 million people. Effects calculations are:

5.83 person-mg/m$^3$ $\times$ 7300 m$^3$/year $\times$ 0.7 effectiveness factor/60 kg
$$= \text{497-mg/kg effective dose per plant-year}$$

497 mg/kg $\times$ (0 to 0.01) lifetime cancer/(mg/kg)
$$= \text{0 to 5 cancer/plant-year.}$$

Uncertainty in the long-range transport model contributes an additional uncertainty factor of ~2 in the result.

### Terrestrial Food Chain

Mass of contaminant in terrestrial food by RAC as a result of air deposition was estimated by ORNL using the TERREX computer code. Only food exposed within 50 km of the plant was considered. Total mass of RAC 15 in leafy vegetables, exposed and protected produce, grain for human consumption, milk, and beef was $5.24 \times 10^6$ μg/year. It was assumed that all of this reaches man. Effects calculations are:

$5.24 \times 10^3$ mg/year $\times$ 0.7 effectiveness factor/60 kg
$$= \text{61-mg/kg effective annual dose}$$

61 mg/kg $\times$ (0 to 0.01) lifetime cancer/(mg/kg)
$$= \text{0 to 0.6 cancer/plant-year.}$$

The results are subject to the uncertainty factor of 2 of the Gaussian plume model plus some additional uncertainty in estimating how much deposited material gets into plants. Losses of contaminant in washing and processing food stuffs are not considered, although in some cases these could be substantial.

The above calculation does not quantify the population exposed. This can be back-calculated from the total food production. ORNL estimated $7 \times 10^6$ kg/year production of vegetables and grains. Applying an estimate of 512 g/person-d of vegetables and cereals yields ~4000 people. This is a full-time-equivalent estimate in that the food may provide part of the total diet for a larger population.

### Drinking Water

Concentrations of each RAC in four downstream reaches extending >1000 km from the site were estimated by ORNL. Source rate to water for RAC 15 was $5.4 \times 10^5$ g/year. The model does not include chemical or biological degradation and so is in some sense an upper-bound estimate of exposure. For the first 50 km, 1150 people/km stream were assumed to drink the water; beyond that, population exposed was taken to be that of the major cities along the Ohio and Mississippi Rivers. Concentrations, population, and mass of contaminant consumed (at 2 L/person-d) are shown in Table VI, totaling 13.3 g/year annual consumption among 3 million people. Effects calculations are:

13,300 mg/year $\times$ 0.7 effectiveness factor/60 kg
$$= 155 \text{ mg/kg effective dose/plant-year}$$

155 mg/kg $\times$ (0 to 0.01) lifetime cancer/(mg/kg)
$$= 0 \text{ to } 1.6 \text{ cancer/plant-year.}$$

For a plant located on the upper Ohio or its tributaries, 1051 km does not take the contamination to sea. By 1000 km, however, dilution has decreased the concentration so that the total mass of contaminant consumed, and thus the total number of induced cancers, are not sensitive to increases in the population at greater distances.

### Aquatic Food Chain

Concentrations in fish were estimated by ORNL at each downstream reach (Table VII). The total annual catch in the Ohio-Mississippi-Red Rock rivers is $4.5 \times 10^7$ kg (although sometimes as little as 40% of this).[9] We assume that 50% of the catch is for human consumption and that the catch is dis-

**Table VI.**  Drinking Water Exposure for RAC 15

| Distance from Site (km) | Estimated Number of People | Concentration (g/L) | Annual Consumption (g) |
|---|---|---|---|
| <2 | $2.3 \times 10^3$ | $6.85 \times 10^{-8}$ | 0.12 |
| 2–51 | $5.6 \times 10^4$ | $6.27 \times 10^{-8}$ | 2.56 |
| 52–551 | $2.0 \times 10^6$ | $6.27 \times 10^{-9}$ | 9.15 |
| 552–1,051 | $2.0 \times 10^6$ | $1.94 \times 10^{-9}$ | 1.42 |
| Totals | $3.0 \times 10^6$ | | 13.25 |

**Table VII.** Aquatic Food Chain for RAC 15

| Distance from Site (km) | Estimated Catch (kg/year) | Concentration in Fish (g/kg) | Total Mass in Catch (g/year) |
|---|---|---|---|
| <2 | $1.2 \times 10^4$ | $4.1 \times 10^{-5}$ | 0.49 |
| 2–51 | $2.9 \times 10^5$ | $3.8 \times 10^{-5}$ | 11.02 |
| 52–551 | $3.0 \times 10^6$ | $3.8 \times 10^{-6}$ | 11.40 |
| 552–1,051 | $3.0 \times 10^6$ | $1.2 \times 10^{-6}$ | 3.60 |
| Totals | $6.3 \times 10^6$ | | 26.51 |

tributed uniformly along the 7550 km length of the combined streams. Estimated catch in each reach is given in Table VI. Effects calculations are:

26,500 mg/year × (0.5) × 0.7 effectiveness factor/60 kg

$$= 155 \text{ mg/kg effective dose/plant-year}$$

155 mg/kg × (0 to 0.02) lifetime cancer/(mg/kg)

$$= 0 \text{ to } 1.6 \text{ cancer/plant-year.}$$

At 26-g fish/person-d, the total catch over the four reaches feeds a full-time-equivalent population of 330,000 people. Similar to the terrestrial food chain, this fish may provide a smaller portion of the diet of a larger population.

As with the drinking water estimates, this is an upper-bound calculation.

## CONCLUSIONS

A method for risk analysis of complex technologies has been demonstrated, carrying the analysis from source term to increased cancer. The results provide a basis for comparing effects from various pathways and considering absolute magnitude of the risk from a synfuels plant. Other synfuels plants may not have the same emission rates, and these conclusions refer only to the specific plant analyzed. Comparison with others can be made on the basis of relative emissions rates.

Effects from air emissions seem greater in Table V since air emissions are 50-fold greater than water emissions; on a unit-emission basis, upper-bound cancer estimates of Table V associated with water emissions are about 12 times greater than those associated with air emissions.

It is not known whether the plant will produce any increase in cancer. This method of analysis produces a nonzero upper bound in any case in which the RAC includes a known or suspected carcinogen. We believe the upper bounds of the ranges are reasonably estimated. Although not exactly comparable, the highest upper-bound estimate is from local direct inhalation—0.6% increase in cancer rate. This may be sufficiently high to warrant further consideration.

The range of uncertainty is large, including zero. Although some aspects of uncertainty can be reduced by using more sophisticated models and better data, the uncertainty largely reflects the current state of knowledge and can be improved significantly only through better understanding of the mechanisms of chemical carcinogenesis.

Risk analysis does not eliminate the problem of how to make decisions concerning new industries that emit pollutants which may cause cancer. It cannot produce better estimates than the data on which it is based. It simply provides a means of bringing existing knowledge to bear on problems in a systematic and useful way. We believe that such quantitative estimates with explicit uncertainties will aid in making both technological and environmental decisions.

## ACKNOWLEDGMENTS

Work reported in this chapter was supported by the U.S. Environmental Protection Agency, Office of Research and Development, Office of Environmental Processes and Effects Research, Energy and Air Division. The authors thank A.A. Moghissi and S. Holtzman for support and encouragement; colleagues at Oak Ridge National Laboratory[2] for their cooperation; J. Van Ryzin, K. Rai, and D. Krewski for providing computer codes and for help and advice in implementing the extrapolation models; C. Conard for technical assistance; and A. Link for typing and organizing this chapter through several drafts.

## REFERENCES

1.  Moghissi, A.A., and G.J. Foley. "Assessment of Environmental Impact of Coal-Conversion and Oil-Shale Technologies," in *Health Impacts of Different Sources of Energy* (Vienna: International Atomic Energy Agency, 1982) pp. 665–673.
2.  Emissions and concentration data were provided by C.F. Baes, L.W. Barnthouse, C.W. Gehrs, S.G. Hildebrand, B.D. Murphy, R. Raridon, G.W. Suter, G.P. Thompson, and A.P. Watson, all of Oak Ridge National Laboratory.
3.  Crouch, E.C., and R. Wilson. "Interspecies Comparison of Carcinogenic Potency," *J. Tox. and Environ. Health* 5:1,095–1,118 (1979).
4.  Krewski, D., and C. Brown. "Carcinogenic Risk Assessment: A Guide to the Literature," *Biometrics* 37:353–366 (1981).
5.  Morris, S.C., H.C. Thode, Jr., J.I. Barancik, H. Fischer, P.D. Moskowitz,

J. Nagy and L.D. Hamilton. "Methods for Assessing Cancer Risks Using Animal and Human Data" (Upton, NY: Brookhaven National Laboratory, 1982).

6. "Ambient Water Quality Criteria for Polynuclear Aromatic Hydrocarbons," PB 81-117806 (Washington, DC: U.S. Environmental Protection Agency, 1980).

7. Schneiderman, M.A., N. Mantel, and C.C. Brown. "From Mouse to Man or How to Get From the Laboratory to Park Avenue and 59th Street," *Ann. NY Acad. Sci.* 246:237–248 (1976).

8. *Report of this Task Group on Reference Man,* ICRP23 International Commission on Radiological Protection (New York: Pergamon Press, 1975).

9. U.S. Bureau of Census, Statistical Abstract of the United States: 1975. Washington, DC, 1975.

10. Pollack, E.S., and J.W. Horm. "Trends in Cancer Incidence and Mortality in the United States, 1969–76," *J. NCI* 64:1,091–1,103, 1980.

## DISCUSSION

*M. Uziel, Oak Ridge National Laboratory:* Your basic assumption is that the dose responses in animals and man are equal in terms of the milligram-per-kilogram relationship. If that were not so, how would that affect your data? For example, rodents seem to be more sensitive in terms of response at the subcellular level to many of these agents, for example the PAHs, than many human tissues. Thus, there might be a considerable difference in response at the animal level compared to the human.

*S. Morris:* There is work going on to further resolve this mouse-to-man relationship. The upper bound of our estimates is determined essentially by the most potent compound within the risk assessment category that we have considered in the animal system and the extrapolation model that together give the highest effect. I'm not really happy with that as the highest end point, but I am not sure of another way to do it that doesn't involve a lot of assumptions. Clearly, differences between animals and humans would make a difference. I tried to use the human data that we have, and there are half a dozen sources of epidemiological data of which I think the coke oven worker data are the strongest. The range from the coke oven worker study overlaps our animal range from the coke oven worker study overlaps our animal results.

*V. Frankos, Clement Associates:* You presented a risk assessment for only category 15 in your list. What would you propose to do once you had risk assessments done for each of the categories as far as combining the risks?

*S. Morris:* We are in the process of doing a similar calculation for every category, and we are still discussing the problem of how we are going to combine them. The plan is to add them all together, but there are a couple of worrisome problems. One is that there may be overlapping effects; there may be synergistic or antagonistic effects. We have been specifically told by our sponsor not to worry about those. In a practical sense, you almost can't worry about them. There are very few specific instances where we have information about synergistic or antagonistic effects that we can apply, and, while we might be concerned about them at this point, there is not a whole lot that we can do about them.

*M.S. Legator, University of Texas:* There has been a certain tendency now, at least for individual chemicals, to get away from the standard risk assessment by the various models. It would be replaced by a ranking system, the kind of approach that was proposed in the Food Safety Council and finally by Bob Squire, where you consider the total animal data. What is your feeling for the ranking kind of approach versus the quantitative risk assessment from modeling?

*S. Morris:* It depends on how much information you have. In many cases, the ranking approach is probably much more appropriate. On the other hand, the ranking approach does not give you what you need to go on to the next step to a benefit/risk analysis. The quantitative approach gives this information but, unfortunately, it may end up giving us a range that is so wide it doesn't help us too much. It does give us a true reflection of the range of uncertainty that exists which might be something we didn't know.

*S.V. Kaye:* It appears that much data lumping was used in this study. Starting with the meteorological calculations for exposure of about 350,000 people, you more or less assumed that they all received the same exposure, they are all adults, and they all have the same physiology and the same susceptibility to cancer induction. Then you use 70 kg for the weight of an adult person so that if there is any particularly susceptible or critically exposed population, they're averaged out and there really is no average individual or average exposure. Have you looked at any of the specific groups in the exposed populations to see if they receive an order of magnitude higher probability of cancer induction, or whatever the number might be, when you consider pathways of exposure that might be unique or critical or are a susceptible age group? Part of your population may have been too old for cancer induction. Others, maybe 25%, were in a younger age group which had a higher probability, and so on. Have you looked at or do you plan to look at any of those specifics?

*S. Morris:* Originally, we made the decision to look first at an average, rather than at maximally exposed people or highly susceptible groups. Obviously these have to be studied, too. You need to be concerned with people that for some reason might have high background exposures, that might have high susceptibilities, or that might have high exposures from the plant itself. This can get into a much more complex study. We decided the first thing to do was to look at averages and then later go back in and see whether we can identify particular groups that are at higher risk.

*S.V. Kaye:* But if you have so many different important competing factors, the overall effect that you calculate may be completely fictitious and doesn't really exist, and it's the individual populations and exposure situations that are the important ones. That is what I was implying.

# CHAPTER 15

## Identifying Problem Compounds in Complex Organic Mixtures: Oil-Shale Retort Water Examples

J.S. Meyer,
G.L. Linder,[1]
M.D. Marcus,[2] and
H.L. Bergman

*Fish Physiology and Toxicology
Laboratory
Department of Zoology and
Physiology
University of Wyoming
Laramie, WY 82071*

Complex chemical mixtures pose difficult challenges for identifying problem compounds. Results of three biological fate-and-effects tests illustrate how these challenges can be approached. First, although it has previously been touted as a useful procedure for identifying toxic components of chemical mixtures, fractional toxicity testing seldom has produced detailed toxicity information about specific problem organics. Fractional toxicity testing would be more cost effective if current approaches were reoriented to mimic routinely used wastewater treatment processes. Second, bioaccumulation studies in which aquatic organisms are exposed to sublethal concentrations of a chemical mixture can be effectively used to monitor uptake and depuration kinetics and bioconcentration factors for individual compounds and classes of compounds. Finally, biodegradation of chemical mixtures is difficult to predict. Laboratory screening studies provide useful qualitative information about transformations in whole mixtures, but laboratory results will have to

---

[1]Linder present address: Patuxent Wildlife Research Center, U.S. Department of Interior, Laurel, MD 20811
[2]Marcus present address: Western Aquatics, Inc., P.O. Box 546, Laramie, WY 82070

be correlated with field studies before reliable quantitative predictions of biodegradation are possible.

## INTRODUCTION

Most products, wastewaters, treated waters, and effluents from synthetic fuel technologies are complex chemical mixtures. Although products and related waters differ within and between process technologies, they usually contain many inorganic compounds (e.g., ammonia, bicarbonate, sulfate, heavy metals) and hundreds of organic compounds (e.g., phenols, nitrogen heterocyclics, sulfur heterocyclics, polyaromatics).[1-3] Identifying all major and trace constituents in these mixtures is a monumental analytical task. Furthermore, predicting environmental fate and effects will be arduous and expensive if the constituents are investigated on a chemical-by-chemical basis. Yet predictions of toxicity, environmental partitioning, and persistence are needed to estimate safe discharge concentrations and to evaluate environmental risks associated with synthetic fuel technologies.

Fortunately, methods are being developed to cost effectively address potential environmental problems of synfuel products and related waters. In this chapter we discuss biological tests that can be used to identify problem compounds in complex organic mixtures without relying on exhaustive chemical analyses of the whole material. We present results for oil-shale retort waters because they represent an extreme of mixture complexity. Despite our emphasis on oil-shale retort waters, methods described for these studies also apply to other complex chemical mixtures (e.g., chemical manufacturing effluents, refinery effluents, solid waste leachates).

In the following sections we first review physical and chemical characteristics of oil-shale retort waters. Then we present examples of three biological test methods that have been used to identify problem compounds in retort waters. These test methods are (1) fractional toxicity, (2) bioaccumulation, and (3) biodegradation. Results from these studies can indicate individual compounds that may have to be targeted for chemical monitoring of discharges or removed during wastewater treatment. Additionally, results of the bioaccumulation and biodegradation tests can be used to predict expected exposure concentrations, which are necessary to conduct hazard assessments of complex mixtures. Details of these studies have been previously reported[3-5] or will be published elsewhere. The purpose of this chapter is to discuss potential applications and problems of each test method and recommend future research and development.

## CHARACTERISTICS OF OIL-SHALE
## RETORT WATERS

Four oil-shale retort waters were tested. These waters and the processes from which they were generated are (1) Omega-9, true in situ retort;

(2) Geokinetics-9, true in situ retort; (3) Occidental-6, modified in situ retort; and (4) Paraho 77-78, above-ground retort. In Table I, chemical characteristics of these waters are listed. Reverse-phase high-performance liquid chromatography (HPLC) gradients appear in Figure 1.

Water quality parameters for Omega-9, Geokinetics-9, and Occidental-6 retort waters are similar. In general, these waters are alkaline and contain a variety of dissolved inorganic and organic compounds. Specifically, alkalinity, organic carbon, conductivity, ammonia, dissolved solids, sulfate, and sodium levels are relatively high. Only hardness, magnesium, and sodium values are considerably lower in Occidental-6 than in Omega-9 and Geokinetics-9 waters. These differences are probably caused by varying compositions of major ions in oil shales from Colorado's Green River Formation.

**Table I.**   Chemical Characteristics of Oil-Shale Retort Waters

| Parameter[a] | Oil-Shale Retort Water | | | |
|---|---|---|---|---|
| | Omega-9[b] | Geokinetics-9[b] | Occidental-6[c] | Paraho 77–78[b] |
| Alkalinity, as CaCO$_3$ | 16,200 | 9,500 | 6,700 | 29,000 |
| Carbon, total organic, as C | 1,000 | 1,600 | 2,900 | 37,000 |
| Chemical oxygen demand | 8,100 | 7,400 | 7,900 | 154,000 |
| Conductivity, μseimens/cm at 25°C | 20,000 | 11,000 | 13,000 | 70,000 |
| Hardness, as CaCO$_3$ | 110 | 1,200 | 10 | 3,400 |
| Nitrogen | | | | |
| Ammonia, as N | 3,100 | 1,200 | 800 | 7,900 |
| Kjeldahl, as N | 3,400 | 2,600 | 1,000 | 28,000 |
| pH, units | 8.7 | 8.8 | 8.9 | 8.4 |
| Solids, total dissolved | 14,000 | 16,000 | 10,200 | 124,000 |
| Sulfate, as SO$_4^{2-}$ | 2,000 | 5,000 | 1,400 | 8,000 |
| Selected elements | | | | |
| Arsenic | 1 | 0.4 | 0.7 | 20 |
| Boron | 20 | 60 | 100 | 30 |
| Calcium | 10 | 5 | 2 | 20 |
| Fluoride | 60 | 20 | 40 | 40 |
| Magnesium | 20 | 70 | 2 | 700 |
| Mercury | <0.02 | 0.06 | <0.1 | <0.03 |
| Potassium | 50 | 90 | 60 | 20 |
| Sodium | 5,300 | 6,100 | 330 | 240 |
| Zinc | 0.3 | 0.5 | 0.1 | 0.5 |

[a]Values reported as mg/L unless otherwise noted.
[b]Values reported by Skogerboe; in Reference 6.
[c]Values reported by Bergman et al.; in Reference 3.

**Figure 1.** Reverse-phase HPLC gradient chromatograms for four oil-shale retort waters: (a) Omega-9; (b) Geokinetics-9; (c) Occidental-6; (d) Paraho 77-78. Chromatographic conditions for all waters are 30-cm $\mu$-$C_{18}$ Bondapak column; 50 $\mu$L injection; 60-min linear gradient programmed from 100% $H_2O$ to 100% $CH_3CN$ at 2.0 mL/min; 254-nm UV detector (note that the sensitivity for the Paraho 77-78 chromatogram is $0.1 \times$ the sensitivity of the other three chromatograms). Retention times of five representative compounds are indicated above each chromatogram: 1 = resorcinol; 2 = phenol; 3 = benzene; 4 = toluene; 5 = naphthalene.

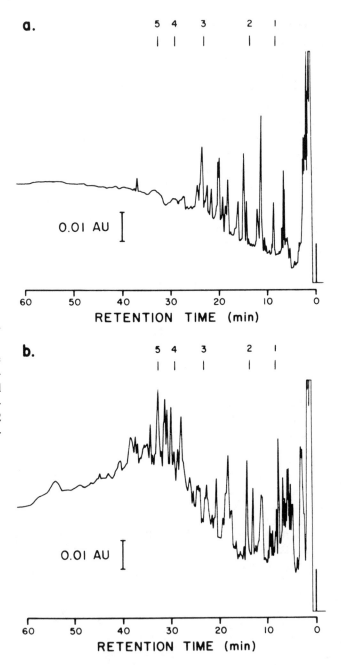

Paraho 77-78 retort water differs considerably from the other three waters. Organic carbon, conductivity, hardness, ammonia, Kjeldahl nitrogen, dissolved solids, arsenic, and magnesium levels considerably exceed values for Omega-9, Geokinetics-9, and Occidental-6. Although shale compositions differ, most of these elevated parameters are probably a

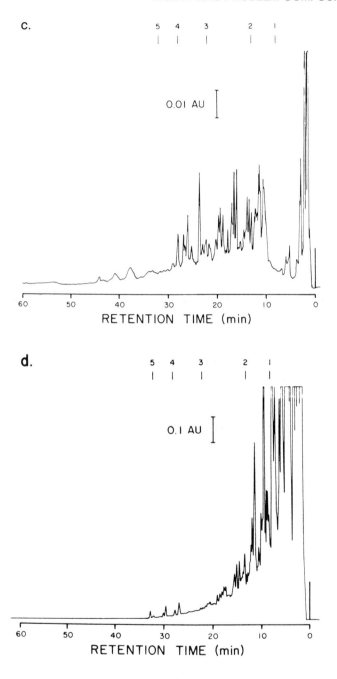

consequence of the aboveground retorting process for Paraho 77-78 compared to underground retorting for the other three waters. Only higher
magnesium and lower sodium concentrations in the Paraho retort water are
probably caused by different shale compositions.

The relatively high organic carbon levels of all four retort waters in-

clude hundreds (possibly thousands) of compounds.[2] For example, Leenheer et al.[7] attributed approximately 40% of the organic carbon in Occidental-
6 retort water to aliphatic monocarboxylic acids. Other compound classes
at relatively high concentrations included aliphatic dicarboxylic acids, aromatic carboxylic acids, thiocyanate, phenols, hydroxypyridines, aliphatic
amides, and lactones. Our HPLC gradient chromatograms (Figure 1) illustrate this variety.

In reverse-phase HPLC gradient elutions, relatively polar and low-
molecular-weight organics, such as phenols, elute earlier than relatively nonpolar and high-molecular-weight organics, such as polynuclear aromatic hydrocarbons (PAH). With the 254-nm ultraviolet (UV) absorbance detector
used for these chromatograms, mostly aromatic and PAH compounds are
detected. Thus, many nonabsorbing organic compounds are not recorded
in Figure 1. Additionally, many high-molecular-weight organics that elute
later in these gradients do not appear at the detector sensitivities used for
these chromatograms.

Although they differ in details, chromatograms for Omega-9, Geoki-
netics-9, and Occidental-6 waters are qualitatively similar. But Paraho 77-
78 water differs considerably. First, as stated before, it contains greater than
10 times as much total organic carbon; note that the Paraho 77-78 chromatogram [Figure 1(d)] was recorded at $0.1 \times$ the detector sensitivity of the
other three chromatograms so that the majority of its peaks would not
deflect off-scale. Second, much more of the total UV absorbance is associated with relatively polar compounds that elute before phenol. This difference is probably caused by various retorting conditions of the aboveground
Paraho process and the belowground processes for Omega-9, Geokinetics-
9, and Occidental-6. Similar concentrations of intermediate- and high-
molecular-weight compounds may be present in all four retort waters. However, Paraho 77-78 contains a greater percentage of relatively polar, low-
molecular-weight organics.

## FRACTIONAL TOXICITY

### Previous Studies

Fractionation is a chemical procedure used to facilitate the biological identification of toxic constituents in complex mixtures.[8] In concept, fractions
are separated according to physical and chemical properties of the mixture
components. Analyzing only the toxic fractions reduces the effort and expense necessary to identify a mixture's toxic constituents. Moreover, physical and chemical characteristics of the toxic fraction and the individual toxic
compounds can be used to reduce or eliminate concentrations of problem
compounds through product upgrading or effluent treatment.

Fractional toxicity testing has been applied to several synfuel products and wastewaters. Parkhurst[8] reviewed aquatic toxicity tests conducted for coal and oil-shale-conversion wastewater fractions. Coal and oil-shale-conversion products have also been fractionated and assayed for mutagenic and carcinogenic activity.[9-12] Generally, these studies have evaluated the effects of primary fractions (e.g., acid, base, and neutral organics and inorganics) or, in some studies, effects of secondary fractions derived from the primary fractions. In most cases, several fractions were relatively toxic, indicating that several potentially hazardous compound classes were present in the product or wastewater.

Other than the tests conducted in our laboratory and discussed in more detail below, we are aware of only one fractional toxicity study of an oil-shale retort water.[13] In that study, retort water from the Paraho above-ground process was divided into the following primary fractions: (1) base tar precipitate, (2) base/neutral organics, (3) acid tar precipitate, (4) acid organics, and (5) residual water. Furthermore, the base/neutral organics were divided into secondary fractions by using reverse-phase HPLC. Genotoxic tests were performed using Ames/*Salmonella* bioassays, Chinese hamster ovary (CHO) bioassays, and CHO photoactivation bioassays. Greater than 90% of the photoactive, genotoxic components partitioned into the base/neutral organics fraction, and two of the secondary HPLC fractions accounted for most of that activity. Several chemical classes including furans, furfurals, pyrazines, pyridines, ketones, and alkylated polynuclear aromatics may have contributed to the observed effects. These results contrast with acute toxicities observed in our laboratory for fish and invertebrates exposed to retort waters in which the hydrophilic fraction was most toxic.

### Aquatic Toxicity of Retort Waters

Geiger[4] tested fractions of oil-shale retort waters produced from the following three processes: Omega-9, Geokinetics-9, and Paraho 77-78. Waters were fractionated by Dr. Rodney Skogerboe, Colorado State University (CSU), using column chromatography separations modified from Leenheer and Huffman (Figure 2).[14] Basically, the four primary fractions separated were hydrophilic organics and all inorganics, hydrophobic organic bases, hydrophobic organic acids, and hydrophobic neutral organics. Each of the first three fractions was collected as four sequential subfractions that eluted from the column; the hydrophobic neutral fraction was collected as two subfractions. Additionally, subsamples of the first two hydrophilic subfractions were vacuum stripped to remove ammonia and other volatile inorganics and organics. All fractions were analyzed at CSU to determine concentrations of inorganic compounds and total organic carbon (TOC).

Toxicity tests were conducted for 24 h at 23°C to determine $LC_{50}$ values. For each subfraction, fathead minnow *(Pimephales promelas)* neonate larvae and *Daphnia pulicaria* adults were exposed to several dilutions of

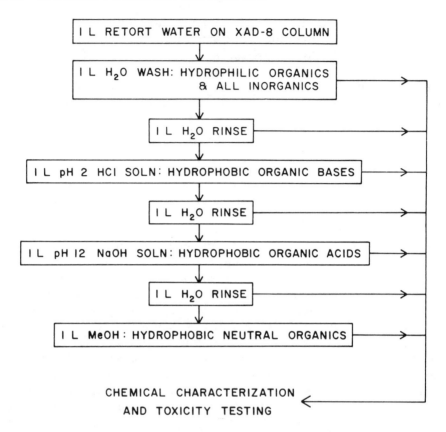

**Figure 2.** Method used to separate fractions of Omega-9, Geokinetics-9, and Paraho 77-78 oil-shale retort waters for toxicity testing (modified from Reference 14).

the subfraction and to a well-water control. Additional methanol controls were tested to evaluate contributions of the methanol carrier solvent to the observed toxicity in the hydrophobic neutral subfractions.

Results of fractional toxicity tests using fathead minnows appear in Figure 3. Also depicted for comparison are ammonia and TOC concentrations of each subfraction. Based on the chemistry and toxicity data collected, it can be concluded that:[4]

1.  Hydrophilic fractions of all three retort waters were the most toxic in acute tests.
2.  Ammonia contributed to hydrophilic fraction toxicities for all three retort waters.
3.  Other major and trace inorganics also contributed to hydrophilic fraction toxicities.

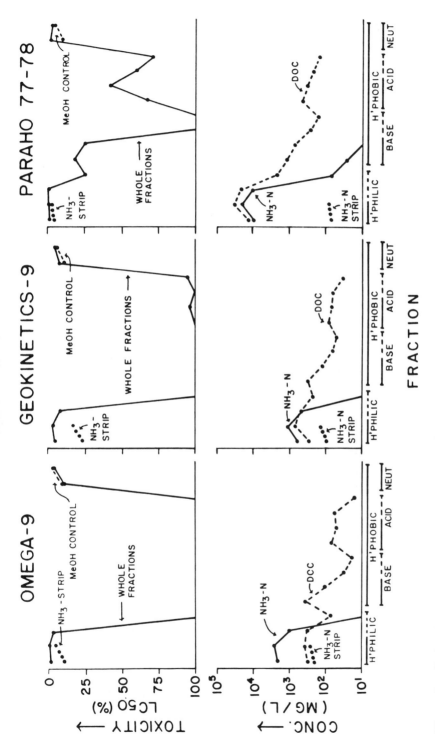

**Figure 3.** Fathead minnow 24-h toxicities and concentrations of ammonia and total organic carbon for Omega-9, Geokinetics-9, and Paraho 77-78 oil-shale retort water fractions.

4. Methanol carrier solvent contributed most of the observed toxicity in the hydrophobic neutrals fraction.
5. Relative importance of ammonia toxicity in the hydrophilic fractions was Geokinetics-9 > Omega-9 > Paraho 77-78.
6. Relative importance of organic chemicals in causing toxicity was greater for Paraho 77-78 than either Omega-9 or Geokinetics-9.
7. Reduction of ammonia and organic compounds in oil-shale retort waters will reduce acute toxicity to aquatic biota.
8. To more precisely identify toxic constituents in hydrophilic fractions, further fractionation and testing are required.

More specific conclusions concerning the organic compounds cannot be made until gas chromatography-mass spectrometry (GC-MS) analyses of these samples are available. Even then, results will be difficult to interpret for the hydrophobic neutral fractions, because the methanol carrier solvent contributed substantially to the observed toxicities.

This study and others noted above have demonstrated the apparent usefulness of fractional toxicity tests. Interestingly, the genotoxic activity tests performed by Strniste et al.[13] identified potential problems caused by organic neutrals in Paraho retort water, whereas Geiger's[4] fish and invertebrate tests implicated the hydrophilic fraction. Obviously, the same compounds that caused acute toxicity would not necessarily cause mutagenesis or carcinogenesis. However, this dichotomy widens the scope of the chemical and biological tests that are necessary and presents several problems that must be addressed in future fractional toxicity testing.

### Problems

Parkhurst[8] discussed several procedural problems that must be pursued to further refine fractional toxicity testing, but three major problems beyond those identified by Parkhurst are apparent from studies conducted to date: (1) carrier solvents can contribute to observed toxicities and confound interpretation of results; (2) few tests have been extended beyond primary fractions, and individual or small groups of toxic compounds have not yet been isolated by the fractionation techniques; and (3) fractionation schemes are not being used beyond the research framework in which they were initially developed.

First, as noted above for the retort-water toxicity studies, carrier solvents, acids, and bases associated with fractionation processes are toxic. This often makes it difficult to separate the toxic contributions of compounds in the original sample from toxic contributions of the fractionation matrix. Acids and bases can be neutralized, but often this produces a high salt concentration in the neutralized fraction. Organic solvents can be evaporated, but often the organics in the fraction that do not evaporate with the carrier solvent are not soluble in water. Thus, these fractions (e.g., hydrophobic neutrals) must always be dissolved in a potentially toxic matrix. New fractionation approaches are needed to circumvent this problem, especially when testing relatively nontoxic whole waters and fractions.

Second, although the virtues of fractional toxicity testing have been extolled by almost all researchers who practice the art, few studies have tested more than a few primary fractions. Even when secondary fractions have been tested, they contained many classes of inorganic or organic compounds. In no case has anyone systematically adhered to sequential fractionation concepts and identified the principal toxic components of a complex chemical mixture using this procedure. Instead, educated guesses have been professed based on results of primary fraction tests. Most likely, these conclusions could have been advanced before the fractions were tested, if analyses of only the major inorganic and organic compounds were available. Thus, fractional toxicity testing has added little to identifying principal toxic components in most studies to date.

This second problem probably results from a trade-off between costs and benefits. Of course, the concept of fractional toxicity testing is scientifically sound, but in many cases study designs cannot always adhere to theoretical procedures. Costs would expand dramatically if fractionation and testing were continued all the way to individual or small groups of toxic chemicals. That procedure might still be more cost effective than testing every major chemical in the mixture, but saving money by only testing the primary fractions often raises as many questions as it resolves. The time, effort, and cost associated with fractional toxicity testing must be decreased considerably, or investigators will continue to conduct only research fractionation studies on relatively few complex chemical mixtures.

Finally, no one in industry appears to be using fractional toxicity to test potential or existing synfuel-related products and waters. Beyond the time, effort, and expense constraints noted above, this last problem probably exists because no one has interpreted the fractions in terms of feasible treatment methods. Of course, hydrophilic/hydrophobic separations can be related to adsorption treatment technology, and acid/base/neutral functional separations can be related to ion exchange treatments. But, the oil-shale industry is pursuing its own treatment processes without consulting fractional toxicity test results. Steam stripping appears to be a requisite first step for treating gas condenser waters. For retort waters, oil separation and sand filtering may precede steam stripping. Following these treatments, activated carbon adsorption, reverse osmosis, or biological treatment (activated sludge) may be employed. To provide more useful results, fractionation procedures should be designed similar to treatment methods most likely to be used by industry.

### Directions

Future research should address fractional toxicity of complex chemical mixtures in a new light. Whenever possible, the product or wastewater should be tested after a fraction has been removed, rather than testing the removed fraction. This should avoid problems associated with testing fractions contained in a toxic chemical matrix. In cooperation with the U.S. Environmental Protection Agency's Environmental Research Laboratory-Duluth, we are currently developing such a subtractive fractionation technique, as opposed to traditional isolative fractionations. We are using column chromatography methods similar to Leenheer,[15] but results are only preliminary. Isolated fractions are still valuable in this scheme, for only through chemical analyses of the compounds retained on columns can we identify compounds responsible for observed toxicity decreases. Additionally, these analyses are necessary to determine further subfractionation strategies.

Perhaps fractional toxicity results could be interpreted more usefully by using alternative fractionation methods. Specifically, we suggest that the following separations might provide more-useful information when treatment recommendations are the objective of fractional toxicity testing:

1.  Volatiles: vacuum stripping; head space analysis by GC-MS would identify the volatilized fraction.
2.  Carbon adsorbers: batch extraction or column chromatography with activated carbon; solvent extraction and GC-MS would identify the adsorbed fraction.
3.  Permeables: dialysis with an appropriate membrane; direct analysis of the dialysate would identify the impermeable fraction.
4.  Ion exchangeables: anion and cation exchange; acid or base elution followed by organic and inorganic analyses would identify the exchangeable fraction.
5.  Biodegradables: a fraction that might be technologically meaningful, but would be difficult to control; constituents in degraded fractions could only be identified by before-and-after comparisons of the water.

Of course, these fractions could be removed sequentially from complex mixtures, or they could be removed in separate experiments to interpret potential treatment effectiveness. Individual compounds still would not be isolated using only these primary separations, but the results would be more useful to industry. If necessary, detailed chemical analyses could be performed to identify the individual compounds and compound classes in the fractions.

## BIOACCUMULATION

### Previous Studies

Bioaccumulation of organic compounds in fish and other aquatic organisms has been studied extensively. In addition to determining realized bioconcentration factors (BCFs) for many individual chemicals, researchers have also developed correlations that use surrogate physical and chemical properties of organics to predict potential bioaccumulation of untested compounds (e.g., octanol-water partitioning and reverse-phase HPLC retention).[16] For some organics, uptake and depuration rates have been determined in short-term exposures and used to predict steady-state bioconcentration factors.[17–18]

Not all organic compounds bioaccumulate as intensively as predicted from partition coefficients. For example, Southworth et al.[19] demonstrated that expected bioconcentration factors of azaarenes were as much as an order of magnitude higher than realized bioconcentration. Fish metabolized these compounds rapidly and thus decreased the steady-state tissue burdens below predicted values. In fact, metabolites of dibenz($a,h$)acridine accumulated four times greater than did the parent compound. This suggests that metabolites of some environmental contaminants may pose greater bioaccumulation hazards than the original compounds if they are not rapidly excreted. More importantly, these metabolites and their effects cannot yet be evaluated using traditional physical-chemical screening procedures for organic compounds.

Relatively little is known about bioaccumulation of organic compounds from chemical mixtures, even though aquatic organisms are seldom, if ever, exposed to only one chemical at a time in natural systems. One approach for predicting bioaccumulation from mixtures is to identify all organics present and use single-compound correlations. However, as discussed above and as demonstrated in exposures to two-compound mixtures,[20] these predictions are not always reliable.

An alternate approach is to expose organisms to a chemical mixture and then identify compounds that accumulate in their tissues.[21] This approach accounts for parent compounds and persistent metabolites, and results can be correlated with individual chemicals in the exposure water. Several researchers have demonstrated this technique for water-soluble extracts of petroleum products accumulated by marine organisms.[22–28] In general, they used GC-MS techniques to identify major alkane and aromatic organics. No attempt was made to calculate bioconcentration factors or to compare predicted and realized bioaccumulation.

Except for a few experiments involving exposures to mixtures of two pesticides,[29–31] bioaccumulation of chemical mixtures by freshwater organisms has been ignored. Consequently, there is almost no information available concerning potential bioaccumulation hazards of synfuel-related waters or water-soluble fractions from synfuel products. In the following section we present preliminary results of bioaccumulation from an oil-shale retort water.

### Bioaccumulation of Retort Water Constituents

We performed two preliminary bioaccumulation experiments using Occidental-6 retort water. These studies were designed to accomplish three objectives:

1.  test whether BCFs of an organic compound are similar when fish are exposed in retort water and in single-compound experiments,
2.  determine uptake and depuration kinetics during these exposures, and
3.  identify whether organic compounds in retort water accumulate at relatively high concentrations in fish.

For the first experiment, rainbow trout were exposed for 3 d to [14]C-anthracene alone and to [14]C-anthracene dosed in a sublethal concentration of Occidental-6 retort water. Following this exposure period, fish were transferred to clean water for an additional 6 d to monitor depuration. Fish and water samples were analyzed during the uptake and clearance phases of the study to determine concentrations of anthracene and its metabolites.[5]

Although this was only a short-term experiment in which steady-state accumulation was not attained, considerable differences occurred during the uptake phase. Specifically, anthracene BCFs in retort water exposures were 45 and 25% less than in anthracene alone after 2 and 3 d exposure respectively (Figure 4). Based on subsequent calculations of uptake and depuration rates, this phenomenon was caused by lower uptake rates in the retort water. Depuration rates were essentially identical for the two exposures. These results suggest there may be important competition for carriers that transport PAH from adsorption sites (e.g., gill) to tissue storage and processing sites (e.g., liver).[5] Metabolic enzyme systems apparently were not induced rapidly enough by the additional organics in retort water to increase the anthracene depuration rate during these relatively short exposures.

In the second experiment, rainbow trout were exposed to sublethal concentrations of Occidental-6 retort water for 15 weeks. Whole fish, livers, and bile were analyzed at 1, 3, 6, 9, 12, and 15 weeks. Whole fish and livers were extracted using exhaustive steam distillation; bile was only deproteinized. These samples were then analyzed using reverse-phase HPLC gra-

**Figure 4.** Bioaccumulation of [14]C-anthracene by rainbow trout in single-compound exposure and in Occidental-6 oil-shale retort water.

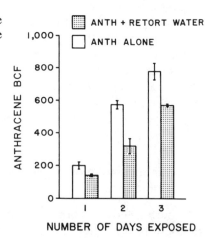

dients to identify accumulated compounds.[5] Peaks appearing in exposed fish but not in controls were compared to the retort water chromatogram [Figure 1(c)] to attempt to identify parent peaks. Because a relatively low sensitivity was used for the UV detector, most organics would not have been detected unless their concentrations were greater than 1 to 5 mg/kg in the whole-fish samples.

Figure 5 illustrates typical chromatograms for whole-fish extracts during the first 3 weeks of this experiment. Only one unique peak was detected in exposed fish, and its retention time (approximately 16 min) occurred between the retention times for phenol and benzene. After 3 weeks no differences were observed between exposed and control whole fish, even though detector sensitivity was increased 10-fold for these chromatograms (i.e., approximately 0.1 to 0.5 mg/kg detectable). This suggests that metabolic and depuration enzyme systems (e.g., mixed function oxygenases) may have been induced after 3 weeks of exposure to retort water.

After 6 weeks, differences between exposed and control chromatograms were observed for both liver and bile extracts. For example, Figure

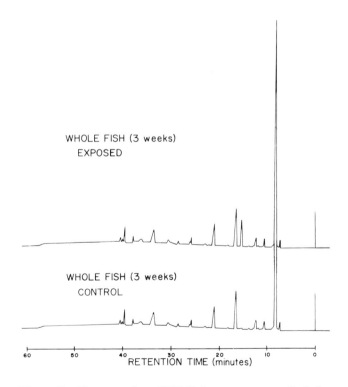

**Figure 5.** Reverse-phase HPLC chromatograms of whole-fish extracts after 3-week exposure to Occidental-6 oil-shale retort water.

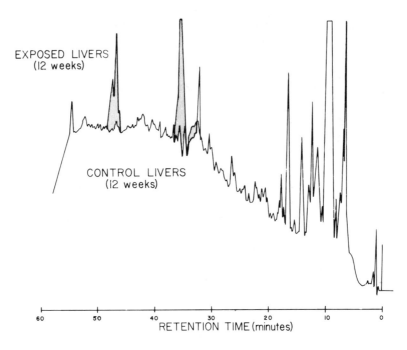

**Figure 6.** Reverse-phase HPLC chromatogram of liver extracts after 12-week exposure to Occidental-6 oil-shale retort water. Stipled areas indicate peaks that were present in exposed liver but not in control liver chromatograms.

6 shows several unique peaks with long retention times in an exposed liver extract at 12 weeks. These peaks may represent high-molecular-weight parent compounds, metabolites, or cellular macromolecules induced by exposure to the retort water. We have not yet attempted to characterize these chromatographic peaks and determine their sources.

In the 12-week chromatogram of exposed bile (Figure 7), at least three distinct peaks appeared at retention times of approximately 16 min. Since these peaks had nearly the same retention time as the peak identified in the whole-fish chromatograms, and since the bile peaks first appeared when the whole-fish peak disappeared, we suspect that the bile peaks are related to this initial peak in the whole fish. If so, then the phenomenon we observed was caused by an initial high concentration of parent compound or intermediate metabolite in the whole fish, followed by transport to the bile and rapid elimination from the fish after 3 weeks of exposure. Again, we have not yet characterized these peaks. However, candidate compounds include phenolic parent compounds or hydroxylated dicyclic and tricyclic aromatics.

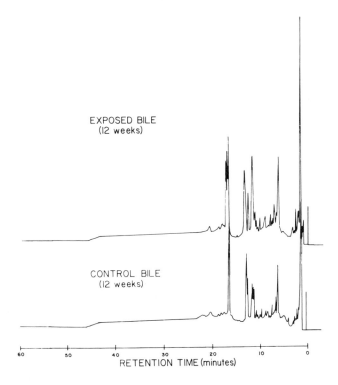

EXPOSED BILE
(I2 weeks)

CONTROL BILE
(I2 weeks)

60      50      40      30      20      10      0
RETENTION TIME (minutes)

**Figure 7.**  Reverse-phase HPLC chromatograms of bile extracts after 12-week exposure to Occidental-6 oil-shale retort water.

## Problems

Quick screening procedures are useful for determining whether complex chemical mixtures pose potential bioaccumulation hazards. For the retort water sample discussed in the previous section, only one chromatographic peak was detected at tissue levels greater than approximately 1 to 5 mg/kg. Whether this peak contained one or several organic compounds, it disappeared after 3 weeks of exposure to Occidental-6. Thus, no compounds that could be detected by UV absorbance were accumulated at relatively high concentrations in fish tissue during long-term exposures. Unfortunately, at this detection limit some PAH (e.g., pyrene, benzo(*a*)pyrene) would have required BCFs greater than 10,000 (mg/kg/mg/L) to have been detected on these chromatograms.

In defense of this relatively high detection limit, the U.S. Food and Drug Administration (FDA) has used 1 ppm (mg/kg) residue concentration as an arbitrary undesirable level not to be exceeded for human consumption.[32] However, these relatively high residue concentrations should only be used as a quick screening criterion in the early tiers of a hazard assessment. More sensitive analyses will be necessary when additional testing in a hazard assessment hierarchy is justified or when concentrations of individual compounds are required.

There are still many problems associated with the prediction and identification of potential bioaccumulation hazards in complex chemical mixtures. First, biologically active compounds can present hazards to human and aquatic organism health at concentrations lower than the arbitrary FDA Action Limits. More-sensitive detection limits than this are advisable for bioaccumulation studies in hazard assessments; however, as detector sensitivity increases, the number of identifiable compounds also increases. For some complex mixtures, this will require extensive and costly analyses to identify each compound. Moreover, this will create a problem for interpreting the potential biological effects of these compounds, many of which may not have been tested before. Obviously, sensitive detectors are needed for bioaccumulation studies, but sensible criteria should be chosen so that complex effluent hazard assessments do not become unmanageable.

Second, HPLC detection systems only record a portion of the organic compounds that occur in synfuel-related waters. Vassilaros et al.[33] discussed these problems and demonstrated how gas chromatography and capillary GC-MS systems can be used to detect PAH, PASH (polyaromatic sulfur heterocycles), and PANH (polyaromatic nitrogen heterocycles) at concentrations less than 1 ppb ($\mu$g/kg) in fish tissue. However, reverse-phase HPLC gradients will still provide useful information concerning relative polarity and relative bioaccumulation potential for organic compounds in complex chemical mixtures.[21] Only a combination of several analytical techniques will supply enough information to evaluate potential bioaccumulation hazards in synfuel-related waters and other complex chemical mixtures.

Third, bioaccumulation kinetics change during exposures to single compounds and chemical mixtures. Mixed function oxygenases, enzyme systems that control metabolism of organic compounds, require variable exposure periods for induction in cold-water fishes.[34-35] For example, Payne and Penrose[34] observed significant increases of liver enzyme activities within 17 d using brown trout *(Salmo trutta)* exposed to a crude oil. This lag period probably accounted for the initial accumulation of a contaminant peak followed by its disappearance in whole-fish samples after 3 weeks of exposure to Occidental-6 retort water. Thus, bioaccumulation can differ considerably between short-term and long-term exposures; not all bioaccumulation curves increase monotonically as exposure time increases. It is important to design bioaccumulation experiments considering potential exposure durations for the aquatic organisms at risk and to monitor bioaccumulation throughout the exposure period if short-term exposures are of concern.

Finally, little is known about the effects of complex mixtures on the bioaccumulation of individual organic compounds. From the few studies reported,[5,29-31] it appears that BCFs in fish decrease by at most a factor of 2 when other organic compounds are present. Additional bioaccumulation tests exposing invertebrates and fish to a range of inorganic and organic synthetic mixtures and industrial effluents spiked with radiolabeled organics will be necessary to correlate realized and potential bioaccumulation. If predicted BCFs do not differ from realized BCFs by more than a factor of 5 to 10, then single-compound bioaccumulation predictions will also be valid for chemical mixtures. Otherwise, mixtures will have to be tested on a case-by-case basis to determine potential bioaccumulation hazards.

## BIODEGRADATION

### Previous Studies

Bacterial degradation of organic compounds has been studied intensively for many years (e.g., see References 36 and 37). In fact, biodegradation test methods and predictive models for bacterial transformation of pollutants have been incorporated into several aquatic ecosystem hazard assessments (see Reference 38). Unfortunately, most bacterial degradation studies have focused on single compounds rather than chemical mixtures. Degradability of mixtures is often difficult to predict on a chemical-by-chemical basis be-cause interactions of organic compounds influence the degradative fate of the individual chemicals.[39] Thus, bacterial degradation of complex mixtures must be approached differently from single compounds.

Despite an emphasis in the literature on single-compound studies, some effort has been devoted to investigating the microbial degradation of petro-leum hydrocarbons associated with oil spills (see review by Atlas[40]). Two important processes that must be considered for these complex organic mix-tures are cooxidation and sparing (diauxie). These processes increase and decrease degradation rates, respectively, compared to rates predicted from single-compound tests. Although a number of rate-limiting factors for oil-spill degradation have been elucidated, the interactions of microorganisms, oil, and environment are still not completely understood.[40]

Even less is known about bacterial degradation of synfuel-related waters. Activated sludge processes have been investigated as potential treatment methods for retort waters,[41-42] but bacterial processing usually follows sev-eral preliminary treatment steps that remove some retort-water components. For example, Torpy et al.[41] steam-stripped Occidental-6 retort water, added phosphorus, and lowered the pH using sulfuric acid before evaluating acti-vated sludge treatment efficiency. They reported that carboxylic acids are readily biodegraded, but several refractory compound classes, including ox-ygenated nitrogen heterocyclics, were not transformed.

Regarding environmental transformations, Williams and coworkers[43] have investigated interactions of soil microorganisms with Omega-9 retort water. Additionally, Gauger[44] reported dissolved organic carbon degradation in retort waters by indigenous bacteria. However, both studies emphasized taxonomy of the bacteria and biological effects caused by retort water, rather than the effects of bacteria on retort-water composition. To more adequately address environmental fate in aquatic systems, we have monitored changes in retort-water composition. In the following section we present results for a laboratory screening method that characterizes bacterial degradation of retort waters exposed to a variety of bacterial inocula.

### Degradation of Retort Waters

To screen complex chemical mixtures for potentially persistent compounds, we use an approach similar to that described for bioaccumulation.[21] Essentially, bacteria degrade easily transformed compounds and thus isolate persistent organics. Compounds that only slowly degrade remain as unchanged peaks on an HPLC chromatogram, whereas persistent metabolites appear as new chromatographic peaks. An important advantage of this approach is that interactions between mixture constituents that might not be predicted from results of single-compound studies are integrated by testing the whole mixture.

All four of the oil-shale retort waters discussed above have been tested in our biodegradation screening system under various experimental conditions. Basically, we conduct two types of experiments. In the first, retort water and bacteria from an oil refinery settling pond are added to a modified basal salts medium[45] contained in 250-mL Erlenmeyer flasks. Flasks are incubated at 25°C under continuous light in the laboratory for up to 20 weeks. We compare chromatograms of control flasks (no bacterial inoculum) and treatments to determine which groups of compounds are slowly degraded under these relatively ideal conditions. Details of these experiments are described by Bergman et al.[3]

Results of preliminary studies for Omega-9 and Geokinetics-9 waters showed similar trends. Briefly, many chromatographic peaks migrated and disappeared, indicating that these compounds were readily degraded. However, other compounds persisted after 20 weeks, suggesting they would be difficult to degrade even in activated sludge treatments. A more complete discussion of these results appears in Reference 3.

The second type of screening experiment is designed to provide information that can be more easily interpreted for environmental hazard assessments. For this scenario, we have degraded Occidental-6 and Paraho 77-78 retort waters using "best-case," "intermediate-case," and "worst-case" bacterial inocula. Best-case degradation is simulated by adding retort water to oil refinery settling pond water; intermediate-case degradation is mimicked by adding retort water to Laramie River water collected directly below a wood-treating plant in Laramie, Wyoming; and worst-case degradation is represented by adding retort water to Laramie River water collected 44 km upstream from Laramie in a relatively pristine ranching valley.

All retort waters are diluted 1:9 with bacterial inoculum (oil refinery settling pond water, downstream river water, or upstream river water) and placed in 250-mL Erlenmeyer flasks. We do not add nutrients or adjust the pH of these inocula. Treatments are continuously shaken at approximately 25°C under a 16-h light/8-h dark photoperiod. Control flasks contain identical retort water and inoculum additions but are stored at 4°C in the dark. After 125 d, flask contents are filtered and injected into an HPLC for reverse-phase gradient analyses.[3]

To evaluate alterations in organic constituents, we superimpose chromatograms for paired treatment and control flasks on a light table. Then we prepare interpretive tracings that indicate where the chromatograms differ. Figures 8(a) and (b) illustrate results for Occidental-6 and Paraho 77-78 degraded by oil refinery settling-pond bacteria. Due to the density of peaks during the first 15 min of the chromatograms and the difficulty of interpreting chromatographic changes in this region of relatively polar compounds, we have omitted the first 15 min of the gradients from these tracings.

In Figures 8(a) and (b), black areas indicate peaks that were present in refrigerated controls but not in treatment flasks after 125 d; unmarked peaks were present in control and treatment flasks. In other words, black peaks represent compounds that were degraded or otherwise altered in treatment flasks. Although in other tests we have observed potentially recalcitrant metabolites in an oil-shale condenser water, as indicated by peaks present in the treatment but not in the control, we did not observe any apparent metabolites for the retort waters reported here.

Chromatograms for treatments inoculated with oil refinery settling pond water showed the most obvious changes in retort-water composition. Numbers of peaks and peak heights were not reduced as much in downstream Laramie River water inocula and were reduced the least of all three treatments in upstream Laramie River water inocula. These results support the hypothesis that gradients of degradation can be expected in natural aquatic systems, depending on upstream anthropogenic activity. Under favorable conditions, considerable degradation of organic compounds will occur, but in relatively pristine waters, little or no bacterial degradation may be expected.

Although we did not characterize persistent peaks in the treatment chromatograms, our qualitative results agree with the conclusions of activated sludge treatments conducted by Torpy et al.[41] First, many organic compounds in retort water are readily biodegraded, yet some appear to be recalcitrant. This is probably an effect of sparing (diauxie), a bacterial process by which some organic compounds are preferentially metabolized.[39]

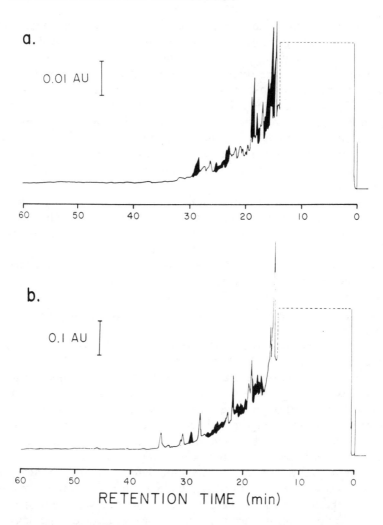

**Figure 8.** Interpretive tracings of 125-d reverse-phase HPLC chromatograms for oil-shale retort waters degraded by oil refinery settling pond bacteria: (a) Occidental-6; (b) Paraho 77-78. Black areas denote peaks that were present in control flasks but not in treatments, indicating that these compounds were degraded by the bacteria. (Note that the Paraho 77-78 chromatogram is 0.1 × the sensitivity of the Occidental-6 chromatogram).

The apparently recalcitrant organics would normally be degraded in single-compound exposures but are not metabolized because of the presence of preferred substrates in the mixture.

Second, retort-water organics throughout the polarity range of our chromatographic gradients were degraded by experimental treatments. This indicates that there is no polarity range above which or below which degradation of process water constituents is prevented. More likely, as Torpy et al.[41] noted, certain classes of organic compounds are more resistant to bacterial transformation because of unique chemical structures and not because of their relative polarity.

Eventually, all organic compounds derived from fossil fuels can be expected to degrade, but an important consideration is whether they degrade rapidly or slowly in natural aquatic systems. The screening method described above can be used to evaluate potential hazards associated with complex chemical mixture discharges and to predict expected exposure concentrations for use in environmental hazard assessments. Predictions based on single-compound degradation kinetics may overestimate or underestimate degradation of mixtures, thus they may not be reliable for predicting the environmental fate of synfuel-related waters.

## Problems

Extrapolating from laboratory results to field conditions poses three problems for biodegradation screening: (1) selecting representative bacterial inocula, (2) evaluating appropriate environmental parameters, and (3) interpreting the observed degradation kinetics.

The first problem can be most readily approached for site-specific assessments by testing potential receiving waters with no supplemental nutrient or bacterial additions. For more generic assessments, a range of potential degradation scenarios can be tested. As we demonstrated in the studies reported above, results may vary from almost no degradation in pristine waters to relatively rapid degradation by bacterial populations acclimated to organic compounds. Since only qualitative results will be generated from these generic tests, professional judgment must be used in assessing the potential persistence hazards.

Although we did not vary experimental conditions in the studies reported above, temperature and aeration gradients might provide important information for extrapolation to field conditions. Other potentially important experimental variables include light intensity and dilution ratio of the mixture, if relatively high concentrations are tested.

And finally, the rates of degradation observed in laboratory studies must be extrapolated cautiously to field conditions. To this end, field validation of laboratory results should be a high priority for future biodegradation studies with complex mixtures. Without solid correlations between laboratory and field studies, hazard assessment screening strategies will not be reliable.

For most degradation studies of complex mixtures, persistent chromatographic peaks must be chemically characterized to identify problem compounds and classes of compounds. Innovative analytical approaches other than GC-MS have been used to monitor degradation of petroleum oils.[46] Rapid scanning approaches that obviate the time and expense of GC-MS analyses might be useful for observing disappearance of chemical classes during the early stages of bacterial degradation.

## CONCLUSIONS

We believe that the most cost-effective approach to evaluate environmental fate-and-effects problems of complex chemical mixtures is to use biological responses and transformation processes for identifying problem compounds. Analytical chemistry is an important component in this identification process but should be used as a monitoring technique rather than as a surrogate for predicting biological processes. This is the most important difference between our proposed hazard assessment strategy for complex mixtures[21] and strategies currently used for single compounds.[47,48]

Based on results of the tests reviewed here, we make the following recommendations:

1. Approaches to fractional toxicity testing should be reoriented to directly address reasonable treatment options. Although complex mixtures can theoretically be separated into individual compound classes, the time and expense of proceeding through several fractionation tiers will seldom be justified by the information gained. Instead, cost-effective fractionation strategies will mimic routinely used wastewater treatment processes such as steam stripping, carbon adsorption, and reverse osmosis. This approach may generate less toxicity information about individual compounds or compound classes but will provide potential users with much more useful information about potential treatment options.
2. Additional research is needed to determine whether bioaccumulation predictions based on single-compound studies and on physical-chemical properties of individual compounds are reliable for individual chemicals in complex mixtures.
3. For evaluating potential bioaccumulation hazards to aquatic organisms, more-sensitive detection limits than the current 1 mg/kg FDA Action Limit (based on safe human exposure levels) are needed. But as more residue chemicals are identified at lower concentrations in tissues, better correlations will have to be developed to interpret the biological significance of these residues.
4. Bacterial degradation of complex chemical mixtures is difficult to predict. Simple laboratory screening tests of whole mixtures provide useful qualitative information about potentially persistent organics. However, additional refinement of procedures and correlation with field validation tests will be necessary before laboratory data can be reliably extrapolated to field exposures.

## ACKNOWLEDGMENTS

Research described in this report was supported by a U.S. Environmental Protection Agency–U.S. Department of Energy Interagency Agreement under DOE Contract No. DE-AT20-80LC10402, and by U.S. Environmental Protection Agency–University of Wyoming Cooperative Agreement No. CR808671020. Deborah Sanchez assisted in many of the experiments; Rodney Johnson, Michael Parker, and Bryan Steadman provided valuable contributions. Since neither the U.S. Environmental Protection Agency nor the U.S. Department of Energy has reviewed this chapter, it does not necessarily reflect the views of either agency, and no endorsement should be inferred.

## REFERENCES

1. Fox, J.P., D.S. Farrier, and R.E. Poulson. "Chemical Characterization and Analytical Considerations for an In Situ Oil Shale Process Water," DOE LETC/RI-78/7 (Laramie, WY: Laramie Energy Technology Center, 1978).
2. Pellizzari, E.D. "Identification of Components of Energy-Related Wastes and Effluents," EPA-600/7-78-004 (Athens, GA: U.S. Environmental Protection Agency, 1978).
3. Bergman, H.L., et al. "Effects of Aqueous Effluents from In Situ Fossil Fuel Processing Technologies on Aquatic Systems, Annual Progress Report, 1 January–31 December 1979," DOE LETC/10058-T1 (Laramie, WY: Laramie Energy Technology Center, 1980).
4. Geiger, D.L. "Identification of Toxic Constituents of Oil Shale Retort Waters Using Chemical Fractionation and Toxicity Bioassays," M.S. Thesis, University of Wyoming, Laramie (1981).
5. Linder, G.L. "Anthracene Bioconcentration in Rainbow Trout in Single-compound and Complex Chemical Mixture Exposures," Ph.D. Thesis, University of Wyoming, Laramie (1982).
6. Skogerboe, R.K., M.M. Miller, and D.L. Dick. "Chemical Characterization of Oil Shale Retort Waters. Part I—Inorganic Constituents" (Fort Collins: Colorado State University, 1981).
7. Leenheer, J.A., T.I. Noyes, and H.A. Stuber. "Determination of Polar Organic Solutes in Oil Shale Retort Water," *Environ. Sci. Technol.* 16(10):714–723 (1982).
8. Parkhurst, B.R. "The Role of Fractionation in Hazard Assessments of Complex Materials," in *Environmental Hazard Assessment of Effluents,* H.L. Bergman, R.A. Kimberle, and A.W. Maki, Eds. (New York: Pergamon Press, in press).
9. Rubin, I.B., M.R. Guerin, A.A. Hardigree, and J.L. Epler. "Fractionation of Synthetic Crude Oils from Coal for Biological Testing," *Environ. Res.* 12:358–365 (1976).
10. Pelroy, R.A. "The Mutagenic and Chemical Properties of SRC-I Materials: A Status Report," PNL-3604 (Richland, WA: Battelle Pacific Northwest Laboratory, 1981).
11. Pelroy, R.A., and B.W. Wilson. "Fractional Distillation as a Strategy for

Reducing the Genotoxic Potential of SRC-II Coal Liquids: A Status Report," PNL-3787 (Richland, WA: Battelle Pacific Northwest Laboratory, 1981).

12. Wilson, B.W., R.A. Pelroy, and D.D. Mahlum. "Chemical Characterization and Genotoxic Potential Related to Boiling Point for Fractionally Distilled SRC-I Coal Liquids," PNL-4277 (Richland, WA: Battelle Pacific Northwest Laboratory, 1982).

13. Strniste, G.F., J.M. Bingham, W.D. Spall, J.W. Nickols, R.T. Okinaka, and D. J-C. Chen. "Fractionation of an Oil Shale Retort Process Water: Isolation of Photoactive Genotoxic Components," presented at the Symposium on the Application of Short-term Bioassays in the Analysis of Complex Environmental Mixtures, Chapel Hill, NC, Jan. 25–27, 1982.

14. Leenheer, J.A., and E.W.D. Huffman. "Analytical Method for Dissolved-Organic Carbon Fractionation," Water-Resources Investigations 79-4 (Lakewood, CO: U.S. Geological Survey, 1979).

15. Leenheer, J.A. "Comprehensive Approach to Preparative Isolation and Fractionation of Dissolved Organic Carbon from Natural Waters and Wastewaters," *Environ. Sci. Technol.* 15(5):578–587 (1981).

16. Veith, G.D., N.M. Austin, and R.T. Morris. "A Rapid Method for Estimating log P for Organic Chemicals," *Water Res.* 13:43–47 (1979).

17. Hamelink, J.L. "Current Bioconcentration Test Methods and Theory," in *Aquatic Toxicology and Hazard Evaluation* ASTM STP 634, F.L. Mayer and J.L. Hamelink, Eds. (Philadelphia: American Society for Testing and Materials, 1977), pp. 149–161.

18. Neely, W.B. *Chemicals in the Environment* (New York: Marcel Dekker, Inc., 1980).

19. Southworth, G.R., C.C. Keffer, and J.J. Beauchamp. "Potential and Realized Bioconcentration. A Comparison of Observed and Predicted Bioconcentration of Azaarenes in the Fathead Minnow *(Pimephales promelas),*" *Environ. Sci. Technol.* 14(12):1529–1531.

20. Bergman, H.L., and J.S. Meyer. "Complex Effluent Fate Modeling," in *Modeling the Fate of Chemicals in the Aquatic Environment*, K.L. Dickson, A.W. Maki, and J. Cairns, Jr., Eds. (Ann Arbor, MI: Ann Arbor Science Publishers, Inc., 1982), pp. 247–267.

21. Bergman, H.L., G.M. DeGraeve, J.S. Meyer, M.D. Marcus, and D.L. Geiger. "Aquatic Ecosystem Hazard Assessment of Underground Coal Gasification Process Waters," in *Proceedings of The Twentieth Hanford Life Sciences Symposium on Coal Conversion and the Environment: Chemical, Biomedical, and Ecological Considerations*, D.D. Mahlum, R.H. Gray, and W.D. Felix, Eds. Richland, WA, Oct. 19–23, 1980, pp. 270–293.

22. Clark, R.C., Jr., and J.S. Finley. "Analytical Techniques for Isolating and Quantifying Petroleum Paraffin Hydrocarbons in Marine Organisms," in *Marine Pollution Monitoring (Petroleum)*, Special Publication 409. (Washington, DC: National Bureau of Standards, 1974), pp. 209–212.

23. Clark, R.C., Jr., J.S. Finley, and G.G. Gibson. "Acute Effects of Outboard Motor Oil Effluent on Two Marine Shellfish," *Environ. Sci. Technol.* 8(12):1009–1014 (1974).

24. Clark, R.C., Jr., and J.S. Finley. "Uptake and Loss of Petroleum Hydrocarbons by the Mussel, *Mytilus edulis,* in Laboratory Experiments," *Fish. Bull.* 73:508–515 (1975).

25. Cox, B.A., J.W. Anderson, and J.C. Parker. "An Experimental Oil Spill: The Distribution of Aromatic Hydrocarbons in the Water, Sediment, and Animal Tissues within a Shrimp Pond," in *Protection and Control of Oil Pollution.* (Washington, DC: American Petroleum Institute, 1975), pp. 607–612.

26. Parker, P.L., K. Winters, C. Van Baalen, J.C. Batterton, and R.S. Scalan. "Petroleum Pollution: Chemical Characteristics and Biological Effects," in *Sources, Effects and Sinks of Hydrocarbons in the Aquatic Environment.* (Washington, DC: American Petroleum Institute, 1976), pp. 256–269.

27. Teal, J.M. "Hydrocarbon Uptake by Deep Sea Benthos," in *Sources, Effects and Sinks of Hydrocarbons in the Aquatic Environment.* (Washington, DC: American Petroleum Institute, 1976), pp. 358–372.

28. Malins, D.C., and H.O. Hodgins. "Petroleum and Marine Fishes: A Review of Uptake, Disposition and Effects," *Environ. Sci. Technol.* 15(11):1272–1278 (1981).

29. Reinert, R.E., L.J. Stone, and H.L. Bergman. "Dieldrin and DDT: Accumulation from Water and Food by Lake Trout *(Salvelinus namaycush)* in the Laboratory," *Proc. 17th Conf. Great Lakes Res.* 1974:52–58 (1974).

30. Matsumura, F. "Absorption, Accumulation, and Elimination of Pesticides by Aquatic Organisms," in *Pesticides in the Aquatic Environment,* M.A.Q. Khan, Ed. (New York: Academic Press, Inc., 1977), pp. 77–105.

31. Mac, M.J., and J.G. Seelye. "Potential Influence of Acetone in Aquatic Bioassays Testing the Dynamics and Effects of PCBs," *Bull. Environ. Contam. Toxicol.* 27:359–367 (1981).

32. Kimerle, R.A., W.J. Adams, and D.R. Grothe. "A Tiered Approach to Aquatic Safety Assessment of Effluents," in *Environmental Hazard Assessment of Effluents,* H.L. Bergman, R.A. Kimerle, and A.W. Maki, Eds. (New York: Pergamon Press, in press).

33. Vassilaros, D.L., P.W. Stoker, G.M. Booth, and M.L. Lee. "Capillary Gas Chromatographic Determination of Polycyclic Aromatic Compounds in Vertebrate Fish Tissue," *Anal. Chem.* 54(1):106–112.

34. Payne, J.F., and W.R. Penrose. "Induction of Aryl Hydrocarbon (Benzo[a]pyrene) Hydroxylase in Fish by Petroleum," *Bull. Environ. Contam. Toxicol.* 14(1):112–116 (1975).

35. Gerhart, E.H., and R.M. Carlson. "Hepatic Mixed-Function Oxidase Activity in Rainbow Trout Exposed to Several Polycyclic Aromatic Compounds," *Environ. Res.* 17:284–295 (1978).

36. ZoBell, C.E. "Action of Microorganisms on Hydrocarbons," *Bacteriol. Rev.* 10:1–49 (1946).

37. Dagley, S. "Catabolism of Aromatic Compounds by Microorganisms," *Adv. Micro. Physiol.* 6:1–46 (1971).

38. Maki, A.W., K.L. Dickson, and J. Cairns, Jr., Eds. *Biotransformation and Fate of Chemicals in the Aquatic Environment* (Washington, DC: American Society for Microbiology, 1980).

39. Atlas, R.M. "Microbial Degradation of Complex Mixtures of Organic Pollutants," in *Environmental Hazard Assessment of Effluents,* H.L. Bergman, R.A. Kimerle, and A.W. Maki, Eds. (New York: Pergamon Press, in press).

40. Atlas, R.M. "Microbial Degradation of Petroleum Hydrocarbons: An Environmental Perspective," *Microbiol. Rev.* 45:180–209 (1981).

41. Torpy, M.F., R.G. Luthy, and L.A. Raphaelian. "Activated-sludge Treatment

and Organic Characterization of Oil Shale Retort Water," in *Fifteenth Oil Shale Symposium Proceedings,* J.H. Gary, Ed. (Golden: Colorado School of Mines, 1982), pp. 487–493.

42.  Jones, B.M., R.H. Sakaji, and C.G. Daughton. "Physicochemical Treatment Methods for Oil Shale Wastewater: Evaluation as Aids to Biooxidation," in *Fifteenth Oil Shale Symposium Proceedings,* J.H. Gary, Ed. (Golden: Colorado School of Mines, 1982), pp. 581–597.

43.  Williams, S.E., W.K. Gauger, M. Christensen, R.P. Jones, B.R. DeVore, and D.S. Farrier. *Interactions of Soil Microorganisms with Aqueous Effluents Derived from In Situ Fossil Fuel Technologies—A Preliminary Report* (Laramie: University of Wyoming, 1979).

44.  Gauger, W.K. "Dissolved Organic Carbon Degradation in Oil Shale Retort Waters by Indigenous Bacteria," Ph.D. Thesis, University of Wyoming, Laramie (1981).

45.  Fannin, T.E., M.D. Marcus, D.A. Anderson, and H.L. Bergman. "Use of a Fractional Factorial Design to Evaluate Interactions of Environmental Factors Affecting Biodegradation Rates," *Appl. Environ. Microbiol.* 42(6):936–943 (1981).

46.  Petrakis, L., D.M. Jewell, and W.F. Benusa. "Analytical Chemistry of Petroleum: An Overview of Practices in Petroleum Industry Laboratories with Emphasis on Biodegradation," in *Petroleum in the Marine Environment,* L. Petrakis and F.T. Weiss, Eds. (Washington, DC: American Chemical Society, 1980), pp. 23–53.

47.  Cairns, J., Jr., K.L. Dickson, and A.W. Maki, Eds. *Estimating the Hazard of Chemical Substances to Aquatic Life* (Philadelphia: American Society for Testing and Materials, 1978).

48.  Dickson, K.L., A.W. Maki, and J. Cairns, Jr., Eds. *Analyzing the Hazard Evaluation Process* (Washington, DC: American Fisheries Society, 1979).

## DISCUSSION

*J.L. Epler, Oak Ridge National Laboratory:* In defense of the work that has been done in rather sophisticated fractionation, one of the key reasons for the effort was that the biological endpoints themselves were not discernible because of the overall toxicity of the material. A fractionation procedure was necessary to remove the toxicity so you could look at your genetic endpoints. Perhaps it has been fortuitous that it has permitted us to identify so many of the actual biologically active components.

*J.S. Meyer:* I agree. I could have included several qualifications, especially for genotoxic or carcinogenic studies. Fractional toxicity may be the way to go because of the problems that Jim talked about.

*M. Uziel, Oak Ridge National Laboratory:* The question of persistent chemicals has been approached at the mechanistic level also, and in many of the studies they find very few persistent derivatives, for example, attached to DNA. For those chemicals that do not leave a residue during their metabolism and disappearance, how do you propose to determine their contribution to this problem? In other words, they disappear in a short period and do not accumulate, but their effects do remain in that the tissues have been affected during the period of metabolism.

*J.S. Meyer:* That would have to be an integrated biological assessment, in which you examine your fish more closely. When we do a long-term exposure, we not only look at the concentrations in the fish, but we also include biochemical and histopathology studies and look for biochemical effects of the long-term exposure. It would be difficult and expensive to worry about every compound out of the hundreds of organics in one complex mixture. I believe it is important initially to look for effects and later, if we have the luxury, to find out what mechanism is involved. I think to solve problems, we have to be satisfied at this time with less detailed information about what is occurring.

*M. Uziel:* I believe there is an inherent assumption here that all retort waters will respond and give the same kind of responses so that you don't have to do all these detailed analyses that you are going to do on every separate retort or every separate water sample. Is that correct? In other words, are you going to have to treat each one separately and independently through the entire procedure?

*J.S. Meyer:* We must establish a data base for chronic effects, including both bioaccumulation and biodegradation, to the extent that it is established for acute toxicity. We can make generalizations about retort waters, but at present we don't know enough about long-term exposures and we believe these fate-and-effect studies should be emphasized.

*M.E. Frazier, Pacific Northwest Laboratory:* While I clearly see the value of these kinds of fish studies, it seems that to underemphasize the chemistry may lead to subsequent repetition each time you get a different retort water. If you have the chemistry as you go, you can make predictions. Further, you are making the assumption that fish reflect everything in the aquatic environment, and you have only one species. In the radiation situation, we found that if you look at only one species and you don't look at causes and chemical constituents, you have to go through the same laborious and costly experiments each time. I believe that adequate chemistry is important.

# CHAPTER 16

## Structure-Activity Relationships: Their Function in Biological Prediction

### T.W. Schultz
*College of Veterinary Medicine*
*University of Tennessee*
*Knoxville, TN 37901*

### L.B. Kier
*Medical College of Virginia*
*Virginia Commonwealth University*
*Richmond, VA 23298*

### J.N. Dumont
*Oak Ridge National Laboratory*
*Oak Ridge, TN 37831*

Quantitative structure-activity relationships provide a means of ranking or predicting biological effects based on chemical structure. For each compound used to formulate a structure activity model, two kinds of quantitative information are required: biological activity and molecular properties. Molecular properties are of three types: (1) molecular shape, (2) physicochemical parameters, and (3) abstract quantitations of molecular structure. Currently, the two best descriptors are the hydrophobic parameter, log 1-octanol/water partition coefficient (log P), and the $^1X^v$ (one-chi-v) molecular connectivity index. Biological responses can be divided into three main categories: (1) nonspecific effects due to membrane perturbation, (2) nonspecific effects due to interaction with functional groups of proteins, and (3) specific effects due to interaction with receptors.

Twenty-six synthetic fossil fuel-related nitrogen-containing aromatic compounds were examined to determine the quantitative correlation between log P and $^1X^v$ and population growth impairment of *Tetrahymena pyriformis*. Nitro-containing compounds are the most active, followed by amino-containing compounds and azaarenes. Within each analog series, activity increases with alkyl substitution and ring addition. The planar model log BR = 0.5564 log P + 0.3000 $^1X^v$ − 2.0138 was determined using mononitrogen-substituted compounds. Attempts to extrapolate this model to dinitrogen-containing molecules were, for the most part, unsuccessful because of a change in mode of action from membrane perturbation to uncoupling of oxidative phosphorylation.

## BACKGROUND

One of the first correlations between molecular structure and biological activity was that reported by Richardson[1] in 1868. He demonstrated a direct linear relationship between the number of carbon atoms in each molecule and the narcotic effect of a series of fatty alcohols. The present status of structure-activity relationships has evolved over the past 20 years from studies in medicinal chemistry and drug design. These investigations have shown the value of describing molecular structure in forms suitable for correlational analyses with biological data. Although still in its infancy, structure-activity analysis has the potential for providing a powerful research tool for ranking and predicting health and environmental hazards from organic compounds. The overall objective of quantitative structure-activity relationships (QSAR) is shown in Equation 1.

$$\text{Biological Activity} = f\ (\text{Molecular Properties}) \tag{1}$$

The basic idea is to find a mathematical model that relates biological activity to (some function of) the molecular properties of the chemicals. Once such a relationship is demonstrated, one can then extrapolate and predict the biological activity of other chemicals.

For each given chemical, two types of information are required to generate a structure-activity model: some measurement of biological activity (e.g., toxicity) that is derived quantitatively from a dose-response correlation and possesses some measure of confidence and one or more molecular properties or descriptors that represent quantitations of chemical structure or physicochemical parameters. Such descriptors are used as predictors in QSAR and are of three types. The first is the shape of the molecule. For specific toxicity or selective activity such as blocking a receptor, shape is the most important determinant. However, for nonspecific toxicity such as narcosis, molecular shape is less critical. Currently, there is no good method of describing shape in mathematical terms. The second descriptor is the overall physicochemical parameters of the molecules. This descriptor reflects free-energy-related properties including hydrophobic, steric, and electronic parameters and has recently been reviewed by Hansch and Leo.[2] Most published literature deals with the correlations of such physicochemical properties, taken separately or in combination, with biological response in one form or another. The leading physicochemical descriptor is the hydrophobic parameter log l-octanol/water partition coefficient (log P).[3] The success in using this predictor has been due in large part to the fact that the rate of movement of organic molecules through biological materials is approximately proportional to their partition coefficients,[4] and to the fact that l-octanol/water partitioning is a good index of partitioning in biological systems in general.[5]

In addition to experimental determination, l-octanol/water partition coefficients can be calculated because of their additivity by the Substituent or $\pi$ method,[2,5,6] where $\pi$ is defined by the expression:

$$\pi_X = \log P_X - \log P_H \tag{2}$$

where $P_X$ is the partition coefficient of the derivative and $P_H$ is the partition coefficient of the parent compound. Partition coefficients can also be calculated by summing appropriate structural fragments. This Fragment method[2,7] is based on a set of molecular fragment values using the following expression:

$$\log P = \sum_1^n x_n f_n \tag{3}$$

where x is the number of times fragment f of structural type n appears in the molecular formula. The personnel of the U.S. Environmental Protection Agency (EPA) research laboratory at Duluth recently developed computer algorithms which optimize the computation of log P values by the Fragment method.

The third and final group of predictors are quantitated molecular-structural descriptors. This category includes atom counts, molecular weight, molecular connectivity, molecular orbital theory, and quantum mechanics; the most often used is molecular connectivity.[8,9] While more sophisticated than simple counts of atoms or molecular weight, molecular connectivity is less rigorous than either molecular orbital theory or quantum mechanics. It describes a molecule by its topological characteristics. The molecular connectivity method results in predictors consisting of numerical indices that are generated with the assumption that it is possible to differentiate molecular structure by abstract numerical means.

Since molecular structure is simply a topological graph (i.e., a set of vertices or atoms connected by edges or bonds), numerical indices (i.e., counts of sigma electrons other than those bonding to hydrogen) can easily be generated. These indices, based on 0-, 1-, 2-, 3-, or 4-bond subgraphs, are numerical encodings of structural information concerning numbers and types of atoms, branching, cyclization, and saturation as well as other parameters. In an effort to minimize redundancy for conformational isomers, a reciprocal square root transformation of the product of the vertex valences is performed in calculating the molecular connectivity indices.

The most often used molecular connectivity index is the $^1X^v$ (one-chi-v) index. The only type of molecular subgraph used is the bond(s) between two atoms. This index is described by the expression:

$$^1X^v = \sum_{S=1}^{Nb} (\delta_i^v \delta_j^v)^{-1/2} \qquad (4)$$

where bond $b_s$ is between atoms $\delta_i$ and $\delta_j$. The number of bonds in the molecule is $N_b$ and $\delta_i^v$ and $\delta_j^v$ (valence delta) is the hydrogen suppressed valence of each atom and an index of multiple bonds. Common $\delta^v$ values include: C, 4; N, 5; O, 6.

At the recent EPA-sponsored workshop[10] held to assess the role of QSAR methods in predicting environmental toxicity, an attempt was made to distill a realistic approach using QSAR techniques to aid in screening industrial chemicals for potential hazards. Several points were brought out that bear repeating. The development of computer-assisted statistical analyses has made the task of generating molecular descriptors and developing quantitative models of toxicological endpoints technically feasible. Since predictive correlations are only as good as the data used to establish them, the procedures used to generate QSAR data bases must assure the highest accuracy for both biological response and molecular descriptors. Predictability is enhanced by increased similarity in molecular structure but requires the molecules in question to elicit a response through the same mode of action. The latter is difficult, if not impossible, to assess prior to testing.

Initially, industrial chemicals should be divided into 60 or so rational groups based on chemical structure. Each group should consist of about 20 representatives selected to include as many substituent variations as possible and as wide a range of descriptors as possible. It is the process of lumping and splitting molecules into toxicologically meaningful groups that provides the greatest challenge before QSAR can be used to rank chemicals. Although it is not possible to group molecules before they are tested, it seems logical that toxic molecules will fall into several categories.

Biological responses to chemical insults can be classified into three general cause-effect categories.

1.  Nonspecific effects may be due to membrane perturbation. These would be expected to result in behavioral alterations, narcosis, and eventually death. This classification may also include effects on specific membrane-bound enzymes and electron transport mechanisms. Such effects are most likely to be correlated with the 1-octanol/water partition coefficient. About 70% of industrial chemicals fall into this category.
2.  Nonspecific effects may be due to a direct action of the compound

with a specific functional group of proteins such as an amino, carboxyl, or mercapto group. Effects of this type would most likely correlate with some index of molecular structure along with the partition coefficient.

3. The third category is the most diverse and consists of effects that may be due to interactions with specific receptor sites or enzyme complexes. Chemicals that produce such specific toxic effects would be analogs of naturally occurring biochemicals. Such toxic results are often unpredictable, as they are not often obvious from molecular structure or physicochemical properties.

The literature suggests that structure-toxicity relationships have been successfully developed for groups of chemicals divided along classical organic chemistry lines into cogeneric series of homologs, analogs, and, in some cases, conformational isomers (for review see Reference 11). From these studies some general trends are available. It appears that many aliphatic compounds have generally low toxicity. The more toxic aliphatic molecules are mostly the small, quite reactive ones. Aromatic molecules, limited at this time to substituted benzenes and naphthalenes, appear generally more toxic than aliphatic compounds. Their toxicity is usually increased by halogens and nitro groups and decreased by amino and thio groups. Few heterocyclic molecules have been studied. Thus, trends concerning their toxicity are less clear. However, azaarenes are certainly less toxic than their corresponding aromatic hydrocarbons. Increased in-ring nitrogen substitution decreases toxicity, whereas the crowding of multiple nitrogen substitution increases toxicity.

## INTRODUCTION

With this general background of QSAR in mind, let us turn to its application to health and environmental studies of synthetic fossil-fuel technologies. Synthetic fossil-fuel crude oils differ markedly in their chemical composition from the naturally occurring, conventional petroleum crude oils. Specifically, synfuel crudes have a higher aromatic content and greater amounts of organic heteroatoms such as nitrogen. Organonitrogen compounds associated with synfuel materials include azaarenes and primary aromatic amines and their alkyl analogs, especially methyl substituents. These differences have sparked our structure-toxicity work with primary aromatic amines and basic and neutral nitrogenous heterocyclics.[12] We have recently expanded these studies to include nitroaromatics because of their involvement in diesel combustion emissions.

We have used the free-living ciliate *Tetrahymena pyriformis* strain GL-C (Figure 1) as our bioassay model. It has been shown to be a rapid, inexpensive, and well-characterized test system that lends itself to quanti-

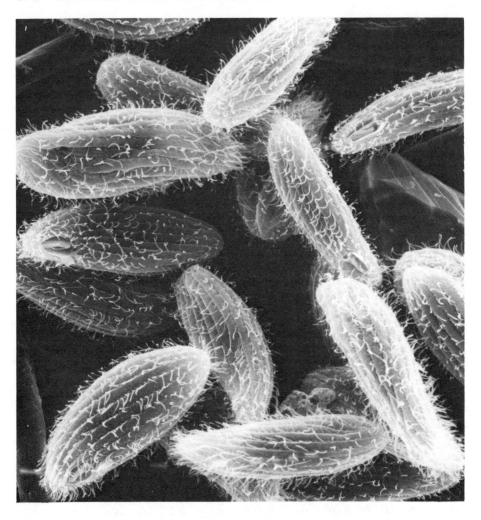

**Figure 1.**  Scanning electron micrograph of *Tetrahymena pyriformis*.

tative concentration-response analysis. Based on studies with acridine[13] the biological response of population growth has been selected as the test end-point and the methodology standardized as a short-term screen.[14] *Tetrahymena* is not only appropriate as a zooplankter aquatic toxicity test system but also as an eucaryotic cytotoxicity model.

In this investigation, we report a correlation between the log P and $^1X^v$ molecular descriptors and toxicity monitored as population growth impairment of *Tetrahymena* using 15 selected azaarenes, primary aromatic amines, and nitroaromatics. Extrapolation of the resulting model is then investigated using dinitrogen-substituted analogs and homologs.

## MATERIALS AND METHODS

Axenic cultures of the amicronucleated strain GL-C of *Tetrahymena pyriformis* were tested at 28°C under acute conditions. The ciliates were cultured in a proteose peptone medium.[11] The tested chemicals were secured from commercial sources (Aldrich Chemical Co., Milwaukee; Pfaltz and Bauer, Inc., Stamford, Connecticut) and were not repurified. The compounds selected form a series of aromatic analogs and homologs that can be subdivided into three categories, (1) azaarenes, (2) primary aromatic amines, and (3) nitroaromatics. Test chemicals were initially dissolved in ACS reagent grade dimethyl sulfoxide (DMSO) to form 10,000-, 50,000-, or 500,000-mg/L stock solutions. Subsequently, aliquots of stock solutions no greater than 300 μL were added to the culture medium. Previously, Schultz and Cajina-Quezada[15] noted that DMSO in concentrations as high as 0.75% (375 μL/50mL) does not affect population growth of *Tetrahymena.*

The biological response of population growth was used to quantify activity. Population growth was monitored using the method of Cooley et al.,[16] with cell density being measured spectrophotometrically as optical density (absorbance) at 540 nm. Cameron[17] noted that the number of *Tetrahymena* in culture is directly proportional to the absorbance. Cultures were grown for 60 h in 50 mL of test solution in 250-mL Erlenmeyer flasks. Flasks for each test molecule were prepared in a five-step graded-concentration series. Flasks without test chemicals served as controls, and each flask was inoculated with 0.2 mL of log-growth-phase culture. Two assays for each concentration were conducted simultaneously in three replicates. Each replicate used freshly prepared stock solutions. For analysis, absorbance values were transformed to percent control absorbance. For each test molecule, the best concentration-response line was fitted by least-squares linear regression. The 60-h $IGC_{50}$ value (concentration that inhibits 50% growth) and 95% confidence limits were determined for each test molecule.

For structure-activity correlations, the $IGC_{50}$ values (mg/L) were converted to mmol/L prior to taking the log of the inverse, hereafter referred to as the log BR (Biological Response). The log P values were secured from Appendix II of Hansch and Leo[2] or calculated by the Substituent method using the substituent constants of Hansch and Leo.[2] The first order valence $^1X^v$ molecular connectivity index values were determined using the one-bond fragment algorithm $C_{ij} = (\delta_i^v \delta_j^v)^{-1/2}$, with the $\delta^v$ values being based upon the equation $\delta^v = Z^v - h$, where $Z^v$ is the number of valence electrons and h is the number of bonded hydrogen atoms.[9] Based on results of previous structure activity analyses,[11,13,15,18,19] QSARs were examined for the 15 alkyl and ring-addition analogs of pyridine, aniline, and nitrobenzene using log P and $^1X^v$ as the independent variables with log BR as the dependent variable. The structure activity models were developed using regression analysis with goodness of fit being compared by the variance. Analyses were conducted using Statistical Analysis Systems software.

## RESULTS AND DISCUSSION

Presented in Table I are the Chemical Abstract Service (CAS) registry number, 60-h $IGC_{50}$ value (mmol/L), and 95% confidence limits for each compound assayed. Biological activity varies between the three main chemical classes, azaarenes (molecules 1 through 5), primary aromatic amines (molecules 6 through 10), and nitroaromatics (molecules 11 through 15). Among each homologous series, the nitro derivatives are the most active, followed by the amines. Within each analog series, activity increases with increased alkyl substitution. The exceptions are compounds 10 and 15, 1-aminoanthracene and 9-nitroanthracene, which, due to aquatic solubility limitations, are not toxic at saturation.

Since log P and the $^1X^v$ index are currently the best molecular descriptors, these parameters were chosen as predictors for QSAR. Presented in Table II are the log P, $^1X^v$, log BR observed and predicted and residual values for each of the initial 13 test compounds. A three-dimensional plot of log P vs log BR vs $^1X^v$ is presented in Figure 2. The planar regression model of these data is:

$$\log BR = 0.5564 \, (\log P) + 0.3000 \, (^1\chi^v) - 2.0138 \quad r^2 = 0.887 \quad (5)$$

**Table I.** Growth Inhibition to *Tetrahymena* of Selected Nitrogen-Containing Aromatics

|  | *Compound* | *CAS Number* | *IGC50* | *95% Confidence Interval* |
|---|---|---|---|---|
| 1. | Pyridine[a] | 110–86–1 | 15.32 | (11.18–20.99) |
| 2. | 3-Picoline[a] | 108–99–6 | 10.41 | (6.27–17.27) |
| 3. | 3,4-Lutidine[a] | 583–58–4 | 3.02 | (2.16–4.21) |
| 4. | Quinoline[a] | 91–22–5 | 0.97 | (0.67–1.41) |
| 5. | Acridine[a] | 260–94–6 | 0.04 | (0.03–0.06) |
| 6. | Aniline[a] | 62–53–3 | 1.69 | (1.34–2.06) |
| 7. | 3-Toluidine[a] | 108–44–1 | 2.59 | (1.93–3.46) |
| 8. | 3,4-Xylidine[a] | 95–64–7 | 1.94 | (1.37–2.75) |
| 9. | 1-Naphthylamine[a] | 134–32–7 | 0.60 | (0.48–0.76) |
| 10. | 1-Aminoanthracene | 610–49–1 |  |  |
| 11. | Nitrobenzene[a] | 98–95–3 | 1.16 | (0.67–1.99) |
| 12. | 3-Methyl-1-nitrobenzene[a] | 99–08–1 | 0.49 | (0.39–0.58) |
| 13. | 3,4-Dimethyl-1-nitro-benzene[a] | 99–51–4 | 0.23 | (0.11–0.46) |
| 14. | 1-Nitronaphthalene[a] | 86–57–7 | 0.10 | (0.09–0.12) |
| 15. | 9-Nitroanthracene | 602–60–8 |  |  |

[a]Denotes listing on EPA Toxic Substance Control Act (TSCA) inventory.

**Table II.**  Comparison of Molecular Descriptors and Biological Response of Selected Nitrogen-Containing Aromatics

|    | Compound | log $P^a$ | $^1X^v$ | log BR | log $BR^b$ | Residual |
|----|----------|-----------|---------|--------|-----------|----------|
| 1. | Pyridine | 0.64 | 1.850 | −1.185 | −1.103 | −0.082 |
| 2. | 3-Picoline | 1.24 | 2.260 | −1.017 | −0.646 | −0.371 |
| 3. | 3,4-Lutidine | 1.68 | 2.677 | −0.480 | −0.276 | −0.204 |
| 4. | Quinoline | 2.04 | 3.264 | 0.013 | 0.100 | −0.087 |
| 5. | Acridine | 3.40 | 4.679 | 1.398 | 1.282 | 0.116 |
| 6. | Aniline | 0.90 | 2.199 | −0.228 | −0.853 | 0.625 |
| 7. | 3-Toluidine | 1.42 | 2.611 | −0.413 | −0.440 | 0.027 |
| 8. | 3,4-Xylidine | 1.98 | 3.028 | −0.288 | −0.004 | 0.284 |
| 9. | 1-Naphthylamine | 2.23 | 3.610 | 0.222 | 0.310 | −0.088 |
| 10. | 1-Aminoanthracene | 3.22 | 5.016 | | −0.283 | |
| 11. | Nitrobenzene | 1.84 | 2.500 | −0.064 | −0.240 | 0.176 |
| 12. | 3-Methyl-1-nitroben-zene | 2.43 | 2.912 | 0.310 | 0.212 | 0.098 |
| 13. | 3,4-Dimethyl-1-nitro-benzene | 2.96 | 3.324 | 0.638 | 0.630 | 0.008 |
| 14. | 1-Nitronaphthalene | 3.19 | 3.911 | 1.000 | 0.934 | 0.066 |
| 15. | 9-Nitroanthracene | 4.17 | 5.317 | | 1.901 | |

$^a$From Reference 2, this chapter.
$^b$Based on Equation 5.

In Equation 5, both log P and $^1X^v$ are significant with p values of 0.0001 and 0.2732 respectively. Statistical analysis of residual values based on Equation 5 reveals that none of the observed log BR values of these compounds are significantly different from their predicted values at the 0.05 level. Attempts were made to extrapolate the Equation-5 model using the more complex dinitrogen-containing compounds, 16 through 26, listed in Table III. Again, due to aquatic solubility, 1,5-dinitronaphthalene does not elicit the measured response at saturation. The log P, $^1X^v$, observed log BR, predicted log BR, and residual values are presented in Table IV. Predicted log BR values are based on Equation 5. The predicted response of compounds 16 through 18 fits well with their corresponding observed activity (Table IV). However, the activity of compounds 19 through 24 is significantly greater than predicted by Equation 5 (Table IV). Structurally, these compounds are dinitrogen-substituted aromatics where the nitrogen is in the diamino form or with at least one nitrogen present as a nitro group.

Equation 5 is very similar to Equation 9, log BR = 0.4446 (log P) + 0.3866 ($^1X^v$) − 2.0282, of Schultz[14] describing the aquatic toxicity of 26 unsubstituted basic and neutral organonitrogen heterocyclic molecules containing one to four nitrogen atoms and one to three rings. Equation 5 represents baseline toxicity due to membrane perturbation. The fact that the

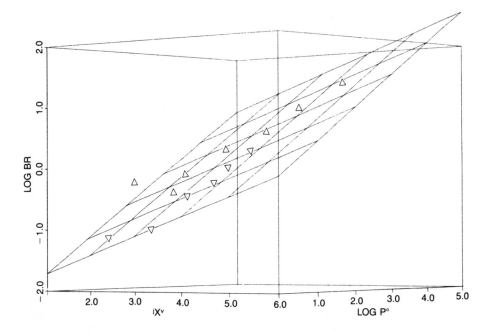

**Figure 2.** Regression analysis of log P vs log BR vs $^1X^v$ for compounds 1-15. The regression equation is Equation 5. Upward pointing triangles are above the plane, downward pointing triangles below the plane.

**Table III.** Growth Inhibition to *Tetrahymena* of Selected Validation Compounds

| | Compound | CAS Number | IGC50 | 95% Confidence Interval |
|---|---|---|---|---|
| 16. | Pyrazine | 290–37–9 | 66.36 | (47.72–92.29) |
| 17. | Quinoxaline[a] | 91–19–0 | 2.01 | (1.23–3.29) |
| 18. | 2-Aminopyridine[a] | 504–29–0 | 3.94 | (3.01–5.16) |
| 19. | 4-Nitropyridine[a] | | 0.38 | (0.27–0.53) |
| 20. | 1,2-Phenyldiamine[a] | 95–54–5 | 0.45 | (0.31–0.68) |
| 21. | 1,5-Diaminonaph-thalene | 2243–62–1 | 0.27 | (0.17–0.41) |
| 22. | 4-Nitroaniline[a] | 100–01–6 | 0.07 | (0.04–0.12) |
| 23. | 4-Nitro-1-naphthyla-mine | 776–34–1 | 0.08 | (0.05–0.11) |
| 24. | 1,4-Dinitrobenzene[a] | 100–25–4 | 0.05 | (0–0.13) |
| 25. | 1,5-Dinitronaphthalene | 605–71–0 | | |
| 26. | 2,4-Dinitrophenol[a] | 51–28–5 | 0.08 | (0.05–0.13) |

[a]Denotes listing on EPA TSCA inventory.

**Table IV.**  Comparison of Molecular Descriptors and Biological Response of Selected Validation Compounds

|     | Compound | log $P^a$ | $^1X^v$ | log BR | log $BR^b$ | Residual |
|-----|----------|-----------|---------|--------|-----------|----------|
| 16. | Pyrazine | −0.22 | 1.699 | −1.822 | −1.627 | −0.195 |
| 17. | Quinoxaline | 1.10$^c$ | 3.545 | −0.303 | −0.338 | 0.035 |
| 18. | 2-Aminopyridine | 0.52 | 2.059 | −0.595 | 1.108 | 0.513 |
| 19. | 4-Nitropyridine | 0.60$^c$ | 2.350 | 0.420 | −0.975 | 1.395 |
| 20. | 1,2-Phenyldiamine | 0.15 | 2.400 | 0.347 | −1.210 | 1.557 |
| 21. | 1,5-Diaminonaphthalene | 1.01$^c$ | 3.816 | 0.569 | −0.307 | 0.876 |
| 22. | 4-Nitroaniline | 1.39 | 2.735 | 1.155 | −0.420 | 1.575 |
| 23. | 4-Nitro-1-naphthylamine | 1.96$^c$ | 4.151 | 1.097 | 0.322 | 0.765 |
| 24. | 1,4-Dinitrobenzene | 1.47 | 3.002 | 1.301 | 0.295 | 1.596 |
| 25. | 1,5-Dinitronaphthalene | 3.89$^c$ | 4.194 |  | 1.409 |  |
| 26. | 2,4-Dinitrophenol | 1.52 | 3.143 | 1.097 | 1.132$^d$ | −0.035 |

[a]From Reference 2, this chapter.
[b]Based on Equation 5.
[c]Calculated by substituent method.
[d]Based on Equation 6.

biological activity of compounds 19 through 24 is greater than that predicted suggests a different mode of action for these compounds.

Regression analysis of log P vs log BR vs $^1X^v$ for compounds 19 through 24 (Figure 3) yields the model:

$$\log BR = 0.7938 \, (\log P) + 0.2870 \, (^1X^v) + 0.8272 \quad r^2 = 0.896 \quad (6)$$

The good correlation between biological response and log P suggests that the rate-limiting factor for both toxicities (i.e., Equations 5 and 6) is passive cellular uptake, that is, the movement of the test chemical by simple diffusion to the intracellular site of action.

As noted in the Introduction, effects on electron transport mechanisms (e.g., uncoupling of oxidative phosphorylation) should correlate with log P. Since compounds 19 through 24 include dinitro-substituted aromatics, a molecular substructure associated with uncoupling agents (i.e., 2,4-dinitrophenol),[20] it is possible that Equation 6 represents a predictive model for compounds which uncouple oxidative phosphorylation. In an effort to lend credence to this idea, we assayed 2,4-dinitrophenol, compound 26. The observed biological response was not significantly different from that predicted based on Equation 6 (Table IV).

Since the biological activity assays were static in design, the abiotic loss of the test compounds, especially the more volatile ones, is a potential variable. Davis and co-workers[21] studied the aquatic persistence of several nitrogen-containing compounds including aniline and pyridine and found them to be persistent under laboratory conditions similar to those employed

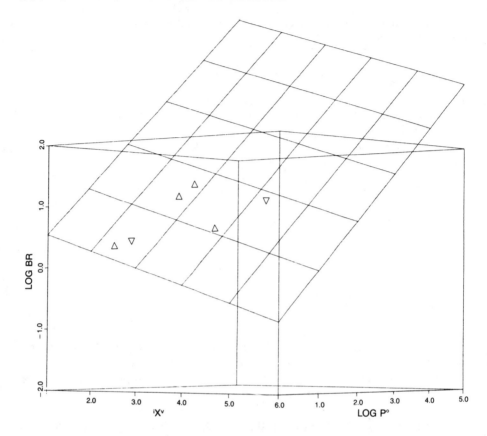

**Figure 3.** Regression analysis of log P vs log BR vs $^1X^v$ for compounds 19-24. The regression equation is Equation 6. Upward pointing triangles are above the plane, downward pointing triangles below the plane.

in these studies. These findings, coupled with the results of this study, suggest that abiotic loss was not a factor in these experiments.

The compounds assayed in the investigation are relatively simple in structure. This fact undoubtedly aids in explaining the high percentage of the biological variability with only two descriptors. We expect that, as the compounds become more structurally complex (e.g., multisubstituted conformational isomers), other descriptors will become important (i.e., steric and/or electron parameters), and the models will become more complex.

Although there is little chance in the foreseeable future that QSAR will be able to predict biological activities with enough reliability to make testing superfluous, it seems clear from the small amount of data available that QSAR modeling can reduce the number of experiments by allowing us to rank compounds and establish some priority for testing. It is also apparent that advancement of the state-of-the art in QSAR will require larger and more diverse data sets and possibly the development of new and more universal descriptors.

## ACKNOWLEDGMENT

This research was sponsored by the Division of Biomedical and Environmental Research, U.S. Department of Energy (DOE), under contract W-7405-eng-26 with the Union Carbide Corporation. Although the research described in this chapter has been funded wholly or in part by the U.S. Environmental Protection Agency (EPA) through Interagency Agreement Nos. 79-D-X0533 and 79-D-X0521 to DOE, it has not been subjected to EPA review and therefore does not necessarily reflect the views of EPA, and no official endorsement should be inferred.

## REFERENCES

1. Richardson, B.W. "Physiological Research on Alcohols," *Med. Times, Gaz.* 2:703–704 (1868).
2. Hansch, C., and A. Leo. *Substituent Constants for Correlation Analysis in Chemistry and Biology* (New York: John Wiley & Sons, Inc., 1979), p. 339.
3. Hansch, C. "A Quantitative Approach to Biochemical Structure-Activity Relationships," *Acc. Chem. Res.* 2:232–239 (1969).
4. Collander, R. "The Permeability of *Nitella* Cells to Non-Electrolytes," *Physiol. Plant* 7:420–445 (1954).
5. Leo, A.J., C. Hansch, and D. Elkins. "Partition Coefficients and Their Uses," *Chem. Rev.* 71:525–616 (1971).
6. Fujita, T., J. Iwasa, and C. Hansch. "A New Substituent Constant, H, Derived from Partition Coefficients," *J. Am. Chem. Soc.* 86:5175–5180 (1964).
7. Leo, A.J. "Calculation of Partition Coefficients Useful in the Evaluation of the Relative Hazard of Various Chemicals in the Environment," in *Symposium on Structure-Activity Correlations in Studies of Toxicity and Bioconcentration with Aquatic Organisms,* G.D. Veith and D.E. Konasewich, Eds. (1975), pp. 151–176.
8. Kier, L.B., and L.H. Hall. *Molecular Connectivity in Chemistry and Drug Research* (New York: Academic Press, Inc., 1976), p. 257.
9. Kier, L.B. "Molecular Connectivity as a Description of Structure for SAR Analysis," in *Physical Chemical Properties of Drugs,* S. Yalvowsky, Ed. (New York, Marcel Dekker, 1980), pp. 277–319.
10. Workshop on Structure Activity Concepts in Environmental Sciences, San Antonio, TX, Feb. 1–4, 1981.
11. Schultz, T.W., M. Cajina-Quezada, and J.N. Dumont. "Structure-Toxicity Relationships of Selected Nitrogenous Heterocyclic Compounds," *Arch. Environ. Contam. Toxicol.* 9:591–598 (1980).
12. Schultz, T.W., and T.C. Allison. "Toxicity and Toxic Interaction of Aniline and Pyridine," *Bull. Environ. Contam. Toxicol.* 23:814–819 (1979).

13. Schultz, T.W., C.S. Richter, and J.N. Dumont. "Cytotoxicity of Acridine, a Synfuel Component, to *Tetrahymena*," *Environ. Pollut. Ser. A.* 26:215–226 (1981).
14. Schultz, T.W. "Aquatic Toxicology of Nitrogen Heterocyclic Molecules: Quantitative Structure Activity Relationships," in *Aquatic Toxicology,* J.O. Nriagu, Ed. (New York: John Wiley & Sons, Inc., 1983), p. 579–612.
15. Schultz, T.W., and M. Cajina-Quezada. "Structure-Toxicity Relationships of Selected Nitrogenous Heterocyclic Compounds II. Dinitrogen Molecules," *Arch. Environ. Contam. Toxicol.* 11:353–361 (1982).
16. Cooley, N.R., J.M. Keltner, Jr., and J. Forester, "Mirex and Aroclor 1254: Effects on and Accumulation by *Tetrahymena pyriformis* Strain W," *J. Protozool.* 18:636–638 (1972).
17. Cameron, I.L. "Growth Characteristics of *Tetrahymena*," in *Biology of Tetrahymena,* A.M. Elliott, Ed. (Stroudsburg, PA: Dowden, Hutchinson and Ross, Inc., 1973), pp. 199–226.
18. Schultz, T.W., L.M. Kyte, and J.N. Dumont. "Structure-Toxicity Correlations of Organic Contaminants in Aqueous Coal-Conversion Effluent," *Arch. Environ. Contam. Toxicol.* 7:457–463 (1978).
19. Schultz, T.W., L.B. Kier, and L.H. Hall. "Structure-Toxicity Relationships of Selected Nitrogenous Heterocyclic Compounds III. Relationships Using Molecular Connectivity," *Bull. Environ. Contam. Toxicol.* 28:373–378 (1982).
20. Lardy, H. A., and H. Wellman. "The Catalytic Effect of 2,4-Dinitrophenol on Adenosinetriphosphate Hydrolysis by Cell Particles and Soluble Enzymes," *J. Biol. Chem.* 201:357–370 (1953).
21. Davis, K.R., T.W. Schultz, and J.N. Dumont. "Toxic and Teratogenic Effects of Selected Aromatic Amines on Embryos of the Amphibian *Xenopus laevis*," *Arch. Environ. Contam. Toxicol.* 10:371–391 (1981).

# CHAPTER 17

## Extrapolation of Ecotoxicity Data: Choosing Tests to Suit the Assessment

### G.W. Suter II and D.S. Vaughan

*Environmental Sciences Division*
*Oak Ridge National Laboratory*
*Oak Ridge, TN 37831*

The test species and test types used in aquatic toxicology should be selected to suit the needs of assessment. Sensitive tests would be desirable in the screening phase of hazard assessment, but none of the standard screening tests are consistently sensitive. A better criterion for test selection is the ability of a particular test to predict the responses of other species and other test types. This predictive ability is shown by correlation analysis. The variance in a correlation can be used to generate the risk in a risk analysis or the cutoff concentrations in a hazard assessment. Examination of a variety of correlations suggests that invertebrate toxicology relative to fish toxicology needs more attention.

### INTRODUCTION

This chapter examines the bases for selection of test organisms and test types for studies of aquatic environmental toxicology. We do not consider purely practical criteria such as availability, ease of handling, or uniformity of response, but rather we examine the ability of the test to fulfill its role in an assessment. The purpose of toxicity testing is assumed to be the determination of the effects of a chemical or complex effluent on organisms in a receiving community. This determination can be accomplished through either hazard assessment or risk assessment.

Hazard assessment is a process of arriving at a yes or no answer concerning the safety of a potential toxicant by an iterative program of testing and quantitative analysis. At each level of hazard assessment, the results of effects tests are compared to the results of fate tests and predicted release rates to decide if the chemical is safe or unacceptably hazardous or if more testing is needed. If more testing is needed, a series of more definitive and more expensive tests is conducted, and the analysis is repeated using the new results. While hazard assessment procedures have received considerable attention,[1-3] there are no generally accepted procedures.

Risk assessment is concerned with estimating the probability of certain undesired events given a particular effluent release.[4] For example, risk assessment could estimate the probability that effluents from a coal liquefaction plant would reduce game-fish biomass in the receiving river by at least 25%. While the application of probabilistic risk assessment techniques to environmental end points is a new field, the demand is great for environmental analogues to human health risk assessment as an aid to decision making.

## CRITERIA

A variety of criteria has been used to justify the choice of test systems. One frequently mentioned criterion is sensitivity. If an inexpensive test system could be shown to be consistently more sensitive than any other, and if it represented an organism and life stage that would be exposed in the field, then it would be the test of choice in hazard assessment. The greatest need for sensitivity is in the first tier or "screening" tests where a false negative result (declaring nonhazardous a chemical that will cause significant toxic effects in the field) would end the hazard assessment and allow a serious toxicant to be released. However, because of the need to screen numerous chemicals, the screening tests must be rapid and inexpensive acute tests; hence, they are usually less sensitive than chronic tests.

Even if an assessment is only concerned with acute toxicity (e.g., only accidental releases), none of the standard test species appears to be reliably most-sensitive. Table I shows an analysis of the relative sensitivity of the

**Table I.** Percentage of Comparisons in the Columbia Data Set[5] in which the Listed Test Species Has the Lowest $EC_{50}$ or $LC_{50}$

| Test Species | Percent Most Sensitive | $n^a$ | Number of Species |
|---|---|---|---|
| *Daphnia* spp.[b] | 67 | 517 | 49 |
| *Gammarus* spp.[b] | 64 | 720 | 50 |
| Rainbow trout | 52 | 834 | 54 |
| Fathead minnow | 24 | 630 | 53 |
| Bluegill sunfish | 42 | 867 | 54 |

[a]Number of pair comparisons with different species and chemicals.
[b]When two species of *Daphnia* (5 cases) or *Gammarus* (8 cases) were tested with the same chemical, the average $EC_{50}$ was used in the comparison.

five most commonly used aquatic test species. The analysis is based on the Columbia National Fisheries Research Laboratory's acute toxicity data set (Columbia data set) which contains tests of 271 chemicals and 57 species of fish and aquatic arthropods.[5] We adapted this data set for species comparisons by deleting alternate formulations of the chemicals and tests of larval fish. The analysis shows that the *Daphnia* spp. $EC_{50}$ is the most consistently sensitive of the standard acute tests. However, it is most sensitive in only 67% of pair comparisons with other invertebrate $EC_{50}$s and fish $LC_{50}$s. Therefore, a sensitive species offers no advantage per se because, at minimum, some safety factor must be applied to screening tests to ensure sufficient sensitivity. However, if a taxon such as the aquatic algae can be shown to be consistently insensitive,[10] then it can be excluded from the set of screening tests, though not from higher levels of testing.

A more important criterion is the ability of one toxicity test to predict the response of other tests. The simplest criterion of prediction is the similarity of response. The similarity of two tests can be expressed as the percent deviation or the absolute magnitude of deviation. When two organisms can be shown to have responses consistently similar to within a factor of 2 or even an order of magnitude, the need to test both species is effectively precluded. A demonstration by McKim[11] of the similarity of response levels of fish in embryo-larval tests to life-cycle tests has led to near abandonment of the latter test in favor of the former. However, this criterion cannot be used for pairs of species or test types that show different levels of sensitivity. In that case, some sort of regression analysis must be performed, even if it is just a correction factor arrived at by "eyeballing" the data.

Regression analysis provides the most powerful tool to determine the utility of a test relative to other potential tests. The parameters of the regression equation provide an indication of the magnitude and significance of differences in sensitivity. The bounds of the 95% confidence interval provide defensible safety factors for the decision points in hazard assessments, and the predicted values and probability distributions are both used in risk analysis.[4] The squared correlation coefficient or coefficient of determination ($r^2$) is the percent of the variance in one variable that can be explained by its linear relation to another variable. It is a powerful and intuitively appealing indicator of the predictive potential of a test.

## SOME CORRELATIONS

### Acute Toxicity

Before performing correlation analyses, it is important to determine what questions must be answered. Most of the published comparisons between tests relate to the question of redundancy between common test types and organisms (Table II).[6-9] These results suggest that there is considerable redundancy between acute toxic responses of common test fish (fathead

**Table II.**   Correlations of Acute Toxicities from Published
Sets of Comparative Data

| Independent Variable/ Dependent Variable | $r^2$ | $n$ | Test Chemicals | Reference |
|---|---|---|---|---|
| Rainbow trout $LC_{50}$/ |  |  | Insecticides + |  |
| Daphnia spp. $LC_{50}$ | 0.31 | 48 | herbicides | 6 |
| Fathead minnow $LC_{50}$ | 0.83 | 20 |  | 7 |
| Bluegill sunfish $LC_{50}$ | 0.92 | 41 |  | 7 |
| Bluegill sunfish $LC_{50}$/ |  |  | Insecticides + | 7 |
| Fathead minnow $LC_{50}$ | 0.74 | 21 | herbicides |  |
| Daphnia pulex $LC_{50}$/ |  |  |  |  |
| Hyalella azteca $LC_{50}$ | 0.95 | 13 | Insecticides | 8 |
| Palaemonetes |  |  |  |  |
| kadiakensis $LC_{50}$ | 0.88 | 5 |  |  |
| Culex restuans $LC_{50}$ | 0.64 | 11 |  |  |
| Daphnia magna $LC_{50}$ |  |  |  |  |
| Fathead minnow $LC_{50}$ | 0.61 | 29 | Nitroaromatics | 9 |

minnow, rainbow trout, and bluegill) and between crustacean test species
(*Daphnia pulex* versus *Hyallela azteca* and *Palaemonetes kadiakensis*). The
three worst correlations between acute responses are for species in different
phyla or classes (*Daphnia* versus rainbow trout, fathead minnow, and *Culex
restuans*). This result suggests the hypothesis that taxonomic similarity implies similar toxicological responses.

This reasonable sounding hypothesis is supported by an examination
of the Columbia data set. Table III shows that when a large number of
species and higher taxa are correlated, $r^2$ declines with increasing taxonomic
distance. Further, at each level, $r^2$ is lower for arthropods than for fish,

**Table III.**   Mean Correlations between Taxa in the Columbia Data Set[5]

| | Fish | | Arthropods | |
|---|---|---|---|---|
| Taxonomic Level | $r^2$ | $n^a$ | $r^2$ | $n^a$ |
| Species within genera | 0.90 | 9/105 | 0.80 | 2/13 |
| Genera within families | 0.89 | 8/243 | 0.87 | 2/51 |
| Families within orders | 0.82 | 2/74 | 0.57 | 3/33 |
| Orders within classes | 0.75 | 10/1518 | 0.31 | 14/370 |
| Classes within phyla |  |  | 0.17 | 1/440 |
| Across phyla (fish versus arthropods) |  |  | 0.07 | 1/2312 |

[a]Number of pairs of taxa correlated/total number of points in the correlations; correlations with <5 points were not included.

suggesting that arthropods are toxicologically more diverse. Finally, the regressions of insects versus crustaceans and of fish versus arthropods result in correlations that are not significantly different from random.

The Columbia data set can also be used to examine the question of how well the standard test species represent major taxa. Table IV shows the mean correlations of each of five common test species with all species of crustaceans, insects, and fish. These results indicate that all three fish are equally good at representing fish in general and are equally poor at representing arthropods. Unfortunately, *Daphnia* and *Gammarus* are not very good representatives of either arthropod class. The mean correlation of *Daphnia* with all fish in this data set is much lower than that for *Daphnia* and fathead minnow (Table II). This analysis agrees with earlier analyses in suggesting that a fish is a fish is a fish, and any of the standard test species of fish is adequate. However, extrapolation to an entire class of arthropods involves considerable error.

## Chronic Toxicity

Considerably less data are available to analyze the predictability of chronic toxicity (Table V).[12-16] As with acute toxicity, the correlation of chronic toxicities of *Daphnia* and fathead minnow, expressed as the no-observed-effects concentration (NOEC), is remarkably good relative to the taxonomic distance involved. The correlation between the fathead minnow life cycle, geometric mean, maximum allowable toxicant concentration (GMATC), and GMATCs for all other fish is somewhat lower than the equivalent acute toxicity correlation (Table IV). This is not surprising, considering the greater number of physiological processes involved in life-cycle toxicity and the greater extraneous error in the chronic correlation due to the use of data from different laboratories.

**Table IV.** Mean Correlations of Standard Test Species with Other Species in the Columbia Data Set Averaged Across Classes

| | Crustaceans | | Insects | | Fish | |
| Test Species | $r^2$ | $n$ | $r^2$ | $n$ | $r^2$ | $n$ |
|---|---|---|---|---|---|---|
| *Daphnia* ssp.[a] | 0.38 | 138 | 0.40 | 68 | 0.10 | 295 |
| *Gammarus* spp.[a] | 0.37 | 146 | 0.28 | 82 | 0.53 | 471 |
| Rainbow trout | 0.20 | 229 | 0.39 | 88 | 0.73 | 494 |
| Fathead minnow | 0.29 | 150 | 0.20 | 61 | 0.76 | 396 |
| Bluegill sunfish | 0.27 | 229 | 0.28 | 88 | 0.72 | 528 |

[a]When two species of *Daphnia* (5 cases) or *Gammarus* (8 cases) were tested for the same chemical, the average $EC_{50}$ was used in the correlation.

**Table V.**   Correlations for the Prediction of Chronic Toxicities

| Independent Variable/ Dependent Variable | $r^2$ | $n$ | References |
|---|---|---|---|
| *Chronic/chronic* | | | |
| *Daphnia* spp. NOEC/ Fathead minnow NOEC | 0.62 | 27 | 12 |
| Fathead minnow GMATC/other fish spp. GMATC | 0.67 | 19 | 13 |
| *Acute/chronic* | | | |
| All fish $LC_{50}$/GMATC | 0.64 | 46 | 13 |
| *Daphnia* spp. $EC_{50}$/ *Daphnia* spp. 3–4 week MATC | 0.81 | 27 | 14–16 (combined) |

Sufficient data are available to examine the relationship between acute and chronic toxicity of *Daphnia* and of freshwater fish in general. The 48-h $EC_{50}$ for *Daphnia* appears to be a very good predictor of the 3- to 4-week reproductive tests (MATC). The correlation of fish $LC_{50}$s with GMATCs used only data pairs for which the same water, fish, and toxicant sources were used in both tests.[13] The resulting correlation ($r^2 = 0.64$) is nearly as high as the correlation of fathead minnow GMATCs with GMATCs of other fish species ($r^2 = 0.67$). It appears that the information gain from running a fathead minnow life-cycle test may not be great relative to running an $LC_{50}$. Definitive analysis of this question would require a much larger data base for species-specific acute/chronic and chronic/chronic correlations.

## Patterns of Correlations

The clearest implication of these correlations is that the responses of fish are relatively predictable. All of the methods of comparing the acute toxicities of fish taxa result in $r^2 > 0.70$ (Tables II–IV). Even life-cycle toxicity to fish is reasonably well explained by either acute toxicity to the same species or chronic toxicity to the fathead minnow (Table V). However, despite the good correlations between *Daphnia* and fathead minnow (Tables II and V), *Daphnia* responses do not appear to be very good predictors of responses of fish in general (Table IV).

Aquatic arthropods appear to be considerably less predictable than fish. The correlations presented in Table III and the results of a recent study of four species of chironomid midges[17] indicate that good predictions can be made between members of arthropod families. However, correlations drop off significantly at higher taxonomic levels (Table III), and neither *Daphnia* nor *Gammarus* results can explain more than 40% of the average variation across chemicals in the $EC_{50}$s of crustaceans and insects (Table IV).

These results suggest that it would be appropriate to expend more toxicological effort on aquatic arthropods than on fish, particularly in view of their role in food chains. These results also raise questions concerning the predictability of other aquatic invertebrate taxa such as mollusks, rotifers, and oligochaetes, which are seldom included in large testing schemes. Finally, more attention should be directed to the relationship between acute and chronic toxicity in invertebrates.

## EXAMPLES OF APPLICATIONS

### Hazard Assessment

As explained earlier, hazard assessment requires a procedure for deciding that a chemical is acceptable, unacceptable, or requires more testing. As an example, we consider the problem of determining the safety of chemicals with respect to acute toxicity to aquatic crustaceans on the basis of *Daphnia* 48-h $EC_{50}$ tests. Figure 1 shows the regression of *Daphnia* $EC_{50}$s against

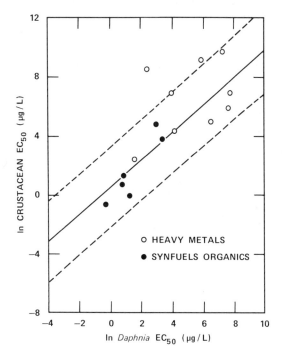

**Figure 1.** Confidence intervals for the prediction of crustacean acute toxicity from a *Daphnia* $EC_{50}$. The regression is derived from all pairs of $EC_{50}$s for *Daphnia* and other crustaceans in the Columbia data set.[5] The plotted points are $EC_{50}$s for *Daphnia* and *Gammarus* from data for metals and synfuel chemicals. (See References 18 and 19, this chapter.)

$EC_{50}s$ for all other crustaceans in the Columbia data set (139 points, not shown).[5] The regression analysis was performed by the major axis method,[18] and the 95% confidence interval is determined for a predicted value rather than for the predicted mean because we are interested in including future observations from the class Crustacea rather than from a typical crustacean.

In this example, the 95% confidence interval extends from approximately 20 to 1/20 times the regression line. The lower boundary of the interval could be used to estimate an acceptable concentration for this criterion, that is, one that would not be acutely toxic to more than 2.5% of crustacean species. Either the upper 95% boundary or the regression line could be used as the bound on the unacceptably toxic concentrations. Predicted environmental concentrations between the acceptable and unacceptable concentrations could trigger additional testing. However, in our example using acute tests to assess acute toxicity, the information gain from additional testing should be slight. Unless the *Daphnia* test was faulty, additional crustacean $EC_{50}$ values would be expected to fall within the confidence interval. Since two species are nearly as small a fraction of all Crustacea as one, little additional predictive power would be gained. The only major advantage would be in assessing specific lower taxa to which the test species belong and which might be of special interest (e.g., test *Gammarus* if amphipods are particularly important).

Use of this decision criterion depends on a number of assumptions: (1) the laboratory-derived $EC_{50}$ or $LC_{50}$ is an acceptable predictor of acute toxicity in the field; (2) the tested species are representative of the higher taxon (e.g., the 12 crustacean species from six orders in the Columbia data set are a random sample of North American crustaceans); and (3) the relative sensitivities of the test organisms to the chemicals in this data set also apply to other chemicals.

The first assumption concerns the validity of current testing procedures, an issue which is beyond the scope of this paper. The second assumption cannot be tested because there is no data set available that addresses a large number of alternate species. However, we do not think it likely that the tested species are a biased sample of the fauna.

The third assumption can be tested by examining the fit of data for chemicals not included in the data set used in the regression. The Columbia data set consists predominantly of organic biocides. We have overlain points on Figure 1 from $EC_{50}s$ of *Daphnia* and *Gammarus* for synfuels chemicals (phenol, B-naphthol, quinoline, acridine, naphthane, and phenanthrene)[19] and heavy metals (Ag, As, Cd, Cu, Hg, Ni, Pb, Se, and Zn).[20] The distribution of points around the line suggests that the regression relationship holds for these other chemical groups. The fact that two of the metals (Ag and Zn) fall above the 95% confidence interval may be attributable to their lower relative toxicity to *Gammarus* or to the higher variability that results from matching data from different laboratories to form the points.

This assumption could be eliminated by developing regressions for individual chemical classes, but few chemicals outside of those in the Columbia data set have been tested under similar conditions with multiple species per class. The assumption could be relaxed by assuming that there is no bias, only variance, in the relationship of *Daphnia* or other test organisms and the taxa they represent. This would be done by calculating the confidence interval for an assumed line with slope 1 and 0 intercept. While this approach makes the analysis less data-set-specific, it throws out potentially useful information about relative sensitivity and increases the width of the confidence interval.

Clearly, in this type of analysis, better correlations mean narrower confidence intervals and fewer inconclusive decisions. In our example of assessing the hazard of acute toxicity to crustaceans, the alternative to *Daphnia* among widely accepted test organisms is *Gammarus*. Neither of these organisms is preferable to the other as a predictor of Crustacea in general (Table IV), and the more convenient of the two can be selected.

## Risk Assessment

Risk assessment uses the uncertainty in the extrapolation from available data to the end point of the assessment to derive probability estimates of exceeding the end point.[4] To the extent that this is a matter of extrapolating between related parameters, regression analysis is the tool of choice.

For example, to assess the risk of chronic toxicity to fish, we must extrapolate between the test species and each of the species of interest and usually between acute toxicity and chronic toxicity.[13] This process is portrayed in Figure 2. The probability distribution of the acute toxicity is based on the inherent variance in the $LC_{50}$. The chronic toxicity (GMATC) has a broader distribution and a shifted centroid due to the variances and biases in the two regressions used to make the extrapolations. The risk of chronic toxicity is the area under the GMATC curve (to the left of the ambient concentration); that is, the probability that the ambient concentration exceeds the GMATC. If the ambient concentration is estimated with error, then the risk is a function of the overlap between the distributions of the ambient concentration and the GMATC.

For risk assessment, test types and species should be chosen so as to reduce the total uncertainty. Uncertainty can be reduced by performing tests that eliminate the need for extrapolations or by using tests and species that are well correlated with the end point. For example, if the assessment concerns direct toxicity to a centrarchid fishery, by testing bluegill (a component of this fishery) rather than fathead minnow (a cyprinid), one could eliminate the taxonomic extrapolation to bluegill and reduce the error in the others. Ideally, a risk assessment should provide not only an estimate of risk but also an estimate of the fraction of the total variance attributable to each

**Figure 2.** Frequency distributions of a measured sunfish *(Lepomis)* $LC_{50}$ and predicted black bass *(Micropterus)* GMATC. The risk that an environmental concentration of 12 $\mu$g/L will be chronically toxic (exceed the GMATC) is the shaded area. (See Reference 13, this chapter.)

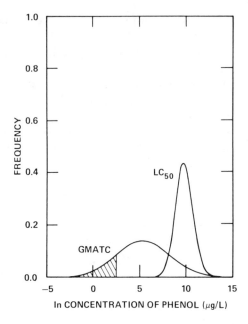

parameter in the source, transport, and effects models and an estimate of the reduction in variance that could be obtained by new parameter measurements. Methods development aimed at this goal is under way.

The concept of creating strings of extrapolations and adding the associated variances could also be applied to hazard assessment. Figure 3 shows the 95% confidence interval on the GMATC for largemouth bass given an $LC_{50}$ for bluegill obtained by combining taxonomic and acute/chronic regressions as discussed above. The confidence interval could be used to establish acceptable, unacceptable, and more-research-needed concentrations as discussed in the previous section. In this case, and in other cases where an extrapolation is made to a higher level of testing, the implication for additional testing is clearer. Because the acute/chronic extrapolation is the major source of variance in this relationship, a predicted concentration that falls between the acceptable and unacceptable bounds would imply the need for chronic testing. However, it should be realized that no amount of testing will eliminate all variance, and some probability of toxicity will have to be accepted.

Because in this case we are interested in estimating the true response concentration of a particular species, the regression is performed by the least-squares method and the confidence interval is calculated for the mean. The typical concern of hazard assessment with protecting entire large taxa can be handled analogously by regressing the bluegill $LC_{50}$ against $LC_{50}$s for all fish (as in the *Daphnia*/Crustacea regression, Figure 1), using the acute/chronic regression to derive a GMATC for the average fish and then adding

**Figure 3.** Regression line and 95% confidence interval for prediction of black bass *(Micropterus)* GMATCs from sunfish *(Lepomis)* LC$_{50}$s.

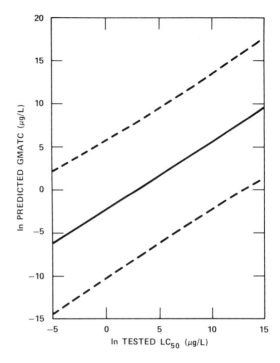

the variances. In that case, the regressions should be performed by the major axis method with the confidence interval calculated for predicted values rather than the predicted means.[18] By combining correlations in this way, it is possible not only to consider the adequacy of a test result to represent all possible results at a given level of testing but also to determine the likelihood that data from higher-level tests will alter the decision concerning acceptability.

At this point, the dichotomy between hazard and risk assessments begins to dissolve. The concern of risk assessment with specific receiving communities is equivalent on the average to hazard assessment concern with biota in general when the receiving community is diverse or when several sites must be considered. The use of a 2.5% probability of effect (one side of the two-tailed 95% confidence interval) as a cutoff point for acceptability in hazard assessments is a special case of risk assessment concern with predicting the probability of an effect. This being the case, test designs and organisms could be selected for both types of assessment on the basis of their correlation with broad taxonomic groups and with realistic exposure durations, life stages, and responses.

The use of correlation analysis in environmental assessment of toxic chemicals is a relatively new activity because only recently have sufficient data been accumulated. Even now, the activity is severely limited by the few species that are regularly used in testing and by the numerous and often unreported sources of variance between testing conditions. It is important to continue to develop and test the necessary correlations for environmental assessments.

## ACKNOWLEDGMENTS

Research sponsored by the Office of Research and Development, U.S. Environmental Protection Agency, under Interagency Agreement 40-740-78 with the U.S. Department of Energy under contract W-7405-eng-26 with the Union Carbide Corporation.

## REFERENCES

1.  Dickson, K.L., A.W. Maki, and J. Cairns, Jr., Eds. *Analyzing the Hazard Evaluation Process* (Washington, DC: American Fisheries Society, 1971).
2.  Cairns, J. Jr., K.L. Dickson, and A.W. Maki, Eds. *Estimating the Hazard of Chemical Substances to Aquatic Life* (Philadelphia: American Society for Testing and Materials, 1978).
3.  Mayer, F.L., and J.L. Hamelink, Eds. *Aquatic Toxicology and Hazard Evaluation* (Philadelphia: American Society for Testing and Materials, 1976).
4.  Suter, G.W., II, L.W. Barnthouse, and R.V. O'Neill. "The Uses of Uncertainty in Environmental Risk Analysis," in *Quantification of Risks: Reducing the Uncertainties* (Washington, DC: American Association for the Advancement of Science, in press).
5.  Johnson, W.W., and M.T. Finley. "Handbook of Acute Toxicity of Chemicals to Fish and Aquatic Invertebrates," Resource Publication 137 (Washington, DC: U.S. Fish and Wildlife Service, 1980).
6.  Kenega, E.E. "Test Organisms and Methods Useful for Early Assessment of Acute Toxicity of Chemicals," *Environ. Sci. Technol.* 12(12):1322–1329 (1978).
7.  Kenega, E.E. "Acute and Chronic Toxicity of 75 Pesticides for Various Animal Species," *Down Earth* 35(2):25–31 (1979).
8.  Bowman, M.C., W.L. Oller, T. Cairns, A.B. Gosnell, and K.H. Oliver. "Stressed Bioassay Systems for Rapid Screening of Pesticide Residues. Part I: Evaluation of Bioassay Systems," *Arch. Environ. Contam. Toxicol.* 10:7–24 (1981).
9.  Pearson, J.G., J.P. Glennon, J.J. Barkley, and J.W. Highfill. "An Approach to the Toxicological Evaluation of a Complex Industrial Wastewater," in *Aquatic Toxicology*, L.L. Marking and R.A. Kimerle, Eds. (Philadelphia: American Society for Testing and Materials, 1977), pp. 284, 301.
10. Kenega, E.E., and R.J. Moolenaar. "Fish and *Daphnia* Toxicity as Surrogates for Aquatic Vascular Plants and Algae," *Environ. Sci. Technol.* 13(12):1479–1480 (1979).
11. McKim, J.M. "Evaluation of Tests with Early Life Stages of Fish for Predicting Long-Term Toxicity," *J. Fish. Res. Board Can.* 34(8):1148–1154 (1979).
12. Maki, A.W. "Correlations Between *Daphnia magna* and Fathead Minnow *(Pi-*

*mephales promelas)* Chronic Toxicity Values for Several Classes of Test Substances," *J. Fish. Res. Board Can.* 36(4):411–421 (1979).

13. Suter, G.W., II, D.S. Vaughan, and R.L. Gardner. "Risk Assessment by Analysis of Extrapolation Error, a Demonstration for Effects of Pollutants on Fish" *Environ. Toxicol. Chem.* 2:369–378 (1983).

14. Biesinger, K.E., and G.M. Christensen. "Effects of Various Metals on Survival Growth, Reproduction, and Metabolism of *Daphnia magna*," *J. Fish. Res. Board Can.* 29:1691–1700 (1972).

15. Buikema, A.L., Jr., and E.F. Benfield. "Effects of Pollutants on Freshwater Invertebrates," *J. Water Poll. Control Fed.* 52(6):1670–1686 (1980).

16. Kenega, E.E. "Aquatic Test Organisms and Methods Useful for Assessment of Chronic Toxicity of Chemicals," in *Analyzing the Hazard Evaluation Process,* K.L. Dickson, A.W. Maki, and J. Cairns, Jr., Eds. (Washington, DC: American Fisheries Society, 1978), pp. 101, 111.

17. Franco, P.J., K.L. Daniels, R.M. Cushman, and G.A. Kazlow. "Acute Toxicity of a Synthetic Oil, Aniline, and Phenol to Laboratory and Natural Populations of Chironomid (Diptera) Larvae" *Environ. Pollut.* (in press).

18. Kendall, M.G., and A. Stuart. *The Advanced Theory of Statistics.* Volume 2, Inference and Relationships (New York: Hafner Publishing Company, 1973).

19. Millemann, R.E., W.J. Birge, J.A. Black, R.M. Cushman, K.L. Daniels, P.J. Franco, J.M. Giddings, J.F. McCarthy, and A.J. Stewart. "Comparative Acute Toxicity to Aquatic Organisms of Components of Coal-Derived Synthetic Fuels," *Trans. Am. Fish. Soc.* 113:74–85 (1984).

20. "Ambient Water Quality Criteria for Arsenic, Cadmium, Copper, Lead, Mercury, Nickel, Selenium, Silver and Zinc," EPA 440/5-80-021, 025,036,057,058,060,070,071, and 079 (Washington, DC: U.S. Environmental Protection Agency, 1980).

## DISCUSSION

*J.S. Meyer, University of Wyoming:* Don Mount analyzed the criteria documents for the priority pollutants and looked at it from a slightly different perspective. Given the five traditional test species that you showed, he looked at the range of toxicity values and found that in almost all cases, these five species covered 80 to 90% of the toxicity values. How well would his technique work with the Columbia data?

*G.W. Suter:* I don't believe that it would do as well. The reason is that the data set that Mount is working with, the criteria documents data set, contain a smaller selection of chemicals and a smaller selection of test species per chemical. Thus, he is seeing a smaller range of taxonomic variance than we are with the Columbia data set.

# SECTION III

# TRANSPORT, TRANSFORMATION, AND FATE

C.W. Gehrs

*Oak Ridge National Laboratory*
*Oak Ridge, TN 37831*

Modification of the structure and concentration of contaminants can result from various physical, chemical, and biological processes and greatly affect the potential hazards of the material. For example, photooxidation, hydrolysis, and metabolism can modify the structure of the parent material, whereas sorption, sedimentation, and bioaccumulation can enhance or decrease the concentrations confronted by biological systems of interest. This section includes chapters on research that describe mechanisms of transport within both the organism and the total ecosystems. It focuses on organismic or ecosystem transport to emphasize analogies in the processes operating in each system.

T. Bidleman discusses the area of atmospheric transport and deposition of organics and explains the difficulties of measuring the materials and determining estimates of the physical-chemical effects on transfer coefficients (for various organics) for model usage. He makes use of data from chlorinated hydrocarbons to show how physical-chemical parameters can be estimated and used in calculating deposition rates. O.J. Schwarz discusses the availability and movement of such deposited organics to terrestrial vegetation. His studies reveal that polycyclic aromatic hydrocarbons are not only taken up by vegetation, but appear to be transferred between components in the food chain leading to man. Dr. Schwarz identifies the need for studies that explain the binding role of various soils to clarify availability and accumulation of organics in terrestrial ecosystems.

The chapters by S.M. Bartell and A.J. Stewart describe investigations of the transport of organic contaminants through natural aquatic ecosystems. Bartell describes an approach that integrates simulation modeling (of basic molecular characteristics) of organics to estimate their transport in, and effects upon, aquatic ecosystems. Utilization of empirical data and Monte Carlo techniques enables not only forecasting for aquatic ecosystems, but it also identifies critical parameters where future data gathering is necessary.

Stewart's investigation demonstrates how naturally occurring organic materials can affect the availability and toxicity of organic materials to biological systems. He emphasizes the need for empirical data gathering to develop an understanding of, and hence predictive ability for, the interactions of dissolved humic materials and organic contaminants.

S. Tong describes research on the binding of two nitrogen-containing polycyclic aromatics to nuclear material. Relationships between chemical structure and binding will require further investigation, although initial data are quite promising for projecting fate within and effects upon specific organisms. In a study of the effects of shale or petroleum-derived jet fuel on rats, W.J. Mehm found visible effects in the liver. Serum chemistry revealed a return to levels similar to controls approximately 5 d after dosage.

The effect of light on the genotoxicity of petroleums is described by G.F. Strniste. His studies demonstrate the need for further research elucidating the role of environmental factors affecting toxicity of materials. All too often, the initial chemical form of a material is used to assess risk and determine "safe" release amounts. His chapter focuses attention on the need to evaluate modifications to chemicals occurring in the environment. Photoactivation may enhance toxicity, whereas abiotic/biotic degradation may decrease toxicity. An explanation of the mechanisms of interaction and modification is required if greater predictive capabilities regarding fate and effects for organic contaminants are to be realized.

# CHAPTER 18

## Possible Biological Fate of Inhaled Pollutants: Interactions with Biological Molecules and Chemical Carcinogens

A.P. Li

*Environmental Health Laboratory*
*Monsanto Company, Mail Zone*
*EHL*
*800 North Lindbergh Boulevard*
*St. Louis, MO 63166*

### J.D. Sun and C.E. Mitchell

*Inhalation Toxicology Research*
*Institute*
*Lovelace Biomedical and Environmental*
*Research Institute*
*P.O. Box 5890*
*Albuquerque, NM 87185*

The possible biological fate of the toxic chemicals associated with environmental pollutants was studied using diesel exhaust particles as an example of a respirable particulate pollutant. Antagonism of the cytotoxicity of the diesel-exhaust particle-associated chemicals by lung and liver cytosols, serum proteins, and sulfhydryl compounds was observed. Both enzymatic and non-enzymatic detoxification processes were probably involved. The chemicals interacted synergistically with benzo($a$)pyrene in the induction of genotoxicity. This synergism was observed using extracts from different cars and with three different endpoints for genotoxicity (mutations at the hypoxanthine-guanine phosphoribosyl transferase gene locus, Na$^+$-K$^+$-ATPase gene locus, and sister-chromatid-exchange inductions). Our findings demonstrate the possible modifications of the toxicity of environmental pollutants by both biological and environmental factors that may influence the potential health hazard of human exposure to environmental pollutants.

## INTRODUCTION

Emissions from the combustion of fossil fuels for energy production may have environmental consequences. The combustion products include toxic gases (e.g., $SO_x$, $NO_x$) as well as respirable particulate matter that may be a potential health hazard. Urban air particles,[1,2] automobile exhaust particles,[3,4] and coal combustion fly ash[5,6,7] have been found to contain cytotoxic and genotoxic chemicals and therefore have the potential to induce functional diseases due to cellular damage as well as cancer. Understanding of the manifestation of the toxicological properties of inhaled pollutants will allow a sound estimation of their risks to the exposed population.

Diesel exhaust particles are an example of a respirable particulate pollutant. The particles consist of a carbonaceous core containing aliphatic and aromatic organic chemicals. The small, respirable size (approximately 0.1 μm) and the association of cytotoxic and genotoxic chemicals with the particles suggest that they can be a potential health hazard. This chapter reviews our findings on the possible biological fate of the toxic chemicals associated with diesel exhaust particles.

## DIESEL EXHAUST PARTICLES AS
## RESPIRABLE POLLUTANTS

Inhaled diesel exhaust particles can have the following biological fates (Figure 1). The particles can be cleared from the lungs through a combination of macrophage and mucociliary actions, or they can be retained in the lungs long enough for the toxic chemicals to dissociate from the inert carbonaceous core. The dissociated chemicals can then interact with surrounding pulmonary tissue, inducing cellular damage, or they can be absorbed from the respiratory tract into blood and transported via the circulatory system to other organs such as the liver where xenobiotics can be metabolized. The toxic chemicals may also interact antagonistically or synergistically with other toxic chemicals in the lung, leading to a lower or higher degree of cellular damage respectively. This chapter deals with the possible biological fates of the toxic chemicals after their dissociation from the core particles. Our findings were obtained using in vitro cytotoxicity[3,8] and genotoxicity[9,10,11] assays with culture Chinese hamster ovary (CHO) cells. Chemicals associated with diesel exhaust particles were studied using an organic extract of the diesel soot.

Because the initial sites of action of the dissociated chemicals may be lung and liver cells, we studied the ability of these cells to alter the cyto-

**Figure 1.** Schematic representation of the possible biological fate of inhaled organic pollutants.

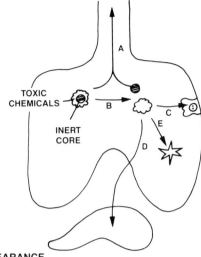

TOXIC CHEMICALS

INERT CORE

A: CLEARANCE
B: DISSOCIATION
C: CELLULAR INTERACTION
D: TRANSPORT
E: XENOBIOTIC INTERACTION

toxicity of the chemicals.[12] We found that although diesel exhaust particle extract was cytotoxic to CHO cells, the addition of liver and lung cytosols could decrease the cytotoxicity. Addition of enzyme cofactors NADP and glucose-6-phosphate further decreased the cytotoxicity, therefore suggesting a possible enzyme-mediated detoxification phenomenon. This detoxification effect was quite dramatic. For instance, using a concentration of extract (100 μg/mL) that would induce almost total cell-killing, the addition of liver or lung cytosol and cofactors increased the survival to almost 50% (Figure 2).

Serum proteins have been found in lung lavage fluid. The chemicals that have dissociated from particles may interact with serum proteins in lungs or, when they are transported in blood, in other organs. We therefore studied the effects of serum on the cytotoxicity of diesel exhaust particle extracts.[12] Sera from five animal species, including that of human, were tested. We found that cytotoxicity was dramatically decreased when CHO cells were treated with the extract in the presence of sera (Figure 3A). This probably is a nonenzymatic detoxification phenomenon involving protein binding, since the sera used were all heat inactivated (56°C, 30 min.), and since purified bovine serum albumin could also exert this detoxification effect (Figure 3B).

Sulfhydryl compounds are present in millimolar quantities in cells and can have a protective function against the possible damaging effects of oxidants. We studied the effects of three sulfhydryl compounds (glutathione,

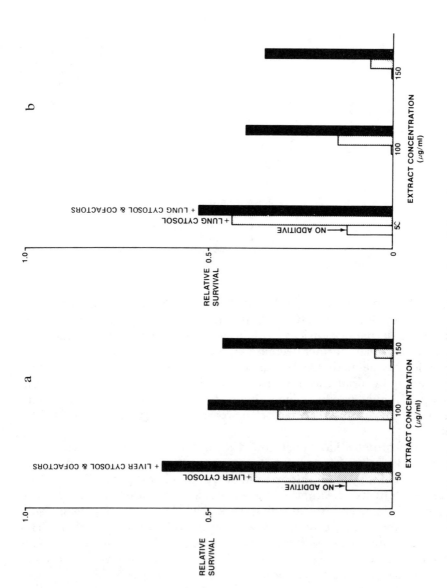

**Figure 2.** Effects of cytosols from liver (a.) or lung (b.) on the cytotoxicity induced by diesel exhaust particle extract. (Source: Reference 12, this chapter.)

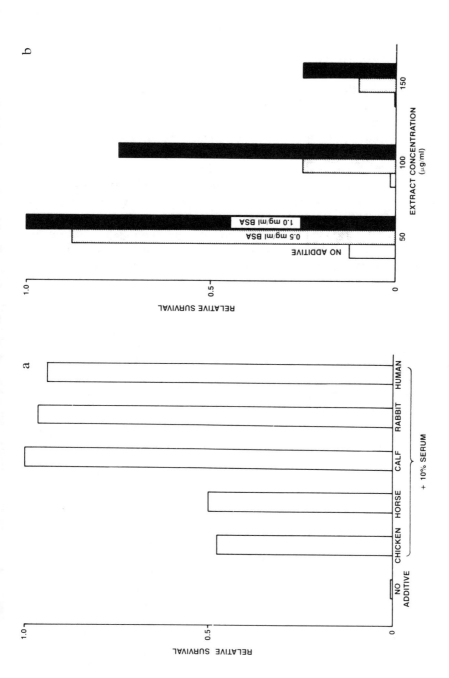

**Figure 3.** Effects of animal sera (10% v/v) of five different animal species (a.) or purified bovine serum albumin (b.) on the cytotoxicity induced by diesel exhaust particle extract. (Source: Reference 12, this chapter.)

cysteine, and β-mercaptoethanol) and their respective nonsulfhydryl analogs (oxidized glutathione, serine, and ethylene glycol) on the cytotoxicity of the diesel particle extract.[12] We found that glutathione, cysteine, and β-mercaptoethanol, as observed with serum and cytosols, could dramatically decrease the cytotoxicity of the extracts. The sulfhydryl moiety was involved in the detoxification as indicated by the ineffectiveness of the nonsulfhydryl analogs to detoxify the extract (Figure 4).

Apparently, although diesel exhaust particles contain cytotoxic chemicals, these cytotoxic chemicals can be readily detoxified. The possible health risk of diesel exhaust particles due to the associated cytotoxic chemicals may be less than predicted from the intrinsic cytotoxicity of the chemicals.

As mentioned earlier, a possible modifier of the activity of pollutant-associated toxic chemicals is their interaction with other toxicants already present in the lung. Such interactions have been observed in the human population exposed to cigarette smoke and asbestos or radiation. Synergism between potential carcinogens is suggested by epidemiological data on the lung cancer incidence of such populations.[13,14] Some chemicals (e.g., pyrene, fluoranthene, catechol) detected in cigarette smoke condensate enhanced the tumor incidence in laboratory animals induced by the known carcinogen,

**Figure 4.** Effect of sulfhydryl compounds or their respective nonsulfhydryl analogs on the cytotoxicity induced by diesel exhaust particle extract. (Source: Reference 12, this chapter.)

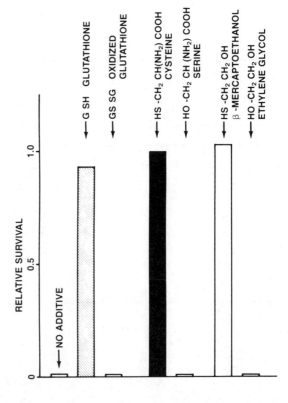

benzo(a)pyrene [B(a)P].[15] Since some of these cocarcinogens (e.g., pyrene and fluoranthene) have also been identified in diesel exhaust particle extract, we studied the possible synergistic effect between diesel exhaust extract and B(a)P in the induction of genotoxicity in CHO cells. It is to be noted that B(a)P is a known environmental pollutant and it is likely that cells exposed to the chemicals associated with diesel exhaust will also be exposed to B(a)P, either from the same diesel exhaust or from other pollutant sources.

CHO cells were treated with diesel exhaust particle extract alone, B(a)P alone, or a combination of B(a)P and diesel exhaust particle extract (Table I). Synergism would be indicated by a mutant frequency higher than the sum of the frequency observed from cells treated with a single agent.[16] This was observed. Using extracts from exhaust particles of 5 cars (each from a different manufacturer), the resulting mutant frequency at the hypoxanthine-guanine phosphoribosyl transferase (HGPRT) gene locus in the CHO cells caused by the combined treatment was approximately three times that expected (Figure 5). To further demonstrate that the observation was not unique to a particular endpoint for genotoxicity, we performed similar experiments using mutation induction at the $Na^+$-$K^+$-ATPase gene locus and induction of sister-chromatid-exchanges as endpoints. Synergism was again observed (Figure 6).[17]

We then studied the possible mechanism of such synergism, because understanding of the mechanism may reveal whether such synergistic interactions can occur in human exposure situations. B(a)P is known to be metabolized by monooxygenases to the 7,8-diol-9,10-epoxide (diol-epoxide) metabolite, which is believed to be the ultimate mutagen/carcinogen. The diol-epoxide can be further metabolized to the 7,8,9,10-tetrol (tetrol), which is believed to be nonreactive, or form a conjugate with reduced glutathione, which is also believed to be nonreactive. We therefore studied the interac-

**Table I.**   Experimental Design for Studying Interactions between Diesel Exhaust Particle Extract and Benzo(a)pyrene [B(a)P] on the Induction of Genotoxicity in CHO Cells

| Treatment | Observed Induced Mutant Frequency |
|---|---|
| Diesel extract only | A |
| B(a)P only | B |
| Diesel extract + B(a)P | C |

Interpretation:
  No interaction: C = A + B
  Synergism:    C > A + B
  Antagonism:   C < A + B

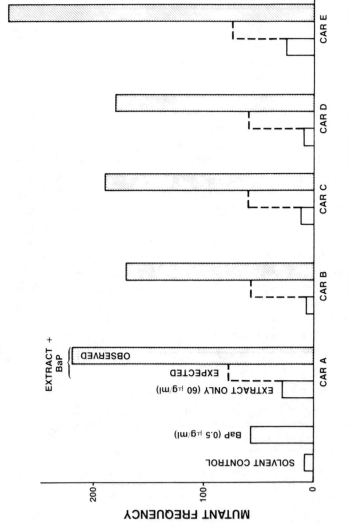

**Figure 5.** Induction of mutation at the HGPRT gene locus in CHO cells by treatment with solvent control (1% DMSO), B($a$)P (0.5 μg/mL), diesel exhaust particle extract (60 μg/mL), or a combination of B($a$)P and diesel exhaust particle extract. Extracts from the exhaust particles were from five cars of different manufacturers. The expected mutant frequency was calculated as the sum of the observed mutant frequency from treatment by B($a$)P alone and diesel exhaust particle extract alone minus that of the solvent control. (Source: Reference 16, this chapter.)

**Figure 6.** Synergism between diesel exhaust extract and B(*a*)P in the induction of genotoxicity as measured by mutation at the Na⁺-K⁺-ATPase gene locus and sister-chromatid-exchange (SCE) induction. (Source: Reference 17, this chapter.)

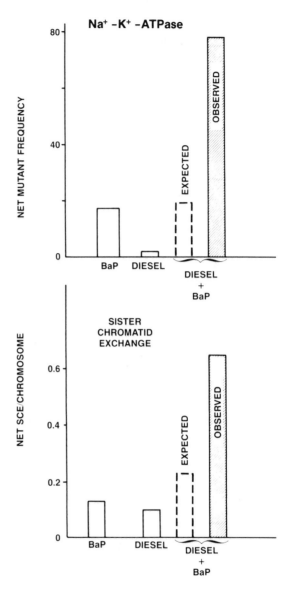

tion of diesel exhaust particle extracts with liver cytosol on B(*a*)P metabolism and with reduced glutathione.

To study the effects of the extract on B(*a*)P metabolism, we incubated ¹⁴C-B(*a*)P with an Aroclor 1254-induced liver cytosol fraction in the presence or absence of diesel exhaust particle extract. Results showed that the diesel extract inhibited the overall metabolism of ¹⁴C-B(*a*)P (Figure 7), which is in contradiction to the observed higher mutant frequency. However, high-performance liquid chromatography (HPLC) analysis of ¹⁴C-B(*a*)P metab-

**Figure 7.** Effect of diesel exhaust particle extract on the metabolism of $^{14}$C-B($a$)P by Aroclor 1254-induced liver cytosol (liver S9). Percent of unmetabolized B($a$)P in medium was plotted vs the amount of liver S9 used. (Source: Reference 17, this chapter.) (♦): no diesel extract; (●) with diesel extract.

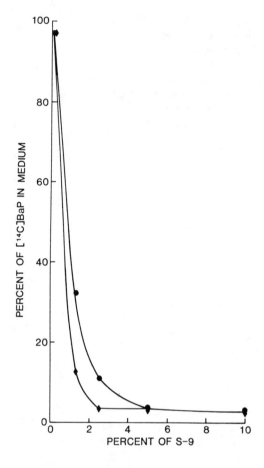

olites revealed a lower amount of the highly polar metabolites when the extract was present (Figure 8). It is possible that the extract could specifically inhibit the conversion of the diol-epoxide to tetrols, therefore allowing a higher level of the diol-epoxide to induce genotoxic effects.

The experiments on the interaction of diesel extract with reduced glutathione yielded more conclusive results. Dose- and time-dependent depletion of reduced glutathione by diesel extract (Figure 9) was observed. Part of the mechanism of the high mutant frequency caused by combined treatment of CHO cells with diesel extracts and B($a$)P may be the depletion of reduced glutathione by the compounds in the extracts, which would then allow the interaction of the reactive diol-epoxide to occur with cellular DNA to produce a higher genotoxic event.

## SUMMARY

Our findings indicate that both biological factors and environmental factors can modify the toxicity of the chemicals associated with diesel exhaust par-

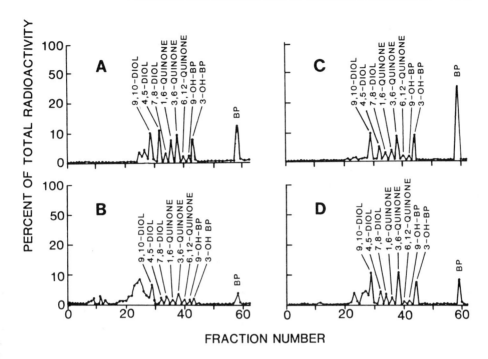

**Figure 8.** HPLC profile of [14]C-B(a)P metabolites after incubation of [14]C-B(a)P with Araclor 1254-induced liver cytosol (liver S9) in the absence (A, B) or presence (C, D) of diesel extract. Liver S9 at two concentrations, 1.25% (A, C) and 2.5% (B, D), were used. (Source: Reference 17, this chapter.)

ticles. The cytotoxicity of the chemicals was shown to be antagonized by liver and lung cytosols, serum proteins, and sulfhydryl compounds. The antagonism possibly involved both enzymatic processes, as indicated by the increased detoxification when cofactors were present with the cytosols, and nonenzymatic processes, as indicated by the ability of purified bovine serum albumin and sulfhydryl compounds to decrease the toxicity of diesel extract. The chemicals associated with diesel exhaust particles may also interact with other environmental pollutants, as exemplified by our findings on the synergism between these chemicals and B(a)P in the induction of genotoxicity. Depletion of reduced glutathione as well as interference with B(a)P metabolism by diesel exhaust, particle-associated chemicals can be part of the mechanisms for the observed synergism.

Our findings also reveal the complexity involved in the research concerning the toxicology of complex environmental pollutants such as diesel exhaust. Besides the difficult task of identifying the specific toxic chemicals in the complex mixture, one is faced with the possible modification of the ultimate toxicity via interactions between chemicals as well as with biological molecules. Our findings only suggest certain possible fates of the toxic chemicals associated with diesel exhaust particles. It remains to be answered

**Figure 9.** Depletion of reduced glutathione by diesel exhaust particle extract as a function of time (a.) and extract concentration (b.); (○ = incubation with solvent control; ● = incubation with diesel extract.

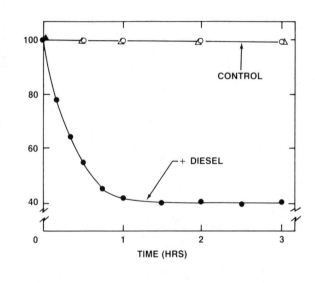

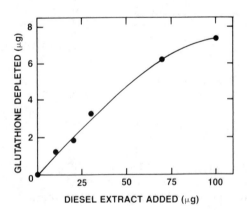

whether such fates actually occur in vivo, especially at realistic doses of exposure. It is certain, however, that information obtained with in vitro systems, such as those presented here, will prove to be useful in the understanding of the observations made in vivo.

## ACKNOWLEDGMENT

Research reported in this chapter was performed at the Inhalation Toxicology Research Institute, Lovelace Biomedical and Environmental Research Institute, under U.S. Department of Energy Contract NO. DE-ACO4-76EV01013.

# REFERENCES

1.  Talcott, R., and W. Harger. "Airborne Mutagens Extracted from Particles of Respirable Sizes," *Mutation Res.* 79:177–180 (1980).
2.  Predecker, B.L.B. "Bacterial Mutagenicity of Particulates from Houston Air," *Environ. Mutag.* 2:75–83 (1980).
3.  Li, A.P., R.E. Royer, A.L. Brooks, and R.O. McClellan. "Cytotoxicity of Diesel Exhaust Particle Extract—A Comparison among Five Diesel Passenger Cars of Different Manufacturers," *Toxicology* 24:1–8 (1982).
4.  Huisingh, J., R. Bradow, R. Jungers, L. Claxton, R. Zweidinger, S. Jejada, J. Bumgarner, F. Duffield, M. Waters, V.F. Simmon, C. Hare, C. Rodriquez, and L. Snow. "Application of Diesel Particle Emission," in *Application of Short-Term Bioassays in the Fractionation and Analysis of Complex Environmental Mixtures,* M. Waters, S. Nesnow, J. Juisingh, S. Sanders and L. Claxton, Eds. EPA 60019-78-027 (Research Triangle Park, NC: EPA Health Effects Research Laboratory, 1978), pp. 1–32.
5.  Fisher, G.L., C.E. Chrisp, and O.G. Raabe. "Physical Factors Affecting the Mutagenicity of Fly Ash from a Coal-Fired Power Plant," *Science* 204:879–881 (1979).
6.  Clark, C.R., and C.H. Hobbs. "Mutagenicity of Effluents from an Experimental Fluidized Bed Coal Combustor," *Environ. Mutag.* 2:101–109 (1980).
7.  Li, A.P., A.L. Brooks, C.R. Clark, R.W. Shimizu, R.L. Hanson, and J.S. Dutcher. "Mutagenicity Testing of Complex Environmental Mixtures with Chinese Hamster Ovary Cells," in *Application of Short Term Bioassays to Complex Environmental Mixtures,* M. Waters, J. Lewtas, L. Claxton, S. Sandhu and N. Chernoff, Eds. (New York: Plenum Press, 1982).
8.  Li, A.P., A.R. Dahl and J.O. Hill. "In Vitro Cytotoxicity and Genotoxicity of Dibutyltin Dichloride and Dibutylgermanium Dichloride," *Toxicol. Appl. Pharmacol.* 64:482–485 (1982).
9.  Hsie, A.W., D.B. Couch, J.P. O'Neill, J.R. San Sebastian, P.A. Brimer, R. Machanoff, J.C. Riddle, A.P. Li, J.C. Fuscoe, N. Orbes, and M.H. Hsie. "Utilization of a Quantitative Mammalian Cell Mutation System, CHO/HGPRT in Experimental Mutagenesis and Genetic Toxicology," in *Strategies for Short Term Testing for Mutagens/Carcinogens,* B.E. Butterworth, Ed. (West Palm Beach, FL: CRC Press, 1979), pp. 39–54.
10. Li, A.P. "Simplification of the CHO/HGPRT Mutation Assay Through the Growth of Chinese Hamster Ovary Cells as Unattached Cultures," *Mutation Res.* 85:165–175 (1981).
11. Li, A.P., and A.L. Brooks. "Use of Chinese Hamster Ovary Cells in the Evaluation of Potential Hazards from Energy Effluents—Application to Diesel Exhaust Emission," in *Proceedings of the International Symposium of Health Impacts of Different Sources of Energy,* M. Lewis, Ed. (Vienna: 1981), International Atomic Energy Agency, pp. 350–355.
12. Li, A.P. "Antagonistic Effects of Animal Sera, Lung and Liver Cytosols, and Sulfhydryl Compounds on the Cytotoxicity of Diesel Exhaust Particle Extracts," *Toxicol. Appl. Pharmacol.* 57:55–62 (1981).
13. Selikoff, I.J., E.C. Hammond, and J. Churg. "Asbestos Exposure, Smoking, and Neoplasia," *J. Am. Med. Assoc.* 204:106–112 (1968).
14. Lundin F.E., Jr., J.W. Lloyd, and E.M. Smith. "Mortality of Uranium Miners

in Relation to Radiation Exposure, Hard-Rock Mining and Cigarette Smoking—1950 through Sep. 1967," *Health Phys.* 16:571–578 (1969).

15.  Hoffman, D., I. Schmeltz, S.S. Hecht, and E.L. Wynder. "Tobacco Carcinogenesis," in *Polycyclic Hydrocarbon and Cancer,* H.V. Gelboin, and P.O.P. Ts'o, Eds. (New York: Academic Press, 1978), Vol. 1, pp. 85–117.

16.  Li, A.P., and R.E. Royer. "Diesel-Exhaust-Particle Extract Enhancement of Chemical-Induced Mutagenesis in Cultured Chinese Hamster Ovary Cells: Possible Interaction of Diesel Exhaust with Environmental Carcinogens," *Mutation Res.* 103:349–355 (1982).

17.  Li, A.P., J.D. Sun, C.E. Mitchell, and A.L. Brooks. "Synergism between Diesel Exhaust Particle Extract and Benzo(*a*)pyrene in the Induction of Genotoxicity in Chinese Hamster Ovary Cells," (in preparation).


## DISCUSSION

*M. Uziel, Oak Ridge National Laboratory:* One of the questions that we always concern ourselves with is whether or not there are any thresholds in terms of toxicity of chemicals to human beings. Your experiment with the glutathione suggests a negative factor in the toxicity, which suggests that maybe there can be a threshold response. Would you comment on that question?

*A.P. Li:* I believe that in the case of glutathione, due to the relative abundance of cellular glutathione as compared to the levels of oxidative toxicants in our body, there may be a threshold effect. The amount of reduced glutathione has to be decreased to a certain level before cellular damage can occur. This threshold effect is important in the manifestation of both toxicity and the synergistic interactions of toxicants, as I described.

*(Unidentified speaker):* In general, do you accept the no-threshold linear relationship between toxicity and exposure?

*A.P. Li:* That is a question that everybody would like answered. We are still discussing a threshold effect for ionizing radiation after many years of research. The dose-response relationship between toxicity and exposure probably is a function of not only the properties of individual agents, but their biological interactions in the exposed cells as well.

# CHAPTER 19

## Collection Methods and Aerial Deposition Predictions for Polycyclic Aromatic Hydrocarbons

### T.F. Bidleman
*Marine Science Program
Department of Chemistry, and
Belle W. Baruch Institute for Marine
  Biology and Coastal Research
University of South Carolina
Columbia, SC 29208*

### C.D. Keller
*Division of Science and Mathematics
Brevard College
Brevard, NC 28712*

Relationships of physical properties to aerial transport and deposition are discussed for two classes of trace organics commonly found in air: polycyclic aromatic hydrocarbons (PAH) and chlorinated hydrocarbons. A sampling method for chlorinated hydrocarbons that uses a glass fiber filter backed up by a polyurethane foam (PUF) trap has recently been applied to PAH collection. Retention of PAH vapors by a PUF bed is influenced by temperature and total air volume sampled. Vapor breakthrough in field experiments can be related to the temperature-weighted air volume, $m^3 p_T/p_{20}$, where $m^3$ is the actual air volume sampled and $p_T$ and $p_{20}$ are the vapor pressures of phenanthrene at the sampling temperature and at 20°C.

The apparent vapor/particle (V/P) ratio for trace organics is operationally defined by the adsorbent-retained and filter-retained quantities. The relationship of this ratio to the true equilibrium distribution in the atmosphere remains unknown. Nevertheless, the operational V/P distribution shows a strong correlation with the subcooled liquid vapor pressure for PAH and PCB. At common ambient temperatures ($\sim$10 to 25°C), the 3- and 4-ring PAH are present mainly as vapors, whereas PAH with $\geq$ 5 rings are largely particulate.

Washout and dry-deposition characteristics for PAH are estimated by

417

analogy to trace elements that have a similar particle-size distribution, and to chlorinated hydrocarbons. Dry-deposition velocities should be highest for PAH that are almost entirely particulate ($\geqslant$ 5 rings) and lower for PAH that are predominantly in the vapor phase (3- and 4-ring). A similar trend should be observed for PAH washout ratios. Based on their Henry's law constants, rainfall scavenging of PAH vapors is estimated to be unimportant compared to particle washout.

Exchange of PAH vapors across the air-water interface is discussed with reference to the two-film diffusion model. Henry's law constants for the 3- and 4-ring PAH are of the order of $10^{-5}$ atm-m$^3$/mol. Most of the resistance to transfer should be in the gas phase; however, the liquid-phase contribution to the total resistance is high enough to be included in exchange calculations. Reference is made to a literature report of PAH volatilization from water, which predicts that evaporation losses of PAH with $\geqslant$ 4 rings would be insignificant due to their low Henry's law constants.

## INTRODUCTION

Within the last 15 years, the importance of aerial transport in dispersing pollutants worldwide has become clearly recognized. Many of the long-range transport investigations for trace organics have been concerned with halogenated hydrocarbons such as chlorinated pesticides and polychlorinated biphenyls (PCB). Initial interest was generated in the late 1960s by findings of DDT and dieldrin on dust carried across the North Atlantic by the trade-winds.[1-3] In the decade following, many more studies of chlorinated hydrocarbon air transport were undertaken, and today we have a reasonably good knowledge of the types of compounds and their concentrations that are found over most of the world's oceans. Figure 1 summarizes DDT measurements over the oceans since 1975.[4-11] Concentrations of DDT over the North Atlantic are low, only a few picograms per cubic meter (pg/m$^3$). Most countries in North America and northern Europe stopped using DDT in the early 1970s, although the higher levels of DDT over the Gulf of Mexico and Baja California may stem from continued DDT use in Central America. By comparison, DDT concentrations over eastern hemisphere oceans are much higher, on the order of tens to hundreds of pg/m$^3$. Countries bordering these oceans are still heavy consumers of DDT and other chlorinated pesticides.[4,12,13]

The intent of this chapter is not to review aerial transport of chlorinated hydrocarbons. Such a review is available for data from the 1960s to the early 1970s,[14] and information up to 1981 is given in the references to Figure 1.[5-11] A summary of aerial transport and deposition of chlorinated organics in the Great Lakes region has also been published recently.[15] Instead, this chapter will discuss some aspects of the atmospheric behavior of "energy-related" organics, particularly polycyclic aromatic hydrocarbons

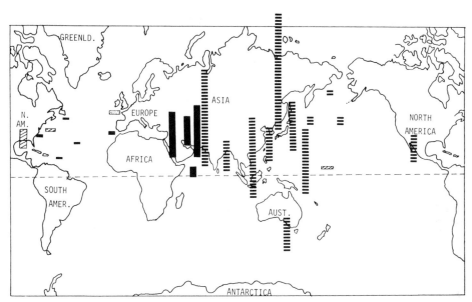

AIRBORNE   DDT   MEASUREMENTS   SINCE   1975

**Figure 1.**  Worldwide measurements of DDT over the oceans since 1975. The bars indicate references: solid, 9 and 10; dotted, 11; slanted, 7 and 8; parallel, 4–6.

(PAH). These compounds are produced in large quantities by fossil-fuel combustion, and some are highly carcinogenic, benzo(a)pyrene being the now-classic example.[16,17] Although many measurements of particulate PAH have been made in urban air, our knowledge of background atmospheric concentrations in remote continental and oceanic environments is very limited. Since the physical properties of PAH are similar to those of chlorinated pesticides and PCB (Table I),[18–31] we can apply some of the chlorinated hydrocarbon air sampling techniques to PAH vapors; perhaps a few years from now another map can be drawn for the global distribution of airborne PAH. We can also draw some parallels about vapor/particle (V/P) ratios in the atmosphere and depositional processes for the two classes of trace organics. Such comparisons, even if speculative, may serve to point out areas of research that are needed to further understand the transport and fate of airborne organics.

## COLLECTION METHODS FOR PAH IN AIR

Like other organics, PAH exist in the atmosphere as vapors and adsorbed to particulate matter. The V/P ratio depends on the PAH vapor pressure

**Table I.** Physical Properties for Chlorinated Hydrocarbons and PAH[a,b]

| | Melting Point (°C) | Vapor Pressure (atm) | Ref.[c] | Water Solubility (mol/m³) | Ref.[c] |
|---|---|---|---|---|---|
| PCB | | | | | |
| Aroclor 1242 | | $5.4 \times 10^{-7}$ | 18 | $2.7 \times 10^{-3}$ | 19 |
| Aroclor 1254 | | $1.0 \times 10^{-7}$ | 18 | $2.1 \times 10^{-4}$ | 19 |
| 2',3,4-TCB | 60 | $1.2 \times 10^{-7}$ | 20 | $3.0 \times 10^{-4}$ | 21 |
| 2,2',5,5'-TCB | 87 | $4.9 \times 10^{-8}$ | 20 | $1.6 \times 10^{-4}$ | 21 |
| 2,2',4,5,5'-PCB | 77 | $1.1 \times 10^{-8}$ | 20 | $9.5 \times 10^{-5}$ | 21 |
| Pesticides | | | | | |
| p,p'-DDT | 109 | $1.9 \times 10^{-10}$ | 22 | $3.4 \times 10^{-6}$ | 23 |
| Dieldrin | 176 | $3.8 \times 10^{-9}$ | 24 | $8.7 \times 10^{-5}$ | 24 |
| Lindane | 113 | $4.1 \times 10^{-8}$ | 24 | $2.0 \times 10^{-2}$ | 24 |
| Hexachloro-benzene | 230 | $2.2 \times 10^{-8}$ | 25 | $1.2 \times 10^{-4d}$ | 26 |
| Toxaphene | | $3.9 \times 10^{-10e}$ | 27 | $1.2 \times 10^{-3}$ | 28 |
| PAH | | | | | |
| Phenanthrene | 101 | $1.6 \times 10^{-7}$ | 29 | $7.2 \times 10^{-3}$ | 30 |
| Anthracene | 216 | $7.9 \times 10^{-9}$ | 29 | $4.4 \times 10^{-4}$ | 30 |
| Fluoranthene | 111 | $1.2 \times 10^{-8}$ | 29 | $1.3 \times 10^{-3}$ | 30 |
| Pyrene | 156 | $5.9 \times 10^{-9}$ | 29 | $6.5 \times 10^{-4}$ | 30 |
| Benzo(a)pyrene | 176 | $7.2 \times 10^{-12}$ | 31 | $1.5 \times 10^{-5}$ | 30 |
| Benzo(e)pyrene | 179 | $7.3 \times 10^{-12}$ | 31 | | |
| Benzo(k)-fluoranthene | 217 | $2.4-3.6 \times 10^{-12}$ | 31 | | |
| Benzo(ghi)-perylene | 276 | $1.3 \times 10^{-13}$ | 31 | $9.4 \times 10^{-7}$ | 30 |
| Coronene | 438 | $1.9 \times 10^{-15}$ | 31 | | |

[a]Different literature reports for some of these physical properties vary by up to an order of magnitude.

[b]Vapor pressures and water solubilities are at 25°C, except for p,p'-DDT, dieldrin, lindane, and toxaphene (20°C). Properties are for solids, except for the Aroclor fluids.

[c]See references at the end of this chapter.

[d]Temperature not reported.

[e]Vapor pressure for Strobane-T, a toxaphene-like mixture.

and the concentration and surface area of suspended particles in air. Most ambient air sampling for PAH has been done by drawing air through glass fiber filters. Pupp et al.[32] suggested that the collection of some PAH might not be complete under these conditions, and in recent years several workers have found that the major portions of the 3- and 4-ring PAH were not filter-retained.[33-37] In our laboratory, polyurethane foam (PUF) has been successfully used as a trapping agent for airborne pesticide and PCB vapors,[38-41] and recently we investigated PAH vapor collection by PUF.[37]

Samples were collected in downtown Columbia, South Carolina, or at the Savannah River Plant, Aiken, South Carolina, by drawing air at 0.4 to 0.5 m³/min through a 20 × 25 cm glass fiber filter followed by two 7.6-cm-diam × 7.5-cm-thick PUF plugs (density = 0.022 g/cm³). After sampling, filters were refluxed with dichloromethane and plugs were soxhlet extracted with petroleum ether. Extracts were cleaned up and separated into "nonpolar" and "polar" fractions on a column of alumina–silicic acid. The extracts were analyzed for total organics by flame-ionization gas chromatography on a 180-cm-long × 0.2-cm-i.d. glass column packed with 3% Dexsil-300, and for PAH by $C_{18}$ reversed-phase high-performance liquid chromatography using acetonitrile-water mixtures and fluorescence detection. Details for preparing and precleaning PUF plugs and glass fiber filters and analytical methods are given elsewhere.[37,38,41,42]

Chromatograms of total organics (Figure 2) and PAH (Figure 3) show that fractionation occurs in the sampling train, with the heaviest components retained by the filter and the more volatile components penetrating into the PUF column. Examination of several gas chromatograms of total organics showed that compounds eluting after n-$C_{19}$ were largely retained by the first PUF plug, with smaller quantities on the second plug. We therefore chose this cutoff point for quantitative analysis of total organics.

A sampling train behaves like a frontal chromatograph, and the movement of a vapor front through the adsorbent column depends on the volatility of the compound as well as on the total air volume.[40] For many high-molecular-weight organics, the vapor pressure approximately doubles for a 5°C rise in temperature. The combined effect of sampling temperature and air volume on the breakthrough from a front to a backup adsorbent trap can be estimated using a temperature-weighted air volume (TWAV). The weighting factor is $pT/p_{20}$, the vapor pressure ratio for the compound of interest at the average sampling temperature to that at 20°C. Billings and Bidleman[41] found that plug 2:plug 1 ratios for PCB vapors correlated better

**Figure 2.**  Gas chromatograms of the non-polar fraction of a Columbia, S.C., air sample, November 1981; 1.0-mL total volumes, 5-µL injections.

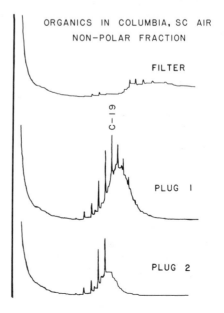

ORGANICS IN COLUMBIA, SC AIR
NON−POLAR FRACTION

FILTER

C-19

PLUG 1

PLUG 2

**Figure 3.** Liquid chromatograms of a Columbia, S.C., air sample, August 1982. Total volumes = 1.0 mL, 20-μL injections. The instrument sensitivity is 10 times higher for the filter chromatogram than for the PUF traps.

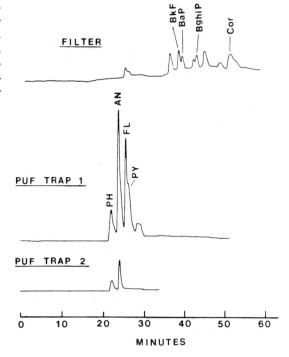

with the TWAV than with air volume alone, due to large day-to-day temperature differences.

Breakthrough of the 3-ring PAH anthracene and phenanthrene with TWAV is shown in Figure 4, where $p_T/p_{20}$ was derived from the temperature dependence of the phenanthrene vapor pressure.[37] In 24 h, our collection system samples about 600 to 700 m³ of air. For a 600-m³ air sample at 20°C, the average trap 2:trap 1 ratios for phenanthrene and anthracene are about 15% (Figure 4) and 25% for total organics heavier than n-$C_{19}$.[37] Under these conditions the 3-ring PAH will be effectively trapped by the foam column. However, at 25°C, the TWAV for a 600-m³ sample is 1140 m³, and the trap 2:trap 1 ratio for 3-ring PAH rises to 40% or more. Yamasaki et al.[36] also observed considerable phenanthrene and anthracene breakthrough with their PUF sampler at temperatures above 25°C. Temperature is thus the most important factor to be considered in designing collection systems for trace organics. Above 20°C, total air volumes should be lowered appropriately to maintain the TWAV below about 700 m³ to reduce the breakthrough of the 3-ring PAH. Less care is needed for the larger PAH fluoranthene and pyrene. Breakthrough of these PAH was less than 10% of the first trap value over the entire TWAV range studied.

Concentrations of organics in the air over Columbia and the Savannah River Plant are given in Table II and include both the filter- and the PUF-retained values. The major portion of total organics $\geq C_{19}$ and the 3- to 4-ring PAH were found on the PUF trap, while over 90% of the higher-ring

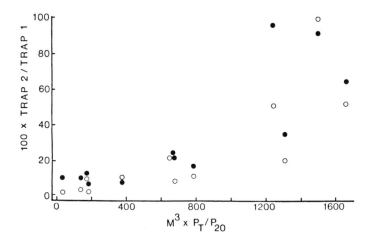

**Figure 4.**  Breakthrough of phenanthrene (●) and anthracene (○) from the first to the second PUF traps as a function of the temperature-weighted air volume.

PAH were collected by the filter. Relationships between volatility and the apparent V/P ratio are considered further in the next section. Blanks for the PUF plugs were very clean, averaging <5% of the quantities of total organics or PAH collected from urban air in a 24-h period.

**Table II.**  Average Concentrations of Airborne Organics in Columbia and at the Savannah River Plant, 1981–82 (ng/m³)[a]

| | Columbia | | | Savannah River Plant | | |
|---|---|---|---|---|---|---|
| | Samples | Range | Mean | Samples | Range | Mean |
| Total organics $\geqslant C_{19}$, nonpolar | 14 | 308–1666 | 641 | 4 | 106–438 | 292 |
| Total organics $\geqslant C_{19}$, polar | 11 | 69–797 | 311 | 4 | 70–223 | 139 |
| Phenanthrene | 11 | 14–140 | 37 | 4 | 6–14 | 10 |
| Anthracene | 11 | 0.3–4.2 | 1.2 | 4 | 0.05–0.2 | 0.11 |
| Fluoranthene | 11 | 2.2–23 | 6.8 | 4 | 0.9–2 | 1.2 |
| Pyrene | 11 | 6–27 | 12 | 4 | 0.5–4 | 2.0 |
| Benzo(k)fluoranthene | 7 | 0.03–0.3 | 0.08 | | | |
| Benzo(a)pyrene | 11 | 0.03–2 | 0.5 | 3 | <0.02 | <0.02 |
| Benzo(ghi)perylene | 11 | 0.2–5 | 1.3 | 1 | 0.02 | 0.02 |
| Coronene | 3 | 0.5–0.6 | 0.6 | | | |

[a]Average (arithmetic) TSP concentrations were 46 µg/m³ in Columbia and 29 µg/m³ at the Savannah River Plant.

## VAPOR:PARTICLE RATIOS FOR AIRBORNE ORGANICS

The apparent V/P distribution is operationally defined by the adsorbent-retained:filter-retained ratio. Yamasaki et al.[36] demonstrated that this ratio for PAH can be described by an equation derived from the Langmuir adsorption concept:

$$\log V(TSP)/P = -A/T + B \qquad (1)$$

where A and B are empirical constants, V and P are the apparent vapor and particulate PAH concentrations ($ng/m^3$), TSP is the total suspended particle concentration ($\mu g/m^3$), and T is the average absolute sampling temperature. A plot of Equation 1 for fluoranthene in Columbia is shown in Figure 5; similar results were obtained for pyrene, total nonpolar and polar fraction organics, and PCB (Aroclor 1254). Parameters for these plots are given in Table III, along with V/P ratios at 0° and 25°C. Concentrations of PAH in Columbia air are low, and for the other PAH we often did not collect enough material to determine the distribution in each phase. For phenanthrene and anthracene, less than 10% was filter retained, and in many cases these quantities approached the detection limit. On the other hand, a vapor-phase component for benzo(a)pyrene and benzo(k)-fluoranthene was usually undetectable.

Yamasaki et al.[36] collected their samples in Tokyo, where the mean TSP concentration was 127 $\mu g/m^3$ and PAH concentrations averaged 3 to 20 times those in Columbia. Considering these differences, it is remarkable that between 0 and 25° C the V/P ratios for fluoranthene and pyrene in the two cities agree within factors of 2 to 3 (Table III). Our data for PCB were obtained in three cities: Columbia, South Carolina, Denver, Colorado, and New Bedford, Massachusetts.[41] It appears that volatility is the most important factor in determining the V/P ratio, with differences in the nature of the TSP from city to city being of secondary importance.

Since the vapor pressure is inversely related to temperature, Equation 1 relates the V/P ratio to the vapor pressure of a single compound at different temperatures. Is the V/P ratio a simple function of vapor pressure for different compounds? Figure 6 shows the relationship between the quantity V(TSP)/P and vapor pressure at 25°C for different PAH and Aroclor 1254, a PCB fluid.[18,31,36,37] V(TSP)/P was calculated from the parameters in Table III and thus represents data from two cities for PAH and three cities for PCB. The vapor pressures used were for the subcooled liquid at 25°C. These can be estimated from solid vapor pressures by[43]

$$\ln p_S/p_L = -6.8(T_M - T)/T \qquad (2)$$

where $p_S$ and $p_L$ are the vapor pressures for the solid and liquid, $T_M$ and T are the absolute melting point and ambient temperatures, and 6.8 is an

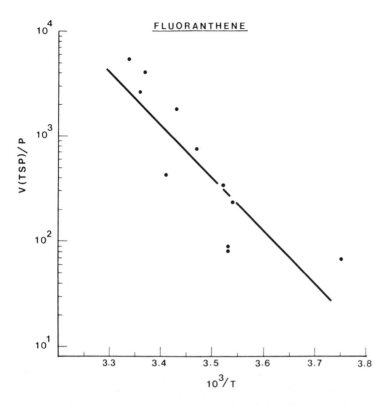

**Figure 5.**  Plot of Equation 1 for fluoranthene.

empirical constant. For high-melting solids, the difference between $p_S$ and $p_L$ is substantial. For example, $p_S$ values for phenanthrene and anthracene at 25°C are $1.6 \times 10^{-7}$ and $7.9 \times 10^{-9}$ atm, a volatility ratio of 20 (Table I). However, the melting point difference for the two compounds is over

**Table III.**  Parameters for Plots of Equation 1

| | A | B | $r^2$ | n | V/P[a] 273 K | 298 K |
|---|---|---|---|---|---|---|
| Total organics, nonpolar | $4.34 \times 10^3$ | 17.85 | 0.681 | 12 | 1.5 | 32 |
| Total organics, polar | $5.30 \times 10^3$ | 21.19 | 0.714 | 8 | 1.0 | 43 |
| Fluoranthene | $5.18 \times 10^3$ | 20.80 | 0.682 | 11 | 1.2 | 44 |
| Fluoranthene[b] | $4.42 \times 10^3$ | 18.52[b] | 0.805 | 27 | 3.6 | 81 |
| Pyrene | $4.51 \times 10^3$ | 18.48 | 0.695 | 11 | 1.5 | 37 |
| Pyrene[b] | $4.18 \times 10^3$ | 17.55[b] | 0.796 | 27 | 2.9 | 57 |
| PCB (Aroclor 1254) | $4.59 \times 10^3$ | 19.11 | 0.810 | 25 | 3.3 | 85 |

[a]For TSP = 60 µg/m³.
[b]Yamasaki et al. (Reference 36, this chapter) reported B values 1000 times greater, with TSP expressed in ng/m³. These B values were recalculated with TSP in µg/m³.

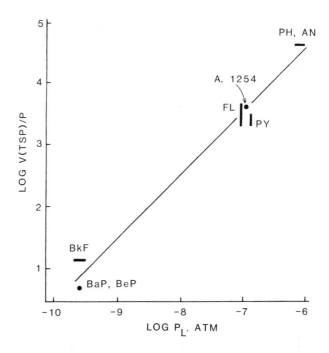

**Figure 6.** Relationship between log V(TSP)/P and liquid vapor pressure at 25°C for PAH and PCB. Symbols: PH = phenanthrene; AN = anthracene; FL = fluoranthene; PY = pyrene; BaP = benzo(a)pyrene; BeP = benzo(e)pyrene; BkF = benzo(k)fluoranthene. Horizontal lines represent the range of vapor pressures for PH and AN and the uncertainty in the BkF vapor pressure (see Reference 31, this chapter). Vertical lines are the range of average V(TSP)/P values at 25°C for FL and PY reported in References 36 and 37, this chapter (also see Table III).

100°C, and $p_L$ values for phenanthrene and anthracene are much closer: 9.1 × $10^{-7}$ and 6.2 × $10^{-7}$ atm, a volatility ratio of only 1.5. For predicting environmental partitioning, vapor pressures and water solubilities for the subcooled liquid may be more accurate than the corresponding constants for the solid phase. Octanol-water partition coefficients and bioconcentration factors for organic compounds are better correlated with subcooled liquid solubilities,[44-46] and breakthrough characteristics of anthracene and phenanthrene on PUF are more similar than would be expected for compounds with a 20-fold volatility difference (Figure 4). The correlation of V(TSP)/P with $p_L$ was very good, $r^2$ = 0.985, suggesting that $p_L$ may be used to accurately predict V/P ratios for nonpolar organics. Whether this simple relationship also holds for more polar organics (e.g., phthalate esters, fatty acids) remains to be tested.

We emphasize again that the V/P ratios discussed above are *operationally defined* by the adsorbent-retained and filter-retained fractions. During collection, air is pulled through the filter at a face velocity of 16 cm/s, and temperature changes occur over a 24-h sampling period. The apparent V/P ratio thus may not reflect an equilibrium situation, and it is surprising that the relationships in Figures 5 and 6 hold as well as they do. How closely the apparent V/P ratio approximates the true equilibrium distribution in the atmosphere is an interesting research problem remaining to be solved.

## ATMOSPHERIC REMOVAL OF TRACE ORGANICS

Aside from destructive processes in the atmosphere, substances are removed by wet and dry deposition of particles and vapors. The theoretical treatment of particle deposition and the exchange of gases across the air/water interface has received much attention,[47-52] and by using various theoretical models, estimates have been made of deposition of trace metals and organics to the Great Lakes.[15,53-59] Input estimates are often made using dry-deposition velocities ($V_d$), washout ratios (W), and Henry's law constants (H). These parameters are derived from atmospheric fluxes (F), concentrations (C), and physical properties, as shown below:

$$V_d = F/C_{air} = \frac{g/cm^2 - s}{g/cm^3} = cm/s \tag{3}$$

$$W = C_{rain}/C_{air} \tag{4}$$

$$H = vapor\ pressure/water\ solubility = atm - m^3/mol \tag{5}$$

Very little field work has been done to investigate wet or dry deposition of trace organics in relation to aerial concentrations. The few washout ratios and deposition velocities that have been measured are for chlorinated hydrocarbons, and no values for PAH in rain or fallout are available. Certainly this situation will change within the next few years. In the meantime, deposition parameters for the chlorinated organics may provide a guide as to what might be expected for PAH.

### Deposition of Particles

Wet and dry removal of particles is strongly influenced by particle size, as discussed by Slinn et al.[47-49] and Sehmel.[51] Theoretical calculations and wind tunnel investigations of monodisperse aerosol deposition show that $V_d$ and W are minimal for particles on the order of 0.6 to 1.2 μm in diameter and increase for smaller and larger particles. Large particles have very high $V_d$. For examples, at wind speeds of 7 to 14 m/s, $V_d$ to a water surface is 0.01

to 0.02 cm/s for a 1-μm-diam particle but 2 to 10 cm/s for a 10-μm-diam particle.[47-49] Thus, a small number of large particles can dominate the flux.

Slinn and Slinn[48,49] pointed out that the mass-average $V_d$ for a polydisperse aerosol can be many times larger than the $V_d$ for a particle of radius equal to the geometric mean. For a log normal distribution with geometric mean radius $r_g$ and standard deviation $\sigma_g$, the mass-average $V_d$ is given by[48,49]

$$\text{mass-average } V_d = \exp\{8(\ln \sigma_g)^2\}V_{d,g} \tag{6}$$

where $V_{d,g}$ is the deposition velocity for a particle of the geometric mean radius. If $\sigma_g = 2$ and $V_{d,g} = 0.01$ cm/s, the mass-average $V_d = 0.5$ cm/s.[49]

In addition, $V_d$ are influenced by meteorological factors and the nature of the receptor surface. Reviews of dry deposition[51,60] reveal an incredible number of field experiments carried out over the last 25 years. Particle $V_d$ vary by three orders of magnitude. Within the same group of experiments some generalities emerge. Pierson et al.[61] and Cawse[62] observed that $V_d$ and W were higher for soil-derived and sea-salt-derived elements having a large particle-size distribution than for other trace elements. A similar relationship for W was found by Gatz.[59] A summary of these flux parameters as related to the element mass median diameter (MMD) is given in Table IV. The W values measured by Gatz[59] in St. Louis are lower than those observed by Cawse[62] in the United Kingdom, but the trend with MMD is the same.

Trace organics are preferentially concentrated on smaller particles, because of their higher surface/volume ratio.[63] Mass median diameters (MMD) for PAH in a few cities are given in Table V.[63-68] These MMD vary greatly among locations, even in the same city, and tend to be lower in the winter than in the summer.[64] However, it appears that in most cases the MMD range from about 0.2 to 1 μm. One might therefore expect depositional parameters for *particulate* PAH to be similar to those for the small-particle trace elements.

What about deposition of the lighter PAH, those having a substantial vapor-phase component? If only the particle-bound PAH are deposited by fallout or scavenged by rain, and if the atmospheric concentration in Equations 3 and 4 is taken as the *sum* of the particulate and vapor-phase components, then $V_d$ and W should be lower for compounds with higher V/P ratios. This was observed for washout and dry deposition of PCB and chlorinated pesticides by various workers (Table VI).[69-72] Deposition parameters tend to be higher for the less volatile organics, reflecting a greater degree of association with particles. In some cases, higher W may also result from vapor scavenging by rain, as discussed in the next section.

Considering that only a small percentage of PCB and chlorinated pesticides are particulate (filter-retained) at temperatures of ~15 to 25°C, the $V_d$ values in Table VI seem altogether too high compared with $V_d$ for particulate trace elements (Table IV). Two possibilities might account for this: (1) the collecting surfaces used to sample organic dry deposition scavenge significant quantities of vapors, or (2) the particle sizes sampled in the or-

**Table IV.**    Variations in $V_d$ and W with Element MMD

| Element | MMD (μm) | $V_d$ (cm/s) | $W^a$ | Reference[b] |
|---------|----------|--------------|-------|--------------|
| Al, Ce, Sc | 3.2–4.2 | 1.2–1.3 | 1000–1600 | 62 |
| Na | 3.1 | 1.2 | | 62 |
| Fe | 2.5 | 1.1 | 1000 | 62 |
| Cl | 2.5 | 0.7 | | 62 |
| Co, Mn, Cr, Zn | 0.9–1.3 | 0.5–0.6 | 650–1100 | 62 |
| Pb, Sb, Br, Cs, V, As | 0.5–0.8 | 0.1–0.4 | 200–700 | 62 |
| Fe | 3.2 | | 250 | 59 |
| Mn | 2.4 | | 370 | 59 |
| Zn | 1.1 | | 180 | 59 |
| Pb | 0.6 | | 76 | 59 |

[a]Here W is on a weight basis, g/kg rain ÷ g/kg air.
[b]See references at the end of this chapter.

ganics dry-deposition studies were larger than those in the trace elements work. The first possibility seems unlikely. Except for McClure,[71] who used mineral-oil-coated glass plates, the workers used pans filled with water or coated with glycerine. Murphy[73] considered the problem of organic vapor sorption by fallout collectors and concluded that hydrophilic fluids, such as water, glycerine, or diols, would not collect appreciable quantities of PCB vapor.

The second explanation is more probable. The trace elements dry-deposition experiments in Table IV were done with a roof over the collector to protect it from rain, and the roof may also have excluded large particles. The significance of large particles in dominating the flux, discussed earlier, was clearly shown for field experiments by Elias and Davidson,[74] who compared trace element deposition to upward- and downward-facing Teflon plates. Fluxes to the upward-facing plate were 3 to 10 times higher than those to the inverted plate, which was shielded from large particle deposition. The fallout pans used by Christensen and Bidleman[69] were open to the sky, and there is no indication that other organics fallout work was done with shielded pans.

Predictions of $V_d$ for PAH are perhaps best made with reference to the chlorinated hydrocarbon data, meager though they might be. For unshielded collectors that can trap large particles, we might expect $V_d$ for fluoranthene and pyrene to be similar to $V_d$ for Aroclor 1254, a few tenths of a centimeter per second, because their vapor pressures are about the same on a liquid-phase basis. The $V_d$ for 3- and 5-ring PAH would be lower and higher, respectively. Fluxes (and $V_d$) would be dominated by the small fraction of PAH on large aerosols. For shielded collectors, $V_d$ should decrease. Totally particulate PAH might then have $V_d$ in the range for small-particle trace elements, 0.1 to 0.4 cm/s, while $V_d$ for PAH with substantial vapor-phase components would be lower. In the end, only field experiments will provide the answer.

**Table V.** Mass Median Diameters for PAH (μm)

| Location | Benzopyrenes | Benzo-fluoranthenes | Benzoperylenes | Dibenzan-thracenes | Coronene | Reference[a] |
|---|---|---|---|---|---|---|
| Toronto, Canada | 0.3–2.6 | 0.3–2.9 | 1.2–2.0 | | 1.4–2.5 | 64 |
| Ottawa, Canada | 0.6 | 0.7 | | | | 67 |
| Pasadena, CA | 0.08–0.12[b] | | | | 0.08–0.12[a] | 63 |
| Tokyo, Japan (tunnel) | 0.17 | | 0.2 | | | 66 |
| Antwerp, Belgium | 0.6–0.7 | | | | | 65 |
| Wilrijk, Belgium | 0.7–0.8 | 0.7 | | 0.8–1.9 | | 68 |
| Botrange, Belgium | 0.9 | 0.8 | | 1.6 | | 68 |
| Petten, Netherlands | 0.7 | 0.7 | | 0.8 | | 68 |

[a]See references at the end of this chapter.
[b]Approximate value; lognormal distribution not followed.

**Table VI.**  Average Deposition Velocities and Washout Ratios for Chlorinated Hydrocarbons

| Compound | Location | $V_d$ (cm/s) | W[a] | Reference[b] |
|---|---|---|---|---|
| Aroclor 1242/1016 | Columbia, SC | ≤0.04 | | 69 |
| | North Inlet estuary, SC | <0.06 | | 69 |
| | Kingston, RI | 0.07 | | 69 |
| | Eniwetok Atoll | <1.3 | | 8 |
| | Lake Michigan | | 14 | 70 |
| Aroclor 1254 | Columbia, SC | 0.43 | | 69 |
| | North Inlet estuary, SC | 0.16 | 94 | 69 |
| | Kingston, RI | 0.11 | | 69 |
| | LaJolla, CA | 1.2 | | 71 |
| | Lake Michigan | | 103 | 70 |
| Aroclor 1242 + 1254 | Minneapolis, MN | 0.13 | | 72 |
| Chlordane | Columbia, SC | 0.07 | | 69 |
| | North Inlet estuary, SC | <0.04 | 8 | 69 |
| | Eniwetok Atoll | <2 | 8 | |
| p,p'-DDT | Columbia, SC | 1.3 | | 69 |
| | North Inlet estuary, SC | 0.28 | 87 | 69 |
| | Kingston, RI | 1.6 | | 69 |
| | Arabian Sea | | 68 | 10 |
| | London | | 65 | 24 |
| Toxaphene | Columbia, SC | ≤0.12 | | 69 |
| | North Inlet estuary, SC | 0.24 | 246 | 69 |
| HCH[c] | Arabian Sea | | 23–41 | 10 |
| | Eniwetok Atoll | | 38 | 8 |
| | London | | 6–13 | 24 |

[a]W = g/kg rain ÷ g/kg air.
[b]See references at the end of this chapter.
[c]$\alpha$-HCH and $\gamma$-HCH (lindane).

## Washout of Vapors

The potential for vapor-phase washout can be determined by considering a raindrop to be in equilibrium with the concentration of vapor in air. Water-air partition coefficients can be calculated from the vapor pressures and solubilities in Table I and expressed as W (Equation 4) or H (Equation 5). These are given in Table VII,[24,75–80] along with some experimental determinations of H. Calculated H values are only as accurate as the physical constants from which they are derived, and in some cases literature values for vapor pressure or water solubility vary by as much as an order of magnitude for the same compound. Despite these uncertainties, the calculated and experimental H agree remarkably well for many compounds.

For most organics in Table VII, washout of vapors is unimportant. The large differences between vapor-phase W and field results for PCB, DDT, and chlordane indicate that wet removal is by washout of particles, not vapors. Liquid-phase vapor pressures of the 4-ring PAH are close to those of Aroclor 1254. The fractions of these PAH on suspended particles should therefore be about the same as for PCB, and their W should be similar—on the order of 100 (Table VI). These W greatly exceed vapor-phase W, so vapor washout would also not be important for 4-ring PAH.

A few compounds with high solubilities and/or low vapor pressures might favorably partition into raindrops. Lindane and toxaphene have vapor-phase W in the 15 to 90 range, which is not too far from field values. Benzo(a)pyrene and benzo(ghi)perylene also have high W for vapors, but at normal temperatures very little of these PAH would be present in air in the unadsorbed state (Figure 6).

### Air-Water Gas Exchange

Gas exchange across the air-water interface has been the subject of many articles in recent years. Theoretical details of the two-film transfer model, along with applications to hydrophobic organic vapors, are presented in several of the references.[15,47,52,53,56,76,78-84] Vapor transfer is controlled by diffusive fluxes in air and water films at the interface. The exchange rate is limited by the resistance to mass transfer in both films, with the ratio of the gas-phase resistance to the liquid-phase resistance given by[79]

$$r_{GL} = RTk_L/Hk_G \qquad (7)$$

Here $k_G$ and $k_L$ are the gas-phase and liquid-phase exchange constants, R is the gas constant (atm$-$m$^3$/deg-mol), T is the absolute temperature, and H is the Henry's law constant (atm-m$^3$/mol). MacKay et al.[79] calculated $r_{GL}$ as a function of H and the $k_G/k_L$ ratio (approximately 150, and usually in the 50 to 300 range). For values of $H > 5 \times 10^{-3}$, the resistance to vapor transfer is almost entirely in the liquid phase; while for $H < 5 \times 10^{-6}$, gas-phase resistance dominates. The resistance to mass transfer in both phases is important in controlling the exchange rate for intermediate H values, with equal resistance in both phases occurring for $H = 1.6 \times 10^{-4}$ ($k_G/k_L = 150$).

Fluxes (positive for water-to-air, negative for air-to-water) through the liquid ($F_L$) and gas ($F_G$) films can be calculated from Equations 8 and 9; for steady-state transfer $F_L = F_G$.

$$F_L = K_{OL} (C_L - p/H) \qquad (8)$$
$$F_G = K_{OG} (C_L H - p)/RT \qquad (9)$$

**Table VII.**  Henry's Law Constants and Washout Ratios for Organic Vapors

| | $H$ (atm-m$^3$/mol) | | | | |
|---|---|---|---|---|---|
| | Calculated[a] | Experimental | Refs[b] | $W^c$ | $r_{GL}{}^c$ |
| **PCB** | | | | | |
| Aroclor 1242 | $2.0 \times 10^{-4}$ | $2.2 \times 10^{-4}$ | 75 | 0.15 | 0.81 |
| | | $7.8 \times 10^{-4}$ | 76 | | |
| | | $7.6 \times 10^{-3}$ | 77 | | |
| Aroclor 1254 | $4.8 \times 10^{-4}$ | $2.0 \times 10^{-4}$ | 75 | 0.061 | 0.33 |
| 2',3,4-TCB | $4.0 \times 10^{-4}$ | $1.5 \times 10^{-4}$ | 75 | 0.073 | 0.40 |
| 2,2',5,5'-TCB | $3.1 \times 10^{-4}$ | $2.2 \times 10^{-4}$ | 75 | 0.095 | 0.52 |
| | | $9.2 \times 10^{-4}$ | 76 | | |
| 2,2',4,5,5'-PCB | $1.2 \times 10^{-4}$ | | | 0.24 | 1.3 |
| **Pesticides** | | | | | |
| p,p'-DDT | $5.6 \times 10^{-5}$ | $1.3 \times 10^{-5}$ | 24 | 0.52 | 2.9 |
| Dieldrin | $4.4 \times 10^{-5}$ | $4.5 \times 10^{-5}$ | 24 | 0.66 | 3.6 |
| | | $2.9 \times 10^{-5}$ | 78 | | |
| Lindane | $2.1 \times 10^{-6}$ | $2.1 \times 10^{-6}$ | 24 | 15 | 76 |
| | | $2.3 \times 10^{-5}$ | 76 | | |
| Hexachlorobenzene | $1.8 \times 10^{-4}$ | $1.3 \times 10^{-3}$ | 76 | 0.16 | 0.88 |
| Chlordane | | $(0.9–1.3) \times 10^{-3}$ | 76 | 0.16–0.23 | 0.12–0.17 |
| Toxaphene | $3.3 \times 10^{-7}$ | | | 90 | 484 |
| **PAH** | | | | | |
| Phenanthrene | $2.2 \times 10^{-5}$ | $3.9 \times 10^{-5}$ | 79 | 1.3 | 7.3 |
| | | $5.5 \times 10^{-5}$ | 80 | | |
| Anthracene | $1.8 \times 10^{-5}$ | $6.5 \times 10^{-5}$ | 80 | 1.6 | 8.9 |
| Fluoranthene | $9.2 \times 10^{-6}$ | | | 3.2 | 17 |
| Benz[a] anthracene | | $8.0 \times 10^{-6}$ | 80 | 3.7 | 20 |
| Pyrene | $9.1 \times 10^{-6}$ | $1.9 \times 10^{-5}$ | 80 | 3.2 | 18 |
| Benzo(a)pyrene | $4.8 \times 10^{-7}$ | $<2 \times 10^{-6}$ | 80 | 61 | 333 |
| Benzo(ghi) perylene | $1.4 \times 10^{-7}$ | | | 209 | 1143 |

[a]From Table I data.
[b]See references at the end of this chapter.
[c]Based on calculated H, except for chlordane and benz(a)anthracene.

Here $C_L$ is the concentration of dissolved constituent in the bulk water reservoir (mol/m$^3$) and p is its partial pressure in air (atm). $K_{OL}$ and $K_{OG}$ are the overall exchange constants and contain contributions from the resistance to transfer in each phase:[52]

$$1/K_{OL} = 1/k_L + RT/Hk_G \quad (10)$$
$$1/K_{OG} = 1/k_G + H/RTk_L \quad (11)$$

Note that for large H, $K_{OL} \sim k_L$, and for small H, $K_{OG} \sim k_G$, as discussed by MacKay et al.[79,81]

Prediction of gas exchange rates requires an accurate knowledge of the exchange constants, $C_L$, p, and H. Liss and Slater[52] suggest that reasonable average open-ocean values for a small molecule like $H_2O$ or $CO_2$ are $k_G \sim 3000$ cm/h and $k_L \sim 20$ cm/h. For large molecules, these values may be adjusted by assuming that molecular diffusion varies inversely with the square root of the molecular weight.[52] The exchange constants also vary with wind speed, linearly for $k_G$ and with the square of speed for $k_L$.[52] The need for specific knowledge of the exchange constants can be circumvented by measuring the exchange of two substances (for example, the evaporation of a chemical and the transfer of oxygen).[76,82,83]

For hydrophobic chemicals, the main limitations are a knowledge of H and $C_L$. Unless these parameters can be defined, we cannot even determine the direction of the flux, let alone its magnitude. As an extreme example, fluxes of PCB in Lake Superior can be calculated from concentrations of PCB in the surface water and the air over the lake. These fluxes range from 48,000 kg/year *out of* the lake to 5,100 kg/year *into* the lake, depending on whether a Henry's law constant of $\sim 10^{-4}$ atm-m$^3$/mol or an "effective partition coefficient" of $\sim 10^{-7}$ atm-m$^3$/mol is used in the flux equations.[57] The latter value was determined by Doskey and Andren,[56] who measured the loss rate of PCB from a liter of water containing 10 mg of fly ash. Partitioning of a chemical between water and suspended solids will thus affect the direction and magnitude of air-water exchange; and if H is used in the flux equations, the truly dissolved concentration $C_L$ must be known.

Unfortunately, $C_L$ has proved very difficult to determine experimentally. Most water sampling techniques that attempt to distinguish "particulate" from "dissolved" species do so by using filters of various porosities. The distinction between materials distributed between the two phases is thus purely operational. Hydrophobic organics have high affinities for submicron particles[85] and humic acid colloids.[86] Recent experiments have shown that organic pollutants are strongly associated with dissolved humics.[87–89] The quantitative aspects of these interactions must be taken into account in modeling air-water vapor transfers.

At this point, it can be noted that Southworth[80] has determined H for a few PAH using the vapor stripping method of MacKay et al.[79] These H agree quite well with H calculated from PAH physical properties (Table VII). For anthracene and phenanthrene, $r_{GL}$ is greater than unity, indicating that most of the resistance to transfer of vapors is in the gas phase. However, the contribution of liquid-phase resistance is great enough that overall exchange constants should be calculated from Equations 10 and 11. For the 4-ring and higher PAH, gas-phase resistance dominates and the flux may be calculated from Equation 9, where $K_{OG} \sim k_G$, or Equation 8, where $K_{OL} \sim Hk_G/RT$.

Southworth[80] considered the rate of PAH volatilization from water as a function of wind and current speed. The first-order rate constant for this process is simply $K_{OL}$/depth.[84] A selection of predicted volatilization half-lives for various PAH in a 1.0-m-deep stream is given in Table VIII. Southworth concluded that evaporation losses of PAH with $\geq 4$ rings would be insignificant in most water bodies due to their low H values.

[*Note added in proof:* Since this chapter was written, three reports on PAH and other heavy hydrocarbons in rain have appeared[90-92]. Kawamura and Kaplan[90] collected rainwater in Los Angeles, California, and identified over 300 organic compounds. Unresolved hydrocarbons and n-alkanes ranged from 25 to 56 μg/L and 0.7 to 2 μg/L, respectively. Sixteen PAH were identified at a total concentration of 0.06 to 0.1 μg/L. The major PAH were phenanthrene, fluoranthene, and pyrene. Wade[91] monitored hydrocarbons in bulk atmospheric deposition (wet plus dry) for over a year in the Chesapeake Bay region. Average total hydrocarbon concentrations at four stations ranged from 42 to 114 μg/L, with about 12 to 25% of the total consisting of n-alkanes.

Paukow et al.[92] collected rain in Los Angeles and in two Oregon cities, Beaverton and Portland. Fifteen PAH were identified, the most abundant ones being naphthalene, acenaphthylene, phenanthrene, fluoranthene, and pyrene. Two keto-PAHs were also identified—fluorene-9-1 and 9,10-anthracenedione. Total PAH in rain ranged from 0.1 to 2 μg/L. One rain sample was collected concurrently with measurements of PAH in air. Based on Henry's law calculations, the rain was supersaturated with respect to the concentrations of PAH in ground-level air.

## ACKNOWLEDGMENTS

This work was supported in part by the American Cancer Society and by the Deparment of Energy under the National Environmental Research Park program. The contribution of the Belle W. Baruch Institute is appreciated.

**Table VIII.**   Predicted Half-lives for PAH in a 1.0-m-Deep Stream[a]

|  | Current (m/s) | Wind (m/s) | $T_{1/2}$ (h) |
|---|---|---|---|
| Naphthalene | 0.1 | 1 | 70 |
|  | 1.0 | 1 | 10 |
|  | 0.1 | 4 | 20 |
|  | 1.0 | 4 | 3 |
| Anthracene | 0.1 | 1 | 130 |
|  | 1.0 | 1 | 40 |
|  | 0.1 | 4 | 40 |
|  | 1.0 | 4 | 20 |
| Benz(a)anthracene | 0.1 | 1 | 700 |
|  | 1.0 | 1 | 350 |
|  | 0.1 | 4 | 250 |
|  | 1.0 | 4 | 150 |
| Benzo(a)pyrene | 0.1 | 1 | 2000 |
|  | 1.0 | 1 | 1000 |
|  | 0.1 | 4 | 600 |
|  | 1.0 | 4 | 500 |

[a]See Reference 80, this chapter.

## REFERENCES

1. Risebrough, R.W., R.J. Huggett, J.J. Griffin, and E.D. Goldberg. "Pesticides: Transatlantic Movements in the Northeast Trades," *Science* 159:1233 (1968).
2. Seba, D.B., and J.M. Prospero. "Pesticides in the Lower Atmosphere of the Northern Equatorial Atlantic Ocean," *Atmos. Environ.* 5:1043 (1971).
3. Prospero, J.M., and D.B. Seba. "Some Additional Measurements of Pesticides in the Lower Atmosphere of the Northern Equatorial Atlantic Ocean," *Atmos. Environ.* 6:363 (1972).
4. Tanabe, S., R. Tatsukawa, M. Kawano, and H. Hidaka. "Global Distribution and Atmospheric Transport of Chlorinated Hydrocarbons: HCH (BHC) Isomers and DDT Compounds in the Western Pacific, Eastern Indian, and Antarctic Oceans," *J. Oceanog. Soc. Japan* 38:137 (1982).
5. Tanabe, S., M. Kawano, and R. Tatsukawa. "Chlorinated Hydrocarbons in the Antarctic, Western Pacific, and Eastern Indian Oceans," *Transact. Tokyo Univ. Fisheries* 5:97 (1982).
6. Tanabe, S., and R. Tatsukawa. "Chlorinated Hydrocarbons in the North Pacific and Indian Oceans," *J. Oceanog. Soc. Japan* 36:217 (1980).
7. Giam, C.S., E. Atlas, H.S. Chan, and G.S. Neff. "Phthalate Esters, PCB and DDT Residues in the Gulf of Mexico Atmosphere," *Atmos. Environ.* 14:65 (1980).
8. Atlas, E.L., and C.S. Giam. "Global Transport of Organic Pollutants: Ambient Concentrations in the Remote Marine Atmosphere," *Science* 211:163 (1981).
9. Bidleman, T.F., E.J. Christensen, W.N. Billings, and R. Leonard. "Atmospheric Transport of Organochlorines in the North Atlantic Gyre," *J. Mar. Res.* 39:443 (1981).
10. Bidleman, T.F., and R. Leonard. "Aerial Transport of Pesticides Over the Northern Indian Ocean and Adjacent Seas," *Atmos. Environ.* 16:1099 (1982).
11. Dawson, R., and J.P. Riley. "Chlorine-Containing Pesticides and PCB in British Waters," *Estuar. Coast. Mar. Sci.* 4:55 (1977).
12. Goldberg, E.D. "Synthetic Organohalides in the Sea," *Proc. Roy. Soc. Lond.* B189:277 (1975).
13. Jalees, K., and R. Vemuri. "Pesticide Pollution in India," *Internat. J. Environ. Studies* 15:49 (1980).
14. *Tropospheric Transport of Pollutants and Other Substances to the Oceans* (Washington, DC: National Academy of Sciences, 1978).
15. Eisenreich, S.J., B.B. Looney, and J.D. Thornton. "Airborne Organic Contaminants in the Great Lakes Ecosystem," *Environ. Sci. Technol.* 15:30 (1981).
16. *Particulate Polycyclic Organic Matter* (Washington, DC: National Academy of Sciences, 1972).
17. Perera, F. "Carcinogenicity of Airborne Fine Particulate Benzo[a]pyrene: An Appraisal of the Evidence and the Need for Control," *Environ. Health Perspect.* 42:163 (1981).
18. MacKay, D., and A.W. Wolkoff. "Rate of Evaporation of Low-Solubility Contaminants from Water Bodies to Atmosphere," *Environ. Sci. Technol.* 7:611 (1973).
19. Lee, M.C., E.S.K. Chian, and R.A. Griffin. "Solubility of PCB and Capacitor Fluid in Water," *Water Res.* 13:1249 (1979).
20. Westcott, J.W., C.G. Simon, and T.F. Bidleman. "Determination of PCB

Vapor Pressures by a Semi-Micro Gas Saturation Method," *Environ. Sci. Technol.* 15:1375 (1981).

21. Haque, R., and D. Schmedding. "A Method of Measuring the Water Solubility of Hydrophobic Chemicals: Solubility of Five Polychlorinated Biphenyls," *Bull. Environ. Contam. Toxicol.* 14:13 (1975).

22. Spencer, W.F., and M.M. Cliath. "Volatility of DDT and Related Compounds," *J. Agric. Food Chem.* 20:645 (1972).

23. Bowman, M.C., F. Acree, Jr., and M.K. Corbett. "Solubility of Carbon-14 DDT in Water," *J. Agric. Food Chem.* 8:406 (1960).

24. Atkins, D.H.F., and A.E.J. Eggleton. "Studies of Atmospheric Washout and Deposition of γ-BHC, Dieldrin, and p,p'-DDT Using Radiolabeled Pesticides," SM/142a/32 (Vienna: International Atomic Energy Agency, 1971), p. 521.

25. Farmer, W.J., M.S. Yang, J. Letey, and W.F. Spencer. "Hexachlorobenzene: Its Vapor Pressure and Vapor Phase Diffusion in Soil," *Soil Sci. Soc. Am. J.* 44:676 (1980).

26. Kenaga, E.E., and C.A.I. Goring. "Relationships Between Water Solubility, Soil Sorption, Octanol-Water Partitioning, and Concentration of Chemicals in Biota," Spec. Tech. Public. 707 (Philadelphia, PA: American Society for Testing and Materials, 1980), p. 78.

27. Spencer, E.Y. *A Guide to the Chemicals Used in Crop Protection*, 6th ed., (Ottawa, Ontario: Agric. Canada, 1973), p. 94.

28. Guyer, G.E., P.L. Adkisson, K. DuBois, C. Menzie, H.P. Nicholson, and G. Zweig. "Toxaphene Status Report," (Washington, DC: U.S. Environmental Protection Agency, 1971), p. 10.

29. Sonnefeld, W.J., W.D. Zoller, and W.E. May. "Dynamic Coupled-Column Liquid Chromatographic Determination of Ambient Temperature Vapor Pressures of PAH," *Anal. Chem.* 55:275 (1983).

30. MacKay, D., and W.Y. Shiu. "Aqueous Solubility of PAH," *J. Chem. Eng. Data* 22:399 (1977).

31. Murray, J.J., and R.F. Pottie. "The Vapor Pressures and Enthalpies of Sublimation of Five PAH," *Can. J. Chem.* 52:557 (1974).

32. Pupp, C., R.C. Lao, J.J. Murray, and R.F. Pottie. "Equilibrium Vapor Concentrations of Some PAH, $As_4O_6$, and $SeO_2$ and the Collection Efficiencies of these Air Pollutants," *Atmos. Environ.* 8:915 (1974).

33. Cautreels, W., and K. Van Cauwenberghe. "Experiments on the Distribution of Organic Pollutants Between Airborne Particulate Matter and the Corresponding Gas Phase," *Atmos. Environ.* 12:1133 (1978).

34. Broddin, G., W. Cautreels, and K. Van Cauwenberghe. "On the Aliphatic and Polyaromatic Hydrocarbon Levels in Urban and Background Aerosols from Belgium and the Netherlands," *Atmos. Environ.* 14:895 (1980).

35. Thrane, K.E., and A. Mikalsen. "High Volume Sampling of Airborne PAH Using Glass Fiber Filters and Polyurethane Foam," *Atmos. Environ.* 15:909 (1981).

36. Yamasaki, H., K. Kuwata, and H. Miyamoto. "Effects of Ambient Temperature on Aspects of Airborne PAH," *Environ. Sci. Technol.* 16:189 (1982).

37. Keller, C.D., and T.F. Bidleman. "Collection of Airborne PAH and Other Organics with Polyurethane Foam," to be published.

38. Simon, C.G., and T.F. Bidleman. "Sampling Airborne Polychlorinated Biphenyls with Polyurethane Foam—A Chromatographic Approach to Determining Retention Efficiencies," *Anal. Chem.* 51:1110 (1979).

39.  Billings, W.N., and T.F. Bidleman. "Field Comparison of Polyurethane Foam and Tenax-GC Resin for High Volume Air Sampling of Chlorinated Hydrocarbons," *Environ. Sci. Technol.* 14:679 (1980).

40.  Burdick, N.F., and T.F. Bidleman. "Frontal Movement of Hexachlorobenzene and Polychlorinated Biphenyl Vapors Through Polyurethane Foam," *Anal. Chem.* 53:1926 (1981).

41.  Billings, W.N., and T.F. Bidleman. "High Volume Collection of Chlorinated Hydrocarbons in Urban Air Using Three Solid Adsorbents," *Atmos. Environ.* 17:383 (1983).

42.  Bidleman, T.F., and C.E. Olney. "High Volume Collection of Atmospheric Polychlorinated Biphenyls," *Bull. Environ. Contam. Toxicol.* 11:442 (1974).

43.  MacKay, D., A. Bobra, D.W. Chan, and W.Y. Shiu. "Vapor Pressure Correlations for Low-Volatility Environmental Chemicals," *Environ. Sci. Technol.* 16:645 (1982).

44.  Banerjee, S., S.H. Yalkowsky, and S.C. Valvani. "Water Solubility and Octanol/Water Partition Coefficients of Organics: Limitations of the Solubility-Partition Coefficient Correlation," *Environ. Sci. Technol.* 14:1227 (1980).

45.  Chiou, C.T., and D.W. Schmedding. "Partitioning of Organic Compounds in Octanol-Water Systems," *Environ. Sci. Technol.* 16:4 (1982).

46.  MacKay, D. "Correlation of Bioconcentration Factors," *Environ. Sci. Technol.* 16:274 (1982).

47.  Slinn, W.G.N., L. Hasse, B.B. Hicks, A.W. Hogan, D. Lal, P.S. Liss, K.O. Munnich, G.A. Sehmel, and O. Vittori. "Some Aspects of the Transfer of Atmospheric Trace Constituents Past the Air-Sea Interface," *Atmos. Environ.* 12:2055 (1978).

48.  Slinn, S.A., and W.G.N. Slinn. "Predictions for Particle Deposition on Natural Waters," *Atmos. Environ.* 14:1013 (1980).

49.  Slinn, S.A., and W.G.N. Slinn. "Modeling of Atmospheric Particulate Deposition to Natural Waters," in *Atmospheric Pollutants in Natural Waters,* S.J. Eisenreich, Ed. (Ann Arbor, MI: Ann Arbor Science, 1981), p. 23.

50.  Scott, B.C. "Modeling of Atmospheric Wet Deposition," in *Atmospheric Pollutants in Natural Waters,* S.J. Eisenreich, Ed. (Ann Arbor, MI: Ann Arbor Science, 1981), p. 3.

51.  Sehmel, G.A. "Particle and Gas Dry Deposition: A Review," *Atmos. Environ.* 14:983 (1980).

52.  Liss, P.S., and P.G. Slater. "Fluxes of Gases Across the Air-Sea Interface," *Nature* 247:181 (1974).

53.  Andren, A.W. "Processes Determining the Flux of PCBs Across Air-Water Interfaces," in *Physical Behavior of PCBs in the Great Lakes,* D. MacKay, S. Paterson, S.J. Eisenreich, and M. Simmons, Eds. (Ann Arbor, MI: Ann Arbor Science, 1983), p. 127.

54.  Eisenreich, S.J. "Atmospheric Input of Trace Metals to Lake Michigan," *Water, Air, and Soil Pollut.* 13:287 (1980).

55.  Dolske, D.A., and H. Sievering. "Trace Element Loading of Southern Lake Michigan by Dry Deposition of Atmospheric Aerosol," *Water, Air, and Soil Pollut.* 12:485 (1979).

56.  Doskey, P.V., and A.W. Andren. "Modeling the Flux of Atmospheric PCB Across the Air-Water Interface," *Environ. Sci. Technol.* 15:705 (1981).

57.  Eisenreich, S.J., and B.B. Looney. "Evidence for the Atmospheric Flux of

PCB to Lake Superior," in *Physical Behavior of PCBs in the Great Lakes,* D. MacKay, S. Paterson, S.J. Eisenreich, and M. Simmons, Eds. (Ann Arbor, MI: Ann Arbor Science, 1983), p. 141.

58. Andren, A.W., and J.W. Strand. "Atmospheric Deposition of Particulate Organic Carbon and PAH to Lake Michigan," in *Atmospheric Pollutants in Natural Waters,* S.J. Eisenreich, Ed. (Ann Arbor, MI: Ann Arbor Science, 1981), p. 459.

59. Gatz, D.F. "Pollutant Aerosol Deposition into Southern Lake Michigan," *Water, Air, and Soil Pollut.* 5:239 (1975).

60. McMahon, T.A., and P.J. Denison. "Empirical Atmospheric Deposition Parameters—A Survey," *Atmos. Environ.* 13:571 (1979).

61. Pierson, D.H., P.A. Cawse, L. Salmon, and R.S. Cambray. "Trace Elements in the Atmospheric Environment," *Nature* 241:252 (1973).

62. Cawse, P.A., AERE-R7669 (Harwell, Oxfordshire: Environmental and Medical Sciences Division, United Kingdom Atomic Energy Authority 1974).

63. Miguel, A.H., and S.K. Friedlander. "Distribution of Benzo[a]pyrene and Coronene With Respect to Particle Size in Pasadena Aerosols in the Submicron Range," *Atmos. Environ.* 12:2407 (1978).

64. Pierce, R.C., and M. Katz. "Dependency of PAH Content on Size Distribution of Atmospheric Aerosols," *Environ. Sci. Technol.* 9:347 (1975).

65. Van Vaeck, L., and K. Van Cauwenberghe. "Cascade Impactor Measurements of the Size Distribution of the Major Classes of Organic Pollutants in Atmospheric Particulate Matter," *Atmos. Environ.* 12:2229 (1978).

66. Handa, T., Y. Kato, T. Yamamura, T. Ishii, and K. Suda. "Correlation Between the Concentrations of PAH and Those of Particulates in an Urban Atmosphere," *Environ. Sci. Technol.* 14:416 (1980).

67. Albagli, A., H. Oja, and L. DuBois. "Size Distribution Patterns of PAH in Airborne Particulates," *Environ. Lett.* 6:241 (1974).

68. Van Vaeck, L., G. Broddin, and K. Van Cauwenberghe. "Differences in Particle Size Distribution of Major Organic Pollutants in Ambient Aerosols in Urban, Rural, and Seashore Areas," *Environ. Sci. Technol.* 13:1494 (1979).

69. Bidleman, T.F., and E.J. Christensen. "Atmospheric Removal Processes for High Molecular Weight Organochlorines," *J. Geophys. Res.* 84:7857 (1979).

70. Murphy, T.J., and C.P. Rzeszutko. "Precipitation Inputs of PCBs to Lake Michigan," *J. Great Lakes Res.* 3:305 (1977).

71. McClure, V.E. "Transport of Heavy Chlorinated Hydrocarbons in the Atmosphere," *Environ. Sci. Technol.* 10:1223 (1976).

72. Eisenreich, S.J., G.J. Hollod, and T.C. Johnson. "Atmospheric Concentrations and Deposition of PCB to Lake Superior," in *Atmospheric Pollutants in Natural Waters,* S.J. Eisenreich, Ed. (Ann Arbor, MI: Ann Arbor Science, 1981), p. 425.

73. Murphy, T.J. "Evaluation of a Technique for Measuring Dry Aerial Deposition Rates of DDT and PCB Residues—Discussion," *Atmos. Environ.* 15:206 (1981).

74. Elias, R.W., and C.E. Davidson. "Mechanisms of Trace Element Deposition from the Free Atmosphere to Surfaces in a Remote High Sierra Canyon," *Atmos. Environ.* 14:1427 (1980).

75. Murphy, T.J., J.C. Pokojowczyk, and M.D. Mullen. "Vapor Exchange of PCBs with Lake Michigan: The Atmosphere as a Sink for PCBs," in *Physical*

*Behavior of PCBs in the Great Lakes,* D. MacKay, S. Paterson, S.J. Eisenreich, and M.S. Simmons, Eds. (Ann Arbor, MI: Ann Arbor Science, 1983), p. 49.

76. Atlas, E., R. Foster, and C.S. Giam. "Air-Sea Exchange of High Molecular Weight Organic Pollutants: Laboratory Studies," *Environ. Sci. Technol.* 16:283 (1982).

77. Paris, D.F., W.C. Steen, and G.L. Baughman. *Chemosphere* 4:319 (1978).

78. Slater, R.M., and D.J. Spedding. "Transport of Dieldrin Between Air and Water," *Arch. Environ. Contam. Toxicol.* 10:25 (1981).

79. MacKay, D., W.Y. Shiu, and R.P. Sutherland. "Determination of Air-Water Henry's Law Constants for Hydrophobic Pollutants," *Environ. Sci. Technol.* 13:333 (1979).

80. Southworth, G.R. "The Role of Volatilization in Removing PAH from Aquatic Environments," *Bull. Environ. Contam. Toxicol.* 21:507 (1979).

81. MacKay, D., and A.T.K. Yuen. "Transfer Rates of Gaseous Pollutants Between the Atmosphere and Natural Waters," in *Atmospheric Pollutants in Natural Waters,* S.J. Eisenreich, Ed. (Ann Arbor, MI: Ann Arbor Science, 1981), p. 55.

82. Smith, J.H., D.C. Bomberger, Jr., and D.L. Haynes. "Prediction of the Volatilization Rates of High Volatility Chemicals from Natural Waters," *Environ. Sci. Technol.* 14:1332 (1980).

83. Matter-Muller, C., W. Gujer, and W. Giger. "Transfer of Volatile Substances From Water to the Atmosphere," *Water Res.* 15:1271 (1981).

84. MacKay, D., and P.J. Leinonen. "Rate of Evaporation of Low Solubility Contaminants from Water Bodies to Atmosphere," *Environ. Sci. Technol.* 9:1178 (1975).

85. Pfister, R.M., P.R. Dugan, and J.I. Frea. "Microparticulates: Isolation from Water and Identification of Associated Chlorinated Pesticides." *Science* 166:878 (1969).

86. Poirrier, M.A., B.R. Bordelon, and J.L. Laseter. "Adsorption and Concentration of Dissolved Carbon-14 DDT by Coloring Colloids in Surface Waters," *Environ. Sci. Technol.* 6:1033 (1972).

87. Carter, C.W., and I.H. Suffet. "Binding of DDT to Dissolved Humic Materials," *Environ. Sci. Technol.* 16:735 (1982).

88. Wijayaratne, R.D., and J.C. Means. "Affinity of Hydrophobic Pollutants for Natural Estuarine Colloids in Aquatic Environments," *Environ. Sci. Technol.* 18:121–123 (1984).

89. Landrum, P.F., S.R. Nihart, B.J. Eadie, and W.S. Gardner. "Reversed-Phase Separation Method for Determining Pollutant Binding to Aldrich Humic Acid and Dissolved Organic Carbon of Natural Waters," *Environ. Sci. Technol.* 18:187–192 (1984).

90. Kawamura, K., and I.R. Kaplan. "Organic Compounds in the Rainwater of Los Angeles," *Environ. Sci. Technol.* 17:497 (1983).

91. Wade, T.L. "Bulk Atmospheric Deposition of Hydrocarbons to Lower Chesapeake Bay," *Atmos. Environ.* 17:2311 (1983).

92. Paukow, J.F., L.M. Isabelle, W.E. Asher, T.J. Kristensen, and M.E. Peterson. "Organic Compounds in Los Angeles and Portland Rain: Identities, Concentrations, and Operative Scavenging Mechanisms," in *Precipitation Scavenging, Dry Deposition, and Resuspension,* Vol. I, H.R. Pruppacher, R.G. Semonin, and W.G.N. Slinn, Eds. (New York, NY: Elsevier, 1983), p. 403.

# CHAPTER 20

## Food Chain Transport of Synfuels: Experimental Approaches for Acquisition of Baseline Data

### O.J. Schwarz
*Botany Department*
*University of Tennessee*
*Knoxville, TN 37996*

### G.R. Eisele
*Oak Ridge Associated Universities*
*Oak Ridge, TN 37831*

Experiments designed to define the extent of uptake, retention, and distribution of radiolabeled naphthalene, $\alpha$-naphthol, and 7-methylbenz(c)acridine in consumable meats, eggs, milk, and plants are described. The data from these experiments demonstrate the retention of variable but significant amounts of these compounds and/or their metabolites, indicating that they have the potential to enter the food chain. The animal experiments with swine, chickens, and dairy cattle include both acute and chronic studies. Plant experiments measured the extent of uptake and transport via a root port-of-entry mechanism in selected vegetable crops (i.e., lettuce, *Lactuca sativa;* onion, *Allium sepa;* pea, *Pisum sativum*). A hydroponic-based system was used to provide "worst case" exposure conditions.

### INTRODUCTION

This chapter describes our approach toward determining the extent of uptake, retention, and distribution of three potentially hazardous synfuel-derived compounds [naphthalene, $\alpha$-naphthol, and 7-methylbenz(c)acridine] in consumable meats, eggs, milk, and plants. Development of risk-benefit decisions requires information on behavior and metabolism of potential environmental pollutants. Coal liquefaction and shale-oil production technologies are being developed as major energy sources and will provide products

441

of great chemical complexity and produce wastes of uncertain composition. Societal concern was aptly expressed by Dr. C.R. Richmond in the opening address to the Third Life Sciences Symposium on Health Risk Analysis:[1]

> There will be demands from many quarters of the scientific and other communities to determine whether or not individual or classes of compounds are hazardous or toxic or carcinogenic or mutagenic, and to what extent these materials may be detrimental to man.

Many of the compounds found in synfuel products and wastes are known toxic substances, and many are closely related chemically to recognized carcinogens and mutagens.[2-3] Major sources of human risk will be food-chain transport of toxic wastes from production plants and spillage during production, transportation, and utilization. We do not know what levels of these substances and their metabolites will reach human populations through foodstuffs. Regulatory agencies charged with estimation of these risks to man may be forced to make this assessment in the face of serious deficiencies in pertinent data. There are few data on how organic components from synfuels impinge on man via the food chain.[4-6] It is not reasonable or accurate to predict these risks by extrapolation from laboratory animals and from experiments that are often unrealistic and peripheral to risks that will occur in real-world situations involving food-producing animals. The uncertainties about source terms, chemical characteristics, and exposure conditions must be recognized when assessing the impact on food-producing animals and plants. Much of the body burden of the animals will come from ingested feed and water, with the primary route of human exposure being the consumption of this contaminated meat, milk, and eggs. The port of entry to food plants may, depending on the route of environmental contamination, be any one or a combination of mechanisms involving root or foliar uptake. It is imperative that studies addressing these questions be initiated prior to the large-scale deployment of this industry so that adequate emission standards can be set to safeguard human foods.

### Rationale

Both proposed and existing coal-conversion processes, designed for various types of fuel production, produce substances that are potentially toxic to man. Although direct exposure of workers to these substances is a concern, the possibility also exists for environmental release of these effluents, which may result in their uptake, transport, and biological concentration in primary foodstuffs directly and indirectly consumed by the public.

The animal studies include the determination of the biological retention of representative compounds following acute and chronic oral administration, the accumulation and loss of these compounds in consumable products following an acute exposure, and the rate of accumulation and their steady-state levels in tissues when they are administered chronically.

Plants are the primary food source for man, either by direct comsumption or as feed for livestock, fish, or poultry. The plant portion of the food-chain research program deals with efforts to determine the extent of uptake and transport via the root port-of-entry mechanism in selected vegetable crop species commonly consumed by man. Test plants were selected for physiological and morphological diversity of the organs consumed by humans.

Radiotracer methodology was used to determine the distribution of compounds and their metabolites in consumable products (i.e., milk, eggs, meat, and plants). The use of radiolabeled ($^{14}$C) compounds allows the determination of total retained label in each tissue of each species studied. Analysis for parent compound remaining in the tissues is underway; these values are reported where available.

## MATERIALS AND METHODS

### Animals, Acute Studies

#### Poultry

Single-comb White Leghorn pullets, approximately 41 weeks of age, were caged individually and received the specific test compound by oral intubation. A complete all-mash laying ration and water were available ad libitum. Eggs were collected daily for analysis of the albumin and yolk. Pullets were killed 1 and 3 d after dosing, and samples of muscle (light and dark meat), liver, and fat were taken.

#### Swine

Male and female swine were maintained in individual metabolism units after receiving the specific compound by oral intubation or in the feed. Feeding and watering were from pans contained in the metabolism unit. At necropsy, 1 and 3 d postexposure, two muscle samples, liver, and fat samples were collected for analysis.

#### Dairy Cattle

Dairy cows, approximately 3 years of age, were maintained in individual metabolism units after receiving the compounds in gelatin capsules via a balling gun. They were fed a balanced concentrate of feed. Roughage and water were available ad libitum. The cows were milked twice daily, and milk and milk fat were evaluated for the parent compound and its metabolites. Automatic milking units were decontaminated after each use. Animals were killed 3 d postexposure, and two muscle samples, liver, and fat were examined.

## Animals, Chronic Studies

In the chronic ingestion studies, the same three species previously described received daily doses of low levels of the same compounds used in the acute studies. Animals were killed 30 d postexposure to determine the bioaccumulation of these compounds. Production data (e.g., milk yield, egg production, feed efficiency, growth rate, and clinical manifestations or pathological conditions) were also evaluated.

### Poultry

Single-comb White Leghorn pullets, approximately 41 weeks of age, were used in these experiments. All eggs were evaluated over the 30-d period. At necropsy, samples of muscle (light and dark meat), liver, and fat were taken for analysis.

### Swine

Male and female swine were used for each experiment. The swine were maintained in confinement units and received a balanced growing ration. Swine were trained to consume a bolus containing the compound under study. After consumption of the contaminated meal, additional feed was offered throughout the day. At necropsy, two muscle samples, liver, and fat were evaluated for accumulation of the respective compounds and their metabolites.

### Dairy Cattle

Dairy cows, approximately 3 years old, were maintained in individual stanchion stalls. A balanced concentrate, good quality roughage, and water were available. The organic compounds were given in a bolus or other media. Cows were milked twice a day and milk profile determinations conducted. At necropsy, two muscle samples, liver, and fat were collected for analysis.

## Plants

The overall experimental design was to provide near-optimal growth conditions to minimize environmental stress during the time of exposure of the plants to the test substances. A hydroponic-based system was designed to provide "worst case" exposure conditions for measuring the contribution of a root mechanism of uptake. The hydroponic system assures a uniform water and nutrient supply and maximal availability of the dissolved test substance (i.e., assuming plant availability is essentially governed by waterborne or mediated uptake systems).

The test plants were chosen for physiological and morphological diversity of the parts eaten by humans. The test plants were lettuce, *Lactuca sativa;* onion, *Allium sepa;* and pea, *Pisum sativum.*

### Test Plant Source

All plants were grown from single batches of certified seed to minimize plant-to-plant variation. Seed (or bulbs in the case of onion) were sown weekly in a synthetic soil mix in standard 24-pocket commercial flats. Plants were thinned to one plant per pocket 2 to 3 weeks after germination, the time depending on the species. The initial germination and early growth of the seedlings were accomplished in a walk-in growth chamber. Irradiation (250 $\mu$E m$^{-2}$ s$^{-1}$) was provided by a mixed, cool-white fluorescent/incandescent light bank (80 and 20% wattage, respectively) timed to a 16-h light/8-h dark photoperiod. Thermoperiodicity was maintained at approximately $22 \pm 2°C$ over the 24-h photoperiod. Humidity levels were reasonably stable at $45 \pm 5\%$. Ambient carbon dioxide concentrations were maintained as a result of continual outside air exchange.

Weekly plantings provided a constant supply of transplant-size seedlings for planting into a hydroponic culture unit located in a greenhouse. The plant support matrix was flooded three times per 24-h d with half-strength Hoaglands nutrient solution, pH 5.7.[7] Plants remained in the hydroponic culture unit until they attained sufficient morphological maturity to be considered "ready for harvest" (i.e., appropriate maturity for human consumption). As needed for testing, plants were transferred from the hydroponic culture unit to the hydroponic root-uptake testing unit.

### Hydroponic Root-Uptake Testing Unit

The hydroponic test chamber is diagramed in Figure 1. The unit shown is a modified version of a more complete unit designed to monitor both root and shoot environments. This version of the test unit isolated the root of the plant from the aboveground shoot, minimizing the possibility of leaf uptake of volatilized test compounds. The unit provided the test plants with a reasonably uniform root environment. The entire hydroponic system has an internal working volume of 18.6 L. The nutrient solution (half-strength Hoaglands, pH 5.7) was continuously pumped from the main chamber into the solution aeration chamber and allowed to gravity syphon back to the main tank. The variable speed pump circulated the nutrient solution so that the entire solution turned over approximately six times an hour. Measurements of the nutrient solution with an oxygen electrode under actual running conditions showed that the test solution maintained ambient saturation levels of oxygen.

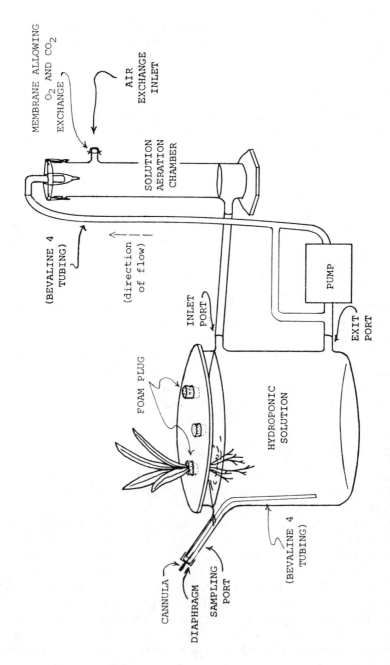

**Figure 1.**   Hydroponic root-uptake testing unit.

The hydroponic unit is constructed of relatively chemically inert materials [e.g., Pyrex glass, Bev-a-line IV tubing (Bev-a-line IV, Thermoplastic Scientifics, Inc., Cole-Parmer Instrument Company, Chicago, IL 60648), stainless steel fittings] to minimize, where possible, interaction between the substance being tested and the unit itself. This type of construction and design also provides for minimal maintenance and downtime between experimental runs. After each complete run, the units were flushed with a 30% ethanol: 2 $N$ HCl-$H_2O$ mixture to facilitate decontamination and general cleaning of the units. Currently, two such units are operational, providing 2,3-plant-replicate capability per run. When necessary, the outer surfaces of the hydroponic units were double wrapped in foil to prevent exposure of the nutrient solution to ambient light.

The entire test unit was placed in a standard laboratory fume hood equipped with a mixed, cool-white fluorescent/incandescent light bank. Irradiation was 300 $\mu E$ $m^2$ $s^{-1}$ at the leaf surface, approximately 85% full sunlight. The plants were provided with a 16-h light/8-h dark photoperiod. The air flow over the plants averaged 50 ft/min providing a moderate air exchange. This rate of air exchange provided for uniform ambient levels of carbon dioxide and oxygen and the necessary temperature stabilization of the nutrient solution and plant environment at 24 ± 2°C.

The length of time the plants were exposed to any particular test substance was 72 ± 2 h. The test substrate concentration of the hydroponic solution was monitored at appropriate intervals during the experiments to determine the kinetics of its removal. Samples of nutrient solution were taken at the end of each run to determine the stability of the parent compound. This approach was dictated because of the wide physical and chemical diversity of compounds to be tested. Data presented for the uptake and distribution of radiolabel within the various plants were derived from a single harvest time. The limitation of this type of experimental design is discussed in the Results and Discussion section.

### Radiometric Analysis

For radioanalysis, three 100-mg samples were placed directly into standard scintillation vials to which was added 1 mL of tissue solubilizer (Unisol, Isolab, Inc.). Vials were capped, mixed, and placed in a 37°C water bath until tissue samples were solubilized. Vials were removed from the water bath, and the following were added in sequence: 0.5 mL methanol, 10 mL Unisol-Complement (Isolab, Inc.), and 0.1 mL 30% hydrogen peroxide. Samples were mixed again and counted (Searle Mark III Liquid Scintillation system). Each counting group included appropriate standards and a background determination. The Mark III has a 70% efficiency for $^{14}C$ under the conditions used.

## RESULTS AND DISCUSSION

### Animal Studies

The results of acute exposure of laying hens to naphthalene (0.443 mg), α-naphthol (0.336 mg), and 7-methylbenz(c)acridine (1.76 mg) are shown in Figure 2. The major sites of deposition for all three compounds were the liver and fat. At 72 h, naphthalene concentration was reduced in all tissues. The two muscle samples, white and dark meat, indicate that naphthalene is readily taken up by these muscles and approximately one-half is removed 72 h later. It is interesting to note that the two types of muscle appear to differ in their retention of naphthalene, the dark meat apparently retaining more of the compound. A similar observation was noted for benzo(a)pyrene (BaP) (work not reported here), the uptake being greater in the white meat. Naphthol was taken up by liver within the first 24 h, approximately one-half being lost by 72 h; little, however, was taken up by meat or fat. After an acute exposure, all three of these chemicals or their metabolites were retained in edible portions of the laying hens. Thus, naphthalene, followed by 7-methylbenz(c)acridine, and, to a lesser extent naphthol, all have the potential to enter the food chain. The postexposure distribution of naphthalene is shown in Table I.

Little work appears in the literature on determination of levels of naph-

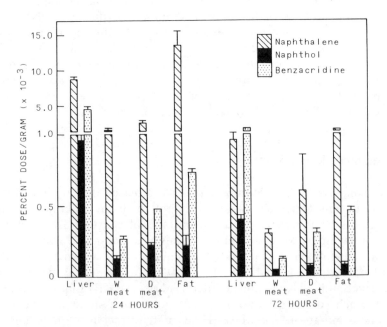

**Figure 2.**   Naphthalene, naphthol, and 7-methylbenz(c)acridine in tissues from laying hens after an acute exposure.

**Table I.** Distribution of Naphthalene and Its Metabolites in Laying Hens, Pigs, and Dairy Cattle After an Acute Exposure

| Tissue | 24 h Postexposure (mg equiv/g Tissue) | 72 h Postexposure (mg equiv/g Tissue) |
|---|---|---|
| Laying hens | | |
| Liver | 3.87 ± 0.175[a] | 0.475 ± 0.051[a] |
| Fat | 6.00 ± 0.878 | 0.710 ± 0.027 |
| Muscle (dark) | 1.17 ± 0.115 | 0.282 ± 0.091 |
| Muscle (white) | 0.74 ± 0.071 | 0.135 ± 0.015 |
| Pig | | |
| Liver | 6.47 ± 1.48[b] | 8.44 ± 5.88[b] |
| Fat | 70.50 ± 60.7 | 53.67 ± 28.40 |
| Muscle (loin) | 2.75 ± 0.763 | 1.33 ± 0.0 |
| Muscle (ham) | 3.04 ± 0.497 | 1.36 ± 0.03 |
| Dairy Cow | c | |
| Liver | c | 4.71[b] |
| Fat | c | 0.38 |
| Muscle (loin) | c | 2.34 |
| Muscle (flank) | c | 4.86 |

[a]Value ± standard error ($10^{-5}$).
[b]Value ± standard error ($10^{-6}$).
[c]No data.

thalene, α-naphthol, or their metabolites in tissues of complex organisms. The most recent efforts at determining these levels are the works of Malins et al.[8] and Roubal et al.[9] in fish tissues. Our studies on the metabolism of naphthalene in food-producing animals used two separate analytical approaches recommended by these authors.

The first method uses a strongly acidic and then a strongly basic digestion that destroys most conjugates but allows an estimate of the levels of unchanged naphthalene and the extent of its metabolism. This method also permits near-complete dissolution of the labeled compounds from the tissues. As shown in Table II, 24 h after dosing, a considerable level of unchanged naphthalene was found in fat and heart; lower levels were found in liver, kidney, and dark and light muscle. Unmetabolized naphthalene could not be detected in egg. In the parallel swine studies, 24 h after dosing, high levels of unchanged naphthalene were found in fat, and lower levels were present in liver, heart, loin, and ham. After 72 h, only fat, among the swine tissues examined, had detectable levels of unchanged naphthalene.

The second method[10,11] uses extensive extraction of the tissues by organic solvents and permits the analysis for individual metabolites by high-pressure liquid chromatography but suffers from incomplete extraction of labeled compounds. This method yielded wide variations in the effectiveness of solubilization of the labeled metabolites (Table III). Very effective sol-

**Table II.** Residue of Unmetabolized Naphthalene[a] in Tissues of Chicken and Swine

| Tissue | Chicken[b] (%) | Swine[c] (%) |
|---|---|---|
| Liver | 12 | 33 |
| Fat | 55 | 63 |
| Kidney | 3 | |
| Heart | 57 | 39 |
| Dark muscle | 16 | |
| Light muscle | 18 | |
| Ham | | 38 |
| Loin | | 45 |

[a]Naphthalene was determined by the method of Roubal et al. (see Reference 9, this chapter).
[b]Chickens were dosed with 0.433 mg of (1-$^{14}$C) naphthalene and sacrificed at 24 h.
[c]Swine were dosed with 2.4 mg of (1-$^{14}$C) naphthalene and sacrificed at 24 h.

**Table III.** Partition of the Metabolic Products of Naphthalene in Chicken[a] Tissues between Soluble and Insoluble Fractions

| Tissue[b] | Soluble (%) | Insoluble (%) |
|---|---|---|
| Light muscle | 59 | 41 |
| Dark muscle | 49 | 51 |
| Heart | 56 | 44 |
| Fat | 98 | 2 |
| Liver | 33 | 67 |
| Kidney | 11 | 89 |
| Egg white | 94 | 6 |
| Egg yolk | 76 | 24 |

[a]Chickens were orally dosed with 0.443 mg (1-$^{14}$C) naphthalene and sacrificed at 24 h.
[b]Tissues were extracted by the organic solvent procedure of Varanski et al. (see References 10 and 11, this chapter).

ubilization was observed in chicken fat and egg white; moderately effective solubilization was observed in egg yolk, heart, and dark and light muscle; and poor solubilization was observed in chicken liver and kidney. Whether the effectiveness of solubilization is related to the proportion of naphthalene metabolites that are present in free vs conjugate form has not yet been determined. However, most conjugates exhibited a solubility preference for aqueous solvents, and the strong acid-base procedure was more effective (Table II) in hydrolyzing and solubilizing the naphthalene metabolites. In any case, the organic solvent extractable portions of these tissues are currently being analyzed for individual metabolites.

The uptake by eggs of naphthalene, naphthol, and 7-methylbenz(c)acridine is shown in Figure 3. Within the first 24 h, a significant amount of naphthalene was incorporated in both the yolk and albumen (white) of the egg. In the internal egg (egg which has been formed but not laid), the yolk was the preferred part for deposition of these compounds. The internal yolks were still on the stalk and ready for ovulation and subsequent egg formation. All three compounds showed preference for yolk, with little deposited in the albumen. It is important to note that the values for internal yolk mean that eggs will still contain residues of these materials after 72 h.

Chronic exposure (30 d, 1.10-mg total dose) of laying hens to naphthalene is shown in Figure 4. Liver and fat are the major deposition sites. The acute 24-h values are higher than the chronic (30-d exposure) values as expected, with rapid absorption of compound and little excretion having occurred by 24 h. The comparison of chronic vs 72 h postacute shows liver values of comparative value (0.75 vs 0.95% dose/g × $10^{-3}$), with the remaining chronic samples having values approximately one-half of those at 72 h. Again, dark meat appeared to retain more naphthalene than white meat. In both the acute and chronic study, no adverse effects were noted

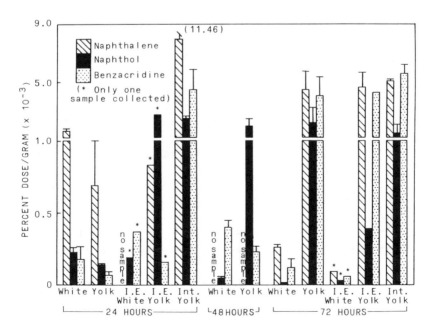

**Figure 3.**   Naphthalene, naphthol, and 7-methylbenz(c)acridine in eggs after an acute exposure.

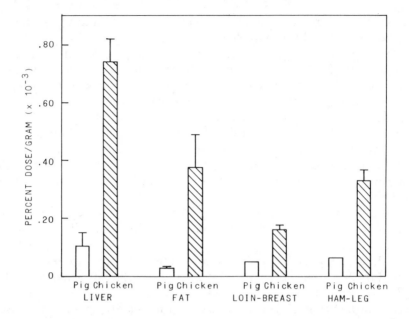

**Figure 4.**   Naphthalene in tissues from pigs and laying hens after a chronic exposure.

in egg production or body weight, suggesting that dose levels were below the toxic level.

The results of an acute exposure of swine to naphthalene (2.40 mg) and α-naphthol (1.34 mg) are shown in Figure 5. The major site of deposition is fat, remaining high at 72-h postexposure, followed by liver. Both loin and ham muscle retained low levels of the compounds, which were reduced even more by 72 h. It appears from these data that naphthalene is first deposited in the fat and then redistributed to the liver for possible subsequent excretion. The metabolism of α-naphthol appears to be slower, increasing slightly only in the liver after 72 h and then possibly excreted from the body. The concentration of naphthalene in swine tissue is shown in Table I. Because the annual consumption of pork is approximately 27 kg/ person in the United States, possible human exposure via meat appears to be low. Pork fat, which is used as an additive in pork products as well as other nonpork meat products, would allow a substantial amount of the material to enter the food chain.

The results of chronic exposure (30 d, 3.46-mg total dose) of swine to naphthalene is shown in Figure 4. All values are below or about the same as the 24- and 72-h acute values. It is interesting to note that with chronic exposure, fat does not appear to be a major site of deposition, which suggests redistribution within the body (fat → liver) and subsequent excretion.

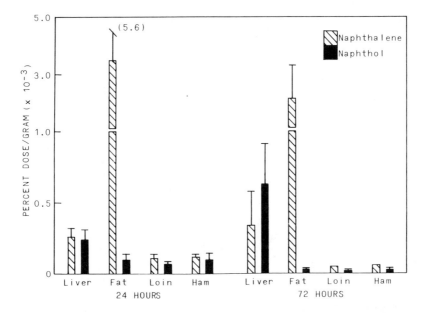

**Figure 5.** Naphthalene and naphthol in tissues from swine after an acute exposure.

The results of the acute naphthalene (30.72 mg) and α-naphthol (13.4 mg) exposures in dairy cows are shown in Figure 6. The liver is, again, one of the major tissues of deposition. The fat, however, is the lowest in retention for both chemicals, which was not the case for the other species. Another interesting finding is, again, a selective difference between muscle (loin and rump). The reason for this is unclear. Even though the dairy cow has relatively little back fat compared to swine, the low concentration in fat is also unusual. The concentration of naphthalene in dairy cattle tissue is shown in Table I. The percent of dose found in the milk is shown in Figure 7. Within 8 h after exposure, the highest levels of labeled naphthalene and α-naphthol were found in milk, decreasing rapidly by 72 h. The first milking (8-h postexposure) showed that α-naphthol was secreted more rapidly than naphthalene; in tissue retention, the reverse was seen in all other species. Both compounds were about equally distributed in milk and milk fat after 24 h, at which time only trace levels were observed.

Samples from chronic exposure of laying hens to α-naphthol and 7-methylbenz(c)acridine are currently being analyzed. Experiments in progress are acute exposure of swine to 7-methylbenz(c)acridine and chronic exposure to α-naphthol and 7-methylbenz(c)acridine; and acute exposure of dairy cattle to 7-methylbenz(c)acridine and chronic exposure to naphthalene, α-naphthol, and 7-methylbenz(c)acridine.

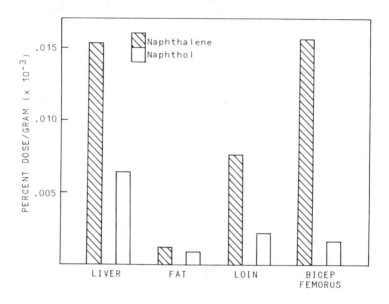

**Figure 6.** Naphthalene and naphthol in tissues from dairy cows after an acute exposure (i.e., 72 h after dosing).

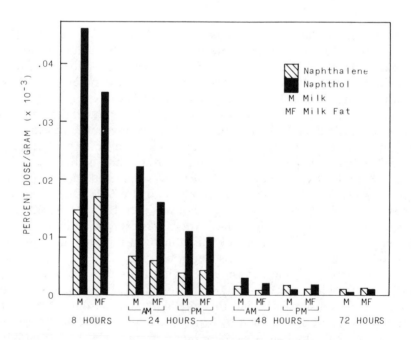

**Figure 7.** Naphthalene and naphthol in milk of dairy cows after an acute exposure.

## Plant Studies

Control runs were performed with each of the three substances to test the hydroponic system's ability to retain a uniform concentration of the test substances over time. Isotopically labeled α-naphthol, naphthalene, or 7-methylbenz(c)acridine was placed in the complete system, minus test plants, for 72 to 100 h. The results are presented in Figure 8. Nutrient solution samples for isotope counting were taken periodically over the entire incubation period. The two test units were run as replicates. The average percent variation between the two units was never greater than ± 5% of the activity (disintegrations per minute) present for all three compounds tested. The ability to obtain reproducible samples of nutrient solution over an extended incubation period is clearly shown in Table IV. These data show that the two hydroponic test units are very similar with reference to their between-unit reproducibility. Of the three substances tested, α-naphthol proved to exhibit the most stable system retention over time; that is, label recovery was essentially 100%. The extent of label recovery decreases as a function of incubation time for the other two compounds. For naphthalene, this decrease may directly reflect its relatively high vapor pressure. Very rapid initial losses were observed for 7-methylbenz(c)acridine followed by a much slower rate of disappearance; however, all of the isotope could be accounted for when adsorption to the unit's inner glass surfaces was taken into account. As a result of these blank runs, the plants were placed in the hydroponic units at varying times after isotope spiking to provide a more stable substrate concentration to the roots (e.g., 45 min for α-naphthol and 24 h for the other two compounds). The initial substrate concentrations for all plant

**Figure 8.** Retention of α-naphthol, naphthalene, and 7-methylbenz(c)acridine in hydroponic nutrient solution during a blank run (i.e., minus plants).

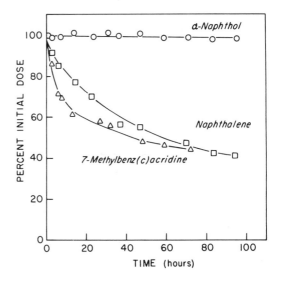

**Table IV.** [14]C-α-Naphthol Blank Run Illustration of Individual Unit Performance and Between-Unit Reproducibility of Nutrient Solution Samples Taken Over a 95-h Control Run

| | DPM/500 μL Nutrient Solution |
|---|---|
| Unit A | |
| Mean | 4529 |
| Standard deviation | 96.4 |
| Standard error | 17.0 |
| Unit B | |
| Mean | 4450 |
| Standard deviation | 148 |
| Standard error | 26.0 |

species and compound combinations given in Table V were calculated at the time the plants were placed in the units and not from the initial delivered isotope dose. Additional control runs were made for each species tested minus the test substance. These incubations were used to provide control nonlabeled tissue for various blank determinations (i.e., fresh weight to dry weight ratios, etc.) and to set control levels for transpiration rates.

The hydroponic units also enable the monitoring of water loss from the system, which translates directly into plant transpirational losses. During the blank runs (i.e., minus plants), water loss was not measurable over the incubation period. No difference in rate of transpirational water loss was ever observed between control runs with plants minus the test compound and complete test runs.

The uptake and distribution of the radiolabeled compounds were determined for pea, onion, and lettuce (Tables VI, VII, and VIII) after 72 h. Plants of similar developmental maturity, grown as described in the Mate-

**Table V.** Initial Concentration (mg/L) and Dose [μCi/18.6 L (Curvette)]

| | Naphthalene[a] | | α-Naphthol[b] | | 7-Methylbenz(c)acridine[c] | |
|---|---|---|---|---|---|---|
| | mg/L | μCi/Curvette | mg/L | μCi/Curvette | mg/L | μCi/Curvette |
| Pea | 0.054 | 39.2 | 0.03 | 74.0 | 0.016 | 20.5 |
| Onion | 0.062 | 45.1 | 0.033 | 81.9 | 0.015 | 19.4 |
| Lettuce | 0.050 | 36.6 | 0.033 | 82.3 | 0.018 | 22.4 |

[a][1(4,5,8)-14C]-Naphthalene (specific activity: 5 mCi/mmole; 39.1 μCi/mg).
[b](1-14 C)-α-Naphthol (specific activity: 19.4 mCi/mmole; 134 μCi/mg).
[c]14C-7-Methylbenz(c)acridine (specific activity: 19.4 mCi/mmole; 79.7 μCi/mg).

**Table VI.**  Distribution of $^{14}C$ Isotope Given as $^{14}C$-Naphthol to Pea, Onion, and Lettuce[a]

| Plant | % of Total $^{14}C$ Recovered in Whole Plant | $\mu Ci/g$ Dry Wt | mg($^{14}C$-Naphthol equiv)/g Dry Wt |
|---|---|---|---|
| Pea | | | |
| Leaf | $0.259 \pm 0.01$[b] | 0.048 | $0.358 \times 10^{-3}$ |
| Stem | $0.297 \pm 0.05$ | 0.114 | $0.847 \times 10^{-3}$ |
| Root | $99.25 \pm 1.07$ | 95.39 | 0.712 |
| Pod | $0.214 \pm 0.11$ | 0.053 | $0.396 \times 10^{-3}$ |
| Onion | | | |
| Leaf | $0.285 \pm 0.07$ | 0.028 | $0.209 \times 10^{-3}$ |
| Stem (bulb) | $0.255 \pm 0.08$ | 0.189 | $1.410 \times 10^{-3}$ |
| Root | $99.46 \pm 0.15$ | 70.670 | 0.527 |
| Lettuce | | | |
| Leaf | $0.041 \pm 0.01$ | 0.011 | $0.080 \times 10^{-3}$ |
| Stem | $0.264 \pm 0.08$ | 0.246 | $1.836 \times 10^{-3}$ |
| Root | $99.69 \pm 0.09$ | 83.24 | 0.621 |

[a] All values given are averages of six plants per species.
[b] Mean $\pm$ standard error.

**Table VII.**  Distribution of $^{14}C$ Isotope Given as $^{14}C$-Naphthalene to Pea, Onion, and Lettuce[a]

| Plant | % of Total $^{14}C$ Recovered in Whole Plant | $\mu Ci/g$ Dry Wt | mg($^{14}C$-Naphthalene equiv)/g Dry Wt |
|---|---|---|---|
| Pea | | | |
| Leaf | $3.04 \pm 0.38$[b] | 0.026 | $0.665 \times 10^{-3}$ |
| Stem | $37.4 \pm 2.99$ | 0.422 | $10.80 \times 10^{-3}$ |
| Root | $59.0 \pm 3.38$ | 1.962 | $50.18 \times 10^{-3}$ |
| Pod | $0.55 \pm 0.08$ | 0.004 | $0.093 \times 10^{-3}$ |
| Onion | | | |
| Leaf | $2.62 \pm 0.45$ | 0.040 | $1.031 \times 10^{-3}$ |
| Stem (bulb) | $2.64 \pm 0.44$ | 0.209 | $5.345 \times 10^{-3}$ |
| Root | $94.8 \pm 0.75$ | 5.439 | 0.139 |
| Lettuce | | | |
| Leaf | $3.87 \pm 0.29$ | 0.041 | $1.038 \times 10^{-3}$ |
| Stem | $4.52 \pm 0.64$ | 0.484 | $12.38 \times 10^{-3}$ |
| Root | $91.6 \pm 0.78$ | 3.254 | 0.083 |

[a] All values given are averages of six plants per species.
[b] Mean $\pm$ standard error.

**Table VIII.** Distribution of $^{14}$C Isotope Given as $^{14}$C-7-Methylbenz(c)acridine to Pea, Onion, and Lettuce[a]

| Plant | % of Total $^{14}$C Recovered in Whole Plant | $\mu Ci$/g Dry Wt | mg [$^{14}$C-7-acridine Equiv/g] Dry Wt |
|---|---|---|---|
| Pea | | | |
| Leaf | 3.030 ± 1.04[b] | 0.040 | 0.584 × 10$^{-3}$ |
| Stem | 4.520 ± 1.16 | 0.091 | 1.342 × 10$^{-3}$ |
| Root | 92.40 ± 2.12 | 5.656 | 83.58 × 10$^{-3}$ |
| Pod | 0.090 ± 0.01 | 0.001 | 0.015 × 10$^{-3}$ |
| Onion | | | |
| Leaf | 5.180 ± 0.62 | 0.042 | 0.313 × 10$^{-3}$ |
| Stem (bulb) | 2.850 ± 0.28 | 0.122 | 1.800 × 10$^{-3}$ |
| Root | 91.90 ± 0.62 | 3.451 | 0.051 |
| Lettuce | | | |
| Leaf | 0.385 ± 0.07 | 0.015 | 0.214 × 10$^{-3}$ |
| Stem | 0.255 ± 0.03 | 0.079 | 1.161 × 10$^{-3}$ |
| Root | 99.40 ± 0.08 | 13.49 | 0.199 |

[a]All values given are averages of six plants per species.
[b]Mean ± standard error.

rials and Methods section, were selected for each experimental run to minimize plant-to-plant variation. In every case, the radiolabel was traceable to all parts of the plant. The values given for the $^{14}$C isotope in the various plant organs may represent a combination of parent compounds plus metabolites (i.e., $^{14}$C-isotope equivalents). Representative samples have been taken from each plant organ to determine the percentage of the isotope that remained as the parent compound. Until these results are obtained, the values listed must be considered as representing parent compound plus metabolites in unknown proportions. These results do confirm the ability of all three species to take up a waterborne compound from the environment and transport it or its metabolites from the root zone to all plant parts. The compound's concentration is greatest in the root (as one would expect from the method of isotope application) and falls in concentration as the distance from the point of application increases. In every combination of test compound and plant species except one, the label was partitioned such that over 90% was found in the root region; the remaining was apportioned between stem and leaves and, in the case of pea, the pods. The one exception was the garden pea (*Pisum sativum*) when exposed to $^{14}$C-naphthalene. Apparently, the parent compound or its metabolites are rapidly transported acropetally into the stem. In any case, a general pattern of distribution of $^{14}$C isotope is found for all compounds tested in all test plant species: (1) the root region is highest in isotope content, followed by the stem, the leaf, and, in the case of the pea, the pod; and (2) all edible portions of these vegetable crops contain measurable levels of isotope and therefore are not isolated from contamination by the parent compound or associated metabolites via a root-uptake mechanism (i.e., port of entry).

No definitive statement can be made about the mechanism of uptake or the initial rate of transport from the root zone to the various aerial portions of the plant. Kinetic analysis is highly amendable to the hydroponic system described in this report. Four additional units would be required to accomplish the analysis. The extent of "risk" to humans implied by these data must await the determination of the parent compound and metabolites present in each of the various plant parts mentioned above and the associated toxicity, mutagenicity, etc. posed by them.

## CONCLUSIONS

In determining the adverse effect of coal liquefaction and shale-oil products on the populace from exposure via the food chain, it is imperative to characterize the materials that could enter the system through spillage during production, transportation, and utilization. These data will allow regulatory agencies to begin to assess the transport through the food chain and, subsequently, derive the appropriate risk to man. Data presented here demonstrate that accumulation of potentially hazardous substances from these energy products are retained in consumable meats, eggs, milk, and plants.

Milk, which is essential for the newborn infant and also plays a vital role throughout early childhood, is a primary pathway for early insult. The neonate, which has the ability to absorb greater quantities of materials via the gastrointestinal tract due to the physiological phenomenon of the "open gut," may be at greatest risk. Butter, butter oils, cheese, and cheese foods are all major food items derived from milk. Eggs are also used extensively in products as an add-in ingredient. Meat is a major staple of our diet, with an annual consumption of approximately 94 kg per person. Fruits (fresh and processed), vegetables (fresh, canned, and frozen), various grains, and other minor commodities are all a part of our total diet. Potential contamination of these foods must be recognized and evaluated so that adequate standards can be set to safeguard human health.

The experiments performed to test the hydroponic exposure system design are very encouraging. The units perform in a similar and reproducible manner with respect to label-retention ability and provide a workable approach to the monitoring of various system and physiological parameters necessary to follow the progress of the experiment (e.g., transpirational losses and plant-mediated isotope removal). The experiments (endpoint analysis) are a part of the preliminary screen that will be performed on all test plants for all selected compounds to determine if uptake and subsequent transport of the substance need to be considered further. Our results show that all three substances are taken up by the three test plant species, and the parent compound or its metabolites reach the edible portion of the plants in a relatively short time after initial exposure. The animal experiments also indicate that material does enter the food chain through meat, milk, and eggs. Even though the material is redistributed and excreted from the body and the remaining levels are relatively low, the potential risk is present.

The data from these experiments demonstrate the retention of variable but significant amounts of the test compounds and their metabolites. Without a thorough study to identify which compounds are associated with the $^{14}$C label, one cannot identify potential or mutagenic compounds and their respective toxic risks. Such a study is beyond the scope of the present program.

## ACKNOWLEDGMENTS

Research supported by the U.S. Environmental Protection Agency under Interagency Agreement 81-D-X0533 and by the U.S. Department of Energy, Contract No. DE-AC05-760R00033, with Oak Ridge Associated Universities.

## REFERENCES

1. Richmond, C.R. "Health Risk Analysis: A Challenge for the 1980s," in *Health Risk Analysis, Proceedings of the Third Life Sciences Symposium,* C.R. Richmond, P.J. Walsh, E.D. Copenhaver, Eds. (Philadelphia: Franklin Institute Press, 1981), pp. 1–9.
2. Epler, J.L., F.W. Larimer, T. Ho, C.E. Nix, A.W. Hsie, and T.K. Rao. "Short-Term Mutagenicity Testing," in *Synthetic Fossil Fuel Technologies: Potential Health and Environmental Effects,* K.E. Cowser and C.R. Richmond, Eds., Conf. 780903, Sept. 25–28, 1978 (Oak Ridge, TN: Oak Ridge National Laboratory, U.S. Department of Energy, 1978), pp. 129–136.
3. Holland, J.M., M.S. Whitaker, and J.W. Wesley. "Carcinogenicity of Syncrudes Relative to Natural Petroleum and Assessed by Repetitive Mouse Skin Application," in *Synthetic Fossil Fuel Technologies: Potential Health and Environmental Effects,* K.E. Cowser and C.R. Richmond, Eds., Conf. 780903, Sept. 25–28, 1978 (Oak Ridge, TN: Oak Ridge National Laboratory, U.S. Department of Energy, 1978), pp. 137–142.
4. Faulkner, J.K., S.K. Figdor, A. M. Monro, M.S. von Wittenau, D.A. Stopher, and B.A. Wood. "The Comparative Metabolism of Pyrantel in Five Species," *J. Sci. Food Agr.* 23:79–91 (1972).
5. Meyer, T., J.C. Larsen, E.V. Hansen, and R.R. Scheline. "The Metabolism of Biphenyl. III. Phenolic Metabolism in the Pig," *Acta Pharmacol. Toxicol.* 39:433–441 (1976).
6. West, C.E., and B.J. Horton. "Transfer of Polycyclic Hydrocarbons from Diet to Milk in Rats, Rabbits and Sheep," *Life Sci.* 19:1543–1551 (1976).

7. Epstein, E. *Mineral Nutrition of Plants: Principles and Perspectives* (New York: John Wiley, 1972).

8. Malins, D.C., T.K. Collier, L.C. Thomas, and W.T. Roubal. "Metabolic Fate of Aromatic Hydrocarbons in Aquatic Organisms: Analysis of Metabolites by Thin-Layer Chromatography and High-Pressure Liquid Chromatography," *Intern. J. Environ. Anal. Chem.* 6:55–66 (1979).

9. Roubal, W.T., T.K. Collier, and D.C. Malins. "Accumulation and Metabolism of Carbon-14 Labeled Benzene, Naphthalene, and Anthracene by Young Coho Salmon *(Oncorhynchus kisutsch),"* *Arch. Environ. Contam. Toxicol.* 5:513–29 (1977).

10. Varanski, U., D.T. Gmur, and W. Reichart. "Effect of Environmental Temperature on Naphthalene Metabolism by Juvenile Starry Flounder *(Platichthys stellatus),"* *Arch. Environ. Contam. Toxicol.* 10:203–14 (1981).

11. Varanski, U., D.T. Gmur, and P.A. Treseler. "Influence of Time and Mode of Exposure on Biotransformation of Naphthalene by Juvenile Starry Flounder *(Platichthys stellatus)* and Rock Sole *(Lepidopsetta bilineata),"* *Arch. Environ. Contam. Toxicol.* 8:673–692 (1979).

## DISCUSSION

*S.M. Bartell, Oak Ridge National Laboratory:* Do you think the initial similarity of uptake of different compounds by the root might have been due to simple adsorption of compound onto the root surface?

*O.J. Schwarz:* My opinion at this point is that much of the uptake, especially with those compounds that are relatively nonpolar, is by simple adsorption. The initial rapid rate of uptake is probably primarily adsorptive. Thereafter, the rate of apparent uptake rapidly decreases. If one does log plots, one gets two intersecting straight lines of different slopes. Adsorption is probably responsible for the initial uptake observed.

*S.M. Bartell:* Do you have any plans to expand your experiments or fit these data to kinetic models to look at different mechanisms of uptake?

*O.J. Schwarz:* Yes, if support becomes available. Use of the hydroponic model system has been proposed as a worst-case system. I plan to try to relate this system to a soils environment by doing KD analysis and soil partitioning analysis of a variety of soils and compounds of interest, thereby providing the modeler with appropriate data.

*S.V. Kaye, Oak Ridge National Laboratory:* The literature is replete with data on small experiments, studies where plants are individually grown in small containers and pots, where the constraints of the root system and their physiology is different than those in a real crop system. A hydroponic system is different in its physiology from plants which are grown in a field or cropped in the usual way. Why didn't you start with the soil system instead of using the hydroponic system in the first place, and what kind of credibility can you give to the data on uptake, which are going to be used in an assessment study?

*O.J. Schwarz:* In my opinion, it is quite credible. After reviewing the literature, we found there was very little data for synfuel technology effluents. Looking at herbicide and pesticide data and various soil-based test systems, and consulting with various investigators, I came to the conclusion that for every system that one might assemble (e.g., pot size and soil type), differing results might be expected. The results obtained seemed to be, to a varying degree, dependent on the soil system and lysimeter setup used, time of year, soil type, methodology of application of the compound, etc. What I set out to do was to provide baseline data—design a standardized test system to refer back to as worst-case water-based mediated uptake. I did some testing and made sure that in this particular test system, for example, the oxygen concentration was at ambient levels all the time. The environmental stresses that might inhibit plant growth and normal physiological processes because of system design are engineered to be minimal. We were looking for an optimal kind of a system, perhaps not one that is often attained in nature; however, it does give one the ability to come back and repeat the experiment and come out with essentially the same results.

*S.V. Kaye:* What would be your guess? Are you within an order of magnitude, two orders of magnitude, from what you might expect in a normal crop system?

*O.J. Schwarz:* That would depend on the compound and the soil type. From a risk assessment point of view, unless I misunderstand the philosophy, if you look at a worst-case condition and you show that the water-based mediated uptake is minimal and not of concern, perhaps you are a bit safer in your judgment as to whether that compound should be considered further. It is as a preliminary screen. I realize that there are various mechanisms of soil transport, activation, etc. of the primary compound, and this system does not address these factors. What it does address is the ability of the plant to take up the compound from a water-based media.

# CHAPTER 21

## Biotransformation of Aromatics: Metabolic Conversion of Nitrogen-Containing Derivatives of Benzo(*a*)pyrene

S. Tong and
J.K. Selkirk
*The University of Tennessee
—Oak Ridge Graduate School
of Biomedical Sciences, and
Biology Division
Oak Ridge National Laboratory
Oak Ridge, TN 37831*

The metabolism of two nitrogen-containing polycyclic aromatic hydrocarbons, 6-nitroB(a)P and 10-azaB(a)P, was studied in an intact cell system consisting of hamster embryonic fibroblasts and a cell-free system employing rat liver microsomes. For both compounds, high-pressure liquid chromatography (HPLC) separation of microsomal metabolites indicated the predominant presence of phenolic products with only small amounts of dihydrodiols formed. In contrast, incubation of the chemicals with hamster cells yielded dihydrodiols as major organic solvent-soluble products. On closer examination, it was found that although phenols were formed, they were conjugated with glucuronic acid to become water-soluble products and, therefore, did not accumulate in their "free" phenolic form.

Studies in the nuclear macromolecular binding of the two compounds showed that 6-nitroB(a)P was bound to DNA, RNA, and proteins with much the same affinity as that exhibited by B(a)P, whereas the specific binding activities for 10-azaB(a)P were several-fold lower in all cases. This may be explained by the substitution of a nitrogen atom in an important metabolic region in the B(a)P molecule, thus altering its potential macro-molecular binding properties.

## INTRODUCTION

Polycyclic aromatic hydrocarbons (PAH) are an important class of environmental pollutants and are widely found in our surrounding air, water, and soil.[1] They are products of the incomplete combustion of fossil fuels and are, therefore, major exhaust components of industrial transportation energy sources and refuse burning.[2] Although a number of these compounds have been shown to be both mutagenic and carcinogenic, the exact biochemical mechanism by which they exert such properties is not completely understood. However, it is generally realized that the binding of potential carcinogens to biological macromolecules such as DNA is a crucial step in the process of chemical carcinogenesis. For PAH, such an interaction occurs when the parent compound is metabolically activated to form electrophilic products that readily attack nucleophilic sites in the cell. The activation of a potential carcinogen to its reactive intermediate is one of the most fundamental steps in chemical carcinogenesis, and metabolism studies leading to the identification of the proximate carcinogenic product are of critical importance in our understanding of the biochemical events leading to malignant transformation.

Among the PAH, benzo(a)pyrene [B(a)P] has been most studied and is often used as a representative for this group of compounds. Figure 1 shows the major oxygenated metabolites of B(a)P that have been isolated intact. In the animal body or in intact cell systems where appropriate enzymes are present, toxic products are effectively converted to more polar metabolites by conjugatory reactions catalyzed by cytoplasmic enzymes such as glucuronyl transferases. This is generally regarded as a detoxification reaction since polar metabolites are more readily excreted from the animal body. The phenolic products, in particular, are known to undergo such reactions, whereas the dihydrodiols (diols) are poorer substrates for the transferases and may, therefore, accumulate, become reactivated, and attack cellular components to produce adverse effects.

Enzymatic studies have shown that aryl hydrocarbon hydroxylase (AHH),[3-5] a mixed-function oxidase, and epoxide hydrase (EH)[6-8] are of great importance in the conversion of B(a)P to its various oxygenated metabolites. It is now known that the critical pathway for B(a)P to exert its carcinogenic properties is via the formation of its 7,8-diol (Figure 2) as catalyzed by AHH and EH. The diol produced is then reactivated by AHH to form the more mutagenic and carcinogenic 7,8-diol 9,10-epoxide.[9-11] This product is relatively unstable and opens to form a triol-carbonium ion, which is the alkylating species of B(a)P with high affinity for the exocyclic N-2 of

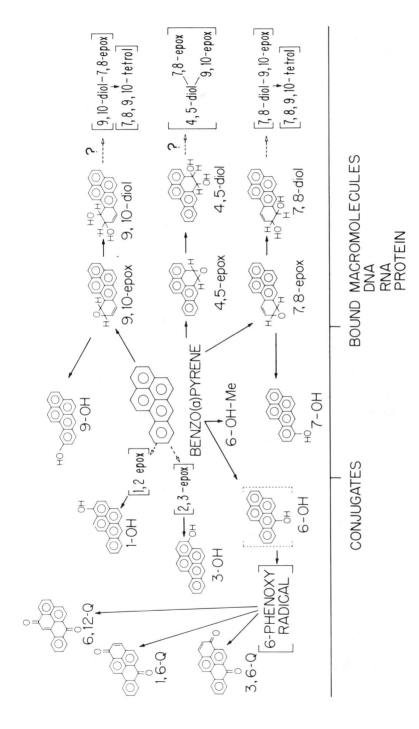

**Figure 1.** Metabolic conversion of benzo(a)pyrene to its oxygenated products. [ ] = Products that have not been unequivocally identified; ? = products that have been hypothesized.

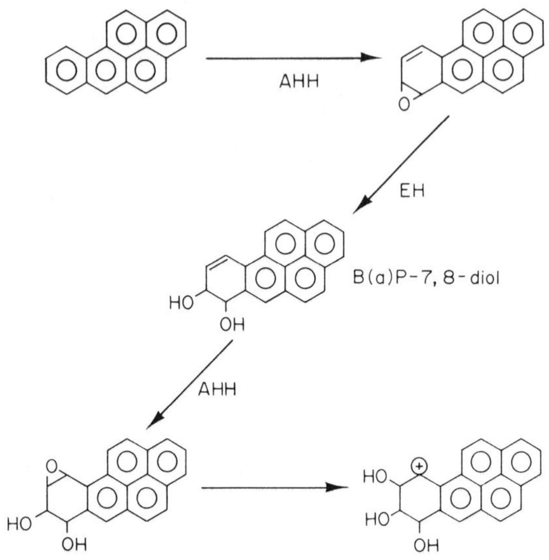

**Figure 2.** Pathway leading to the formation of B(a)P 7,8-diol 9-10 epoxide as catalyzed by microsomal aryl hydrocarbon hydroxylase and epoxide hydrase.

guanine in DNA.[12] However, a plausible mechanism by which this alkylation initiates the process of malignant transformation has not been forthcoming.

## EXPERIMENTAL PROTOCOL

### Nitrogen-Containing Polycyclic Aromatic Hydrocarbons

In recent years, much attention has been given to nitrogen-containing PAH because of their presence as environmental contaminants in a variety of sources including automobile exhaust,[13] cigarette smoke,[14] and shale-oil fractions.[15] Similarly, mutagenic[16,17] and carcinogenic[18] properties exhibited by some of these compounds have aroused major concern. We have studied the metabolism of two nitrogen-containing derivatives of B(a)P, namely 6-nitroB(a)P and 10-azaB(a)P. The chemical structures of these compounds are shown in Figure 3. Occupation of the "bay-region" of the B(a)P molecule with a nitrogen atom, as in 10-azaB(a)P, is particularly noteworthy since this site is metabolically important for the formation of the active 7,8-diol 9,10-epoxide of B(a)P as described in the previous section.

The systems for studying the metabolism of these compounds were that of an intact cell system using hamster embryonic fibroblasts (HEF) to reflect metabolism in the animal body, and a cell-free system using rat liver microsomes. The latter model was also chosen, because similar systems are often used in routine short-term mutagenicity testing as sources for metabolic activation. In addition, nuclear macromolecular interaction of these compounds was investigated.

**Figure 3.** Chemical structures of B(a)P, 6-nitroB(a)P and 10-azaB(a)P indicating the "bay-region" area in the B(a)P molecule.

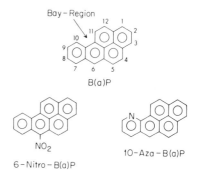

B(a)P

6 - Nitro - B(a)P

10-Aza - B(a)P

## Metabolic Conversion of 6-NitroB(a)P

### Microsomal Metabolism

Organic solvent-soluble metabolites produced by incubation of 6-nitroB(a)P with hepatic microsomes from 3-methylcholanthrene pretreated rats were extracted with ethyl acetate and separated by high-pressure liquid chromatography (HPLC). Figure 4 indicates that microsomal metabolism of the compound produced a major phenolic peak (peak 5) that was identified by the characteristic red-shift exhibited by phenols when their UV-visible spectra were obtained under alkaline conditions.[19] In addition, small amounts of dihydrodiols were produced between fractions 20 and 60, because their formation was inhibited in the presence of 1,1,1-trichloropropene 2,3-oxide, a specific inhibitor of epoxide hydrase,[20] the enzyme responsible for the formation of dihydrodiols.

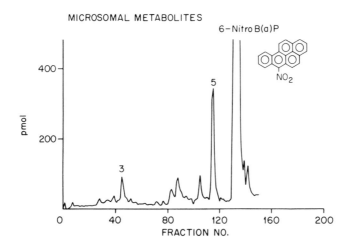

**Figure 4.** Separation of metabolites by HPLC after microsomal metabolism of 6-nitroB(a)P.

### Cellular Metabolism

The experimental protocol used in the study of cellular metabolism is outlined in Figure 5. After incubation of 6-nitroB(a)P with HEF, organic solvent-soluble products were extracted by ethyl acetate from the cultural medium. The remaining aqueous phase consisted of metabolites that had undergone conjugatory reactions (e.g., glucuronidation) to become water-soluble products. However, dissociation of metabolites with glucuronic acid could be achieved by treatment with β-glucuronidase. Once in their "free" form, these metabolites may be extracted with ethyl acetate for analysis. To understand the relative distribution of metabolites during cellular processing of the compound, we also determined in this study products that were present in the cytoplasm and radioactivity that was associated with macromolecules in the nuclei.

After an incubation period of 24 h, the majority of radioactivity was found to be present in the extracellular medium, with about 10% associated with the cytoplasm and only 0.12% bound to the nuclei (Table I). HPLC analysis of the organic solvent-soluble metabolites in the extracellular medium showed that metabolites were mainly those of the dihydrodiols (peaks 1–4) with comparatively little phenolic products present (Figure 6A). This differed markedly from microsomal metabolism where a major phenol peak was observed. The metabolites formed in the two systems were, however, qualitatively similar, as indicated by their identical UV-visible and fluorescence spectra and retention time through the HPLC column.

Analysis of the water-soluble products revealed an important aspect of

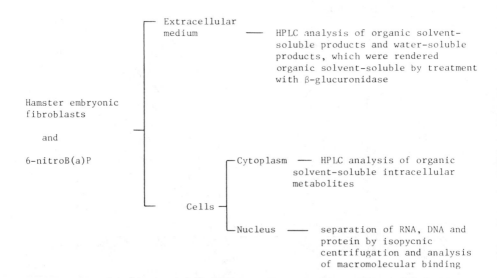

**Figure 5.**   Scheme used for the analysis of metabolites produced after metabolism of PAH by hamster embryonic fibroblasts.

**Table I.**   Distribution of Radioactivity After 24 h Incubation of 6-NitroB(a)P with Hamster Embryonic Fibroblasts

|  | *Original Radioactivity (%)* |
| --- | --- |
| Extracellular Medium | |
|    Organic solvent soluble | 31 |
|    Water soluble | 49 |
| Cytoplasm | |
|    Organic solvent soluble | 6.5 |
|    Water soluble | 3.4 |
| Nucleus | 0.12 |

**Figure 6.**  HPLC separation of metabolites resulting from the metabolism of 6-nitroB(a)P by hamster embryonic fibroblasts. A. Organic solvent-soluble products in extracellular medium; B. water-soluble products; C. cytoplasmic products.

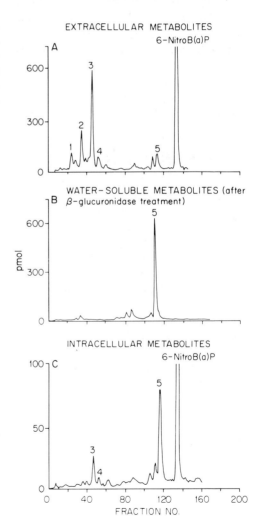

intact cell metabolism. For 6-nitroB(a)P, the main glucuronide conjugate was found to be that of the phenolic product (Figure 6B), previously observed as the major microsomal metabolite (peak 5). It becomes clear that, although the phenol was produced in cells, it was effectively being conjugated with glucuronic acid and, therefore, did not accumulate substantially in its free form in the medium. Since microsomal preparations are deficient in conjugatory enzymes, phenols once produced remained in their free unconjugated form. Analysis of intracellular metabolites in the cytoplasm showed the predominant presence of the phenol (peak 5) with some dihydrodiol formation.

The significance of the above findings became obvious when it was recently observed that the major microsomal product, identified as 3-hydroxy-6-nitroB(a)P, was suggested to be the proximate mutagen of 6-nitroB(a)P due to its high mutagenicity in the *Salmonella typhimurium* test.[21] Since we found that this metabolite can be effectively converted to a glucuronide conjugate by cellular metabolism, it may not accumulate in the animal body to any extent great enough to result in adverse cellular changes. Similarly, the positive result obtained for 6-nitroB(a)P in mutagenic testing may not necessarily reflect its carcinogenic properties, since cell-free systems were employed in these tests for metabolic activation.

### Metabolic Conversion of 10-azaB(a)P

As with 6-nitroB(a)P, microsomal metabolism of 10-azaB(a)P resulted in the production of phenolic peaks, and only small amounts of dihydrodiols were formed (Figure 7). In cellular metabolism, a major dihydrodiol peak was produced, whereas phenols were not significantly present (Figure 8). Analysis of metabolites after treatment of the aqueous phase with β-glucuronidase showed that significant amounts of the phenols were recovered (Figure 9); therefore, conjugation with glucuronic acid had again prevented

**Figure 7.** Microsomal metabolites of 10-azaB(a)P as separted by HPLC.

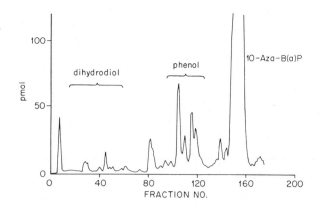

**Figure 8.** Extracellular organic solvent-soluble metabolites of 10-azaB(a)P after metabolism by hamster embryonic fibroblasts.

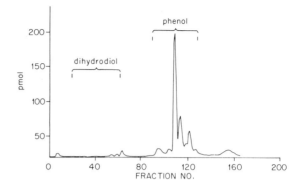

**Figure 9.** Extracellular water-soluble metabolites of 10-azaB(a)P after metabolism by hamster embryonic fibroblasts.

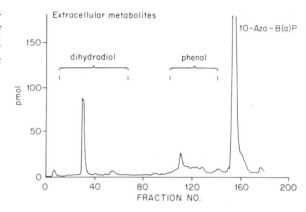

phenolic products to accumulate in the free form in extracellular medium. Such properties in the metabolism of 10-azaB(a)P were previously observed for 6-nitroB(a)P and further demonstrate an important difference between metabolic conversion of PAH by a cell-free system and intact cells.

## Nuclear Macromolecular Binding of PAH

To study macromolecular binding, nuclei were isolated from HEF that were separately incubated with radiolabeled B(a)P, 6-nitroB(a)P and 10-azaB(a)P. RNA, DNA, and nuclear proteins were then separated by isopycnic centrifugation, and radioactivity covalently associated with these nucleus macromolecules was determined.[22] Noncovalently bound materials were removed prior to centrifugation by repetitive extraction with ethyl acetate.

The specific binding activities of B(a)P, 6-nitroB(a)P, and 10-azaB(a)P are summarized in Table II. Note that both B(a)P and 6-nitroB(a)P interacted with the three classes of macromolecules, but their affinity for nuclear protein was particularly high, especially for the latter compound. Of interest

**Table II.** Binding of B(a)P, 6-NitroB(a)P, and 10-AzaB(a)P to Nuclear Macromolecules

| | PAH/mg Nucleic Acid or Protein (pmol) | | |
| --- | --- | --- | --- |
| | B(a)P | 6-NitroB(a)P | 10-AzaB(a)P |
| RNA | 99 | 83 | 19 |
| DNA | 93 | 78 | 20 |
| Protein | 302 | 443 | 91 |

is that 10-azaB(a)P differed from the other two chemicals in that its binding to macromolecules in all three cases was several-fold lower. For B(a)P, we know that the formation of 7,8-diol-9,10-epoxide is required for its interaction with DNA; therefore, the presence of a nitrogen atom at the 10-position of 10-azaB(a)P may affect the compound's ability to bind macromolecules. This may be due to an inhibition of the formation of the reactive diol-epoxide or metabolism shift to an alternate region of the molecule. At present, it is difficult to relate our results with existing data in the literature. Since both 6-nitroB(a)P[23] and 10-azaB(a)P[24] have been found to be mutagenic in the *Salmonella typhimurium* test, their roles as potential carcinogens are not clear. The B(a)P derivative, 10-azaB(a)P, was demonstrated to be carcinogenic[25] in one study, but in another case the compound was essentially inactive.[26] Recently, 6-nitroB(a)P was found to have weak tumor-initiating activity because small numbers of skin tumors were produced in mice.[27] Apparently, these nitrogen-containing PAH have considerably weaker carcinogenic properties than B(a)P, which has conclusively been proven to be tumorigenic.

Further studies are required to reveal the exact chemical structure of the various metabolites produced from 6-nitroB(a)P and 10-azaB(a)P. Identification of the positions of function groups on the parent molecule, particularly with the dihydrodiols, would help explain an important part of the mechanism underlying the biological activities of these nitrogen-containing PAH.

## ACKNOWLEDGMENTS

Research sponsored by the Office of Health and Environmental Research, U.S. Department of Energy, under contract W-7405-eng-26 with the Union Carbide Corporation and by NCI Grant No. RO1-CA3055. Research by S. Tong was supported by subcontract No. 3322 from the Biology Division of Oak Ridge National Laboratory to the University of Tennessee.

# REFERENCES

1. Committee on Biologic Effects of Atmospheric Pollutants, "Particulate Polycyclic Organic Matter" (Washington, DC: National Academy of Sciences, 1972), pp. 13–35.
2. Badger, G.M. "Mode of Formation of Carcinogens in Human Environment," *Natl. Cancer Inst. Monogr.* 9:1–16 (1962).
3. Conney, A.H. "Pharmacological Implications of Microsomal Enzyme Induction," *Pharmacol. Rev.* 19:317–366 (1967).
4. Gelboin, H.V. "Carcinogen, Enzyme Induction and Gene Action," *Adv. Cancer Res.* 10:1–81 (1967).
5. Nebert, D.W., A.R. Boobis, H. Yagi, D.M. Jerina, and R.E. Kouri. "Genetic Differences in Benzo(a)pyrene Carcinogenic Index In Vivo and in Mouse Cytochrome $P_1$-450-Mediated Benzo(a)pyrene Metabolite Binding to DNA In Vitro," in *Biological Reactive Intermediates,* D.J. Jollow, J.J. Kocsis, R. Synder, and H. Vainio, Eds. (New York: Plenum Press, 1977), p. 125.
6. Oesch, F., P. Bently, and H.R. Glatt. "Epoxide Hydratase Purification to Apparent Homogeneity as a Specific Probe for the Relative Importance of Epoxides Among Other Reactive Metabolites," in *Biological Reactive Intermediates,* D.J. Jollow, J.J. Kocsis, R. Snyder, and H. Vainio, Eds. (New York, NY: Plenum Press, 1977), p. 181.
7. Selkirk, J.K. "Benzo(a)pyrene Carcinogenesis: A Biochemical Selection Mechanism," *J. Toxicol. Environ. Health* 2:1245–1258 (1977).
8. Sims, P., and P.L. Grover. "Epoxides in Polycyclic Aromatic Hydrocarbon Metabolism and Carcinogenesis," *Adv. Cancer Res.* 20:165–274 (1974).
9. Huberman, E., L. Sachs, S.K. Yang, and H.V. Gelboin. "Identification of Mutagenic Metabolites of Benzo(a)pyrene in Mammalian Cells," *Proc. Nat. Acad. Sci. USA* 73:607–611 (1976).
10. Sims, P., P.L. Grover, A. Swaisland, K. Pal, and A. Hewer. "Metabolic Activation of Benzo(a)pyrene Proceeds by a Diol-Epoxide," *Nature* 252:326–328 (1974).
11. Slaga, T.J., A. Viaje, D.L. Berry, W.M. Bracken, S.G. Buty, and J.D. Scribner. "Skin Tumor Initiating Ability of Benzo(a)pyrene 4,5'-, 7,8- and 7,8-Diol-9,10-Epoxide and 7,8-Diol," *Cancer Lett.* 2:115–122 (1976).
12. Weinstein, I.B., A.M. Jeffrey, K.W. Jennette, S.H. Blobstein, R.G. Harvey, C. Harris, H. Autrup, H. Kasai, and K. Nakanishi. "Benzo(a)pyrene Diol-Epoxides as Intermediates in Nucleic Acid Binding In Vitro and In Vivo," *Science* 193:592–595 (1976).
13. Sawicki, E., J.E. Meeker, and M.J. Morgan. "Polynuclear Aza-Compounds in Automobile Exhaust," *Arch. Environ. Health* 11:773–775 (1965).
14. Dong, M., I. Schmeltz, E. Jacobs, and D. Hoffman. "Aza-Arenes in Tobacco Smoke," *J. Anal. Toxicol.* 2:21–25 (1978).
15. Anders, O.E., F.G. Doolittle, and W.E. Robinson. "Polar Constituents Isolated from Green River Oil Shale," *Geochim. Cosmoch. Acta* 39:1423–1430 (1975).
16. Mizusaki, S., H. Okamoto, A. Akiyamas, and Y. Fukuhara. "Relation Between Chemical Constituents of Tobacco and Mutagenic Activity of Cigarette Smoke Condensate," *Mutat. Res.* 48:319–326 (1977).

17. Chiu, C.W., L.H. Lee, C.Y. Wang, and G.T. Bryan. "Mutagenicity of Some Commercially Available Nitro Compounds for *Salmonella typhimurium*," *Mutat. Res.* 58:11–22 (1978).

18. Van Duuren, B.L., J.A. Bilbao, and C.A. Joseph. "The Carcinogenic Nitrogen Heterocyclics in Cigarette-Smoke Condensate," *J. Natl. Cancer Inst.* 25:53–61 (1960).

19. Harvey, D., and G.E. Penketh. "The Determination of Small Amounts of o-Phenylphenol," *Analyst* 82:498–503 (1957).

20. Oesch, F., D.M. Jerina, J.W. Daly, and J.M. Rice. "Induction, Activation and Inhibition of Epoxide Hydrase: An Anomalous Prevention of Chlorobenzene-Induced Hepatotoxicity by an Inhibitor of Epoxide Hydrase," *Chem. Biol. Interact.* 6:189–202 (1973).

21. Fu, P.P., M.W. Chou, S.K. Yang, F.A. Beland, F.F. Kadlubar, D.A. Casciano, R.H. Heflick, and E.E. Evans. "Metabolism of the Mutagenic Environmental Pollutant 6-Nitrobenzo(a)pyrene: Metabolic Activation via Ring Oxidation," *Biochem. Biophys. Res. Commun.* 105:1037–1043 (1982).

22. MacLeod, M.C., G.M. Cohen, and J.K. Selkirk. "Metabolism and Macromolecular Binding of the Carcinogen Benzo(a)pyrene and Its Relatively Inert Isomer Benzo(e)pyrene by Hamster Embryo Cells," *Cancer Res.* 39:3463–3470 (1979).

23. Tokiwa, H., R. Nakagawa, and Y. Ohnishi. "Mutagenic Assay of Aromatic Nitro Compounds with Salmonella Typhimurium," *Mutat. Res.* 91:321–325 (1981).

24. Kitahara, Y., H. Okuda, K. Shudo, T. Okamoto, M. Nagao, Y. Seino, and T. Sugimura. "Identification of an Ultimate Mutagen of 10-Azabenzo(a)pyrene: Microsomal Oxidation of 10-Azabenzo(a)pyrene to 10-Azabenzo(a)pyrene-4,5-oxide," *Chem. Pharm. Bull.* 25:1950–1953 (1978).

25. Lacassagne, A., N.P. Buu-Hoi, F. Zajdela, and P. Mabille. "Activité Cancérogène de Quelques Isostéres Azotès d'Hydrocarbures Pentacycliques Cancérogènes," *C. R. Acad. Sci. Paris* 258:3387–3389 (1964).

26. Shear, M.J., and J. Leiter. "Studies in Carcinogenesis. XVI. Production of Subcutaneous Tumors in Mice by Miscellaneous Polycyclic Compounds," *J. Natl. Cancer Inst.* 2:241–258 (1941).

27. El-Bayoumy, K., S.S. Hecht, and D. Hoffmann. "Comparative Tumor Initiating Activity on Mouse Skin of 6-Nitrobenzo(a)pyrene, 6-Nitrochrysene, 3-Nitroperylene, 1-Nitropyrene, and the Parent Hydrocarbons," *Cancer Lett.* 16:333–337 (1982).

# CHAPTER 22

## Light Activation of Genotoxic Components in Natural and Synthetic Crude Oils

### G.F. Strniste

*Los Alamos National Laboratory*
*Los Alamos, NM 87545*

The correlation between increasing mortality from malignant melanoma and decreasing latitude gives credence to the hypothesis that solar ultraviolet (UV) radiation is a principal cause of skin cancer in man. However, a recent examination of data concerning the incidence of malignant melanoma in areas of the United States for which there were adequate UV radiation records showed that no statistically significant relationship existed between the amount of UV radiation received and the frequency of melanoma mortality.[1] It is reasonable to believe that other factors (e.g., environmental chemical pollutants) contribute in an additive or synergistic manner with UV radiation in the induction of skin melanoma.

The role of various chemicals as sensitizers to UV light has been well documented.[2] Photochemotherapy of various skin ailments is based on the skin-photosensitizing activities of treatment chemicals such as furocoumarins. However, it has also been shown for certain classes of environmental pollutants (e.g., polycyclic aromatic hydrocarbons) that light can photochemically transform them into direct-acting genotoxic agents.[3-7]

Several recent studies have examined the role of light in the photochemical transformation of a variety of complex mixtures derived from various energy technologies.[8-14] The results of these studies strongly suggest that environmental and health risk assessment pertaining to many of these industrial effluents must include factors concerning their photochemical-activating and transforming potentials. In this chapter, I review the results of a variety of in vitro cellular experiments performed in my laboratory during the past 5 years that concern the process of photoactivation. I limit the discussion to the subject matter of photochemical transformation of components in natural petroleum and synfuel-related products into geno-toxic agents. For comparison, the genotoxic potentials of these light-acti-vated complex mixtures are related to the measured genotoxic potential of the potent skin carcinogen, far UV (FUV) light, in the various cellular assays discussed.

The latter part of this chapter is devoted to a discussion of some pre-liminary data concerning our attempt to adapt the Ames *Salmonella* assay[15] using near UV (NUV) light in lieu of a metabolic enzyme mixture as the activation source. This modified, short-term bioassay is currently facilitating the bioassessment of chemically fractionated oil-shale retort process water. The goal of this particular study is the identification of those classes of chemical components present in the process water that are responsible for its photoactivity.

## MATERIALS AND METHODS

### Test Materials

The natural crude petroleum samples used in this study were American Petroleum Institute reference oils for biological studies and are referred to as KCO, Kuwait natural crude oil (3FEB78-1); and LCO, Louisiana natural crude oil (3FEB78-2). The three shale oils used were obtained from the Oak Ridge National Laboratory Fossil Fuel Repository. These are designated as PRHO 601, aboveground retorted shale oil (29MAY79-601); PRHO 602, hydrotreated PRHO 601 crude shale oil (29MAY79-602); and LETC, simulated, modified in situ retorted shale oil, run No. 13 in the 150-ton retort at the Laramie Energy Technology Center (24FEB81-2). The dated reference numbers are those used in cataloging samples at the Los Alamos Synfuel Repository. All oils were extracted with dimethylsulfoxide (DMSO), and nontoxic dilutions of these extracts were used in the various bioassays.[13] Preparation and characterization of the oil-shale retort process water de-scribed in this chapter have been previously reported.[11,14] Dilutions of this particular process water of 1:100 (v/v) or greater were necessary to eliminate the toxic effect in mammalian cell cultures.

Primary fractionation of the oil-shale process water was accomplished by an acid/base extraction scheme.[16] The base neutral fraction (5 g in 25 mL methanol) was applied and eluted through a Waters Prep-PAK $C_{18}$ reverse-phase, radial compression column (Waters Associates, Milford, Mass.) using a Perkin-Elmer Series 3 liquid chromatography system (Perkin-Elmer Corp., Norwalk, Conn.). The material was eluted with a linear gra-dient of water:acetonitrile (100:0 to 0:100%, v/v) followed by washes of tetrahydrofuran and *n*-hexane. The resulting 471 fractions (12.5 mL each) were pooled into 17 samples according to their residual solids (RS) distribution.

Aliquots of these 17 samples were diluted into DMSO and assessed for biological activity in the Ames *Salmonella* assay as described below.

Benzo(a)pyrene [B(a)P] was purchased from Aldrich Chemical Company (gold label, 99%+ pure) and used without further purification. Samples were prepared in DMSO and the concentration of B(a)P determined spectrophotometrically. Other chemicals used were of the highest grade available.

### Cell Cultures

*Salmonella typhimurium* strains TA98 and TA100 were obtained from Dr. B. Ames, University of California, Berkeley. Strain UTH8413, constructed from the plasmid-bearing donor strain TA98 and recipient strain TA1978, was obtained from Dr. T.S. Matney, University of Texas Health Science Center, Houston. Characteristics of these strains and their use in biotesting are published elsewhere.[15,17]

Chinese hamster ovary (CHO) cells (line AA8-4) were obtained from Dr. L. Thompson, Lawrence Livermore National Laboratory, Livermore, Cal. Culture conditions for this cell line are described elsewhere.[11,14] Low-passage human skin fibroblast cultures were purchased from either the American Type Culture Collection (Rockville, Md) or the Human Genetic Mutant Cell Repository (Camden, N.J.). Cultures discussed in this chapter are NF, normal skin fibroblasts (GM10), and $XP_A$, $XP_C$, and $XP_G$ (CRL1295, GM3616, and GM677, respectively), xeroderma pigmentosum fibroblasts. A description of their culturing conditions is reported elsewhere.[12,18]

### Irradiation

The source of FUV (primarily 254-nm wavelength) was a single 15-W General Electric germicidal lamp (G15T8). The incident fluence was 0.5 J m$^{-2}$ s$^{-1}$. The source of NUV (300 to 400 nm) was a pair of 15-W General Electric blacklights (F15T8-BLB). Incident fluences of these lights ranged from 7.5 to 13.5 J m$^{-2}$ s$^{-1}$. The calibration of these light sources and a description of the protocol using natural sunlight as the radiation source are described elsewhere.[6,11,12,19]

### Ames/*Salmonella* Bioassay

The standard plate protocol described by Ames and colleagues[15] was modified to incorporate NUV light as the activation source. As shown in Figure 1, bacteria from an overnight culture are mixed in the 0.6% top agar solution

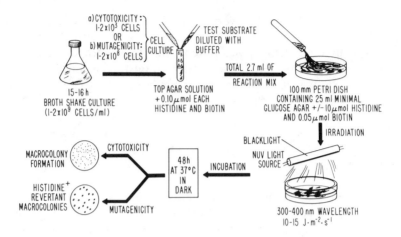

**Figure 1.** Protocol used for determining genotoxic potential of light-activated compounds in a modification of the Ames *Salmonella* bioassay.

containing a dilution of the test substance and 0.10 μmol each biotin and histidine. This reaction mix (2.7 mL total) is applied to a 100-mm plastic petri dish containing 25 mL minimal glucose agar (1.5%) with or without the addition of 10-μmol histidine and 0.05-μmol biotin for cytotoxicity or mutagenicity determinations, respectively. Within 5 min after application of the top agar solution, the plates with lids attached are exposed to the NUV source. Irradiated plates are incubated for 48 h at 37°C in the dark before scoring macrocolony formation. Assays incorporating metabolic activation were performed essentially as described by Ames et al.[15] with the exception that only 15-μL S9 fraction was added per plate.[20] S9 fraction from Aroclor 1254-induced male Sprague/Dawley rat livers was purchased from Litton Bionetics (Kensington, Md).

## CHO Cell Bioassays

The protocols used for measuring cytotoxicity (colony forming ability) and mutagenicity [at the hypoxanthine-guanine phosphoribosyl transferase (HPRT) locus] using CHO AA8-4 are reported in detail elsewhere.[11,14] Irradiation of attached, plated cells with NUV or FUV light was accomplished by exposure of plates to the source with or without lids attached, respectively. Cytotoxicity data are normalized to plating efficiencies (EOP) for control, nontreated cells. The numbers of 6-thioguanine (6-TG^R) mutants induced have been corrected for EOP determined for each dose point at time of selection.

## Human Cell Bioassays

Cultures of human skin fibroblasts were maintained in medium containing 20% fetal calf serum (FCS; Reheis Chemical Co., Scottsdale, Ariz.) and subcultured weekly as previously described.[6,18] For cytotoxicity measurements, between 100 and 5000 cells per 60-mm dish were allowed to attach in medium with 20% FCS for 18 h. This medium was removed and replaced with medium containing only 1% FCS plus appropriate dilution of test material. After 1 h incubation at 37°C (dark), the treatment medium was removed and the plates exposed to NUV light. Medium plus 20% FCS was then added, and the plates were incubated for 9–12 d before staining and scoring of colonies (clusters of >30 cells each). All data are normalized to EOP for untreated control dishes that were 25 to 40% for NF and 10 to 25% for $XP_A$, $XP_C$, and $XP_G$. Irradiation with FUV was accomplished by exposure of plated cells minus lids to the germicidal lamp for selected times.

## RESULTS AND DISCUSSION

Exposure of the procarcinogen B(a)P to NUV light in the presence of oxygen results in its chemical transformation into a variety of products including phenols, diols, tetrols, and quinones.[6] Photochemical-induced formation of B(a)P-DNA adducts has been observed.[21,22] Cytotoxic effects of concomitant exposure of various polycyclic aromatic hydrocarbons and NUV light in mammalian cells have been reported.[6,7] In Figure 2, survival data are shown for the colony-forming ability of cultured human fibroblasts exposed to B(a)P and NUV light. The role of excision repair in modulating the photochemical-induced toxic response is evident from the increased sensitivity of $XP_A$ cells, which are severely deficient in excision repair,[23,24] compared to the response seen for NF cells. However, the magnitude in the difference of the cytotoxic effect in $XP_A$ compared to NF cells is not as great as that observed for FUV light (see insert, Figure 2). Cytotoxic lesions in cellular targets other than DNA induced by B(a)P-sensitized singlet oxygen formation[25] could account for a significant amount of cell killing. Since this damage would presumably be unaffected by DNA excision repair capacity, the two cell types might be expected to respond in a more similar fashion. A similar observation concerning photodynamic cytotoxicity has been reported for mammalian cells exposed to 7,12-dimethylbenz(a)anthracene and NUV.[7]

Phototoxic components are formed in petroleum products,[8,10,26] fossil-fuel combustion effluents,[9] and synfuel-related by-products[11–14,16,19] upon exposure to solar-simulated and NUV radiation. The magnitude of the potential risks to humans or to the environment by exposure to photochemically transformed complex mixtures is unassessed at present.

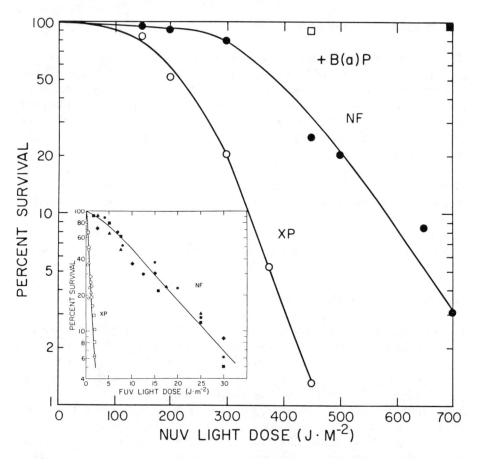

**Figure 2.** Loss of colony-forming ability in normal human skin fibroblast (NF) cells (closed circles) and in xeroderma pigmentosum (XP$_A$) cells (open circles) after 1 h exposure to B(a)P at 5 µg/mL and subsequent exposure to NUV light. The open and closed squares are surviving fractions of XP$_A$ and NF, respectively, after exposure to NUV light only. The insert graph shows the loss of colony-forming ability in these two cell types after exposure to FUV light only.

In Figure 3, we show results of an experiment in which both cytotoxic and mutagenic end points were measured in CHO cells exposed to dilutions of DMSO extracts of natural and synthetic crude oils and subsequently irradiated with NUV light. The D$_{37}$ values (dose of NUV light required to reduce colony-forming ability to 37% of control values) were between 1200 and 2400 J m$^{-2}$. An upgraded (hydrotreated) shale oil was consistently more phototoxic than the corresponding parent crude shale oil. The two natural petroleums elicited as great a phototoxic response in CHO cells as did the synthetically produced shale oils. However, the photoinduced mutagenic potentials of these various oils differed significantly. The crude shale oil had

**Figure 3.** Loss of colony-forming ability (A), and the induction of mutations at the HPRT locus (B) in CHO cells pretreated with dilutions of natural or synthetic crude oils and subsequently irradiated with NUV light. (See Reference 13, this chapter, for additional details.) Symbols used in graph B are defined in graph A.

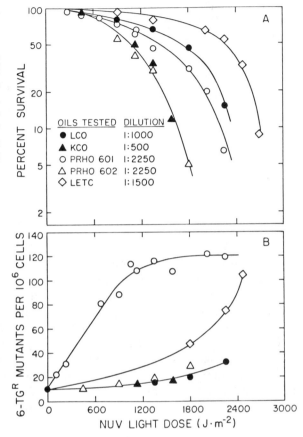

the highest mutagenic potential. Hydrotreatment of this oil, however, reduced its photomutagenic potential to a level comparable to that seen for the two natural petroleums tested.

We have also examined the photoactivity of a variety of oil-shale retort process waters.[11,12,14,16,19] In the retorting of oil shale, it is estimated that as much as 2 bbl of process water will be generated for each barrel of crude shale oil produced. These waters are heavily contaminated with organic and inorganic compounds. In Figure 4, data are presented that show photoinduced mutations at the HPRT locus in CHO cells pretreated with a 1:300 dilution of an aboveground oil-shale retort process water and subsequently irradiated with artificial NUV light (blacklights) or natural sunlight. For comparison, the induced-mutation frequencies are plotted vs $\log_{10}$ cell survival (colony-forming ability). From the data, we conclude that sunlight and artificial NUV light, at equitoxic doses, induce comparable mutations in the process-water-treated CHO cells. These data suggest that the NUV component of natural sunlight is responsible for photoactivating the process

**Figure 4.** Induction of mutations at the HPRT locus in CHO cells pretreated with an oil-shale retort process water and subsequently exposed to artificial NUV light (blacklights) or natural sunlight.

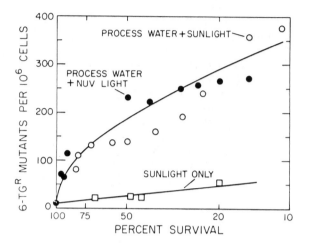

water. This observation has been further documented in experiments using natural sunlight and various optical cutoff filters.[19] Process-water-treated CHO cells are approximately seven times more sensitive to the photomutagenic power of natural sunlight than are untreated cells.

Similar to our findings concerning a cell's response to photoactivated PAH,[6] we have noted that DNA-excision repair capacity modulates a cell's response to the effects of photoactivated retort process water.[12] In Figure 5, data are shown comparing colony-forming ability in normal and XP human skin fibroblasts pretreated with 1:700 dilution of retort process water and exposed to NUV light. As is seen for the response of these cell types to FUV light where survival capacity is dictated by excision repair capacity (graph A), a similar reduction in sensitivity to photoactivated process water is seen in cell types with increasing capacities for excision repair (graph B).

A specific aim of our research is the chemical fractionation and identification of photoactive components residing in retort process waters. The chemical composition of these process waters is extremely complex, and, although physical/chemical methods exist for fractionation and identification, a simple bioassay scheme has not been available to assess photoinduced genotoxicity. Mammalian cell assays described above are very time consuming, expensive, and present logistical problems for bioassessment of multifractionated samples.

Recently, we have succeeded in adapting the standard Ames *Salmonella* plate assay with photoactivation replacing metabolic activation. Our preliminary observations using this assay are reported here, including coupling it to a chemical fractionation scheme currently in use for a particular retort process water. Details in the execution of this assay are described in the Materials and Methods section and are outlined in the schematic shown in Figure 1.

In Figure 6, data are shown for the photoinduction of cytotoxicity and

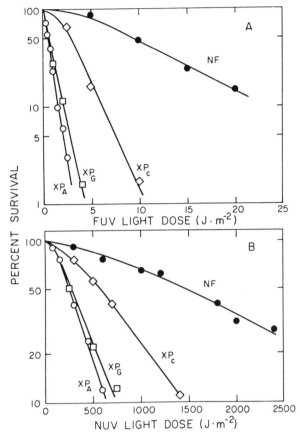

**Figure 5.** Loss of colony-forming ability in cultured normal human skin fibro-blasts (NF) and in xeroderma pigmentosum fibroblasts (complementation groups A, C, and G) after exposure to FUV light (A) or an oil-shale retort process water plus NUV light (B).

mutagenicity in strain TA98 as a function of varying amounts of process water added per plate or dose of NUV light. A similar response is seen in process-water-treated strain TA100 (data not shown). It is estimated from the survival curves that a 1:100 dilution of process water induces a cytotoxic response in cells exposed to NUV approximately 30 times that seen in untreated cells exposed to NUV light only (comparing $D_{37}$ values). Although the kinetics of induced mutation vary as a function of amount of process water added, the maximal response seen is regularly about five times the average number of background mutational events for untreated cells (25 ± 3 his+ revertants per $10^8$ cells).

In Figure 7, results are shown comparing cytotoxicity induced in TA98 (uvr−) vs the repair proficient strain UTH8413 (uvr+) after exposure to FUV light only (graph A) or combinations of process water and NUV light (graph B). Sensitization to the effects of photoactivated process water seen in the UV repair-deficient strain is similar in magnitude to the responses of TA98 compared to UTH8413 for FUV radiation.

**Figure 6.** Loss of colony-forming ability (A) and the induction of histidine⁺ revertants (B) in *Salmonella typhimurium* TA98 after exposure to an oil-shale retort process water and NUV light. Aliquot sizes noted represent the amount of process water added to the 2.7-mL top agar mixture.

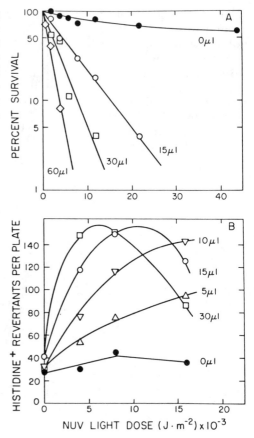

The application of the Ames *Salmonella* light activation bioassay to assess photoactivity of pooled fractions from reverse-phase high-pressure liquid chromatography (HPLC) of a base/neutral fraction of this retort process water is shown in Figure 8. For comparison, the mutagenic potential of each fraction when assessed in TA98 with metabolic activation is also shown. At least three significant photoactive peaks are discernible: fraction 1, which contains highly polar components; and fractions 8 and 13, containing components of intermediate and low polarity. A considerable amount of activity is eluted in fraction 17, which constitutes the column wash with *n*-hexane. Apparently, there are both qualitative and quantitative differences in the elution of photoactive components of this base/neutral fraction compared to the elution of components activated by microsomal enzymes. The significance of these differences is uncertain because of the poor recovery of applied activity (~30% for both photo- and enzyme-activated). Experiments in progress are addressing this problem.

Gas chromatographic/mass spectrophotometric analysis of the highly

**Figure 7.** Loss of colony-forming ability in *Salmonella* strains TA98 (open circles) and UTH8413 (closed circles) after exposure to FUV light (A) or 15 μL per plate oil-shale retort process water plus NUV light (B). The open and closed squares in graph B are surviving fractions of TA98 and UTH 8413, respectively, after exposure to NUV light only.

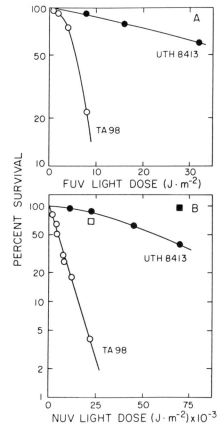

polar and photoactive HPLC peak indicates the presence of a variety of chemical species including pyrazines, pyridines, furans, furfurals, anilines, ketones, nitriles, thiophenes, and various alkylated derivatives of each noted class.[16] Within the classes of pyridines, anilines, ketones, and nitriles, 2,4,6-trimethylpyridine, N,N-dimethylaniline, methyl vinyl ketone, and isobutyronitrile, respectively, are most predominant (1 to 10 ppm in the original water). Additional fractionation of this photoactive sample employing an NH$_2$-μBondapak column (Waters Associates, Milford, Mass.) is in progress to better resolve the photoactive components.

## SUMMARY

Undefined components in natural and synthetically produced petroleums elicit a genotoxic response in cultured mammalian cells after exposure to light. The NUV component of the solar spectrum is the radiation responsible

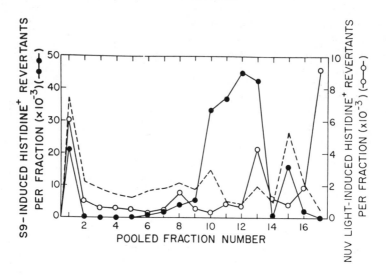

**Figure 8.** Mutagenicity of an HPLC effluent of a base/neutral fraction of an oil-shale retort process water. The mutagenic potential of the 17 pooled-HPLC fractions was determined in the Ames *Salmonella* assay using strain TA98 with NUV light or enzyme-mediated activation. The relative residual solids per pooled fraction are indicated by the dashed line. For metabolic activation, 15 µL of S9 mixture plus cofactors were added per plate. For light activation, plates with lids attached were exposed for 5 min to NUV light at an incident fluence of 13.5 J m$^{-2}$ s$^{-1}$. The number of his$^+$ revertants per fraction was calculated from the slopes of dose response curves using linear regression analysis.

for photochemical transformation. The type(s) of lesion(s) induced in DNA by the photoactivation process is mimetic of FUV light-induced genotoxic lesions (bulky adduct-like) due to the similar sensitizing abilities of either insult in cells deficient in excision repair.

Because of their intimate contact with the oil in the various stages associated with the production of shale oil, process waters contain significant quantities of UV-absorbing organic materials. Chemical fractionation of a process water has been achieved using an acid/base extraction scheme and reverse-phase HPLC. Resulting fractions have been assessed for photoinduced genotoxicity using a modification of the Ames *Salmonella* bioassay in which NUV light is the source of activation in place of metabolic enzymes. Chemical identification of components in a photoactive peak fraction is in progress employing an additional class fractionation scheme and GC/MS methods.

## ACKNOWLEDGMENTS

Several of the experiments were done in collaboration with Drs. Richard T. Okinaka and David J. Chen of the Genetics Group, and Dr. W. Dale Spall of the Toxicology Group, Life Sciences Division, Los Alamos National Laboratory. I am indebted to Ms. Judy M. Bingham and Ms. Joyce W. Nickols for their excellent technical assistance. I also thank Ms. Monica H. Fink for typing this manuscript. This work was funded by the Office of Health and Environmental Research of the Department of Energy and the Office of Research and Development of the Environmental Protection Agency.

## REFERENCES

1. Baker-Blocker, A. "Ultraviolet Radiation and Melanoma Mortality in the United States," *Environ. Res.* 23:24–28 (1980).
2. Ito, T. "Cellular and Subcellular Mechanisms of Photodynamic Action: The $^1O_2$ Hypothesis as a Driving Force in Recent Research," *Photochem. Photobiol.* 28:493–508 (1978).
3. Issaq, H.F., A.W. Andrews, G.M. Janini, and E.W. Barr. "Isolation of Stable Mutagenic Photodecomposition Products of Benzo[a]pyrene by Thin-Layer Chromatography," *J. Liq. Chrom.* 2:319–325 (1979).
4. Pitts, J.N., K.A. Van Couwenberghe, D. Grosjean, J.P. Schmid, D.R. Fritz, W.L. Belser, Jr., G.B. Knudson, and P.M. Hynds. "Atmospheric Reaction of Polycyclic Aromatic Hydrocarbons: Facile Formation of Mutagenic Nitro Derivations," *Science* 202:515–519 (1978).
5. Santamaria, L., G.C. Giordano, M. Alfisi, and F. Cascione. "Effects of Light on 3,4-Benzpyrene Carcinogenesis," *Nature (Lond.)* 210:824–825 (1966).
6. Strniste, G.F., and R.J. Brake. "Cytotoxicity in Human Skin Fibroblasts Induced by Photoactivated Polycyclic Aromatic Hydrocarbons," in *Polynuclear Aromatic Hydrocarbons: Fifth International Symposium on Chemical Analysis and Biological Fate,* M. Cooke and A.J. Dennis, Eds. (Columbus, OH: Battelle Press, 1981), pp. 109–118.
7. Utsumi, H., and M.M. Elkind. "Photodynamic Cytotoxicity of Mammalian Cells Exposed to Sunlight—Simulating Near Ultraviolet Light in the Presence of the Carcinogen 7,12-Dimethylbenz(a)anthracene," *Photochem. Photobiol.* 30:271–278 (1979).
8. Callen, D.F., and R.A. Larson. "Toxic and Genetic Effects of Fuel Oil Photoproducts and Three Hydroperoxides in *Saccharomyces cerevisiae*," *J. Toxicol. Environ. Health* 4:913–917 (1978).
9. Lankas, G.R., D.A. Haugen, and M.M. Elkind. "Enhanced Near-Ultraviolet Sensitivity Induced by Coal Combustion Effluents in Cultured Mammalian Cells," *J. Toxicol. Environ. Health* 6:723–729 (1980).
10. Larson, R.A., L.L. Hunt, and D.W. Blankenship. "Formation of Toxic Products from a No. 2 Fuel Oil by Photooxidation," *Environ. Sci. Technol.* 11:493–496 (1977).

11. Strniste, G.F., and D.J. Chen. "Cytotoxic and Mutagenic Properties of Shale Oil Byproducts. I. Activation of Retort Process Waters with Near Ultraviolet Light," *Environ. Mutagenesis* 3:221–231 (1981).

12. Strniste, G.F., D.J. Chen, and R.T. Okinaka. "Genotoxic Effects of Sunlight-Activated Waste Water in Cultured Mammalian Cells," *J. Nat. Cancer Inst.* 69:199–203 (1982).

13. Strniste, G.F., J.M. Bingham, R.T. Okinaka, and D.J. Chen. "Genotoxicity Induced in Cultured Chinese Hamster Cells Exposed to Natural and Synthetic Crude Oils and Near Ultraviolet Light," *Toxicol. Lett.* 13:163–167 (1982).

14. Chen, D.J., and G.F. Strniste. "Cytotoxic and Mutagenic Properties of Shale Oil Byproducts. II. Comparison of Mutagenic Effects at Five Genetic Markers Induced by Retort Process Water Plus Near Ultraviolet Light in Chinese Hamster Ovary Cells," *Environ. Mutagenesis* 4:457–467 (1982).

15. Ames, B.N., J. McCann, and E. Yamasaki. "Methods for Detecting Mutagens with the *Salmonella*/Mammalian—Microsome Mutagenicity Test," *Mutat. Res.* 31:347–364 (1975).

16. Strniste, G.F., J.M. Bingham, W.D. Spall, J.W. Nickols, R.T. Okinaka, and D.J. Chen. "Fractionation of an Oil Shale Retort Process Water: Isolation of Photoactive Genotoxic Components," in *Application of Short-term Bioassays in the Analysis of Complex Environmental Mixtures,* M.D. Waters, S.S. Sandhu, J. Lewtas, L. Claxton, N. Chernoff, and S. Nesnow, Eds. (New York: Plenum Press, 1983), pp. 139–151.

17. Matney, T.S. "Mutagenic Assays in Gram-Negative Bacteria for the Detection of Potential Carcinogens: Activation by Mammalian Microsomal Fractions," in *Microbial Testers: Probing Carcinogenesis,* I.C. Felkner, Ed. (New York: Marcel Dekker, Inc., 1981), pp. 121–129.

18. Hildebrand, C.E., and G.F. Strniste. "Ultraviolet Light Inactivation of Zinc-Mediated Metallothionein Induction in Normal and Repair-Deficient Human Cells," *Mutat. Res.* 95:417–426 (1982).

19. Strniste, G.F., D.J. Chen, and R.T. Okinaka. "Sunlight Activation of Shale Oil Byproducts as Measured by Genotoxic Effects in Cultured Chinese Hamster Cells," in *Polynuclear Aromatic Hydrocarbons: Sixth International Symposium on Chemical Analysis and Biological Fate,* M. Cooke, A.J. Dennis, and G.L. Fisher, Eds. (Columbus, OH: Battelle Press, 1982), pp. 773–778.

20. Nickols, J.W., and G.F. Strniste. "Optimizing Mutagenicity of Complex Mixtures in the Ames/*Salmonella* Bioassay," *Environ. Mutagenesis* 4:318 (1982).

21. Strniste, G.F., E. Martinez, A.M. Martinez, and R.J. Brake. "Photo-induced Reactions of Benzo(a)pyrene with DNA In Vitro," *Cancer Res.* 40:245–252 (1980).

22. Hoard, D.E., R.L. Ratliff, J.M. Bingham, and G.F. Strniste. "Reactions Induced In Vitro Between Model DNA and Benzo(a)pyrene by Near Ultraviolet Radiation," *Chem. Biol. Inter.* 33:179–194 (1981).

23. Robbins, J.H., K.H. Kraemer, M.A. Lutzner, B.W. Festaff, and H.G. Coon. "Xeroderma Pigmentosum: An Inherited Disease with Sun Sensitivity, Multiple Cutaneous Neoplasms and Abnormal DNA Repair," *Ann. Intern. Med.* 80:221–248 (1974).

24. Friedberg, E.C., U.K. Ehmann, and J.I. Williams. "Human Diseases Associated with Defective DNA Repair," in *Advances in Radiation Biology,* Vol.

8, J.T. Lett and H. Adler, Eds. (New York: Academic Press, 1979), pp. 85–174.

25. Inomata, M., and C. Nagata. "Photoinduced Phenoxy Radial of 3,4-Benzopyrene," *Gann* 63:119–130 (1972).

26. Larson, R.A., and L.L. Hunt. "Photooxidation of a Refined Petroleum Oil: Inhibition by β-Carotene and Role of Singlet Oxygen," *Photochem. Photobiol.* 28:553–555 (1978).

## DISCUSSION

*H.L. Ketcofsky, Pittsburgh Energy Technology Center:* My question should not, perhaps, be answered by this particular speaker, but I think he prompts it. I can certainly see the rationale for studies of this type, but I am a little concerned. During this symposium, we have been given a lot of generalizations based on, I think, good scientific evidence about why we proceed with studies of this type. I have spent most of my professional life looking at free radicals in coals and in coal liquefaction products and would like to cite a few findings. One is that the free radicals are concentrated in high boiling fractions. If you take high boiling fractions and do a chemical separation, you'll find that those free radicals are most highly concentrated in the nitrogen bases as opposed to the phenolics. If you do other types of functional group separations, you look at the fractions, but you don't see free radicals. If you hydrotreat these materials, you find that the free radical content decreases significantly. I find a lot of correlations that are essentially the same as those you have found associated with mutagenesis. There is a line of demarcation in this room—on one side we have people who have one view of the surgeon general's warning and on the other side of the room we have other people with other views. It's well known that cigarette tars contain benzo[a]pyrene. However, also in that cigarette tar you have approximately one free radical electron for every three or four thousand carbon atoms. It's known that cancerous tissue contains free radicals. It's known that many biological processes proceed through free radical type mechanisms. But my question is really the following. Are we so concerned with benzo[a]pyrene and the nitrogen-containing PNAs that we exhibit tunnel vision towards other possibilities? It's not fair for me to direct that to the speaker, but I'd like anybody in this room to respond to that.

*A. Stewart, University of Oklahoma Biological Station:* Later in the session I will be talking about humic materials in aquatic systems, and those have stable free radicals, which I'm going to implicate as being important. I think we do need to pay some consideration to that.

*C.W. Gehrs, Oak Ridge National Laboratory:* I think your question is excellent. It is one that people working in the area of synfuels have wrestled with for a while. It also shows what we're attempting to do in this symposium: that is, bring in individuals from diverse backgrounds and also talk at different levels, such as the presentation which you just had, which was very specific science, as well as some of the more general studies such as that which will be presented by Dr. Stewart later this morning.

*M. Uziel, Oak Ridge National Laboratory:* I would like to make one addition. To assess the relative contributions of radical or specific metabolism, or any other chemistry which may lead to a mutagenic situation or carcinogenesis, we must have some way of quantitating results and correlations in such a way that at some point we can know whether we have considered all the toxic reactions that are available and contributing to the ultimate toxicity. This is not an easy subject, but I think this is another area which deserves attention.

*J.M. Giddings, Oak Ridge National Laboratory:* We have been studying the effects of water-soluble fractions of coal liquids, shale oils, and petroleum on aquatic organisms for some years. Dr. E. Herbes has looked at the effects of exposing the oil and water system to light while the water is extracting the water-soluble fractions from the oil on the subsequent toxicity of that water-soluble fraction to *Daphniea magna* and to algae. For both natural and synthetic oils, he has found the toxicity increases. I believe he has implicated quinones and hydroperoxides as the probable agents for that increase in toxicity.

*R.H. McKee, Exxon:* In your early slides, you seemed to show a fairly clear separation between the cytotoxic and mutagenic end points. Would it be fair to assume that different molecules are responsible for the two events and what molecules are they likely to be?

*G.F. Strniste:* I'll give an example in an attempt to answer the first part of your question and I'll speculate on the second part. On the first part, I would say yes. From recent data generated in my laboratory, it would appear that there are at least two types of lesions induced in the DNA and possibly other classes of lesions induced elsewhere in the cell (membrane damage, for example). These observations are based on results of experiments in which both repair-deficient and repair-proficient cultured Chinese hamster (line CHO) cells were used as targets. We found that the magnitude of the cytotoxic response was definitely influenced by the presence of the UV excision repair pathway. However, mutagenicity did not vary to any appreciable degree in cells with or without excision repair capacity. As to the second part of your question, I must rely on the experimental data of others (notably R.A. Larson and colleagues). They have shown that addition of the singlet oxygen scavenger, β-carotene, results in a substantial reduction of hydroperoxides in a UV-irradiated complex mixture (natural petroleum). Peroxides and related free radicals are known cytotoxins.

# CHAPTER 23

## Biological Analysis of Progressive Toxicity of Shale-Derived vs Petroleum-Derived Fuels in Rats

W.J. Mehm[a] and C.L. Feser

*Physiology, Veterinary Medicine, and*
*Experimental Hematology*
*Departments*
*Armed Forces Radiobiology Research*
*Institute*
*Bethesda, MD 20814*

Rats were gavaged with either petroleum-derived or shale-derived JP5 jet fuel (24 mL per kg of body weight) and killed at selected intervals between 3 h and 15 d after gavage. Samples of liver tissue and blood were taken and examined for evidence of hepatocellular damage. Lesions produced from both fuels occurred in the periportal region of the hepatic lobule, showing extensive vacuolization (fatty change) and increases in binucleated cells, mitotic figures, and pyknotic nuclei. Visible hepatic lesions appeared 6 h earlier and lasted approximately 1 d longer in the shale-treated rats than in the petroleum-treated rats. No difference was noted in the nature of the lesions induced by the two fuels. Serum chemistry analyses substantiated evidence for hepatocellular damage, with elevated levels of serum glutamic pyruvic transaminase (SGPT) and serum glutamic oxaloacetic transaminase (SGOT), also know as alanine and aspartate amino transferases. Significant differences in these values, dosed versus controls, occurred as early as 6 h and lasted up to 5 d postgavage. Peak levels for both enzymes were seen in animals killed 12 h after gavage. These findings suggest the biologic effects of both shale-derived and petroleum-derived JP5 to be the same, with trends that may indicate differences.

---

[a]Present address: DFB, USAF Academy, Colorado Springs, CO 80840.

## INTRODUCTION

In view of presently decreasing petroleum reserves, the military is assessing the suitability of shale-derived fuels for practical use. In accordance with the Toxic Substance Control Act of 1976 (which states that the biological effects of new and potentially toxic substances must be determined), the U.S. Navy has requested a histological study of the toxicity of shale-derived and petroleum-derived jet fuel, specifically jet propulsion fuel No. 5 (JP5).

Recently, Parker et al.[1] found that the LD50/14 was more than 60 mL per kg of body weight for petroleum-derived JP5 and 39 mL per kg for the Sohio refined shale-derived JP5. Using a constant dose of 24 mL per kg, a 3-d uniform-dose study showed that microscopically visible changes in the liver were not apparent until day 2. Despite differences in lethality, both fuels produced similar liver lesions.

Before the work of Parker et al.,[1] very little histological information was available on the long-term toxic effects of high-performance aircraft fuels.[2] Available information on conventional distillates dealt primarily with generalized neurological and behavioral abnormalities. Toxicity from kerosene was reported by Jacobziner and Raybin[3] to cause depression of the central nervous system. They proposed that petroleum distillates may also damage the liver, kidney, spleen, brain, heart, and bone marrow, but they did not describe the nature of that damage. Lethal doses of kerosene and other petroleum distillates were not determined. In a series of articles, Knave et al.[4–6] reported on the toxic effects to the nervous system of petroleum-derived jet fuel. In those studies, surveys of occupationally exposed industrial workers revealed chronic neurological symptoms such as numbness in the extremities and psychological dysfunctions including mild depression and apathy. These findings and anorexia were also found by Rowe et al.,[7] who fed crude oil and kerosene-treated feed to cattle.

While histological evidence for the hepatotoxicity of petroleum distillates has been sparse, histopathological work on a variety of hepatotoxic chemicals, particularly carbon tetrachloride, has been extensive. Carbon tetrachloride and chloroform both produced centrilobular fatty change (accumulation of lipid within cells around the central vein) and necrosis.[8,9] This contrasts with the effects of ethionine and ethanol, which induce fatty change without necrosis.[9,10] In cases of phosphorus poisoning, periportal lesions appear consisting of fatty change and necrosis.[9,10]

The purpose of this investigation was to evaluate more completely the toxic effects of shale-derived vs petroleum-derived JP5 on the liver in rats. The damaging effects of these fuels were assessed from as early as 3 h posttreatment through 15 d. This allowed examination of the initial stages of toxicity, the period of maximum effect, and a posttoxicity phase. Correlations were made between the serological evidence of hepatic damage and the histological evidence of cellular damage.

## METHODS

Male Sprague-Dawley rats [Tac:N(SD)fBR (Taconic Farms, Germantown, N.Y.)], weighing 250 to 500 g, were used for the study. Rats were housed in plastic cages, 48.3 × 26.7 × 44.5 cm. Fuel-treated rats were kept two per cage (one shale-treated and one petroleum-treated), and control rats were kept one per cage. Control rats were separated from fuel-treated rats to prevent contamination from fuel vapors in urine and from exhaled gases. A 12-h light (6 am to 6 pm) and 12-h dark cycle was maintained for all animals. Food (Wayne Lab-Blox, Allied Mills, Inc., Chicago) and chlorinated (10 ppm) (Everchlor chemical feeder, Everpure, Inc., Westmont, Ill.) water were available ad libitum. Room temperature was kept at 22°C, and humidity was kept from 60% to 70%.

Two types of JP5 were studied. The first, a petroleum-derived JP5, was refined by Hess St. Croix from a crude mixture containing primarily Iranian stock (55%) and Nigerian crude (25%). The second fuel, a shale-derived crude, was extracted by the Paraho aboveground retorting process from a shale deposit at Anvil Points, Colorado. It was then refined by Sohio from shale crude produced in 1978–1979.

Rats were divided into two groups of 84 animals each. Gavaging was accomplished by using a plastic syringe (Monoject, Sherwood Medical Industries, Inc., Deland, Fla.) and feeding tube (Premature Infant Feeding Tube, Cutter Laboratories, Berkeley, Calif.). The first group was gavaged with petroleum-derived JP5, 24 mL per kg of body weight. The second group was gavaged with an equal amount of shale-derived JP5. Twenty-four milliliters of fuel per kilogram of body weight was selected as the experimental dose because it had been shown to produce significant liver lesions while being considerably below the LD50/14 in the rat.[1] Two groups of 70 rats each served as water-dosed controls for the petroleum-derived and shale-derived JP5-treated groups, respectively.

Six rats from each experimental and five from each control group were killed at the following times after gavage: 3, 6, 9, 12, and 18 h and 1, 2, 3, 4, 5, 7, 10, 12, and 15 d. While the animal was anesthetized with methoxyfluorane (Metofane, Pitman-Moore, Inc., Washington Crossing, N.J.), its abdominal cavity was opened, and 6 mL of blood was drawn from the abdominal aorta with a plastic syringe (Sherwood) and an 18-gauge needle. The blood was allowed to clot in a glass tube (evacuated, Vacutainer, Becton-Dickinson and Co., Rutherford, N.J.). Serum was obtained after centrifugation and stored at −16°C for a maximum of 5 d before analysis on an automated analyzer (Gilford System 3500 computer directed analyzer, Gilford Instrument Laboratories, Inc., Oberlin, Ohio). Serum was analyzed for levels of serum glutamic pyruvic transaminase (SGPT) and serum glutamic oxaloacetic transaminase (SGOT). These enzymes are also known as alanine aminotransferase and aspartate aminotransferase, respectively. Significant effects of treatment were tested by a one-way analysis of variance (ANOVA). Differences between groups were tested by a t-statistic for multiple comparison using the pooled variance from ANOVA. Statistical significance was set at the 95% confidence level.

Necropsy was also performed at the time intervals designated above. Tissue samples were taken from the liver and immediately fixed in 10% phosphate-buffered formalin. Tissues were processed and embedded in paraffin, cut at 6 μm, and stained with hematoxylin and eosin (H & E) for light microscopy. In addition to formalin-fixed sections, frozen sections of liver were cut at approximately 20 μm and stained with Oil-Red-O for neutral lipids.[11]

## RESULTS

Significant treatment effects were observed in rats gavaged with 24 mL of petroleum-derived or shale-derived JP5 per kg of body weight. Both morphological changes and elevated serum enzyme levels were noted.

### Morphology

Prior to the removal of blood for serum chemistry analysis, necropsy revealed swollen livers with extensive surface mottling in rats killed at 1, 2, and 3 d after gavage. No congestion in the lungs or epicardium was identified in any of the treatment groups. Examination of the abdominal cavity revealed that up to 50% of the original treatment dose was retained in the stomach at 3 h postgavage. By 6 h, complete emptying of the stomach had occurred.

As early as 12 and 18 h after treatment, visible microscopic liver lesions appeared in shale- and petroleum-gavaged rats, respectively. These lesions consisted of numerous fine cytoplasmic vacuoles (ranging from 0.5 to 3.0 μm in diameter) evident in periportal hepatocytes (Figures 1 and 2). Frozen sections of liver, stained with Oil-Red-O, demonstrated lipid material within these vacuoles, which was fatty change (Figure 3). Fatty change was lacking in the control animals, as evidenced by the absence of cytoplasmic vacuoles and the Oil-Red-O reaction. An increased number of binucleated cells was also present in fuel-treated animals, where up to four or five binucleated cells per single portal area were evident. Conversely, binucleated hepatocytes in controls averaged one or two per three periportal areas. This was interpreted as evidence of regeneration and paralleled the substantial increases in dividing hepatocytes identified by mitotic figures (Figure 4).

At subsequent intervals, liver lesions exhibited increases in the size and number of cytoplasmic vacuoles (up to 5 μm in diameter) and in the number of binucleated cells. In addition, frequent mitotic figures (Figure 4) and occasional pyknotic nuclei were observed (Figure 5). These changes

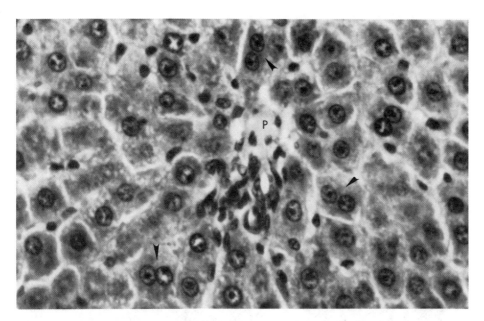

**Figure 1.** Cytoplasmic vacuolization surrounding portal tract (P) in rats killed 12 h after gavage with shale-derived JP5. Vacuoles 0.5 to 2.0 μm in diameter occur throughout cytoplasm. Note frequent appearance of binucleated cells (arrows). Paraffin embedded, H & E, ×400.

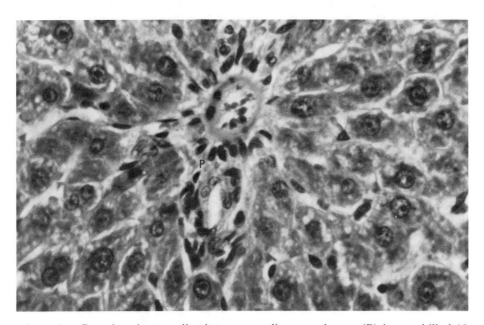

**Figure 2.** Cytoplasmic vacuolization surrounding portal tract (P) in rats killed 18 h after gavage with petroleum-derived JP5. Vacuoles 1.0 to 3.0 μm in diameter occur throughout cytoplasm. Paraffin embedded, H & E, ×400.

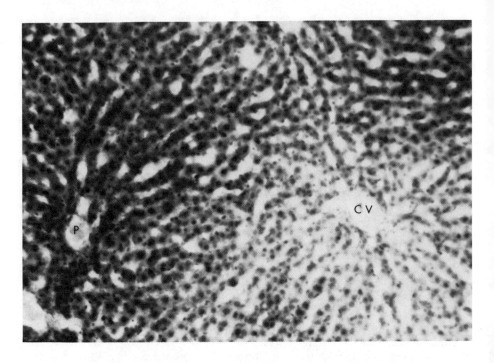

**Figure 3.**   Oil-Red-O stain demonstrating lipid material (dark areas) within hepatocytes surrounding portal tract (P) in rats killed 48 h after gavage with petroleum-derived JP5. Note absence of hepatocellular lipid in proximity to central vein (CV). Frozen section, ×100.

culminated in maximum visible lesions at 2 and 3 d posttreatment in both petroleum- and shale-gavaged rats, respectively.

Visible liver damage appeared to be less severe on days 3 and 4 post-gavage in petroleum-treated rats and on day 4 in shale-treated rats. This was evidenced by the small number and size of cytoplasmic vacuoles, reduced number of binucleated cells, and absence of mitotic figures and pyknotic nuclei. Essentially normal tissue was observed from day 5 through day 15 in both treatment groups. The nature of histological damage was identical in both petroleum- and shale-treated groups. The degree of damage varied only as a function of the interval at which the animals were killed after gavage.

### Serum Chemistries

Significant differences from controls in SGOT and SGPT levels were recorded in both petroleum- and shale-treated groups. Both groups had SGOT

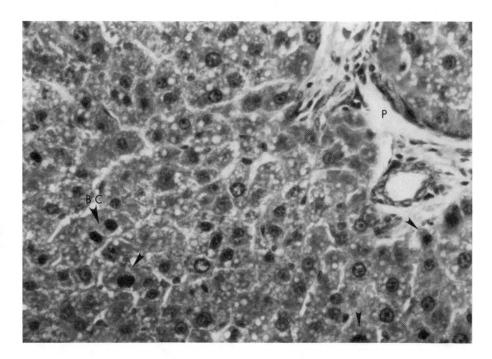

**Figure 4.**   Generalized pattern of maximum periportal vacuolization (fatty change) characteristic of lesions induced by petroleum-derived JP5. Hepatocellular vacuoles, 2.0 to 5.0 μm in diameter, surround portal tract (P). Mitotic figures frequently appear (arrows), and a postmitotic binucleated cell (BC) can be seen. 48-h petroleum-gavaged rat, paraffin embedded, H & E, ×250.

levels significantly different from controls 9 h through 2 d postgavage (Figure 6). SGPT levels appeared significantly different from controls at 6 and 9 h postgavage for petroleum- and shale-treated groups, respectively. SGPT levels remained significantly different from controls through day 3 for shale-treated animals and through day 5 for petroleum-treated animals (Figure 7). There were no significant differences in enzyme levels between fuel groups.

## DISCUSSION

Hepatic changes identified in this study were similar in part to those reported by Parker et al.[1] Those authors found swollen and mottled livers with cytoplasmic vacuolization (fatty change), mitotic figures, and occasional pyknotic nuclei in the periportal region of the hepatic lobule. Our study substantiates these findings as well as those identifying no differences in the

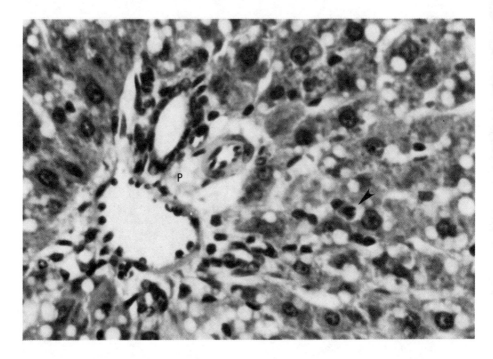

**Figure 5.**   Extensive cytoplasmic vacuolization in periportal hepatocytes in rats killed 3 d after gavage with shale-derived JP5. Vacuoles, 1.5 to 3.0 μm in diameter, occupy majority of cytoplasm in a few cells. Note presence of pyknotic nucleus in degenerating cell (arrow). P, portal tract. Paraffin embedded, H & E, ×400.

nature of hepatic lesions induced by either shale- or petroleum-derived fuel. However, contrasting with observations made in this study, Parker et al.[1] did not comment on an increase in the number of binucleated cells associated with the lesion. Further, with the exception of an occasional observation in rats killed 1 d after gavage, those authors did not report periportal cytoplasmic vacuolization (fatty change) until the second day after dosing. They also identified more severe fatty change occurring in the rats treated with the shale-derived fuel.

The zonal occurrence of periportal hepatic lesions from JP5 found in this study and by Parker et al.[1] contrasted sharply with the regional distribution of lesions induced by classical hepatotoxins. These toxins, including carbon tetrachloride, ethionine, ethanol, chloroform, etc., cause centrilobular fatty change.[8,9] Classical hepatotoxins are thought to produce centrilobular lesions because this region, being at the distal end of the lobular blood supply, is most hypoxic and therefore highly susceptible to stress.[9] Smith et al.[12] suggested that potent hepatotoxins induce periportal lesions by destroying the first cells they encounter as they enter the lobule. Evidence

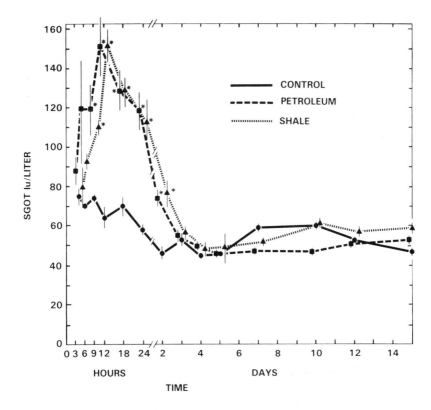

**Figure 6.** Mean SGOT levels ± standard errors for three treatment groups at times indicated (n = 5). Asterisk denotes significant treatment effect by analysis of variance (p<0.05). Note broken time scale between 24 h and day 2.

collected to date suggests that JP5 falls into this category. However, Robbins[9] states that no physiological evidence has been established to adequately explain why hepatic lesions occur in the midzonal or periportal region.

This study showed visible JP5-induced lesions occurring 6 h earlier in the shale-treated rats than in the petroleum-treated rats (12 h and 18 h, respectively). These data may suggest a more rapidly acting toxicity from the shale-derived fuel. Further, the earlier disappearance of visible lesions in the petroleum-treated rats may suggest a longer lasting toxicity from the shale-derived fuel. These findings agree with Parker et al.,[1] who observed a greater degree of lethality and severity in the lesions resulting from treatment with the shale-derived fuel. The absence of visible microscopic lesions after 5 d postgavage in either shale- or petroleum-treated animals may indicate that hepatocellular recovery has occurred.

The longer lasting toxicity of shale-derived JP5 may be attributed to

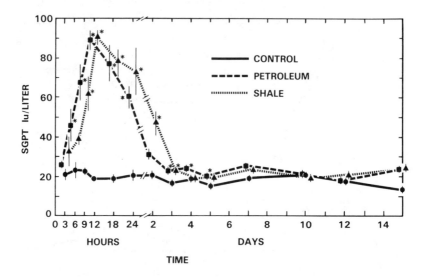

**Figure 7.** Mean SGPT levels ± standard errors for three treatment groups at times indicated (n = 5). Asterisk denotes significant treatment effect by analysis of variance (p<0.05). Note broken time scale between 24 h and day 2.

particular constitutents after refining is complete. It must be made clear, however, that the exact chemical properties of either shale- or petroleum-derived JP5 tend to remain elusive. Petroleum-derived JP5 consists primarily of straight-chain hydrocarbons between $C_{10}$ and $C_{15}$. This mixture frequently contains higher-boiling components than specified by the military, in addition to substituted phenols and amines added to inhibit oxidation.[13,14] The specific characteristics of petroleum fuels depend highly on the source of the original crude or the specific refining process used. Thus, definitive biological research is most difficult with these products, due to their highly variable chemical constituency. Differences in the final product of shale-derived JP5 result from the shale deposit from which the fuel is extracted, specific retorting techniques, and from variations in refining techniques.[15] The work of Hazlett et al.,[16] however, has shown that, although both fuels are chemically similar, shale products contain higher amounts of normal alkanes, hydrogenated polynuclear aromatics, and nitrogen. It is possible, therefore, that some or all of the additional components in shale fuels may lead to increased duration of toxic effects. Further study into the various chemical constituents of shale-derived JP5 and their toxic properties is needed.

The serum chemistry analyses substantiated evidence for hepatocellular damage in rats when gavaged with JP5. Rats treated with either the petroleum- or the shale-derived fuel demonstrated SGOT or SGPT levels significantly different from controls (p < 0.05), from as early as 6 h after gavage through 5 d postgavage. Maximum levels of both SGOT and SGPT were recorded in animals killed 12 h after gavage (Figures 6 and 7). It is evident, therefore, that release of hepatocellular enzymes preceded the appearance of earliest visible damage by 9 h and the maximum visible damage by as much as 60 h. Because the release of SGOT and SGPT from hepatocytes indicates breakdown of cellular membranes,[17] the evidence suggests that events beyond the range of the light microscope are occurring at the subcellular level before the visualization of hepatic lesions. A planned investigation of this phenomenon with the electron microscope may elucidate these subcellular events and relate them more clearly to formation of lesions and release of enzyme.

## SUMMARY

The administration of petroleum-derived and shale-derived JP5 to rats resulted in hepatocellular damage characterized by periportal fatty change, increase in binucleated cells, mitotic figures, and cellular necrosis. Elevated levels of SGOT and SGPT were also evident. These hepatocellular changes correlated with damage to cellular membrane systems and fatty change. Therefore, it is suggested that JP5 exerts its toxic effects on the liver by initially damaging cytoplasmic membranes. This results in the release of intracytoplasmic enzymes into the bloodstream. Histologically, hepatocellular damage becomes evident as marked periportal fatty change.

These findings suggest that the biological effects of both shale-derived and petroleum-derived JP5 apparently function by the same mechanism. While visible hepatic lesions appear earlier and last slightly longer in rats treated with the shale-derived fuel, the differences between these fuels are slight. The only statistical differences are in relation to the controls and not between fuel groups. Therefore, the biological effects of shale-derived and petroleum-derived JP5 appear to be the same, with trends that may indicate differences.

## ACKNOWLEDGMENTS

We are sincerely grateful to Dr. James Nold for his assistance in the interpretation of histological data, Ms. June Egan for the serum analyses, Mr. Steven Hargett for technical assistance in necropsy and histological preparation, and Dr. Charles Bonney, Behavioral Sciences Department, for his initial encouragement and support throughout the project.

Research was conducted under work unit No. MJ 00067, according to the principles enunciated in the "Guide for the Care and Use of Laboratory Animals," prepared by the Institute of Laboratory Animal Resources, National Research Council.

## REFERENCES

1.  Parker, G., V. Bogo, and R. Young. "Acute Toxicity of Conventional Versus Shale-Derived JP5 Jet Fuel: Light Microscopic, Hematologic, and Serum Chemistry Studies," *Toxicol. Appl. Pharmacol.* 57:302–317 (1981).
2.  "Criteria for a Recommended Standard—Occupational Exposure to Refined Petroleum Solvents," (Washington, DC: National Institute of Occupational Safety and Health, 1977).
3.  Jacobziner, H., and H.W. Raybin. "Accidental Chemical Poisonings. Kerosene and Other Petroleum Distillate Poisonings," *N.Y. State J. Med.* 3428–3430 (1963).
4.  Knave, B., P. Mindus, and G. Struwe. "Neurasthenic Symptoms in Workers Occupationally Exposed to Jet Fuel," *Acta Psychiatr. Scand.* 60:39–49 (1979).
5.  Knave, B., B.A. Olson, S. Elofsson, F. Gamberale, A. Isaksson, P. Mindus, H.E. Persson, G. Struwe, A. Wennberg, and P. Westerholm. "Long-Term Exposure to Fuel. II. A Cross-Sectional Epidemiological Investigation on Occupationally Exposed Industrial Workers with Special Reference to the Nervous System," *Scand. J. Work Environ. Health* 4:19–45 (1978).
6.  Knave, B., H.E. Persson, J.M. Goldberg, and P. Westerholm. "Long-Term Exposure to Jet Fuel. An Investigation on Occupationally Exposed Workers with Special Reference to the Nervous System," *Scand. J. Work Environ. Health* 3:152–164 (1976).
7.  Rowe, L.D., J.W. Dollahite, and B.J. Camp. "Toxicity of Two Crude Oils and of Kerosene to Cattle," *J. Am. Vet. Med. Assoc.* 162:61–66 (1973).
8.  Recknagel, R.O. "Carbon Tetrachloride Hepatotoxicity," *Pharmacol. Rev.* 19:145–208 (1967).
9.  Robbins, S.L. *Pathologic Basis of Disease* (Philadelphia: Saunders Co., 1974).
10.  Plaa, G. "Toxic Responses of the Liver," in *Toxicology: The Basic Science of Poisons,* L.J. Casarett and J. Doull, Eds. (New York: Macmillan, 1980), pp. 206–231.
11.  Luna, L.G. *Manual of Histologic Staining Methods of the Armed Forces Institute of Pathology* (New York: McGraw-Hill, 1968).
12.  Smith, H.A., T.C. Jones, and R.D. Hunt. *Veterinary Pathology* (Philadelphia: Lea and Febiger, 1972).
13.  "Turbine Fuel, Aviation Grades JP4 and JP5," Military Specification, MIL-T-5624K (1976).
14.  "Annual Report of Research: Nov. 1976–31 Oct. 1977" (Naval Biosciences Laboratory, 1968).
15.  Maugh, T.H., "Oil Shale: Prospects on the Upswing . . . Again," *Science* 198:1023–1027 (1977).
16.  Hazlett, R.N., J.M. Hall, and J. Solash. "Properties and Composition of Jet Fuel Derived from Alternative Energy Sources. I. Background and N-Alkane Content," presented at the American Chemical Society Division of Fuels Chemistry, August 29–September 3, 1976; *Am. Chem. Soc. Div. Fuel Chem. Prepr.* 21:219 (1976).
17.  Wroblewski, F., and J.S. LaDue. "Serum Glutamic Pyruvic Transaminase in Cardiac and Hepatic Disease," *Proc. Soc. Exp. Biol. Med.* 91:569–571 (1956).

## DISCUSSION

*A. Stewart, University of Oklahoma:* Can you conclude from this that the fuel handlers' lackadaisical attitude did originate from the fuels they were handling?

*W.J. Mehm:* No, we can't conclude that, but it does indicate a hepatocellular response to the fuel. We believe fuel workers are exposed to vapor concentrations up to 1000 ppm under operational conditions. A study conducted at the Armed Forces Radiobiology Research Institute after my departure exposed rats to approximately this concentration. Preliminary results have failed to demonstrate hepatocellular effects. Possibly, work with the central nervous system might be more productive in linking human performance with fuel toxicity.

# CHAPTER 24

## Interactions between Dissolved Humic Materials and Organic Toxicants

### A.J. Stewart

*University of Oklahoma Biological Station and*
*Department of Botany and Microbiology*
*Star Route B*
*Kingston, OK 73439*

Dissolved humic materials (DHM) are important constituents of the dissolved organic carbon pools in most lakes and streams and often occur in concentrations of 5 to 50 mg/L. DHM exists as a heterogeneous complex with a molecular weight spectrum of a few hundred to many thousands. The molecular weight spectrum of DHM is clearly dependent upon environmental factors (pH, ionic strength of the medium, light intensity, etc.), and differential shifts in the molecular weight spectrum of DHM will alter the types of reactions that predominate between DHM and organic toxicants. However, quantitative data regarding seasonal shifts in the molecular weight spectra of DHM in different lake or stream types are unavailable. DHM bears electron-acceptor and -doner groups and possesses stable free radicals; these features enhance DHM chemical reactivity. In the presence of sunlight, DHM generates singlet oxygen ($^1O_2$) from ground-state dissolved oxygen; $^1O_2$ is extremely reactive and promotes both the alteration of organic toxicants and the formation of peroxides. High-molecular-weight DHM demonstrates colloidal properties and can adsorb relatively insoluble pesticides; the transport and fates of the adsorbed toxicants are subsequently modified to an unknown extent. The toxicities of selected organic compounds were assessed in the presence and absence of a low-molecular-weight DHM using an acute (4-h) algal bioassay. When DHM was present, compounds in an aniline methylation series became more toxic (1.1- to 40-fold). DHM similarly increased the toxicity of o-cresol, 2,4-dimethylphenol, and 2,3,6-trimethylphenol (2- to 5.4-fold) but reduced toxicity of p-benzoquinone and quinoline by factors of 6.1 and 1.2, respectively. Evaluation of the importance of DHM to the transport, fate, and ecological effects of organic toxicants will be greatly enhanced by recent trends in methodology, several of which are discussed.

## DISSOLVED HUMIC MATERIALS—
## AN OVERVIEW

The rudimentary physical and chemical properties of humic compounds were initially determined from studies of soil organic matter.[1,2] Preliminary characterization of humic compounds present in soils was based on the solubilities of the compounds in acidic and basic solution (Figure 1).[3] Compounds that could be precipitated from basic soil extracts by acidification were referred to as humic compounds, while substances remaining in solution under acidic conditions were arbitrarily defined as fulvic compounds. Since humic and fulvic materials possess weak acidic groups, they can be called humic and fulvic acids. Although the soil-derived nomenclature persists, one should bear in mind that the acid-base solubility distinction between humic and fulvic acids *is* largely arbitrary. It is frequently much more useful to conceptualize humic compounds as consisting of a heterogeneous collection of

**Figure 1.** Fractionation scheme used for isolating soil humic and fulvic acids (redrawn from Reference 3, this chapter). "S" and "P" designate soluble and particulate phases, respectively. "C" refers to positions at which "S" and "P" phases are separated using centrifugation. The dashed line indicates an iterative route for "purifying" the humic acid fraction. XAD-8 and dialysis steps (terminal) can be used for final "purification" of fulvic and humic acids, respectively.

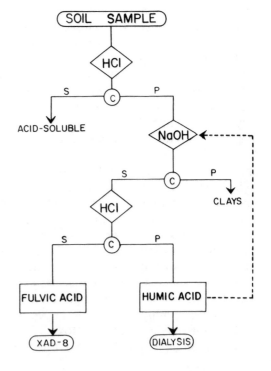

poorly defined organic materials exhibiting a broad molecular weight distribution. Humic acids are predominately of high molecular weight (up to about 300,000), whereas fulvic acids are commonly believed to have molecular weight values of less than about 1,000.[4] Other characteristics of the humic compounds, such as acidity, color, and oxygen content, similarly vary in a consistent fashion along the humic-fulvic molecular weight spectrum (Figure 2).

In aquatic habitats, the humic and fulvic acids can be collectively and most appropriately referred to as dissolved humic materials (DHM). DHM originates predominately from decaying terrestrial and aquatic vegetation. In a given lake, the relative proportions of DHM from terrestrial (allochthonous) and aquatic (autochthonous) sources will depend upon morphological characteristics of the lake and its drainage basin and the types and quantities of vegetation present.[5] In many cases, DHM dominates the dissolved organic pool of lakes and streams simply because more labile organic compounds (amino acids, simple sugars, etc.) are rapidly degraded by the native microbiota; the more recalcitrant DHM remains relatively unaltered. Concentrations of DHM are frequently in the range of 5 to 25 mg/L. In heavily stained systems such as bogs, bog lakes, swamps and "blackwater" streams, much higher concentrations (50 to 70 mg/L) are possible.[6-9]

The molecular weight spectrum of DHM in a given system of necessity results from a balance between inputs and losses of specific molecular weight fractions. Factors regulating the types and quantities of DHM input into

**Figure 2.** Normalized molecular weight spectrum of DHM showing relationship between DHM and soil humic and fulvic acids. The colloidal fraction of DHM (shaded area) is a variable portion of the total (indicated by wide clear arrows). Color, acidity (above), and oxygen content (below) are DHM characteristics that are dependent on molecular weight.

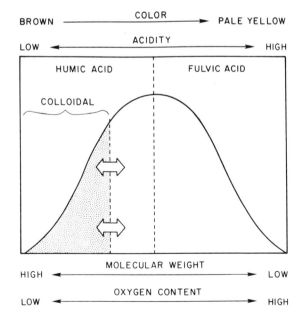

and lost from natural bodies of water are very poorly known, but in all likelihood they include considerations of pH and ionic strength of the water,[10-14] photolysis,[14-18] biotic and abiotic polymerization reactions,[19-21] and selective use of portions of the DHM by microbiota[18,22-25] (Figure 3). Most of the data available for estimating the relative importance of the various processes in controlling the molecular weight distribution of DHM in natural systems have been obtained under laboratory conditions.

A large share of the scientific effort in the realm of humic materials has been devoted to a more complete elucidation of their chemical structure.[9,26-30] The rationale for this approach seems sound: A complete understanding of the chemical character of humus could indeed allow powerful insights into its role and behavior in natural systems. The recent spectacular successes of a similar reductionist approach in the areas of enzymology, biochemistry, and genetic engineering following elucidation of the structure of DNA, however, may have contributed to unrealistic expectations. Although numerous different "type structures" for humic materials have been proposed (Figure 4),[2] it is important to understand that no single structure can be universally valid. DHM is fundamentally detrital, and aspects of its production and alteration within aquatic systems are less tightly constrained by thermodynamic limitations than are the processes and reactions that occur within living cells. The rather dreary outcome of even the most exhaustive structural characterization of DHM to date—the identification of some

**Figure 3.** Regulation of the molecular weight (mol. wt) spectrum of DHM by biotic and abiotic factors. Inputs (high- and low-mol.-wt fractions) are balanced by outputs (sediments, loss as $CO_2$); selective loss of low-mol.-wt DHM (microbial activity, photolysis) or high-mol.-wt DHM (salts, acidic pH, metals, photolysis, freezing) will tend to skew the DHM mol. wt distribution away from normal (dashed lines). The colloidal fraction (shaded area) is particularly vulnerable. Biotic and abiotic polymerization reactions (arrow) can increase high-mol.-wt DHM content at the expense of low-mol.-wt DHM fractions.

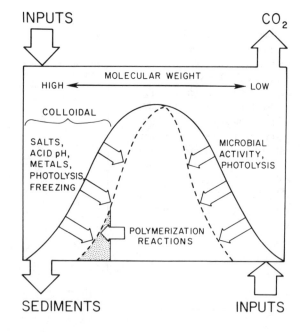

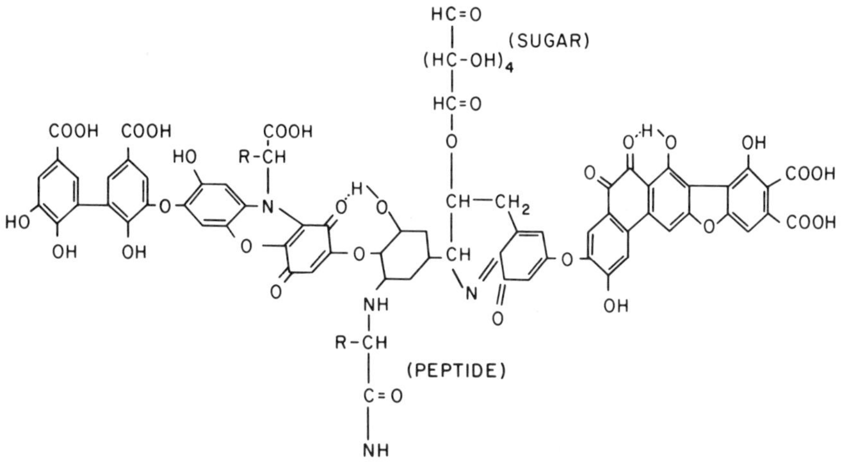

**Figure 4.** "Type structure" for DHM. Note that most functional groups are oxygen-dependent (redrawn from Stevenson[2]).

75 methylated degradation products, which collectively accounted for about 25% of the starting material—does not bode well for this approach.[30]

On the brighter side, however, chemical analyses of humic materials have identified functional groups that probably account for the dominant interactions between DHM and various organic and inorganic materials in aqueous systems.[2,8,9,31] DHM bears both electron-donor ($-$OH, $-$NH$_2$, $-$OCH$_3$, and $-$SH) and -acceptor (carbonyl, carboxyl, and quinone) groups, the activities of which are predictably modified by the proximity of adjacent groups, pH, and the types and concentrations of neutral salts in the medium. The donor-acceptor duality of DHM allows a wide variety of interactions with metals, pesticides, and toxic pollutants. Stevenson[2] points out that adsorption of herbicides to humans can occur via ion exchange, H-bonding, van der Waal forces, and coordination through one or more attached metal ions. The high density of functional groups in humus can further enhance the stability of interactions with pesticides by allowing multiple binding sites (Figure 5).

A unique feature of both humic and fulvic acids is their relatively high content of stable free radicals, particularly of the semiquinone type[2,32–34] (Figure 6). The high stable free radical content allows extensive participation in oxidation-reduction reactions with pesticides and toxic pollutants. Senesi,[35] for example, has shown that single-electron transfer processes take place between ring or chain donor groups of herbicides (particularly s-triazines and substituted ureas) and acceptor quinone units of humic materials. At

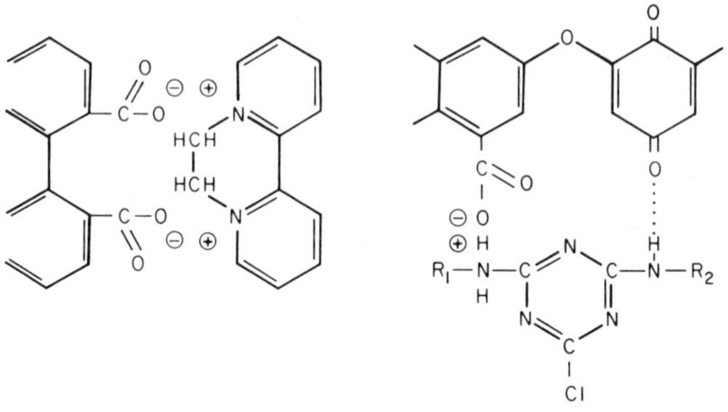

DIQUAT                    s-TRIAZINE

**Figure 5.** Multiplie binding sites on DHM (carboxyl and quinone in this example) efficiently sequester various herbicides, pesticides, and other organic toxicants. Binding of the herbicides diquat (left) and s-triazine (right) are shown. (Redrawn from Reference 2, this chapter.)

alkaline pH values, spin contents for both humic and fulvic acids are maximal due to the stabilization of semiquinone radicals; the compounds tend to be chemically least reactive when neutral salt concentrations are high and at pH values of 5.0 to 6.5.[33]

DHM photochemistry is an area of recent investigation that seems to be especially promising with regard to understanding interactions between DHM and organic toxicants. Baxter and Carey[7] and Zepp et al.,[6] for example, have shown that naturally occurring DHM can photochemically generate singlet oxygen ($^1O_2$) from dissolved ground-state oxygen through coupled reactions:

$$^1DHM \longrightarrow {}^1DHM^* \longrightarrow {}^3DHM^* \qquad (1)$$
$$^3DHM^* + {}^3O_2 \longrightarrow {}^1DHM + {}^1O_2(^1\Delta) \qquad (2)$$

where $^1DHM$ designates the ground state and $^1DHM^*$ and $^3DHM^*$ represent singlet and triplet excited states of DHM, respectively. Singlet oxygen ($^1O_2(^1\Delta)$) is extremely toxic and reactive; it readily deactivates enzymes and oxidizes cell membranes and amino and nucleic acids. There is every reason to suspect that DHM-mediated production of singlet oxygen would similarly cause major chemical alterations in dissolved organic toxicants. Other studies[8,36,37] implicate Fe(II)-Fe(III) transformations as being important components in the consumption of dissolved oxygen; however, the precise relationship(s) between DHM-mediated photochemical reactions and cyclic Fe(II)-Fe(III) transformations remains unknown.

The role of DHM molecular weight in determining the types and rates of reactions that occur between DHM and organic toxicants is still obscure. The proportion of humus in a given system that demonstrates colloidal char-

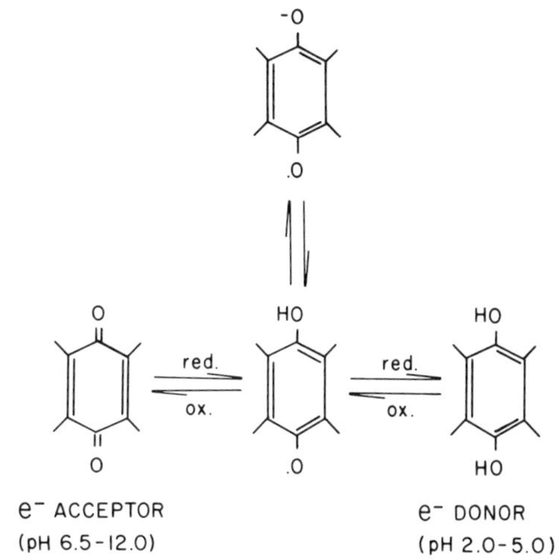

**Figure 6.** Semiquinone units facilitate DHM's ability to act as an electron donor or an electron acceptor. Acceptor and donor roles are favored by high- and low-pH regimes, respectively (redrawn from Reference 33, this chapter).

e⁻ ACCEPTOR
(pH 6.5-12.0)

e⁻ DONOR
(pH 2.0-5.0)

acteristics is quire variable,[38,39] and transitions between colloidal and truly dissolved phases of high-molecular-weight DHM can occur in response to changes in pH, salinity, or concentrations of transition metals.[10,40,41] When colloidal humic materials are abundant, toxicants such as diquat, paraquat, DDT, and 2,4,5-T are rapidly sorbed from solution.[42,43] Humic colloids apparently promote the "solubilization" of relatively insoluble toxicants largely through adsorptive (coulombic) reactions; the increase in proportion of "soluble" toxicant (often on the order of $10^3$- or $10^4$-fold) almost certainly markedly alters their transport and fates. Presumably the adsorbed compounds are transported with the colloids until various precipitation reactions (such as changes in pH or salinity) deposit the colloidal aggregates upon the sediments. Alternatively, increases in ionic strength or decreases in pH may cause the competitive release of the chemically unaltered toxicant into the dissolved phase.[43] In general, I suspect that low-energy DHM-toxicant interactions, such as adsorption and precipitation, predominate when colloidal or high-molecular-weight DHM is most abundant, and that higher-energy DHM-toxicant interactions (such as covalent bonding and photooxidation) become increasingly important when low molecular weight DHM is more abundant (Figure 7).[14] Straightforward experimental designs can be used to test these ideas.

## EXPERIMENTAL APPROACH

The experiments described in this section were designed to evaluate the potential significance of a low-molecular-weight DHM to the toxicity of selected organic toxicants. The experiments were performed under laboratory conditions; changes in toxicity of each organic compound were quan-

**Figure 7.** A conceptual model of the roles of adsorption (above shaded area), microbial degradation (shaded area), and photolysis (below shaded area) in controlling loss of DHM from aquatic ecosystems. Representative types of aquatic systems (dashed ovals) are positioned with respect to salinity ("Y" axis) and pH ("X" axis). The relative importance of each of the three processes involved with DHM loss depends upon ecosystem position (in bogs, for example, microbial degradation is a minor loss). In calcareous systems (top right), precipitation of $CaCO_3$ is a seasonal phenomenon that can selectively remove DHM from surface waters (see Reference 14, this chapter). Salinity variations may shift relative importance of loss processes in estuarine systems (vertical arrows).

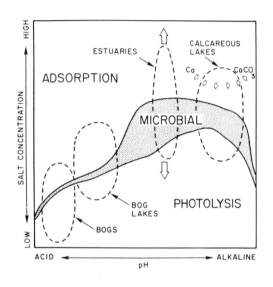

tified using disparities in dose-response curves caused by a 15 mg/L concentration of DHM.

The bioassay used for the tests reported here was the 4-h acute algal assay, which uses as an endpoint the inhibition of photosynthesis.[37] Although somewhat less sensitive than tests using *Daphnia* sp., this assay is advantageous in that replication is excellent, test volumes are small, and the entire test can be completed in about 6 h. The test alga (*Selenastrum capricornutum* Printz) was cultured in EPA medium and was used only during log-phase growth. All assays were performed at 25°C under a light intensity of about 1,200 ft-c (cool white fluorescent lamps). The algae were exposed to the toxicants for 4 h; during the last 2 h, photosynthesis was determined by measuring rate of incorporation of inorganic $^{14}C$. Precise details of the test are given in Reference 37.

The humic material was a commercially available, purified, metal-free fulvic acid isolated from a podzol soil on Prince Edward Island (Contech, E.T.C. Limited, Ottawa). The fulvic acid, which has a reported molecular weight of 643 to 951,[44,45] was used at a concentration of 15 mg/L in all cases. Appropriate quantities of the fulvic acid were dissolved into the required volume of algal culture immediately before the start of an assay. Between experiments, the fulvic acid was stored under desiccant.

Toxicants selected for the experiments included an aniline methylation series (aniline, o-toluidine, 2,3-dimethylaniline, and 2,4,6-trimethylaniline), a phenol methylation series (o-cresol, 2,4-dimethylphenol, and 2,3,6-trimethylphenol), two quinolines (quinoline, 8-methylquinoline), and $p$-benzoquinone. I additionally tested a water-soluble fraction of a coal liquefaction product (an 8:1 water:oil extract), which contained a diverse array of organic compounds. Each toxicant was tested at ten concentrations; three replications were used at each concentration. Within replications, the coefficient of variation was consistently less than 8%. In all experiments, pH values were buffered to 8.5 with Tris-(hydroxymethyl)-aminomethane to a final concentration of 9.9 m$M$.

## RESULTS AND DISCUSSION

The fulvic acid markedly altered the toxicity of most of the compounds tested. In the aniline methylation series, the quantity of toxicant required to reduce algal photosynthesis by 50% declined by factors of 1.1 to 45 when the fulvic acid was present (Figure 8, A through D). Increases in toxicity caused by the fulvic acid were not related simply to the degree of alkalation; o-toluidine (a $C_1$ aniline) became 40 to 45 times more toxic when fulvic acid was present, while 2,4,6-trimethylaniline increased in toxicity only slightly (Figure 8, B and D). Matters were further complicated in the case of o-toluidine because the fulvic material caused a change in slope of the dose-response line, which may be indicative of a change in the mode by which the toxicant interferes with the normal metabolism of the test organism.

Toxicity of the three tested phenols increased by factors of 2.0 to about 5.4 in the presence of fulvic acid (Figure 9, A through C). As with anilines, there was no clear tendency for increases in toxicity to be related to the degree of methylation. In all three phenols, dose-response slopes appeared to be affected by the presence of fulvic material; for o-cresol, interpretation was additionally confounded because even the lowest concentration tested (32 mg/L) reduced photosynthesis by more than 50% (Figure 9, A).

Toxicity of the coal-liquid water-soluble fraction was increased by a factor of 2.2 at the point of 50% inhibition when the fulvic acid was present (Figure 9, D). At dilutions causing less than a 50% reduction in photosynthesis, fulvic acid increased toxicity much more (about 4-fold when photosynthesis was inhibited by 5 to 20%).

The toxicity of 8-methylquinoline was not affected by the fulvic acid, whereas toxicity of quinoline was decreased slightly (Figure 10, A and B). $p$-Benzoquinone became much less toxic to *Selenastrum* when fulvic acid was present (a 6.1-fold decrease; Figure 11). $p$-Benzoquinone is known to interfere with noncyclic electron flow (photosystem II) during photosynthesis[46] and can be reduced to hydroxyquinone easily.[47] A DHM-

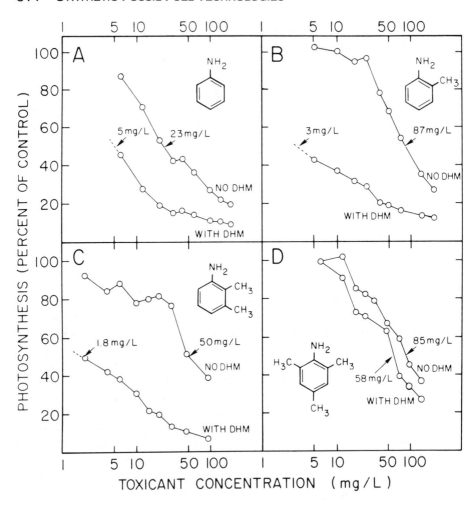

**Figure 8.** Dose response curves for the green alga, *Selenastrum capricornutum,* obtained in the presence an absence of a purified DHM (5 mg/L concentration). Arrows indicate positions at which photosynthesis was reduced by 50%; values adjacent to arrows are toxicant concentrations required to cause 50% inhibition. Toxicants include compounds in an aniline methylation series: aniline, (A); o-toluidine, (B); 2,3-dimethyl aniline, (C); and 2,3,6-trimethyl aniline, (D).

photomediated reduction of ρ-benzoquinone to a less toxic phenol or diphenolic compound appears to be a likely explanation for the observed decrease in toxicity in this instance.

The specific modes of action of the toxicants used in the experiments reported here, with the sole exception of ρ-benzoquinone, are unknown. Consequently, changes in toxicity of the various tested compounds caused

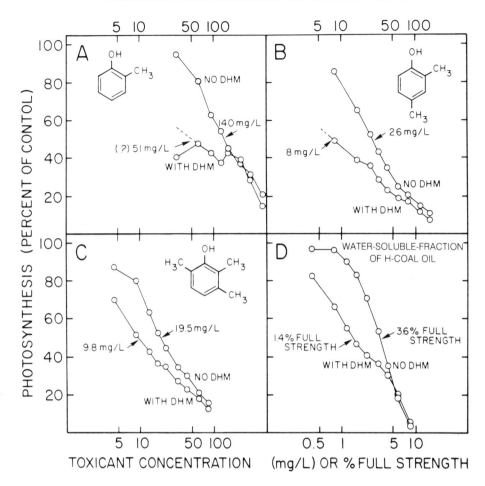

**Figure 9.**  Same as for Figure 8, but for compounds in a homologous phenolic series. Toxicants include: o-cresol, (A); 2,4-dimethyl phenol, (B); 2,3,6-trimethyl phenol, (C); and an 8:1 water-soluble fraction of an H-coal oil, (D).

by the presence of DHM are currently without firm theoretical basis. Several possibilities exist:

1.  DHM facilitates or hinders entry of the compounds into cells of *Selenastrum capricornutum* by interfering with membrane permeability.
2.  DHM mediates one or more (photo)chemical changes in the toxicants, resulting in daughter products that are individually of greater or lesser toxicity to *S. capricornutum*.
3.  DHM preferentially binds to the organic toxicant in question and effectively lowers the quantity of toxicant available for interacting with *Selenastrum*.

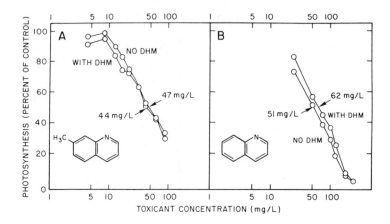

**Figure 10.** Same as for Figure 8, but for 8-methylquinoline (A) and quinoline (B).

**Figure 11.** Same as for Figure 8, but for ρ-benzoquinone.

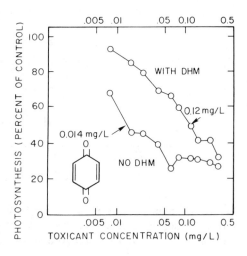

4. DHM adsorbs to the cell surface of *Selenastrum,* and thereby alters toxicant partitioning from the dissolved phase.

The relative importance of these possibilities can be distinguished only by additional, appropriately designed experiments.

In the experiments reported here, changes in toxicity of various compounds caused by the presence of a single concentration of fulvic acid were determined at a fixed pH (8.5). The consequences of changes in pH, light intensity, or concentration of fulvic acid were not addressed. Additionally, these experiments were not designed to examine relationships between changes in toxicity and DHM molecular weight. Each of these interactions, however, can be readily examined using slight modifications of the procedures described in the section of this chapter on experimental approach. If we are to deduce the types of interactions that predominate between organic toxicants and DHM in natural environments, effects of DHM molecular weight, pH, DHM concentration, salt concentration, and the role of photogenerated free radicals must be examined.

## RECENT ADVANCES IN METHODOLOGY

The development of an appreciation of the importance of DHM in natural aquatic systems has understandably been closely tied to improvements in methodology. In my opinion, recent advances in DHM acquisition, high-performance chromatography, fluorescence polarization, and radiolabeling of natural or model DHM will play significant roles in future investigations on DHM-organic toxicant interactions.

The widespread use of highly polymerized soil humic acids (e.g., Aldrich humic acid) as model DHM is to be strongly discouraged, particularly since Thurman and Malcolm[48] have introduced specific, simple procedures for the near-quantitative recovery of gram quantities of DHM. Their procedure, which utilizes a macroporus resin (XAD-8), has numerous advantages, chiefly the relatively mild conditions required for DHM collection; polymerization artifacts are largely avoided. Any investigator who anticipates working with DHM should become familiar with this collection procedure.

Although high-performance liquid chromatography (HPLC) and gas chromatography (GC) may be unable to resolve the specific nature of DHM per se, one can easily envision their use in the elucidation of organic toxicant daughter products, for example, during DHM-mediated photodegradation of a selected toxicant. The types of daughter products formed and the rates of their formation may yield clues as to the types of DHM-organic toxicant interactions involved. HPLC or GC analyses of toxicant degradation products before and after selective methylation of specific DHM functional groups could similarly be very instructive in revealing the functional moieties involved in the photodegradation of toxicants in the presence of DHM.

The fluorescence polarization procedures recently used for examining DHM-organic toxicant interactions by Seitz[49] and Grant and Seitz[50] are quite promising; DHM demonstrates a natural fluorescence, and measurements of fluorescence are much more sensitive (approximately $10^2$ to $10^3$ times) and selective than measurements based on absorbance. Additionally, fluorescence polarization allows detection of DHM-toxicant binding under relatively unadulterated conditions and precludes artifacts that commonly result from imperfect particulate-soluble separations. If the toxicants themselves are fluorescent, fluorescence polarization can similarly be used to study binding of the toxicants to colloidal particles, such as high-molecular-weight DHM or clay.[51] Significant progress in this area seems certain.

Finally, procedures are being developed for radioisotopically labeling natural forms of particulate detritus.[52,53] Very likely, simple modifications of these techniques can be used to append $^3H$ or $^{14}C$ units to high- or low-molecular-weight fractions of DHM collected using the XAD-8 procedure.[48] Since liquid scintillation spectrometry allows extremely sensitive and simultaneous detection of $^3H$ and $^{14}C$, and since a wide variety of labeled organic toxicants are commercially available, toxicant-DHM binding can be followed with liquid scintillation analysis, after any one of several postreaction fractionation methods (dialysis, gel permeation chromatography, selective precipitation of unreacted toxicant, etc.). Alternatively, one might use stepwise methylation of DHM with $^{14}C$ acetic anhydride, with attendant measurements of $^{12}C$:$^{14}C$ in different molecular-weight fractions of the partially methylated DHM. This would allow calculation of the "methylation reactivity" of different DHM molecular weight fractions. Although $^{14}C$-labeled "model" DHM has been used advantageously in some cases (e.g., to examine relationships between DHM molecular weight and its spectral characteristics,[54] one is always left with the quiet certainty that "model" DHM is not the same as DHM in a natural system. The ability to isotopically label natural DHM would help alleviate this encumbrance to a very large degree.

No single technique will yield definitive answers to all aspects of toxicant-DHM interactions in natural systems; the gaps in our knowledge are too great, and the roles of DHM in natural systems are too diverse. However, with judicious application of new methods and thoughtful experimental design, we can begin to understand how organic toxicants, DHM, and aquatic biota interact in natural systems.

## ACKNOWLEDGMENTS

The fulvic acid used in the experiments reported here was generously donated by R.G. Wetzel. I wish to thank collectively members of the Environmental Sciences Division, Oak Ridge National Laboratory, for useful discussions on many aspects of this work. H. de Haan provided a helpful critique of the manuscript in an earlier form.

This work was supported by a postdoctoral fellowship from the Oak Ridge Associated Universities.

## REFERENCES

1. Kononova, M.M. *Soil Organic Matter* 2nd ed. (New York, NY: Pergamon Press, Inc., 1976).
2. Stevenson, F.J., "Role and Function of Humus in Soil with Emphasis on Adsorption of Herbicides and Chelation of Micronutrients," *BioScience* 22:643–650 (1972).
3. Khairy, A.H., and W. Ziechmann. "Die Veranderung von Huminsauren in Alkalischer Losung," *Z. Pflanzen. Bodenkd.* 144(4):407–422 (1981).

4.  Dawson, H.J., B.F. Hrutfiord, R.J. Zasoski, and F.C. Ugolini. "The Molecular Weight and Origin of Yellow Organic Acids," *Soil Science* 132(3):191–199 (1981).

5.  Wetzel, R.G. *Limnology* 2nd ed. (Philadelphia, PA: Saunders College Publishing, 1983), p. 767.

6.  Zepp, R.G., N.L. Wolfe, G.L. Baughman, and R.C. Hollis. "Singlet Oxygen in Natural Waters," *Nature* 267:421–423 (1977).

7.  Baxter, R.M., and J.H. Carey. "Reactions of Singlet Oxygen in Humic Waters," *Freshwater Biol.* 12:285–292 (1982).

8.  Miles, C.J., and P.L. Brezonik. "Oxygen Consumption in Humic-Colored Waters by a Photochemical Ferrous-Ferric Catalytic Cycle," *Environ. Sci. Technol.* 15(9):1089–1095 (1981).

9.  Gjessing, E.T. *Physical and Chemical Characteristics of Aquatic Humus* (Ann Arbor, MI: Ann Arbor Science Publishers, Inc., 1976), p. 120.

10. Ghosh, K., and M. Schnitzer. "Macromolecular Structures of Humic Substances," *Soil Sci.* 129(5):266–276 (1980).

11. Mulholland, P.J. "Formation of Particulate Organic Carbon in Water from a Southeastern Swamp-Stream," *Limnol. Oceanogr.* 26(4):790–795 (1981).

12. Preston, M.R., and J.P. Riley. "The Interactions of Humic Compounds with Electrolytes and Three Clay Minerals under Simulated Estuarine Conditions," *Est. Coastal Shelf Sci.* 14:567–576 (1982).

13. Davis, J.A., and R. Gloor. "Absorption of Dissolved Organics in Lake Water by Aluminum Oxide. Effect of Molecular Weight," *Environ. Sci. Technol.* 15(10):1223–1229 (1981).

14. Stewart, A.J., and R.G. Wetzel. "Dissolved Humic Materials: Photodegradation, Sediment Effects, and Reactivity with Phosphate and Calcium Carbonate Precipitation," *Arch. Hydrobiol.* 92(3):265–286 (1981).

15. Stearns, R.H. "Decolorization of Water by Storage," *J. N. Engl. Water Works Assoc.* 5:115–123 (1916).

16. Kramer, C.J.M. "Degradation by Sunlight of Dissolved Fluorescing Substances in the Upper Layers of the Eastern Atlantic Ocean," *Neth. J. Sea Res.* 13:325–329 (1979).

17. Gjessing, E.T. "Reduction of Aquatic Humus in Streams," *Vatten* 1:14–23 (1970).

18. Strome, D.J., and M.C. Miller. "Photolytic Changes in Dissolved Humic Substances," *Verh. Internat. Verein. Limnol.* 20:1248–1254 (1978).

19. Wang, T.S.C., and S.W. Li. "Clay Minerals as Heterogeneous Catalysts in Preparation of Model Humic Substances," *Z. Pflanzen. Bodenkd.* 140:669–676 (1977).

20. Wang, T.S.C., M.-M. Kao, and P.M. Huang. "The Effect of pH on the Catalytic Synthesis of Humic Substances by Illite," *Soil Sci.* 129:333–338 (1980).

21. Larson, R.A., and J.M. Hufnal, Jr. "Oxidative Polymerization of Dissolved Phenols by Soluble and Insoluble Inorganic Species," *Limnol. Oceanogr.* 25(3):505–512 (1980).

22. Steinberg, C., and A. Herrmann. "Utilization of Dissolved Metal Organic Compounds by Freshwater Microorganisms," *Verh. Internat. Verein. Limnol.* 21:231–235 (1981).

23. Sederholm, H., A. Mauranen, and L. Montonen. "Some Observations on the Microbial Degradation of Humous Substances in Water," *Verh. Internat. Verein. Limnol.* 18:1301–1305 (1973).

24. Dahm, C.N. "Pathways and Mechanisms for Removal of Dissolved Organic Carbon from Leaf Leachate in Streams," *Can. J. Fish. Aquat. Sci.* 38:68–76 (1981).

25. DeHaan, H. "Effect of a Fulvic Acid Fraction on the Growth of a *Pseudomonas* from Tjeukemeer (The Netherlands)," *Freshwater Biol.* 4:301–309 (1974).

26. Povoledo, D., and H.L. Golterman, Eds. *Humic Substances; Their Structure and Function in the Biosphere,* Proceedings of the International Meeting on Humic Substances, Nieuwersluis, Pudoc, Wageningen, 1972.

27. Stabel, H.H., and C. Steinberg. "Cleavage of Macromolecular Allochthonous Soluble Organic Matter," *Naturwissenschafften* 63(11):533 (1976).

28. Steinberg, C. "Vergleich der Gelosten Organischen Stoffe Verschiedener Holsteinischer Seen," *Arch. Hydrobiol.* 80(3):297–307 (1977).

29. Hama, T., and N. Handa. "Molecular Weight Distribution and Characterization of Dissolved Organic Matter from Lake Waters," *Arch. Hydrobiol.* 90(1):106–120 (1980).

30. Liao, W., R.F. Christman, J.P. Johnson, D.S. Millington, and J.R. Hass. "Structural Characterization of Aquatic Humic Material," *Environ. Sci. Technol.* 16(7):403–410 (1982).

31. Schnitzer, M. "Humic Substances: Chemistry and Reactions," in *Soil Organic Matter,* M. Schnitzer and S.U. Khan, Eds. (Amsterdam: Elsevier, 1978).

32. Zimmerman, A.P. "Electron Intensity, the Role of Humic Acids in Extracellular Electron Transport and Chemical Determination of pE in Natural Waters," *Hydrobiologia* 78:259–265 (1981).

33. Ghosh, K., and M. Schnitzer. "Effects of pH and Neutral Electrolyte Concentration on Free Radicals in Humic Substances," *Soil Sci. Soc. Am. J.* 44(5):975–978 (1980).

34. Senesi, N., Y. Chen, and M. Schnitzer. "The Role of Free Radicals in the Oxidation and Reduction of Fulvic Acid," *Soil Biol. Biochem.* 9:397–403 (1977).

35. Senesi, N. "Free Radicals in Electron Donor-Acceptor Reactions Between a Soil Humic Acid and Photosynthesis Inhibitor Herbicides," *Z. Pflanzen. Bodenkd.* 144(6):580–586 (1981).

36. Francko, D.A., and R.T. Heath. "UV-Sensitive Complex Phosphorus: Association with Dissolved Humic Material and Iron in a Bog Lake," *Limnol. Oceanogr.* 27(3):564–569 (1982).

37. Giddings, J.M., A.J. Stewart, R.V. O'Neill, and R.H. Gardner. "An Efficient Algal Bioassay Based on Short-Term Photosynthetic Response," In: *Sixth ASTM Symposium on Aquatic Toxicology,* pp. 445–459 (1983).

38. Lock, M.A., P.M. Wallis, and H.B.N. Hynes. "Colloidal Organic Carbon in Running Waters," *Oikos* 29:1–4 (1977).

39. Pennanen, V. "Seasonal and Spatial Distribution of Humus Fractions in a Chain of Polyhumic Lakes in Southern Finland," *Hydrobiologia* 86:73–80 (1982).

40. Koenings, J.P. "In Situ Experiments on the Dissolved and Colloidal State of Iron in a Acid Bog Lake," *Limnol. Oceanogr.* 21(5):674–683 (1976).

41. Koenings, J.P., and F.F. Hooper. "The Influence of Colloidal Organic Matter on Iron and Iron-Phosphorus Cycling in an Acid Bog Lake," *Limnol. Oceanogr.* 21(5):684–696 (1976).

42. Poirrier, M.A., B.R. Bordelon, and J.L. Laseter. "Adsorption and Concen-

tration of Dissolved Carbon-14 DDT by Coloring Colloids in Surface Waters," *Environ. Sci. Technol.* 6(12):1033–1035 (1972).

43. Narine, D.R., and R.D. Guy. "Binding of Diquat and Paraquat to Humic Acid in Aquatic Environments," *Soil Sci.* 133(6):356–363 (1982).

44. Weber, J.H., and S.A. Wilson. In Research Report No. 14 (Durham: Water Resource Research Centre, University of New Hampshire, 1977).

45. Gamble, D.S., and M. Schnitzer. In *Trace Metals and Metal Organic Interactions in Natural Waters,* P.C. Singer, Ed. (Ann Arbor, MI: Ann Arbor Science Publishers, 1973), pp. 265–302.

46. Levine, R.P. In *Algal Physiology and Biochemistry,* W.D.P. Stewart, Ed. (Berkeley, CA: University of Berkeley Press, 1974), p. 428.

47. Morrison, R.T., and R.N. Boyd. *Organic Chemistry,* 3rd ed. (Boston, MA: Allyn and Bacon, Inc., 1973), p. 878.

48. Thurman, E.M., and R.L. Malcolm. "Preparative Isolation of Aquatic Humic Substances," *Environ. Sci. Technol.* 14(4):463–466 (1981).

49. Seitz, W.R. "Fluorescence Methods for Studying Speciation of Pollutants in Water," *Trends Anal. Chem.* 1:79–83 (1981).

50. Grant, C.L., and W.R. Seitz. "The Potential of Fluorescence Polarization for Measuring Sorption Isotherms of Organics," *Soil Sci.* 133(5):289–294 (1982).

51. von Wandruszka, R.M.A., and S. Brantley. "A Fluorescence Polarization Study of Polyaromatic Hydrocarbons Absorbed on Colloidal Kaolin," *Anal. Lett.* 12(A10):1111–1122 (1979).

52. Banks, C.W., and L. Wolfinbarger, Jr. "A Rapid and Convenient Method for Radiolabelling Detritus with $^{14}C$ Acetic Anhydride," *J. Exp. Mar. Biol. Ecol.* 53:115–123 (1981).

53. Lopez, G.R., and M.A. Crenshaw. "Radiolabelling of Sedimentary Organic Matter with $^{14}C$-Formaldehyde: Preliminary Evaluation of a New Technique for Use in Deposit-Feeding Studies," *Marine Ecol.* 8:283–289 (1982).

54. Stewart, A.J., and R.G. Wetzel. "Asymmetrical Relationships Between Absorbance, Fluorescence, and Dissolved Organic Carbon," *Limnol. Oceanogr.* 26(3):590–597 (1981).

# CHAPTER 25

## Forecasting Fate and Effects of Aromatic Hydrocarbons in Aquatic Systems

### S.M. Bartell

*Oak Ridge National Laboratory*
*Oak Ridge, TN 37831*

Statistical regressions were used to estimate parameters in transport and effects models from basic molecular characteristics of organic hydrocarbons. Uncertainties associated with parameter estimates were carried through forecasts of fate of naphthalene, anthracene, and benzo(*a*)pyrene by means of repeated simulation with parameter sets selected randomly from distributions defined by the regression statistics. Effects of phenol on algal production were similarly forecast.

The combined use of structure-activity regressions, transport or effects models, and Monte Carlo simulation might provide a partial solution to the problem of screening a large number of potential toxic chemicals.

### INTRODUCTION

Society's increasing reliance on chemicals such as pesticides, nutrient additives, preservatives, industrial catalysts, detergents, fertilizers, complex organic compounds, and petroleum-based synthetic materials has increased man's arsenal of commonly used chemicals to approximately 63,000.[1] Cairns[2] points out that the computer registry of the American Chemical Society contains more than 4 million entries and is growing. As the number of chemicals in use increases, so does their potential for harm to man and his ecological life-support systems.

Ecological risk is the probability of occurrence of an adverse effect on the environment in relation to society's activities. Evaluation of risk posed by individual chemicals requires estimates of exposure of natural systems to the chemical. Exposure and, subsequently, dose depend on reliable forecasts of transport and accumulation of the chemical in the target environment. Estimates of accumulation by the biota must then be translated into projections of mortality rates or other physiological end points with the use of toxicological information.

The large number of potential toxicants precludes chemical-by-chemical determinations of risk. Although screening protocols have been suggested,[2,3] the associated cost and small numbers of adequate test facilities and trained personnel combine to defeat experimentally based screening protocols for all but a small number of high-priority pollutants. The magnitude of the problem is forcing a reliance on the development of models that forecast probable fate and effects of chemicals in terrestrial and aquatic ecosystems. Even here, the large number of potential toxicants and the data necessary to estimate parameters needed by models for each new chemical still overwhelm our ability to collect and interpret relevant information.

This chapter will explore a possible solution to the problem concerning the large inventory of chemicals that require evaluation. This solution rests on the premise that much of the necessary information for forecasting fate and effects already exists as familiar pharmacological relationships between molecular structure and chemical behavior of compounds. Recent research[3-6] indicates that toxicological behavior can be inferred from detailed structural analysis of chemicals for a homologous series of aromatic hydrocarbons. Yuan and Jurs[4] established relationships between 28 molecular descriptors and carcinogenic assay results and correctly classified 191 of 200 polycyclic aromatic hydrocarbons (PAHs) as carcinogens or noncarcinogens. Descriptors used by Yuan and Jurs[4] are conveniently divided into three categories: topological, geometric, and environmental. Examples of topological descriptors include sigma electron distribution, presence and distribution of particular molecular substructures, and molecular connectivity. Geometrical descriptors include principal radii, volume, and other characteristics that describe the three-dimensional shape of the molecules. The third class comprises whole-molecule functional descriptors, of which partition coefficients are an example.

Figure 1 outlines the scheme used here to forecast fate and effects of toxicants. Parameters required by separate transport and effects models are estimated from structure-activity relationships derived from published data and results of experiments with individual compounds representative of homologous series. As depicted by the confidence intervals (Figure 1), there are uncertainties associated with model parameters estimated from structure-activity relationships. These uncertainties are carried through the analyses by repeated simulation with values selected at random from distributions defined by statistics of the regression models. As a result, forecasts of transport, accumulation, and toxic effects can be stated in probabilistic terms amenable to interpretation as estimates of risk, constrained by the assumptions implicit in the models. Results of using this approach to forecast fate of naphthalene, anthracene, and benzo(*a*)pyrene (BaP) are presented. Fore-

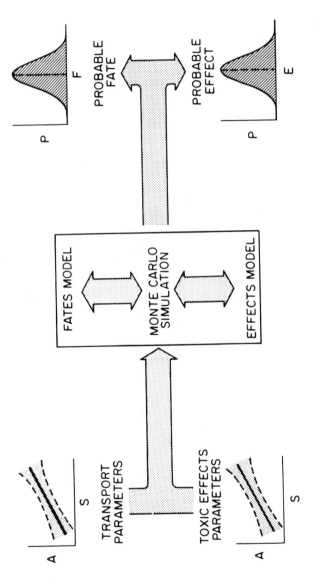

**Figure 1.**   Monte Carlo simulation with fate or effects models can translate structure (S)-activity (A) relationships to probable (P) fate (F) or probable (P) effects (E) of toxicants.

casts of effects of phenol on simulated algal production in culture are also reported.

## MODEL DESCRIPTION

The transport model used in this study is a modification of the Fates Of Aromatics Model (FOAM).[7] FOAM was developed specifically to simulate the transport and accumulation of single PAHs in aquatic ecosystems. The model was originally designed to evaluate the hypothesis that the fate of PAHs could be forecast from basic chemical descriptors of PAHs. Briefly, FOAM tracks the dissolution of PAH from a surface oil slick and simulates the time-varying concentrations of the compound in water, sediments, suspended particulates, and an aquatic food web. The food web includes phytoplankton, periphyton, rooted macrophytes, zooplankton, bacteria, benthic insects, benthic invertebrates, a carnivorous fish, and a benthic detritus-feeding fish. Transport processes include dissolution and evaporation of PAHs from the surface slick, losses to photolytic degradation, sorption, volatilization, and food-web accumulation. Food-web components accumulate PAHs directly from the water and by eating other organisms already contaminated with PAHs. Temporal changes in biomass described by energetics-based growth equations permit examination of accumulation of PAHs introduced to the system at different times of the year and permit simulation of changes in accumulation that result from dilution or concentration of inputs by changing biomass. Surface-light intensities, wind velocities, current velocities, and water temperatures are external forcing functions.

## STRUCTURE-ACTIVITY RELATIONSHIPS FOR PAHs

Table I lists the processes in FOAM that employ structure-activity relations for purposes of parameter estimation. Individual PAHs are defined in FOAM

**Table I.** List of Model Processes that Rely on Structure-Activity Relationships to Estimate Model Parameters

| Process | Parameter | Molecular Descriptors |
|---|---|---|
| Dissolution | S | Melting point, molecular weight |
| Photolysis | $\phi$ | Molecular weight |
| Sorption | $G_{max}$ | Octanol:water partition coefficient |
| Desorption | DSP | Molecular weight |
| Volatilization | H | Molecular weight |
| Bioaccumulation | Q | Molecular weight, octanol:water partition coefficient |
| Depuration | D | Octanol:water partition coefficient |

by their molecular weights (mol. wt), melting points (mp), octanol:water partition coefficients ($K_{o:w}$), and light absorption spectra. Molecular surface area, estimated from the number of aromatic rings, can be used to interpolate a light-absorption spectrum if one is unavailable. Regression models, some described below, were used to estimate model parameters from the above molecular descriptors.

## Physical-Chemical Parameters

### Photolysis

Yield coefficients, $\phi$, for photolytic degradation of PAHs were estimated from molecular weight from data presented in Zepp and Schlotzhauer[8] (Figure 2). The uncertainty associated with estimates of log $\phi$ takes the form of large confidence intervals about the estimates. Log $\phi$ varies as much as 24% for naphthalene, 31% for anthracene, and 34% for BaP.

**Figure 2.** Structure-activity relationship between photolytic yield coefficient and molecular weight for PAHs (see Reference 8, this chapter).

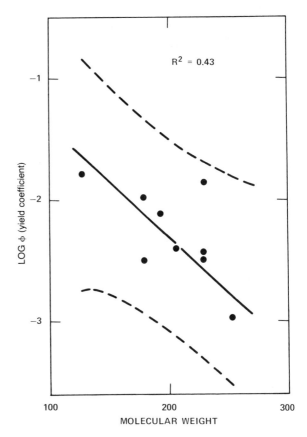

### Solubility

Published estimates[9] of the water solubility of individual PAHs were regressed against melting point and molecular weight:

$$\log(S) = -0.21 - 0.0093(mp) - 0.023(mol. wt) \tag{1}$$

FOAM uses solubilities estimated from this regression to prevent dissolved concentrations from exceeding solubility limits. PAH concentrations in excess of S are shunted to the sediments.

### Sorption

To model PAH sorption to suspended particulate matter and sediments as a dynamic process, partition coefficients estimated from octanol:water partitioning and the organic matter content of the sorbent[10] were divided by the measured time required to reach equilibrium. Calculation of sorption rate constants by this method assumes linear uptake until steady state is achieved.

### Desorption

With data presented in Karickhoff et al.,[10] rates of PAH desorption from suspended and settled sediments were related to molecular weight:

$$DSP = 49.2 \exp[-0.05(mol. wt)] \tag{2}$$

### Volatilization

The Henry's Law constant and gas- and liquid-exchange coefficients can be estimated for PAHs as a function of current velocity, wind velocity, and molecular weight. Southworth[11] derived the specific regression equations used in FOAM to estimate volatilization parameters for PAHs.

## Biological Transport Parameters

Instead of estimating steady-state PAH concentrations from partition coefficients, FOAM uses kinetic parameters to characterize uptake and depuration by food-web components. Published data and results of laboratory experiments with radiolabeled PAHs were used to relate uptake and depuration kinetics to PAH descriptors.

For example, data that quantify accumulation of several PAH by *Daphnia pulex*[12] can be related to molecular weight if the initial dissolved PAH concentrations in the uptake experiments are standardized to their maximum water solubility (Figure 3). As described by this figure, higher-weight, more-hydrophobic PAHs are taken up at a faster rate than the more

**Figure 3.** Structure-activity relationship between rate of PAH accumulation by *Daphnia magna* and molecular weight of PAHs.

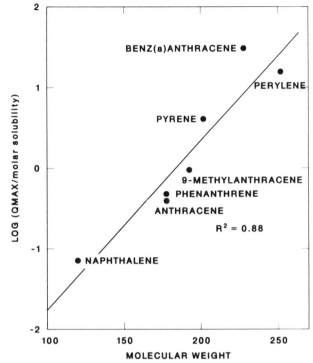

soluble, lower-weight compounds. From these data, the uptake rate of any PAH can be estimated from molecular weight:

$$\log(Q) = 0.021(\text{mol. wt}) - 3.87 \tag{3}$$

where Q has units of grams of PAH per gram of zooplankton per hour, relative to maximum water solubility of the compound. With similar regression models, uptake parameters for phytoplankton, periphyton, rooted aquatic plants, benthic insects, and fish are estimated for individual PAHs from octanol:water partition coefficients and molecular weight.

## FATE OF NAPHTHALENE, ANTHRACENE, AND BaP IN PONDS

FOAM previously forecast concentrations of dissolved anthracene and anthracene concentrations in papershell clams *(Anodonta imbecilis)* with reasonable accuracy.[7] Sediment concentrations of anthracene were consistently lower than measured concentrations, although the observed downstream gradient was predicted by the model. The present simulations were performed to examine FOAM's forecasts for PAHs whose descriptors lie at extremes of the regressions used to estimate transport parameters (Table I). Molecular descriptors for anthracene lie near the mean values for the independent variables in the structure-activity regressions. Uncertainty in the form of regression error is minimal in this region. Naphthalene and BaP represent extremes in molecular weight, solubility, and octanol:water partitioning.

Physical, chemical, and biological parameters for transport and accumulation of naphthalene, anthracene, and BaP were estimated from structure-activity relationships (Table II). Ninety-five percent confidence intervals about the structure-activity regressions were used to calculate coefficients of variation (CV) for model parameters assumed to be normally distributed (Table II). Where confidence intervals were not available, $R^2$ values were used to estimate 95% confidence intervals.[13] To be conservative, these estimated confidence intervals were used to define end points of triangular distributions. Two hundred simulations were performed for each of the three PAHs, with separate parameter sets drawn at random from distributions defined by the data in Table II. To facilitate comparison of the fate of these three PAHs, the same initial concentration (5.4 µmol/L) of each in the surface slick was used. This value was 90% of the maximum water solubility of the least soluble compound, BaP.

## MODELING THE EFFECTS OF PHENOL

The energetics-based growth equations used to simulate changes in biomass in relation to changes in light, temperature, and trophic interactions[7] can be modified to include the effects of dissolved toxicants on growth.[14] For example, the effects of phenol on the photosynthetic rate of the green algae, *Selenastrum capricornutum,* were related to the octanol:water partition coefficient and the concentration of phenol (P)[15]:

$$E = 120.1 - 18.9(K_{o:w}) - 82.2(P) \tag{4}$$

where E is a fractional multiplier of the photosynthesis rate. At no effect, E equals 1.0. Values less than 1.0 reduce the photosynthetic rate used in the growth equation for phytoplankton in FOAM. Other physiological processes that influence growth can be similarly modified in relation to toxicant concentration.[14] Regression statistics for Equation 4 were used to assign a CV to the E value. In this approach, both the magnitude of E and the uncertainty associated with its estimate can contribute to an overall estimate of risk.[14]

A separate algal growth model was isolated from FOAM and used to simulate algal growth under the culture conditions used in bioassays. To include natural variability in the basic growth parameters, CVs of 10% were

**Table II.** Parameter Values, Uncertainties, and Distributions for Monte Carlo Simulations of PAH Fate

| Process | Parameter | Units | Naphthalene | CV[a] | Anthracene | CV | Benzo(a)pyrene | CV | Distribution |
|---|---|---|---|---|---|---|---|---|---|
| Dissolution | S | $\mu$mol/L | −0.409 | 0 | 5.01E-7 | 0 | −2.45E-7 | 0 | Normal |
| Photolysis | $\phi$ | Unitless | 0.022 | 24 | 0.0076 | 31 | 0.0016 | 34 | Triangular[b] |
| Sorption | $G_{max}$ | $g^{-1}g^{-1}d$ | 0.730E-3 | 15 | 0.016 | 10 | 0.771 | 15 | Normal |
| Desorption | DSP | L/d | 0.082 | 100 | 0.67E-2 | 100 | 0.17E-3 | 100 | Normal |
| Volatilization | H | Unitless | −0.020 | 9.6 | −0.002 | 10.3 | −9.35E-5 | 10 | Triangular |
| Bioaccumulation[c] | $Q_z$ | $g^{-1}g^{-1}d$ | 0.457E-6 | 216 | 0.520E-5 | 174 | 0.189E-3 | 102 | Triangular |
| Depuration[c] | $D_z$ | L/d | 0.35 | 100 | 0.35 | 100 | 0.35 | 100 | Normal |

[a] Coefficient of variation (mean/standard deviation × 100).
[b] CVs used to calculate end points of the triangular distribution.
[c] Values for zooplankton only.

arbitrarily assigned. Two-hundred simulations of the basic growth model were performed with independent parameter sets to simulate "control" conditions. Two-hundred simulations were repeated to include the effects of a saturation concentration of phenol in the growth medium. Final biomass after 20 d of simulated algal growth was recorded for each model run.

## RESULTS

### Fates of PAHs

The model forecasts the time-varying PAH concentration for each of 16 possible system components. Output reported here was selected to indicate the nature of results produced by the approach illustrated in Figure 1 and to compare forecasts of the fate of three different PAHs. Concentration of dissolved compounds decreased exponentially to near steady state by day 20 of the 60-d simulations. Steady-state concentrations of naphthalene, anthracene, and BaP were $2.2 \times 10^{-6}$, $1.8 \times 10^{-6}$, and $0.2 \times 10^{-6}$ $\mu mol/L$, respectively.

Figure 4 summarizes the results of 200 simulations of the concentration of dissolved naphthalene on day 10 of the simulations. While the concentrations are low because of the low initial naphthalene content of the surface slick, the central tendency of the distribution suggests minimal model bias, given the values, uncertainties, and distributions of model parameters. Random selection of model parameters does not lead consistently to high or low values of dissolved naphthalene. One utility of expressing model output in this form is that values of toxic concentrations can be superimposed on the distribution to indicate the frequency of model runs that exceeds acceptable dose levels. This frequency can serve as an initial estimation of risk. For

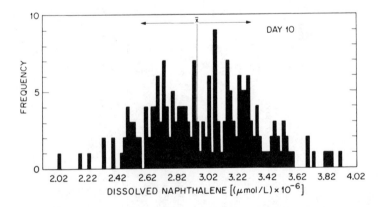

**Figure 4.** Frequency histogram for forecast of dissolved naphthalene concentration on day 10 of simulations (N = 200). Mean and 1 SD indicated.

the FOAM simulations it is possible to construct individual distributions for all system components for each day of the 60-d simulations.

Variation in the concentrations of the PAHs in sediments over time is shown in Figure 5. The rank order of PAHs in sediments agrees with the

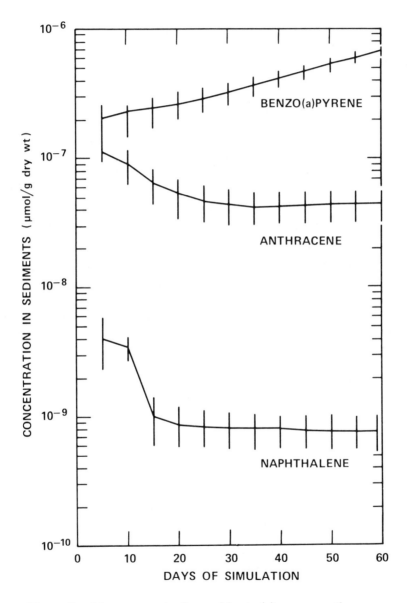

**Figure 5.**   Mean concentrations of benzo(*a*)pyrene, anthracene, and naphthalene in sediments for 200 simulations with FOAM. Vertical lines are 1 SE.

calculations of Herbes et al.[16]: BaP > anthracene > naphthalene. Similarly, Lee et al.[17] recovered 39% of the initial dissolved concentration of BaP in sediments of a large pelagic enclosure, while only 11% of the naphthalene was found in sediments. The different pattern of PAH sedimentation results from differences in parameters that determine sorption and desorption rates. Higher rates of sorption combined with lower desorption rates and low water solubility to generate a time-dependent increase in BaP in sediments. Initial peaks in sediment uptake of anthracene and naphthalene are followed by subsequent decreases as a result of higher desorption rates. Lee et al.[17] observed a similar pattern for naphthalene in microcosm sediments. Sediment concentrations approach steady state after day 20, similar to the steady-state behavior of the dissolved concentrations.

Variance about the mean values of sedimented PAH is similar for all three compounds and results from the similar coefficients of variation assigned to the sorption, desorption, and metabolism parameters for all three PAHs. Desorption parameters for all three PAHs were conservatively assigned CVs of 100% due to absence of data. This variation is approximately 10-fold greater than estimates of uncertainty assigned to sorption rates and explains the high and nearly constant variation about the mean values in Figure 5.

A pattern similar to that of sediments was forecast for PAH accumulation by zooplankton (Figure 6). The depuration rate constant was identical for all three compounds; therefore, the difference in accumulation results from the values in the uptake parameters estimated from Equation 3 (Table II). The rank order of accumulation is consistent with expectations based on measurements of Southworth et al.[12] In contrast to sediment concentrations, the magnitudes of uncertainty about the zooplankton PAH forecasts differ. The relationship between molecular weight and the magnitude of the confidence intervals for estimates of Q (Equation 3), amplified by the log scale, produced very different distributions from which Q values were selected (Table II).

To evaluate the realism of the predicted accumulation, zooplankton bioconcentration factors (BCF) were calculated for BaP. BCF values were calculated for days 2 to 4 to compare with the 24-h BCF values reported for BaP accumulation by *Daphnia magna*.[18] Values calculated from means of the 200 simulations ranged between 670 on day 2 to 2800 on day 4. Leversee et al.[18] measured a zooplankton BCF for BaP of 2800 with a standard error of 580. Comparison with the model BCFs must be interpreted cautiously, even though the simulated value agrees with measured values. First, the measured values are extremely imprecise. Second, the equilibrium concentrations implicit in BCF calculations do not occur in the simulations (Figure 6), and BCF values simulated beyond day 10 are orders of magnitude greater than the Leversee et al.[18] measurements. The simulation results suggest that under conditions of PAH dissolution from a surface oil slick,

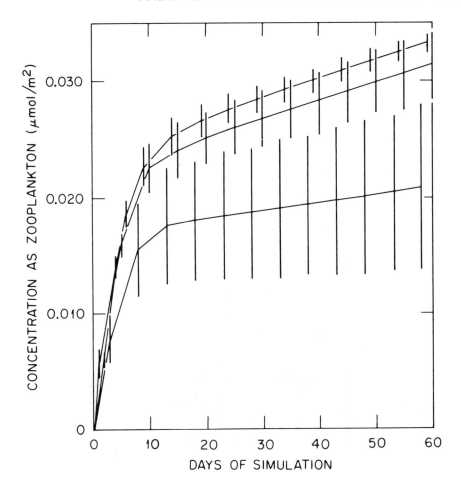

**Figure 6.**   Mean concentration of benzo(*a*)pyrene (upper curve), anthracene (middle curve), and naphthalene (bottom curve) as zooplankton versus time from FOAM simulations (N = 200). Vertical lines represent +1 SD.

necessary equilibrium concentrations of BaP in water and zooplankton are unlikely for the first 60 d.

### Effects of Phenol

Figure 7 compares frequency distributions of algal biomass for 20 d of simulated growth in culture. Growth under the simulated exposure to phenol produced a biomass distribution more positively skewed than that which resulted from simulation of normal culture conditions. Mean biomass of

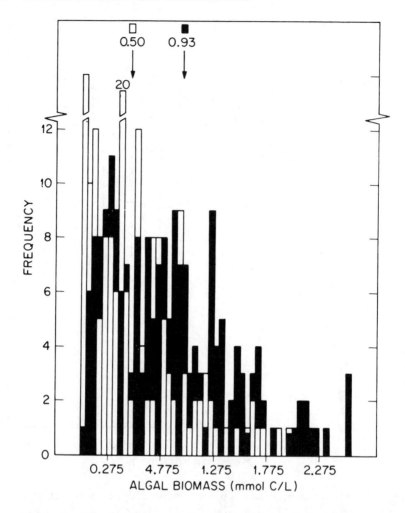

**Figure 7.** Combined frequency distributions for algal biomass simulated in the presence (open bars) and absence (filled bars) of phenol.

algae exposed to phenol was nearly 50% less than that of the control cultures. Maximum biomass values in the presence of phenol were less than maximum values of the control cultures. The frequency of phenol simulations that produced biomass values less than 50% of the mean control cultures was 0.42. This frequency can be interpreted as an initial estimate of risk of decreased algal production under exposure to phenol. The results demonstrate that algal toxicological data can be extrapolated to forecasts of chronic effects on growth.

## DISCUSSION

Available data that quantify rates of transport along environmental pathways can be translated into estimates of FOAM parameters with the use of the regression models. FOAM represents a set of connected hypotheses that extrapolates information summarized by the structure-activity regressions to forecasts of PAH accumulation in system components of interest. As additional data become available, they can be incorporated into the regressions and evaluated in the context of FOAM. CVs assigned to parameters in FOAM and the algal growth model are calculated from residual variance about the structure-activity regressions.[19] Thus, additional data have a direct, measurable effect on these CVs. The CV is partially a function of the square root of the sample size. Therefore, acquisition of sufficient data that meaningfully reduce CVs can be costly. Detailed examination of error propagation by FOAM and the algal growth model will identify structure-activity relationships that should be the focus of additional data gathering. As uncertainties are reduced by the addition of new data, forecasts of transport and effects can be updated to refine estimates of risk.

Through the use of a small number of molecular descriptors and FOAM, forecasts of transport and accumulation consistent with available data were possible for three very different PAHs. Of the 28 descriptors used by Yuan and Jurs,[4] geometrical descriptors were among the most useful for correctly classifying carcinogens. Similarly, Cohen et al.[20] used calculations of molecular geometry to relate relative asymmetry to the toxicity of organic chemicals. According to results of simulations with FOAM, molecular weight, melting point, number of rings, and molecular surface area are useful for forecasting PAH transport and accumulation, which involve very different processes and mechanisms. The three-dimensional configuration of the molecule appears to contain important information concerning chemical behavior in processes that span orders of magnitude in temporal and spatial scale.

The approach outlined in Figure 1 appears useful for extrapolating available information to estimates of the fate and effects of chemicals in aquatic systems. Further derivation of structure-activity relationships for other homologous series of compounds should help reduce the dimensionality of the problem addressed by Maugh.[1]

The probabilistic estimates of dissolved naphthalene concentration (Figure 4) and algal biomass reduction (Figure 7) certainly depend on the simplifications and assumptions embodied by FOAM and the algal growth model. The purpose here is to emphasize the coupling of the structure-activity relationships with the models and the direct inclusion of parameter uncertainty in model forecasts. Models appropriate for other chemicals and ecosystems could be substituted. At the very least, further evaluation of the utility of this approach to fate and effects forecasting will force an inventory, collation, and evaluation of existing data in risk analysis. Identification of classes of chemicals that are amenable to structure-activity-based forecasts, as well as classes that are not, should result in economized future data collection and reduced costs associated with experimental screening of society's chemical arsenal.

## ACKNOWLEDGMENTS

Research supported in part by the Office of Health and Environmental Research, U.S. Department of Energy, under contract W-7405-eng-26 with Union Carbide Corporation, and in part by the U.S. Environmental Protection Agency under Interagency Agreement 40-740-78.

I especially thank R.H. Gardner for derivation of methods for estimation of coefficients of variation from $R^2$ values. Comments from R.H. Gardner and J.F. McCarthy helped improve the manuscript, and I graciously recognize their contribution. I also acknowledge C.W. Gehrs and F.J. Wobber for continued support and encouragement in the development of FOAM.

## REFERENCES

1. Maugh, T.H., II. "Chemicals: How Many Are There?" *Science* 199:162 (1978).
2. Cairns, J., Jr. "Estimating Hazard," *BioScience* 30:101–107 (1980).
3. Duthie, J.R. "The Importance of Sequential Assessment in Test Programs for Estimating Hazard to Aquatic Life," in *Aquatic Toxicology and Hazard Evaluation,* F.L. Mayer and J.L. Hammelink, Eds. ASTM STP 634 (Philadelphia, PA: American Society for Testing and Materials, 1977), pp. 17–35.
4. Yuan, M., and P.C. Jurs. "Computer-Assisted Structure-Activity Studies of Chemical Carcinogens: A Polycyclic Aromatic Hydrocarbon Data Set," *Toxicol. and Appl. Pharmacol.* 52:294–312 (1980).
5. Brugger, W.E., A.J. Stuper, and P.C. Jurs. "Generation of Descriptors from Molecular Structures," *J. Chem. Inf. Comput. Sci.* 16:105–110 (1976).
6. Stuper, A.J., and P.C. Jurs. "ADAPT: A Computer System for Automated Data Analysis Using Pattern Recognition Techniques," *J. Chem. Inf. Comput. Sci.* 16:99–105 (1976).
7. Bartell, S.M., P.F. Landrum, J.P. Giesy, and G.J. Leversee. "Simulated Transport of Polycyclic Aromatic Hydrocarbons in Artificial Streams," in *Energy and Ecological Modelling,* W.J. Mitch, R.W. Bosserman, and J.M. Klopatek, Eds. (New York: Elsevier, 1981), pp. 133–143.
8. Zepp, R.G., and P.F. Schlotzhauer. "Photoreactivity of Selected Aromatic Hydrocarbons in Water," in *Polynuclear Aromatic Hydrocarbons,* P.W. Jones and P. Leber, Eds. (Ann Arbor, MI: Ann Arbor Science Publishers, Inc., 1979), pp. 141–148.
9. Yalkowsky, S.H., and S.C. Valvani. "Solubilities and Partitioning. 2. Relationships Between Aqueous Solubilities Partition Coefficients, and Molecular Surface Areas of Rigid Aromatic Hydrocarbons," *J. Chem. Eng. Data* 24(2):127–129 (1979).

10. Karickhoff, S.W., D.S. Brown, and T.A. Scott. "Sorption of Hydrophobic Pollutants to Natural Sediments," *Water Res.* 13:241–248 (1979).

11. Southworth, G.L. "Transport and Transformation of Anthracene in Natural Waters," in *Aquatic Toxicology*, L.L. Marking and R.A. Kimerle, Eds. ASTM STP 667 (Philadelphia, PA: American Society for Testing and Materials, 1979), pp. 359–380.

12. Southworth, G.L., J.J. Beauchamp, and P.K. Schmieder. "Bioaccumulation Potential of Polycyclic Aromatic Hydrocarbons in *Daphnia pulex*," *Water Res.* 12:973–977 (1978).

13. Gardner, R.H., Oak Ridge National Laboratory. Personal communication.

14. O'Neill, R.V., R.H. Gardner, L.W. Barnthouse, G.W. Suter, S.G. Hildebrand, and C.W. Gehrs. "Ecosystem Risk Analysis: A New Methodology," *Environ. Toxicol. Chem.* 1:176–177 (1982).

15. Giddings, J.M. "Acute Toxicity to *Selenastrum capricornutum* of Aromatic Compounds from Coal Conversion," *Bull. Environ. Contam. Toxicol.* 23:360–364 (1979).

16. Herbes, S.E., G.R. Southworth, D.L. Shaeffer, W.H. Griest, and M.P. Maskarinec. "Critical Pathways of Polycyclic Aromatic Hydrocarbons in Aquatic Environments," in *The Scientific Basis of Toxicity Testing*, H. Witshi, Ed. (New York: Elsevier/North-Holland Biomedical Press, 1980), pp. 113–128.

17. Lee, R.F., W.S. Gardner, J.W. Anderson, J.W. Blaylock, and J. Barxwell-Clarke. "Fate of Polycyclic Aromatic Hydrocarbons in Controlled Ecosystem Enclosures," *Environ. Sci. Technol.* 12(7):832–838 (1978).

18. Leversee, G.J., J.P. Giesy, P.F. Landrum, S.M. Bartell, S. Gerould, M. Bruno, A. Spacie, J. Bowling, J. Haddock, and T. Fannin. "Disposition of Benzo(*a*)pyrene in Aquatic Systems Components: Periphyton, Chironomids, *Daphnia*, Fish," *Chemical Analysis and Biological Fate: Polynuclear Aromatic Hydrocarbons*, M. Cooke and A.J. Dennis, Eds. (Columbus, OH: Battelle Press, 1981), pp. 357–366.

19. Hoel, P.G. *Elementary Statistics.* (New York: John Wiley & Sons, Inc., 1969), p. 218.

20. Cohen, J.L., W. Lee, and E.J. Lien. "Dependence of Toxicity on Molecular Structure: Group Theory Analysis," *J. Pharm. Sci.* 63:1068–1072 (1974).

# SECTION IV

## RESEARCH OPPORTUNITIES FOR THE FUTURE

# CHAPTER 26

## The United States Synthetic Fuels Corporation and Its Requirements for Environmental and Health Protection

### C.A.W. Di Bella

*U.S. Synthetic Fuels Corporation*
*2121 K Street, N.W.*
*Washington, DC 20037*

This chapter describes the purpose, organization, financing, and responsibilities of the United States Synthetic Fuels Corporation (SFC) and the environmental and health protection and monitoring requirements incurred by each recipient of financial assistance from the SFC. The chapter includes a tabulation of some major provisions of the Energy Security Act, a chronology of the SFC, a summary of the status of SFC projects, and a brief discussion of the evaluation of proposed synthetic fuels projects.

### CREATION OF SFC, DEFINITIONS, AND PRODUCTION GOALS

The Energy Security Act, Public Law 96-294, June 30, 1980, created the SFC and defined, for the purposes of the act, the term synthetic fuel (Table I). A synthetic fuel is produced from coal (including, in a broad sense, lignite and peat), shale, tar sands (which I do not believe have been mentioned in this symposium), and certain categories of heavy oil. Eligible categories of heavy oil resources are those for which extraction and processing are not economical under applicable pricing and tax policies and for which costs and economic and technical risks are comparable to those for a coal or shale project under the act. Significant amounts of heavy oil are being produced today, some 300,000 to 350,000 bbl/d, mostly in California. Other categories include water to make hydrogen, coal-oil mixtures, and magnetohydrodynamic topping cycles; I will not dwell on those last three categories.

543

The act defined a synthetic fuel project as one with the purpose of *commercial* production of synthetic fuel. We are not in the pilot plant business. We are in the business of supporting *commercial* synthetic fuel plants.

Production goals were also set in the act: 500 thousand bbl of oil (equivalent) per day by 1987, and 2 million by 1992 (Table I). The act authorized some $14 billion to carry out our task.

## FINANCIAL ASSISTANCE TO SYNTHETIC FUELS PROJECTS

The act also authorized the SFC to provide the following kinds of financial assistance to synthetic fuel projects (Table I): (1) the preferred category includes price guarantees, purchase agreements, and loan guarantees; (2) if the preferred category of financial assistance does not succeed, we are au-

**Table I.** Some Major Provisions of Public Law 96-294, the Energy Security Act, June 30, 1980, Part B

| Type of Provision | Effect of Provision |
| --- | --- |
| Creation of SFC | Created the United States Synthetic Fuels Corporation (SFC) |
| Definitions | Defined "synthetic fuel" as any solid, liquid, or gas produced from any of the following domestic sources:<br>Coal (including lignite and peat)<br>Shale<br>Tar sands (including certain heavy oil resources)<br>Water (but only to produce hydrogen via electrolysis)<br>Mixture of coal and combustible liquids<br>Magnetohydrodynamic topping cycles<br>Defined "synthetic fuel project" as a project with the purpose of commercial production of synthetic fuel |
| Production goals | Established national synthetic fuel production goals:<br>500 thousand bbl of oil (equivalent) per day (boepd) by 1987<br>2 million boepd by 1992 |
| Size of staff | Limited SFC employment to no more than 300 full-time professionals |
| Operating expenses | Authorized $35 million annually for SFC administrative expenses; authorized $10 million annually for SFC "generic studies" |
| Advisory committee | Established an advisory committee to review SFC solicitations and give advice on request, consisting of the Secretaries of Treasury, DOD, DOI, and DOE and the Administrator of EPA |

**Table I.**    *(continued)*

| *Type of Provision* | *Effect of Provision* |
|---|---|
| Financial assistance | Authorized the SFC to provide "financial assistance" to synthetic fuels projects in the following decreasing order of priority:<br>Price guarantees, purchase agreements, loan guarantees<br>Loans<br>Joint ventures<br>Authorized an initial amount of approximately $14 billion for such financial assistance<br>Required the submission by the SFC no later than June 30, 1984, of a "comprehensive strategy" for Congressional approval. After approval, the SFC may make requests for additional appropriations up to a cumulative amount of $68 billion<br>Required the SFC to consider the following, among other things, when awarding financial assistance:<br>Diversity of technologies for each domestic resource<br>Potential for replication<br>Potential of a technology to meet regulatory requirements<br>Required the development of a plan for monitoring environmental and health emissions by each recipient of financial assistance |

thorized to make direct loans; (3) if a direct loan does not work, we can even go into business with a private sector partner, with the SFC being a silent partner in a joint venture. Our board of directors and our management have made it quite clear that we vastly prefer the first-priority category.

In deciding to award financial assistance, the SFC must consider many factors (Table I), including the diversity of technology on a diversity of resources, the amount of liability that we undertake per unit of production, the potential for replication, and the potential of a technology to meet regulatory requirements. In June 1982, our board made a policy statement that we would trade off near-term production for increased diversity. Another important thing that the act required was the development of a plan for monitoring environmental and health emissions by each project supported by the SFC.

## SIZE OF STAFF, OPERATING EXPENSES, AND ADVISORY COMMITTEE

The act limited us to 300 professionals. Our board has said that we want to stay at many fewer than 300 professionals. In fact, we are at 115 professionals today, and I expect that we will not grow very much. The act also authorized funding for SFC operating expenses (Table I).

The act established an advisory committee of Treasury, DOE, EPA, DOD, and DOI for the specific purpose of reviewing the solicitations for proposals that we would issue and for the more general purpose of providing advice to the SFC on request.

## CHRONOLOGY OF SFC THROUGH SEPTEMBER 1982

We have had, like some of the others of you associated with the energy business, an unsettled couple of years. Our first year featured some accomplishments, but was not as productive as many, including ourselves, had hoped initially. Our chronology since the corporation was created is shown in Table II. The SFC was created in June 1980. Within a month or so, President Carter nominated for Congressional consideration a chairman and a board of directors; the Congress, however, adjourned for the 1980 elections without taking action on the nominations. The President then made recess appointments of a chairman and several members of the board of directors. Of course, a new administration was elected. The new administration accepted on or very shortly after inauguration day, January 1981, the resignations of the yet unconfirmed interim board of directors. A new chairman, Ed Noble, was nominated in April 1981 and confirmed in May. Reportedly, during 1981 there was a lot of soul-searching by the administration about just exactly what they wanted the SFC to do and to be. In February 1982, the President declared the Synthetic Fuels Corporation operational, an important psychological boost for the SFC and its supporters.

**Table II.**  Chronology of SFC through September 1982

| 1980 | June | Enactment of Energy Security Act |
|---|---|---|
|  | November | National elections; initial solicitation for proposals released |
| 1981 | March | Closing date for submission of proposals from initial solicitation |
|  | May | Ed Noble confirmed as SFC Chairman |
|  | September | Confirmation of four more board members |
|  | December | Second solicitation for proposals issued |
| 1982 | February | President declares SFC operational |
|  | March | SFC Board selects five projects from initial solicitation to pass strength review |
|  | June | Closing date for second solicitation |
|  | August | Final two SFC board members confirmed by Senate |
|  | September | Eleven projects pass strength review of second solicitation; third solicitation issued (will close January 1983—last of the "nontargeted" solicitations) |

Our first solicitation for proposals had been issued in November 1980, but no final decisions were made regarding their status as late as January 1982. At the first board meeting after having been declared operational, the SFC decided to advance 5 projects, of 63 proposed in the first solicitation, into a negotiation phase. In September 1982, an additional 11 projects from our second solicitation were advanced, and we issued a third solicitation, which will close in January 1983.

## STATUS OF SFC PROJECTS

In SFC parlance, phase II means that a project has been reviewed by the SFC and has passed to the stage where actual negotiations regarding financial assistance are in progress, and we are doing more detailed evaluation of the proposal. Phase III means that a contract for financial assistance has been awarded and the project is actually in construction. As shown in Table III, the only project in phase III at this time is the Union oil shale project, inherited from DOE in February 1982 when the SFC was declared operational. That project is in construction and will start up in late 1983.

All of the other projects are from our first or second solicitations (Table III). There is one oil shale project, Paraho, which has a well-known technology. There is one coal gasification project, Coolwater. There are five coal liquefaction projects. Four of these are indirect liquefaction projects: Hampshire, First Colony, New England Energy Park, and North Alabama.

**Table III.**   SFC Project Status

| Phase | Category | Project | Solicitation(s) from which Advanced |
|-------|----------|---------|-------------------------------------|
| III | Oil shale | Union[a] | |
| II | Oil shale | Paraho-Ute | Second |
| | Coal gasification | Coolwater | Second |
| | Coal liquefaction | Hampshire | Initial |
| | | Breckinridge | Initial |
| | | First Colony | Initial & second |
| | | New England Energy Park | Second |
| | | North Alabama | Second |
| | Tar sands/heavy oil | Calsyn | Initial & second |
| | | Kensyntar | Second |
| | | Sunnyside | Second |
| | | Hop Kern River | Second |
| | | Enpex-Syntaro | Second |
| | | Santa Rosa | Second |

[a]Transferred from DOE in February 1982 under DPA.

One is a direct liquefaction project: Breckinridge. The First Colony project is based on peat feedstock. There are six tar sands/heavy oil projects. Calsyn is a project to upgrade heavy oil to marketable products. The Kensyntar project and the Enpex-Syntaro project are based on in situ recovery of bitumen; the others are based on surface mining, with solvent extraction of the bitumen.

I would like to remark on the mix of projects that we have. The papers presented earlier in this symposium are focused largely on life sciences issues for oil shale, coal liquefaction projects, or coal gasification. However, except for the Union oil shale project and the Great Plains project (a DOE project, not an SFC project), the projects that we suspect are most likely to come on line soonest are in the area of tar sands and heavy oil. These projects tend to be relatively small and relatively quick to get on line, because they are based on surface mining or a development of relatively small patterns of wells. I think there is a very legitimate issue as to whether there are significant or unusual health, safety, and environmental emissions questions associated with these projects. It could be argued perhaps, because of the analogy with conventional oil production and processing, that maybe there are not. Nevertheless, these projects will be coming on line sooner than projects based on resources that perhaps have more strategic significance, such as coal and shale.

## REQUIREMENTS FOR ENVIRONMENTAL AND HEALTH PROTECTION

In the environmental area (Table IV), we have a number of responsibilities that are rather specifically defined in the act. They are broad from one point of view and narrow from another. For example, in the preamble or the findings and purposes clause of the Energy Security Act, it is stated that synthetic fuels should be developed in a manner consistent with the protection of the environment and, similarly, that they should be produced in an environmentally acceptable manner. The act also specifies that, in awarding financial assistance to a synthetic fuels project, we must consider the potential of a particular technology to meet regulatory requirements. We must

**Table IV.** Major Environmental and Health Protection and Monitoring Provisions of the Energy Security Act

Synfuels projects to be consistent with protection of environment and environmentally acceptable

Potential of a technology to meet regulatory requirements a factor in award of financial assistance

Development of a plan for monitoring environmental- and health-related emissions also require the development of a plan for monitoring environmental emissions. I would like to quote that part of the act [Sect. 131(e)]:

> Any contract for financial assistance shall require the development of a plan, acceptable to the board of directors, for the monitoring of environmental and health related emissions from the construction and operation of the synthetic fuel project. Such plan shall be developed by the recipient of financial assistance after consultation with the administrator of the EPA, the Secretary of Energy, and appropriate state agencies.

It is very clear that the *recipient* develops this monitoring plan, not the Synthetic Fuels Corporation; our role is to approve it. It is also clear that there is a very positive obligation put on both EPA and DOE to consult on the development of this plan in order to assure its ultimate acceptability.

Our main business to date in the SFC has been the evaluation of projects proposed to us via our solicitation process. We have not yet reached the stage of approving environmental monitoring plans or of monitoring for other purposes, so I can only describe what we do in the project evaluation phase from an environmental point of view.

## EVALUATION OF PROJECTS

As illustrated in Table V, each proposed project's schedule for permit acquisition is reviewed by the SFC to make sure that it is complete, that the proposer is aware of all of the permits required, and that the schedule for permit acquisition is consistent with the schedule proposed for the project. To aid in verifying this schedule and the permits that are involved, we meet with the appropriate local, state, and Federal officials to evaluate which permits are required and to help verify the accuracy of the permit acquisition plan. In fact, the States Relations Group of the SFC has already met with the environmental authorities of some 20 states.

We also require a socioeconomic impact assessment and mitigation plan. This is required for every project and is very important. However, for some projects, for example a multibillion-dollar project in a sparsely pop-

---

**Table V.**   Project Evaluation

Regulatory compliance
    Each project's schedule for permit acquisition is reviewed for completeness and consistency with overall project schedule
    Meet with appropriate local, state, and Federal officials to evaluate permit acquisition plan accuracy
Socioeconomic impact assessment and mitigation plan
Pollution control technology

---

ulated area, one would expect that the socioeconomic impact assessment and mitigation plan would be detailed and extensive. On first analysis, for some other projects, say a small project in an area with a surplus of skilled labor, it could verge on being minimal. In any case, we do not accept generalizations from sponsors that there are no socioeconomic problems.

In our evaluation of proposed projects, we look very carefully at the pollution control technology. In particular, we look at the basis for the design of pollution control technology: whether the sponsors have identified the amount, the level, and the frequency of the pollutants that they need to control.

The next step in SFC operations will be approval of a plan, developed by each recipient of financial assistance, for the monitoring of environmental- and health-related emissions.

# CHAPTER 27

## Status of and Prospects for Synthetic Fuels Research and Production

### J.V. Dugan

*House Committee on Science
and Technology
Subcommittee on Energy
Research and Production*

Environmental, health, and safety research in support of synthetic fuels technology and other aspects of synthetic fuels research and production are discussed in this chapter from the perspective of the House Science and Technology Committee and from the specific perspective of Rep. Marilyn Lloyd Bouquard, Chairman of the Energy Research and Production Subcommittee, which is relatively supply oriented. The approach I would like to take is to discuss the history of the Committee's interest in synthetic fuels and the environmental research aspects of their production, the status of those activities as Mrs. Bouquard sees them, and their prospects. I think I can provide a somewhat unique perspective, in the sense that when the bill was drafted I was the Republican energy staff person on the Committee and now I am serving the House Majority on the Subcommittee. I hope to relate some "corporate memory" of what has happened in formulating environmental research policy for synthetic fuels development. Throughout the chapter, "Chairman" refers to Mrs. Bouquard, chairman of the subcommittee, and "Committee" refers to the parent committee.

The Committee's various views of environmental research are, of course, somewhat mixed. Even the most environmentally oriented members of the Committee had great concerns several years ago about the EPA research after the CHESS scandal, in which preemptive environmental standards on sulfates resulted without very much of a data base. The Committee had to investigate that incident, in one of the few investigative activities it had ever undertaken. My Chairman perceived throughout the Carter years a lack of technical leadership in environmental research in DOE at the very top levels. The Chairman's position is very supportive of synthetic fuels development, but she is clearly most interested in having environmental, health, and safety research well done, since the very future of such industrial development in the United States clearly hinges on adequate environmental research. From a broader perspective, in the House during the last Congress, the synthetic fuels question was seen as a national defense issue; therefore, the production goals in the Energy Security Act, although somewhat hortatory, were specifically intended to spur the utilization of a variety of resources through a diversity of technologies, with the idea of developing a U.S. industrial potential for replicating plants.

In terms of Synthetic Fuels Corporation (SFC) project criteria, strong management capability, technical diversity, soundness of project management arrangements, and environmental acceptability were paramount. Another aspect on which each project is to be judged is financial maturity or project strength, and this I think is an issue on which my Chairman has a somewhat different view from that of the SFC. There was an idea also, at least on the House side, to make the Department of Energy (DOE) a strong technical arm for the SFC. Various sections of the act refer to that role specifically, and Section 131(e) is an example in point. There was the conscious assumption that the DOE would conduct in parallel a strong technology demonstration program. The Energy Security Act was devised, from our Committee's perspective, on that basis. In fact, there was a tacit assumption that the DOE higher-risk program would complement the SFC effort. I will allude to that later, when I discuss the fact that now the SFC must look at higher-risk projects, since there is no technology demonstration program. Mr. Stockman has successfully managed to kill it.

There was also a sense among the conferees of the House-Senate Conference Committee that there should be an allowance for high-leverage funding through cost sharing for refinement of design, to obtain better cost estimates of plants, including the environmental equipment. Thus, Section 131(u) is one the Committee was specifically interested in, having written it in the conference. There was the tacit assumption that pioneer plants would be built (and built relatively expeditiously) to allow for technology improvement, environmentally and otherwise, so that we would indeed have integrated technology and/or commercial demonstrations at full or prototype scale. Finally, the credit-elsewhere test in terms of financial support for the project was devised specifically to avoid there being any subsidies for Exxon. It is curious to my Chairman that, in fact, the SFC seems to have used that as almost a basis for proving that if any company (not simply Exxon) can get funding other than from the Federal government, they should not receive SFC support.

The DOE demonstration program is gone. This program was a major assumption of the legislation. There have been no project awards yet made by the SFC, either. From the aerospace heritage of the Committee, my Chairman expected that if any organization, government, quasi-public or otherwise, truly intended to build something, they would sit down and negotiate with that end item in mind. They would get capable project managers interested in building the project and then go ahead to build the plants. That is not happening. The proposals before the SFC also now include some riskier projects. I think that is healthy, in that to some degree the SFC has recognized now that it has a hybrid responsibility and cannot simply try to live with the words of the statute, because certain tacit assumptions of the Energy Security Act have been invalidated.

The DOE support role, of course, remains vague and undelineated, whether it be in materials technology, environmental research and development, or whatever; and my Chairman is concerned because, I think, she sees the DOE/SFC relationship as a two-way street. In other words, she asks whether the SFC is telling the DOE enough so that the DOE has an idea what its own focus, initiative, and emphasis should be in the research and technology program that it is presumably to carry out to provide a base for the synthetic fuel plants of tomorrow. I think we see little evidence of that mutual interaction thus far.

The private sector's ability to fund these projects, if the Exxon withdrawal from Battlement Mesa is any indication, is dramatic evidence for the need for continued Federal involvement. The interpretation of foes of the SFC about the very idea of government participation is 180 degrees out of phase with that of my Chairman. They take the position that if Exxon is not going to do it, it certainly is not worth doing. The cost sharing provisions of Section 131(u) have not been implemented or encouraged by the SFC.* In fact, if my Chairman had not pressed the SFC on this issue, I doubt that the SFC would have mentioned these provisions. The SFC has indicated passively that there would be funds available under 131(u) if it had some applications for such awards. These provisions are virtually ignored, and we see strong technical teams all around the country virtually disbanding because they have not passed all the strength and maturity tests and cannot afford to spend several million dollars a month with very vague and uncertain prospects of ever getting an award.

The financial-strength test has become a Catch-22. That reminds me of the old Harry Truman phrase. Take this in a bipartisan sense if you will. Mr. Truman characterized bankers as "the kind of people who will lend you money only if you can prove you do not need it." The tragic thing I see on the House side is that the "corporate memory," except for the Majority Leader and some other principals, particularly in our Committee, for synthetic fuels development as a national security program has been lost. There also have been some senators who still express this view, but it has been virtually lost. I think that strong testimony to this is the sad fact that some of the most strongly pro-defense people in the House side (some conservative Republicans and conservative Democrats) have been involved in attacks on the SFC. The whole approach that the House had in the Defense

---

*Implemented months later through a $4.56 million award to the First Colony Project.

Production Act has become blurred, and my Chairman believes that even people who voted for the Defense Production Act on that basis, in her view, have forgotten that national security is not supported solely through the DOD budget.

Let me turn to the prospects. I certainly think there are many members of the Committee and of the House and Senate leadership who would like to see some awards made, and made soon, to enable projects to go ahead. I think that many members of the Committee feel that the DOE role of providing a research and technology base for the SFC must be reaffirmed. At this point, because we are in Oak Ridge territory, I might mention that the Committee's perspective is that the national laboratories, of which Oak Ridge and Argonne are two marvelous examples, have a solid capability to support fossil energy programs and the Office of Health and Environmental Research in the OER is providing a strong technical base and arm for the SFC. It is also necessary that the SFC recognize that DOE, the national laboratories, and other elements of the organization have a great capability; and it is critical to ensure that this capability is employed properly to complement and support the SFC in the spirit of the Energy Security Act [e.g., Section 131(e)]. Environmental monitoring plans and the supporting research that underpins those plans are key items.

I know that my Chairman, Mrs. Bouquard, and the Chairman of our Environmental Research and Development Subcommittee, Mr. Scheuer, feel that environmental, health, and safety research is the key to the prospects for developing and building environmentally acceptable synthetic fuels plants. In turn, it is important that the SFC recognize our Committee's important stake in this activity, since clearly the role of the SFC must be much more than simply a "commercialization" role, whatever that word was intended to mean. My Subcommittee Chairman would also like to see some implementation of the provisions of Section 131(u). This implementation would include some support for industrial teams to refine cost estimates, to do additional research and development, or even to operate pilot plants to make sure that we can get a better estimate of the cost of these full-scale plants. Mrs. Bouquard has been fairly critical of and impatient with the SFC. We have had discussions with Mr. Schroeder, the SFC President, and others on that point over the past year, but she has not seen the kind of movement that she would like to see. One major solution to alleviate these concerns would be to revisit the Energy Security Act. I think, given the diversity of Congressional views and controversy attendant to that, it is not likely in the next Congress, although it is still a possibility. If we have another oil supply disruption, you might see that kind of legislative activity in either or both bodies. At the moment I would not consider it very probable.

These are chiefly perspectives of my Chairman and to some extent those of other members of our Committee and additional members in the House and Senate. More regulatory-minded committees who share the environmental concerns of our Committee but from a different, nonresearch and development, perspective, have a somewhat different view of the merits of synthetic fuels development. Such committees, of course, have some joint jurisdiction over the activities of the SFC, and have been and will be providing different inputs to the SFC. Some of these inputs will possibly be constructive in my Chairman's view; others will be less benign, as the SFC has already experienced in terms of disruptions of its day-to-day business. The prospects for synthetic fuels are somewhat chancy, but my Chairman hopes to see some tangible action in the form of building plants, and then the Committee can begin to focus more carefully on the DOE support role, including a strong involvement in environmental research and development.

# CHAPTER 28

## Opportunities for Health and Environmental Research from an Industrial Perspective

### G.K. Vick

*Exxon Research and Engineering Company*
*P.O. Box 101*
*Florham Park, NJ 07932*

This chapter considers research requirements and priorities in the area of health and environmental studies in synthetic fuel technologies from the perspective of industry. A conceptual framework is developed for examining the kinds of decisions with which industry is faced and the kinds of health and environmental R&D data needed for those decisions. Some of the more obvious knowledge gaps are then identified within this framework.

This panel discussion deals with research; therefore, I would like to propose what I consider the first and second laws of research. The first law is probably already known to many of you as Kelly's law: "Nothing is ever as simple as it seems." With Kelly's law to guide me, I have formulated Vick's law, which I propose as the second law of research: "Research always raises more questions than it answers." It follows that the more research is done, the greater the need becomes for even more; we all have a lot of empirical evidence for that.

The subject of this panel discussion is "Research Opportunities for the Future." Vick's law predicts that those opportunities, measured in terms of unanswered questions, must already be substantial and growing rapidly. The organizers of this session recognized another fundamental law: "How it looks depends on where you are." They have wisely invited people who are in different places to say how it looks from there. I am in industry, and from my perspective some of the unanswered questions appear more important to industry than others.

When a synthetic fuels industry is built, it seems obvious to me that just about everyone will want it to be safe and cost effective. They will want it to be safe not only to workers, but to customers, the environment, and the general public. Of course, it needs to be cost effective if the products are to be acceptable to its customers. Industry's challenge is how to design, build, and operate such an enterprise. I would like to take this challenge as my starting point and examine the kinds of decisions that have to be made and the kinds of knowledge and data needed to make those decisions. I make the simplifying assumption that we are not concerned with the question of whether there should be a synthetic fuels industry but rather, if there is to be one, what do the designers, builders, and operators need to know to make it safe in a cost-effective manner.

Figure 1 illustrates a conceptual framework for defining the kinds of knowledge needed. Obviously, if we are to have an industry, we need hardware to produce the fuels, to transport them to the customers, and to use them, and we need operating practices that tell us how to use that hardware. Decisions have to be made by decision makers in industry that define the hardware and operating practices. The decision makers need many different kinds of input in order to make those decisions effectively. For the goal of safety, they clearly need some reasonable estimates of the health and environmental impacts that derive from various options, so that they can select the hardware and operating practices that meet society's standards and that do so at the lowest cost. Those impacts must come from some kind of data base and model that can do three things: first, identify the potential hazards; second, quantify those hazards somehow; and third, transform those quantitative estimates of hazards into estimates of risks to man and environment. As input to the environmental and health exposure-response model, an

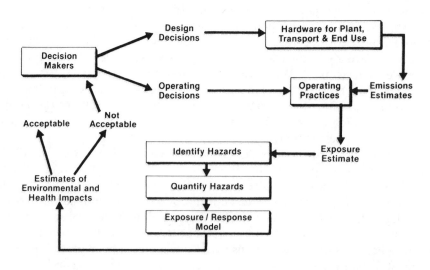

**Figure 1.** Generalized model for decision making.

exposure estimate is needed. This estimate must, in turn, be derived from an estimate of the emissions and some knowledge of what I have called operating practices—the way things are done. The emissions estimate must be derived from some sort of definition of the hardware, and that definition and the operating practices spring from decisions made by the decision makers. We have come full circle, back to where we started. Clearly, this is an iterative process in which many options are examined until an acceptable answer emerges.

Within this framework, I would like to share my thoughts on which health and environmental impacts we can estimate well enough and which we cannot, and which gaps in knowledge and data separate us from our goal. Of necessity, I will be generalizing; to quote another law, "All generalizations (including this one) have exceptions," and so will mine.

As far as synthetic fuels are concerned, I believe that we know enough about the kinds and amounts of materials we will encounter and their acute toxicities to know how to design and operate the industry in order to control the acute hazards. This is not to say that acute toxic hazards are not important, but rather that acute toxicity is not a prime candidate for future research.

Chronic hazards to man are a different matter. I think that there are some prime candidates for research here; carcinogenicity is one. Carcinogenicity has clearly been identified as a potential hazard in the liquids produced by direct coal liquefaction and shale retorting. Furthermore, we now know quite a bit about the carcinogenicity of synthetic fuels. We know that synthetic fuels contain high-boiling aromatics, which include hydrocarbons, hydrocarbons with heteroatom substitution, and heterocycles. We know how boiling range and hydrogenation affect carcinogenicity, and we know that the potency is within current industrial experience. We also know that there are many different compounds that contribute to carcinogenicity, and it is likely that not all of them have been identified as carcinogens. Some compounds act as initiators and some as promoters, and synergisms and antagonisms are believed to complicate matters even more. The situation is so complicated, in fact, that even if we had a perfect analysis of a synthetic fuel, we still could not predict its carcinogenicity; I suspect that we are decades rather than months or years away from that goal.

This problem of relating the carcinogenicity of synthetic fuels to their composition provides many of the unanswered questions I spoke of earlier. But, this knowledge gap is not one, in my opinion, that is of much interest to industry. The kinds of process controls industry has available for controlling composition and, therefore, potency are not calibrated in terms of individual compounds but rather in terms of boiling range and kind and degree of processing.

I am not arguing that there is no value to research aimed at elucidating the relationship between composition and carcinogenicity. Rather, I would argue that while such research will advance us toward a goal of a solid scientific foundation for understanding the phenomenon, it will not advance us toward the goal of a safe industry as fast as research on some other unanswered questions.

To my mind, the crucial data gaps with respect to carcinogenicity are in our ability to quantify the potency and in our ability to relate that measure of potency to risk in man. For filling the quantification gap, I can think of two strategies: mouse skin painting and inhalation. I see mouse skin painting emerging as a tool for quantifying carcinogenicity as a result of testing at multiple dose levels and the application of sophisticated statistical techniques, such as the Kaplan-Meyer and the Weibull distribution, to the analysis of the data. I would encourage that development. However, that still leaves a concern about differences between the skin on the backs of mice and systemic cancers such as lung and liver cancer. A second strategy would be to develop and validate an animal model capable of measuring the tendency of complex mixtures to induce systemic cancers by inhalation, and I would also encourage research with that aim. The key goal here is a method or methods that can measure the potency of complex mixtures from synthetic fuels processes and relate that potency to complex mixtures for which we have some data in man, such as coke oven emissions and cigarette smoke.

Even if we fill the quantification gap, that still leaves a big gap between animals and man. Filling that gap is another prime candidate for research. This research is going to be a very demanding undertaking, because it will require a synthesis of knowledge from a number of areas as diverse as pharmacokinetics on the one hand and epidemiology on the other. One rather simplistic strategy would be to develop some dose-response models for coke oven emissions and cigarette smoke in man. The goal should be a model to use in the very low dose range. This is where the synthesis of a number of disciplines will be needed. Another goal should be a model with broad acceptability in the scientific community. If we had such a model, it could be used with data on the potency of a synthetic fuel relative to coke oven emissions or cigarette smoke, as the case may be, to estimate risk in man. Admittedly, such a procedure still leaves us with the uncertainty about the preservation of relative potency from animals to man. This is another gap to be filled, but until it is, I would prefer to use even the feeble candles I have just described to guide my steps than to sit and curse the darkness.

There are probably other strategies for filling the quantification and dose-response gaps, and they also are prime candidates for research.

Let us assume for the moment that the gaps I have been discussing will get filled. Two obvious questions come to mind: Do we have the input in terms of exposure estimates we need? Can we use a quantitative estimate of risk in man after we get it? We will consider the second question first.

What does a decision maker do when someone hands him a quantitative estimate of risk associated with a proposed design? It seems to me the only thing he can do is compare it with some standard, that is, with some risk level that society has decided is acceptable. This drops us into the middle of that treacherous swamp of "How Safe is Safe Enough?" A chart for finding our way out of the swamp[1] is simply this: the risk level that is acceptable is that associated with the next best alternative. The point is that every course of action has some risks associated with it, including the course of not doing something, because the world goes on, and if A is not done, B, C, or D comes along to fill the gap. The problem is that we either do not know or cannot agree on the alternatives or on the risks associated with them. This issue of acceptable risk has been and will probably continue to be decided politically rather than rationally for some time to come. Political and rational are not necessarily mutually exclusive, although perhaps they are not seen keeping company as often as we would desire. I happen to think that we would be better off if we could put more rationality into the political process when dealing with risk, but to do this we need, among other things, a better data base on alternatives and their risks. This is surely an opportunity for research. Data bases are what research is all about.

Can we estimate the exposures that are the inputs to a dose-response model? This is another area in which I see a knowledge gap. The estimating models for fugitive emissions of vapors and gases are only fair, and models for estimating fugitive aerosol emissions are virtually nonexistent. There are certainly research opportunities here.

What about other hazards associated with chronic exposures? Feto-toxic and teratogenic effects have been seen in rats in tests on synthetic fuels, but the data base is very limited. Data are needed on a broader range of materials. Assuming that the rest of the data looks like what we have now, I do not think that this will be a critical hazard. At this point, the dose levels required to produce these effects appear to be high relative to the dose levels that produce carcinogenesis; therefore, I would expect these hazards to be controlled by what is done to control the carcinogenicity hazard.

There are some other potential hazards to human health that need to be checked out, such as effects on the male and female reproductive systems. My perception is that programs now under way will tell us whether more research is needed.

My discussion thus far has focused on toxic hazards that are presented fairly directly to people through skin contact or through inhalation of dusts, vapors, or aerosols. There is another area of concern: the impact on the environment itself and the impact on people of materials that have been transported through and possibly changed by the environment. Questions seem to outnumber answers in this area by orders of magnitude.

I personally find this area a very troublesome one from the standpoint of trying to decide which of the unanswered questions should be tackled first. For one thing, I have not had the opportunity to delve as deeply into it as I have into the areas I have already discussed. Therefore, on the matter of recommendations, I would like to pass. Instead, I would like to close by suggesting some of the criteria that determine whether a research project is likely to be of value to industry. These criteria will summarize what I have said about research opportunities and perhaps also serve to illuminate the question of research on environmental fate and effects. First, research should address the critical hazards, those that are likely to be controlling. It may be very interesting to study a particular hazard in depth, but if the exposure levels required are an order of magnitude greater than the maximum exposure dictated by the critical hazard, the results are not likely to impact on control decisions. Second, as I have already discussed, we need knowledge and data extending through a long chain of causal relationships from hardware to emissions to transport and exposure, and dose-response. Research priorities should be given to the weak links in that chain, not to the strong ones. Third, there is a dimension one can use to describe research which ranges from the macroscopic, such as the effect of complex mixtures on a whole organism, to the microscopic, such as the interaction of a single compound at the cellular or molecular level in the organism. For the immediate concerns of what to control, how to control it, and how much to control it, research at the macroscopic level is more likely to yield results that are immediately useful than research at the microscopic level.

Finally, let me reemphasize a point I made at the beginning. What is important is relative; it depends on where you are and what you are trying to do. I have tried to confine myself to research which could be of fairly immediate utility to industry. Other perspectives will undoubtedly reveal other opportunities.

## REFERENCE

1.  Derby, S.L., and R.L. Keeney. "Risk Analysis: Understanding 'How Safe is Safe Enough?' " *Risk Analysis* 1:217–224 (1981).

# CHAPTER 29

## Synthetic Fuels Technologies in Health and Environmental Research

### R.W. Wood

*U.S. Department of Energy*
*Washington, DC 20545*

This chapter begins with a brief historical overview of health and environmental research conducted by the U.S. Department of Energy and its predecessor agencies. A summary of recent and current health and environmental research in support of synthetic fuels technologies is presented. Program directions for the future are outlined, including a brief discussion of the evolving interface with the U.S. Synthetic Fuels Corporation.

## HISTORICAL PERSPECTIVE

The health and environmental research program of the U.S. Department of Energy (DOE) had its origins with the creation of the U.S. Atomic Energy Commission (AEC) in 1946. Section 3(a) of the Atomic Energy Act of 1946 provides the legislative authority for the conduct of this research:

> . . . the commission is . . . directed to make arrangements . . . for the conduct of research and development activities related to . . . (3) utilization of fissionable and radioactive materials for medical, biological, health . . . purposes. . . . (5) the protection of health during research and production activities.

This authority was reaffirmed in the Atomic Energy Act of 1954, as amended.

To implement this mandate, the Division of Biology and Medicine was established within the AEC. The scope of the research program was deliberately broad, encompassing basic as well as applied research activities, and ranging in disciplinary makeup from physics, chemistry, and engineering, through environmental and biological sciences, to medical research programs. Thus, radiation dosimeter development, environmental fate and transport of radionuclides, acute and chronic animal exposure, and human epidemiology studies fell within the purview of the biology and medicine research program. This multidisciplinary, integrated approach to health and environmental research has been a consistent research philosophy over the years and continues today as our present mode of operation.

## SYNTHETIC FUELS RESEARCH

In January of 1975, the research and development arm of the AEC, together with several other Federal energy-related agencies or components, were consolidated into the Energy Research and Development Administration (ERDA). Since the only health and environmental research program carried into ERDA was the former AEC activity, a very substantial expansion of our research scope was required. From a program that had exclusively addressed health and environmental issues associated with nuclear energy, we now found ourselves responsible for the health and environmental research in support of many energy technology developments (e.g., coal conversion, shale retorting, geothermal, solar, and various conservation options), as well as sustaining the nuclear energy activities, including fusion energy technology. There ensued some new initiatives, substantial reprogramming of nuclear-related into nonnuclear-related health and environmental research, and no little amount of trauma as our laboratories realigned a very significant portion of their health and environmental research activities.

Two-and-a-half years later, a further consolidation of Federal energy activities took place with the creation of DOE. In each case, the legislation contained specific language calling for a health and environmental research program. Our mandate is stated in Sect. 203(a) of the DOE organization act:

> . . . The functions which the Secretary shall assign to the Assistant Secretaries include . . . (3) . . . conducting a comprehensive program of research and development on the environmental effects of energy technologies and programs.

The requirement for a comprehensive research program was, of course, consistent with our research philosophy and served to reinforce the breadth of research activities that had become established during 1975 and 1976, most notably in the synthetic fuels area.

We have maintained a multidisciplinary approach in the development of our synthetic fuels research program, as is evidenced by the wide range of DOE-supported research presented at this symposium. We also have established a program that ranges from the basic to the applied end of the spectrum. Thus, our program encompasses fundamental research into the basic mechanisms whereby energy-related agents interact with biological or environmental systems as well as short-term, sharply focused studies to define the biological activity that may exist in energy-related materials.

At the inception of the DOE program, the lack of health and environmental data on nonnuclear-energy-related materials placed high priority on short-term studies in order to expand, as rapidly as possible, our data base. Joint research efforts were established with several fossil energy technology program offices within DOE to take advantage of available laboratory and pilot-scale facilities. Extensive interactions took place with industry, and a close interface was maintained with other Federal agencies, such as the Environmental Protection Agency (EPA), the Department of Defense, and the National Institute for Occupational Safety and Health. These collaborative programs included high- and low-Btu gasification, direct coal liquefaction, and aboveground as well as in situ oil shale retorting. Much of this symposium consists of presentations from these synthetic fuels research programs.

## FUTURE RESEARCH DIRECTIONS

During the past five years, we have, I believe, very substantially broadened our synthetic fuels health and environmental data base, particularly for the shorter-term studies. In order to "take stock" of where we were and where we should be going, a major program review was held at Airlie House in January of 1982.[1] In addition, during the past several months, a number of laboratories have prepared comprehensive documents summarizing the status of health and environmental research relative to coal combustion, coal gasification, direct coal liquefaction, and solid wastes. These reports, as well as the Airlie House proceedings, have been published. Based upon these reviews, we anticipate that our synthetic fuels health and environmental research program will be modified somewhat as we move forward.

The process-specific research that utilized samples from specific pilot plant operations was quite comprehensive and extensive. Ongoing activities will be completed, and additional research related to specific processes will be carefully selected in the future. Based on information developed in the program, we can conclude that only a few classes of organic compounds are responsible for most of the mutagenic and carcinogenic activity of coal- and shale-derived synthetic fuel materials. Moreover, the most active classes of coal-related complex materials seem to be the same regardless of the process.

The biological research program, to date, has given primary emphasis to mutagenesis and carcinogenesis studies. Future research will emphasize delayed effects other than cancer production. Long-term, late effects of chronic low-level exposure have not constituted a major component of the program to date and should be investigated more intensively. Finally, we intend to increase efforts on the biophysical and biochemical mechanisms that underlie the biological responses that have been observed. An ad hoc laboratory/DOE group has been established to develop specific recommendations and priorities.

In the environmental area, investigations into food chain transfer of energy-related materials will be emphasized. We also anticipate an expanded effort on the atmospheric transformation of organic materials. A special workshop in atmospheric organic chemistry was conducted last spring, and the proceedings will be published soon. Research relative to solid wastes is an area of high priority, and an enhanced effort is planned to determine the fate and effect of materials emanating from landfills containing synthetic fuels wastes.

Industrial hygiene research will address the need for improved techniques and instrumentation to measure worker exposure to emissions or other materials. In addition, improved cleanup and decontamination techniques are needed, and research in this area will receive high priority.

A continuing risk-analysis program is anticipated, in order to provide an evaluation of information in all of these technical areas and to formulate an assessment relative to health or environmental impact from a commercial-scale industry.

## SYNTHETIC FUELS CORPORATION

The Energy Security Act, which created the Synthetic Fuels Corporation (SCF), places a requirement on each applicant to develop a comprehensive environmental monitoring plan. The EPA and DOE are specifically required to provide consultation to SFC on such plans. A formal interface has been established between DOE and SFC, which includes participation by our health and environmental research arm. We fully recognize that a commercial-scale synthetic fuel operation will provide a unique opportunity to obtain valuable health and environmental data. The SFC recognizes this opportunity equally well, and we will continue to work with them in an effort to make this opportunity become a reality.

## SUMMARY

In conclusion, I believe that we have made a great deal of progress over the past several years. A very substantial knowledge based on the health and environmental aspects of synthetic fuels development has been developed. This, I believe, is due in no small measure to the scientific expertise largely in our national laboratories and to their ability to rapidly realign technical resources in order to address new DOE responsibilities. We have appreciated the dedication of these scientists and will continue to need their assistance in maintaining a strong synthetic fuels health and environmental research program in the future.

## REFERENCE

1. Duhamel, A.P. "Overview and Findings from Airlie House Retreat: Health and Environmental Research Programs Related to Coal Conversion Technologies and Their Future Directions," Chapter 10, this volume.

# INDEX